T0329783

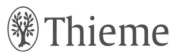

Controversies in Spine Surgery, MIS versus OPEN

Best Evidence Recommendations

OPEN

Alexander R. Vaccaro, MD, PhD, FACS, MBA
Richard H. Rothman Professor and Chairman
Department of Orthopaedic Surgery
Professor of Neurosurgery
Thomas Jefferson University and Hospitals
President, The Rothman Institute
Philadelphia, Pennsylvania

Jason C. Eck, DO, MS
Orthopedic Spine Surgeon
Center for Sports Medicine and Orthopedics
Chattanooga, Tennessee

Christopher K. Kepler, MD, MBA
Associate Professor
Orthopaedic Spine Surgeon
Department of Orthopaedic Surgery
Thomas Jefferson University and Hospitals
The Rothman Institute
Philadelphia, Pennsylvania

MIS

Richard G. Fessler, MD, PhD
Professor
Department of Neurosurgery
Rush University Medical Center
Chicago, Illinois

Faheem A. Sandhu, MD, PhD
Professor of Neurosurgery
Director of Spine Surgery
Co-Director
Center for Minimally Invasive Spine Surgery
Department of Neurosurgery
MedStar Georgetown University Hospital
Washington, DC

Jean-Marc Voyadzis, MD
Co-Director
Center for Minimally Invasive Spine Surgery
Associate Professor of Neurosurgery
MedStar Georgetown University Hospital
Washington, DC

51 illustrations

Thieme
New York • Stuttgart • Delhi • Rio de Janeiro

Executive Editor: William Lamsback
Managing Editor: Elizabeth Palumbo
Associate Managing Editor: Haley Paskalides
Director, Editorial Services: Mary Jo Casey
Production Editor: Naamah Schwartz
International Production Director: Andreas Schabert
Editorial Director: Sue Hodgson
International Marketing Director: Fiona Henderson
International Sales Director: Louisa Turrell
Director of Institutional Sales: Adam Bernacki
Senior Vice President and Chief Operating Officer: Sarah Vanderbilt
President: Brian D. Scanlan

Library of Congress Cataloging-in-Publication Data

Names: Vaccaro, Alexander R., editor.
Title: Controversies in spine surgery, MIS versus open : best
    evidence recommendations / [edited by] Alexander R. Vaccaro
    [and 5 others].
Other titles: Controversies in spine surgery (Vaccaro)
Description: Second edition. | New York : Thieme, [2018] |
    Preceded by Controversies in spine surgery / [edited by]
    Alexander R. Vaccaro, Jason C. Eck. c2010. | Includes
    bibliographical references and index.
Identifiers: LCCN 2017045100| ISBN 9781604068818 (print) |
    ISBN 9781604068825 (ebook)
Subjects: | MESH: Spine–surgery | Minimally Invasive Surgical
    Procedures | Orthopedic Procedures | Evidence-Based Medicine |
    Spinal Fractures–surgery | Spinal Neoplasms–surgery
Classification: LCC RD768 | NLM WE 725 | DDC 617.5/6059–dc23
LC record available at https://lccn.loc.gov/2017045100

© 2018 Thieme Medical Publishers, Inc.

Thieme Publishers New York
333 Seventh Avenue, New York, NY 10001 USA
+1 800 782 3488, customerservice@thieme.com

Thieme Publishers Stuttgart
Rüdigerstrasse 14, 70469 Stuttgart, Germany
+49 [0]711 8931 421, customerservice@thieme.de

Thieme Publishers Delhi
A-12, Second Floor, Sector-2, Noida-201301
Uttar Pradesh, India
+91 120 45 566 00, customerservice@thieme.in

Thieme Revinter Publicações Ltda.
Rua do Matoso, 170
Rio de Janeiro, RJ, CEP 20270-135, Brasil
+55 21 2563 9700

Cover design: Thieme Publishing Group
Typesetting by Thomson Digital, India

Printed in India by Replika Press Pvt Ltd.   5 4 3 2 1

ISBN 978-1-60406-881-8

Also available as an e-book:
eISBN 978-1-60406-882-5

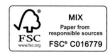

Important note: Medicine is an ever-changing science undergoing continual development. Research and clinical experience are continually expanding our knowledge, in particular our knowledge of proper treatment and drug therapy. Insofar as this book mentions any dosage or application, readers may rest assured that the authors, editors, and publishers have made every effort to ensure that such references are in accordance with **the state of knowledge at the time of production of the book.**

Nevertheless, this does not involve, imply, or express any guarantee or responsibility on the part of the publishers in respect to any dosage instructions and forms of applications stated in the book. **Every user is requested to examine carefully** the manufacturers' leaflets accompanying each drug and to check, if necessary in consultation with a physician or specialist, whether the dosage schedules mentioned therein or the contraindications stated by the manufacturers differ from the statements made in the present book. Such examination is particularly important with drugs that are either rarely used or have been newly released on the market. Every dosage schedule or every form of application used is entirely at the user's own risk and responsibility. The authors and publishers request every user to report to the publishers any discrepancies or inaccuracies noticed. If errors in this work are found after publication, errata will be posted at www.thieme.com on the product description page.

Some of the product names, patents, and registered designs referred to in this book are in fact registered trademarks or proprietary names even though specific reference to this fact is not always made in the text. Therefore, the appearance of a name without designation as proprietary is not to be construed as a representation by the publisher that it is in the public domain.

I would like to dedicate this book to my two little angels Mia age one, and Christian age two. It is a joy for our family watching them grow up and truly enjoying the gift of life.

Alex R. Vaccaro

This book is dedicated to my patients, who have honored me with their trust.

Richard G. Fessler

To my wife Henna and children Zain, Rafae and Sabrina who make all things possible for me with their unwavering love and support. And to my patients who inspire and challenge me to find the best treatments for their spinal problems.

Faheem A. Sandhu

To my wife Nitsa for her unconditional love, understanding and support and for giving me the greatest gift of all: my children Alexandra and Olivia.

Jean-Marc Voyadzis

To Laurie, Katie and Caroline for their love and support during this project.

Jason C. Eck

I dedicate this book to Alana, an incredible wife, mother and surgeon.

Christopher K. Kepler

Contents

Part I: Degenerative

Foreword

Controversies in Spine Surgery, MIS versus Open: Best Evidence Recommendations is a phenomenal book. In this book, readers will find a combination of a 'duel' and a 'duet' – the former as it relates to the evidence provided by authors and editors with differing opinions and philosophies, and the latter as it relates to a synchronous collection of pros and cons (MIS vs Open), etc.

The 'duel/duet' notion is masterfully accomplished in each chapter by the authors and then equally masterfully summed up by the book's editors – each harboring differing opinions on the subject at hand. The strength of the literature and level of evidence is presented and rationalized in each chapter.

MIS (minimally invasive surgery) and Open approaches are repetitively compared and contrasted in each chapter. The two approaches are analyzed in an objective manner with 'opposing sides' presenting the evidence and rationale. After the assimilation of the information, the reader can then draw his/her own conclusions – after enjoying the balanced harmony between the 'duel' and the 'duet'.

The book covers 24 subjects, each with a dedicated chapter. The topics range from discectomy to cost and value. The book is extraordinarily comprehensive and complete. There were absolutely no stones left unturned here.

I cannot comprehend the amount of work the authors and editors must have put into this book. We, the readers, can reap the benefits of their toils. If your allegiance lies with either the Open or the MIS side of the 'duel', this book is for you. It will open your eyes to the other side and to the facts as best we know them.

Edward C. Benzel, MD
Neurosurgeon and Chairman
Department of Neurosurgery
Center for Spine Health
Cleveland Clinic
Cleveland, Ohio

Preface

There are many controversial topics in spine surgery but one area that is widely debated as it now touches all areas of our field is the emergence of minimally invasive techniques to treat common spinal disorders. When first introduced, minimally invasive approaches seemed like sensationalistic procedures that would be done by a few surgeons daring or foolish enough to try them. Fortunately that is not the case and a sizable body of literature has amassed to support the use of minimally invasive techniques. However, minimally invasive techniques are far from being recognized as the standard of care, and when and whether to use a minimally invasive approach remains unclear.

Controversies in Spine Surgery: Best Evidence Recommendations, published in 2010 by Vaccaro and Eck, gave spine surgeons an excellent resource to base clinical treatments on the highest level of evidence from the literature. While there remains a paucity of level I evidence in the field of spine surgery, evaluation of all the best literature still frames a rational approach to clinical treatments.

It is clear that minimally invasive approaches are here to stay but whether they are truly superior to traditional open approaches for different spinal pathologies remains unknown. This body of work attempts to address these questions using the best evidence approach. Topics and authors were carefully selected to help clarify common debates that exist between MIS and open approaches. At least one open and one minimally invasive author were involved in the production of every chapter. Each chapter presents an important topic, an illustrative case demonstrating the minimally invasive and open surgical techniques, and the supporting literature for each approach in a best evidence format. Summary tables of the literature and complications by approach are provided. Finally, Drs. Vaccaro and Fessler end each chapter with remarks on the open and MIS approaches, respectively.

It is not our goal to convince readers that one approach is better than the other but to provide the necessary supportive information for readers to draw their own conclusions and provide their patients with the best evidence-based treatments. We hope to also encourage continued research efforts in clarifying topics we all find controversial.

Alexander R. Vaccaro, MD, PhD, FACS, MBA
Richard G. Fessler, MD, PhD
Faheem A. Sandhu, MD, PhD
Jean-Marc Voyadzis, MD
Jason C. Eck, DO, MS
Christopher K. Kepler, MD, MBA

Acknowledgments

A collaborative body of work of this breadth and magnitude takes years of preparation and the concerted efforts of many. Drs. Sandhu, Voyadzis, Eck, and Kepler would like to thank Drs. Vaccaro and Fessler, internationally recognized clinician scientists and pioneers, for their wisdom and significant contributions to the world of spine surgery. Of the many challenges inherent to this ambitious project, the most important was the invitation to authors to collaborate on each chapter, thus creating the open versus MIS perspective. This could not have been achieved without the enthusiastic efforts of our Georgetown residents, Drs. Anthony Conte, Hasan Syed and Rory Petteys, who were instrumental in contributing chapters, editing others, and bringing this project to fruition.

The Editors

Contributors

Tim Eugene Adamson, MD
Neurosurgeon
Carolina Neurosurgery & Spine Associates
Charlotte, North Carolina

Todd J. Albert, MD
Surgeon-in-Chief, Chief Medical Officer
Chairman Department of Orthopaedics
Hospital for Special Surgery
Weill Cornell Medical College
New York, New York

Marjan Alimi, MD
Senior Clinical Research Fellow in Spine
Weill Cornell Brain and Spine Center
New York-Presbyterian Hospital
Weill Cornell Medical College
New York, New York

Richard Todd J. Allen, MD, PhD
Associate Professor of Orthopaedic Surgery
Director, Spine Surgery Fellowship
UC San Diego Health System
Department of Orthopaedic Surgery
San Diego, California

Navid R. Arandi, MD
Emergency Medicine Resident Physician
Aventura Hospital and Medical Center
Aventura, Florida

John D. Attenello, MD
Orthopaedic Surgery Resident
University of Hawaii Orthopaedic Surgery
  Residency Program
Honolulu, Hawaii

Bryce A. Basques, MD
Orthopaedic Surgery Resident
Rush University Medical Center
Chicago, Illinois

Amandeep Bhalla, MD
Assistant Professor
David Geffen School of Medicine at UCLA
Harbor-UCLA Medical Center
Department of Orthopaedic Surgery
Torrance, California

Oheneba Boachie-Adjei, MD
Professor
Orthopedic Surgery
Weill Cornell Medical College
Accra, Ghana

Daniel D. Bohl, MD
Resident
Rush University Medical Center
Chicago, Illinois

Christopher M. Bono, MD
Chief
Orthopaedic Spine Service
Associate Professor of Orthopedic Surgery
Brigham and Women's Hospital
Harvard Medical School
Boston, Massachusetts

Saad B. Chaudhary, MD, MBA
Assistant Professor
Icahn School of Medicine
Mount Sinai
New York, New York

Michelle J. Clarke, MD
Associate Professor of Neurosurgery
Mayo Clinic
Rochester, Minnesota

Anthony Conte, MD
Resident Physician
Medstar Georgetown University Hospital
Department of Neurosurgery
Washington, DC

Scott D. Daffner, MD
Associate Professor
Department of Orthopaedics
West Virginia University
Health Sciences Center
Morgantown, West Virginia

Vedat Deviren, MD
Professor
Clinical Orthopaedic
UCSF Department of Orthopaedic Surgery
San Francisco, California

Jason C. Eck, DO, MS
Orthopedic Spine Surgeon
Center for Sports Medicine and Orthopedics
Chattanooga, Tennessee

Kurt M. Eichholz, MD, FAANS, FACS
Neurosurgeon
St. Louis Minimally Invasive Spine Center
St. Louis, Missouri

Randa El Mallah, MD
University of Mississippi Medical Center
Jackson, Mississippi

Richard G. Fessler, MD, PhD
Professor
Department of Neurosurgery
Rush University Medical Center
Chicago, Illinois

Jeremy Fogelson, MD
Assistant Professor or Neurological Surgery
Assistant Professor of Orthopaedic Surgery
Mayo Clinic
Rochester, Minnesota

Anthony K. Frempong-Boadu, MD, FACS, FAANS
Associate Professor of Neurosurgery
NYU Langone Medical Center
New York, New York

Gurpreet S. Gandhoke, MD
Chief Resident
Department of Neurological Surgery
University of Pittsburgh Medical Center
Pittsburgh, Pennsylvania

Steven R. Garfin, MD
Distinguished Professor and Chair
UC San Diego
San Diego, California

Joanna Gernsback, MD
Neurosurgery Chief Resident
Jackson Memorial Hospital/University of
   Miami Miller School of Medicine
Miami, Florida

Nicholas S. Golinvaux, MD
Orthopaedic Surgery
Vanderbilt Orthopaedics
Nashville, Tennessee

Jonathan N. Grauer, MD
Professor
Department of Orthopaedics and Rehabilitation
Yale School of Medicine
Yale University
New Haven, Connecticut

Roger Härtl, MD
Professor
Neurological Surgery
Director
Spinal Surgery
Weill Cornell Medical College
New York, New York

Andrew C. Hecht, MD
Chief, Spine Surgery
Mount Sinai Hospital and Mount Sinai Health System
Director, Mount Sinai Spine Center
Associate Professor Orthopaedic and Neurosurgery
Mt. Sinai Medical Center and Icahn School of Medicine
New York, New York

Christopher Clayton Hills, DO
Orthopaedic Surgeon
Teton Orthopaedics
Jackson, Wyoming

Robert E. Isaacs, MD
Associate Professor
Department of Neurosurgery
Duke University Medical Center
Durham, North Carolina

S. Babak Kalantar, MD
Associate Professor
Chief
Division of Spinal Surgery
Department of Orthopaedics
Medstar Georgetown University Hospital
Washington, DC

Adam S. Kanter, MD
Associate Professor
University of Pittsburgh Medical Center
Pittsburgh, Pennsylvania

Jonathan M. Karnes, MD
Resident
Department of Orthopaedics
West Virginia University
Morgantown, West Virginia

Christopher K. Kepler, MD, MBA
Associate Professor
Orthopaedic Spine Surgeon
Department of Orthopaedic Surgery
Thomas Jefferson University and Hospitals
Rothman Institute
Philadelphia, Pennsylvania

John D. Koerner, MD
Spine Surgeon
Hackensack Univesity Medical College
Glen Rock, New Jersey

Joseph Paul Letzelter III, MD
Resident
Georgetown Orthopaedic Surgery
Delray Beach, Florida

John C. Liu, MD
Professor of Neurosurgery and Orthopaedic Surgery
University of Southern California
Los Angeles, California

Luis Marchi, PhD
Director of Clinical Research
Instituto de Patologia da Coluna (IPC)
São Paulo, Brazil

Steven Joseph McAnany, MD
Assistant Professor
St. Louis School of Medicine
Washington University
St. Louis, Missouri

Matthew J. McGirt, MD
Neurosurgeon
Carolina Neurosurgery and Spine Associates
Department of Surgery
University of North Carolina
Charlotte, North Carolina

Ankit I. Mehta, MD
Assistant Professor of Neurosurgery
Director of Spinal Oncology
Associate Neurosurgical Program Director
University of Illinois at Chicago
Chicago, Illinois

Paul W. Millhouse, MD
Spine Research Fellow
Rothman Institute
Department of Orthopaedic Research
Philadelphia, Pennsylvania

Ralph J. Mobbs, MD
Neurospine Research Group
Prince of Wales Private Hospital
University of New South Wales
Sydney, New South Wales, Australia

Troy I. Mounts, MD, MA
Spine Surgeon
Troy I Mounts MD INC
San Luis Obispo, California

Gregory M. Mundis Jr., MD
Co-Director San Diego Spine Fellowship
Scripps Clinic San Diego
San Diego Spine Foundation
La Jolla, California

Ahmad Nassr, MD
Consultant and Associate Professor
Orthopedic Surgery and Biomedical Engineering
Mayo Clinic
Department of Orthopedic Surgery
Rochester, Minnesota

Venu M. Nemani, MD, PhD
Cervical and Reconstructive Spine Surgeon
Raleigh Orthopaedic Clinic
Raleigh, North Carolina

Eric W. Nottmeier, MD
Neurosurgeon
St. Vincent's Spine and Brain Institute
Adjunct Associate Professor of Neurosurgery
Mayo Clinic College of Medicine
St. Vincent's Spine and Brain Institute
Jacksonville, Florida

Alfred T. Ogden, MD
Assistant Professor
Columbia University Medical Center-New York Presbyterian
    Hospital
New York, New York

David O. Okonkwo, MD
Professor
Executive Vice Chair
Department of Neurological Surgery
University of Pittsburgh Medical Center
Pittsburgh, Pennsylvania

Leonardo Oliveira, BS
Researcher
Instituto de Patologia da Coluna (IPC)
São Paulo, Brazil

John E. O'Toole, MD, MS
Professor of Neurosurgery
Rush University Medical Center
Chicago, Illinois

Sylvain Palmer, MD, FACS
Neurosurgeon
Orange County Neurosurgical Associates
Mission Viejo, California

Scott L. Parker, MD
Assistant Professor
Department of Neurosurgery
Vanderbilt University Medical Center
Nashville, Tennessee

Rory J. Petteys, MD
Chief of Neurosurgery
William Beaumont Army Medical Center
El Paso, Texas

Martin H. Pham, MD
Neurosurgery Resident
Department of Neurosurgery
Keck School of Medicine of USC
Los Angeles, California

Luiz Pimenta, MD, PhD
Medical Director
Instituto de Patologia da Coluna (IPC)
University of California San Diego (UCSD)
São Paulo, Brazil

Mark L. Prasarn, MD
Chief
Division of Spine Surgery
Department of Orthopedic Surgery
University of Texas
Houston, Texas

Kristen E. Radcliff, MD
Associate Professor
Rothman Institute
Department of Orthopedic Surgery
Thomas Jefferson University
Egg Harbor, New Jersey

Prashanth J. Rao, MD
Neurospine Research Group
Prince of Wales Private Hospital
University of New South Wales
Sydney, New South Wales, Australia

Peter S. Rose, MD
Associate Professor
Orthopaedic Surgery
Mayo Clinic
Rochester Minnesota

Faheem A. Sandhu, MD, PhD
Professor of Neurosurgery
Director of Spine Surgery
Co-Director
Center for Minimally Invasive Spine Surgery
Department of Neurosurgery
MedStar Georgetown University Hospital
Washington, DC

Daniel M. Sciubba, MD
Professor of Neurosurgery
Oncology & Orthopaedic Surgery
Johns Hopkins University
Baltimore, Maryland

David L. Scott, MD
Surgeon
Gulf Coast Orthopaedic Center
Hudson, Florida

Christopher I. Shaffrey, MD
Professor
Department of Neurological Surgery
University of Virginia
Charlottesville, Virginia

Steven M. Spitz, MD
Assistant Professor
Department of Neurosurgery
Medstar Georgetown University Hospital
Washington, DC

Russell G. Strom, MD
Associate Neurosurgeon
Geisinger Health System
Wilkes-Barre, Pennsylvania

Brian W. Su, MD
Spine Surgeon
Mt Tam Orthopedics Spine Center
Larkspur, California

Hasan R. Syed, MD
Assistant Professor
Department of Neurological Surgery
University of Virginia Health System
Charlottesville, Virginia

Alexander A. Theologis, MD
Resident Physician
University of California – San Francisco (UCSF)
San Francisco, California

Trent L. Tredway, MD
Founder and Neurosurgeon
Tredway Spine Institute
Seattle, Washington

P. Justin Tortolani, MD
Chief
Spine Service and Fellowship Director
Medstar Union Memorial Hospital
Baltimore, Maryland

Jose M. Torres-Campa, MD
Neurosurgeon
Centro Medico de Asturias
Oviedo, Spain

Alexander Tuchman, MD
Clinical Instructor
Department of Neurosurgery
University of Southern California
Los Angeles, California

Juan S. Uribe, MD
Associate Professor
Department of Neurological Surgery
University of South Florida
Tampa, Florida

Alexander R. Vaccaro, MD, PhD, FACS, MBA
Richard H. Rothman Professor and Chairman
Department of Orthopaedic Surgery
Professor of Neurosurgery
Thomas Jefferson University and Hospitals
President, The Rothman Institute
Philadelphia, Pennsylvania

Michael J. Vives, MD
Associate Professor
Orthopaedics
Chief
Spine Division
New Jersey Medical School
Rutgers University
Newark, New Jersey

Jean-Marc Voyadzis, MD
Co-Director
Center for Minimally Invasive Spine Surgery
Associate Professor of Neurosurgery
MedStar Georgetown University Hospital
Washington, DC

Michael Y. Wang, MD, FACS
Professor of Neurological Surgery
Division Chief
Spine Medical Director
Spine JMH
Spine Fellowship Director
UMH Medical Director
Minimally Invasive Spine UMH
UMH Chief of Neurosurgery
University of Miami
Miami, Florida

Peter G. Whang, MD, FACS
Associate Professor
Department of Orthopaedics and Rehabilitation
Yale School of Medicine
Yale University
New Haven, Connecticut

Chun-Po Yen, MD
Associate Professor
Department of Neurological Surgery
University of Virginia
Charlottesville, Virginia

Jonathan Yun, MD
Resident
Columbia University Medical Center-NewYork
  Presbyterian Hospital
New York, New York

Alp Yurter, BS
Medical Student
Yale School of Medicine
New Haven, Connecticut

Part I

Degenerative

1 Lumbar Discectomy: Is Tubular or Endoscopic Discectomy Better Than Traditional Microdiscectomies?

MIS: Martin H. Pham, Alexander Tuchman, and John C. Liu
Open: John D. Attenello, Steven R. Garfin, and Richard Todd J. Allen

1.1 Introduction

Mixter and Barr[1] described the first discectomy for lumbar disc herniation in 1934, where they performed a laminectomy with a transdural approach to remove the intervertebral disc. A few years later, Love[2,3] described an intralaminar, extradural approach to disc removal. This procedure serves as the basis for open discectomy (OD) today and remained largely unchanged until the 1970s when the introduction of the surgical microscope gave rise to less invasive approaches with smaller incisions, less tissue dissection, and decreased surgical manipulation and trauma to the musculature and nerve roots. Yasargil[4] and Caspar[5] were the first to independently describe their use of the operating microscope to refine the previous approach into the open microdiscectomy, which is currently the most common surgical procedure for lumbar disc herniation worldwide.[6,7,8,9] Continued advancements in visualization technology prompted an increase in minimally invasive discectomy (MID) techniques[10] designed to minimize postoperative pain and hospital stays and allow for quicker mobilization and resumption of daily activities.

In 1997, Foley and Smith[11] described microendoscopic discectomy (MED) as a transmuscular technique to gain access to the disc via dilators of increasing diameter and a tubular retractor, whereby simultaneous visualization and removal of disc can be performed through a single portal. This replaced the conventional subperiosteal approach. These minimally invasive techniques were introduced to speed up recovery rates and decrease morbidity while achieving comparable clinical outcomes; however, studies evaluating functional outcomes and complications, comparing MID and OD, have not shown consistent benefit.

1.2 Indications

Lumbar discectomy is an effective surgical treatment for lumbar disc herniation causing nerve root compression and presenting with radiating leg pain, paresthesias, and back pain. Severe symptoms refractory to conservative treatment for ≥ 6 weeks commonly necessitate the removal of all or part of the offending intervertebral disc fragment, to decompress the nerve root. Other indications for surgery include intractable pain, new or progressive weakness, saddle anesthesia, or bowel/bladder symptoms suggesting cauda equina syndrome. In cases of congenital stenosis requiring decompression, to minimize iatrogenic neural injury, and possibly in cases of cauda equina syndrome, an open approach may be favored to expand the bony decompression and access the disc/stenosis at multiple angles (sometimes limited by endoscopic and tubular approaches).

1.3 Advantages of Minimally Invasive Surgery

Traditional open surgery requires muscle dissection and retraction, of which the iatrogenic morbidity of soft-tissue injury has been well established.[12,13,14] Minimally invasive surgery (MIS) approaches involve a less traumatic approach with tubular retractors to temporarily expand a surgical corridor through the soft tissue, which then falls back in place at the completion of the operation. The use of a tubular retractor for MIS discectomy minimizes tissue injury and ensures that deeper tissues are less exposed to potential pathologic organisms as a result of the restricted surgical field.[15,16,17] The advantages of minimally invasive surgical techniques also include smaller incisions with reduced soft-tissue damage and faster immediate postoperative recovery. This in effect allows for a shorter hospital stay and an earlier return to work.

1.4 Advantages of Open Surgery

A commonly cited advantage of OD is the historical success of the procedure. OD is well known to spine surgeons and has been developed and refined since the 1930s with consistently favorable results demonstrated in numerous studies since then.[18,19,20,21,22,23,24,25] Furthermore, many of the most powerful or highest level studies evaluating patient outcomes in microdiscectomy are those primarily employing open techniques. The ubiquitous nature of the open approach avoids the steep learning curve of MIS techniques, which can be associated with unfavorable outcomes and increased risk of complications particularly early on and when extension to open is needed. Additional advantages of OD include greater visualization of the dural sac/neural elements and surrounding structural relationships, direct visualization of all anatomic structures, ability to access extruded/migrated fragments safely by extending the decompression or obtaining the optimal angle for disc removal, and lower costs for instrumentation.

1.5 Case Illustration

A 36-year-old man with a history of low back pain developed worsening left leg pain into the foot that failed anti-inflammatory medications, muscle relaxants, physical therapy, and activity modifications. Despite three epidural steroid injections over a 4-month period, he continued to have worsening leg pain and mild ankle dorsiflexion weakness. Imaging studies showed a left L4–L5 paracentral disc herniation (▶ Fig. 1.1a,b) without evidence of instability on flexion and extension lateral lumbar radiographs.

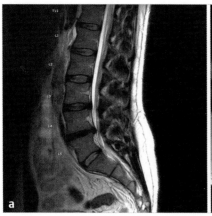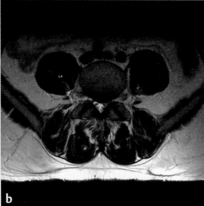

Fig. 1.1 (a) Sagittal and (b) axial magnetic resonance imaging of the lumbar spine demonstrating a broad central disc herniation at L4–L5 compressing the left L5 nerve root.

1.6 Surgical Technique in Minimally Invasive Surgery

After general endotracheal intubation is obtained, the patient is positioned prone onto a Jackson table with a Wilson frame. Arms are positioned up by the head, the neck is checked to be in appropriate neutral position, and all pressure points are appropriately padded. The bed attachment for the tubular arm is placed on the contralateral side of the planned MIS discectomy. The area is then prepped with antiseptic solution and draped in standard surgical fashion.

Anteroposterior fluoroscopy is used to confirm that the patient is not rotated, and then lateral fluoroscopy is used with a 22-gauge needle to mark the appropriate level and trajectory to the intended disc space. An 18-mm incision is made in the skin, which is then dissected down with monopolar electrocautery until fascia is reached. The fascia is then also opened with electrocautery. A Kirschner wire is then carefully docked on the lamina, and serial tubular dilation is used around the wire until the appropriate-sized tubular retractor is reached. Lateral fluoroscopy is used to confirm the correct level, and anteroposterior fluoroscopy can be used to confirm that the tube is medialized toward the spinous process. This last fluoroscopy film is especially important in patients with large facet joints, given the facet joint may be mistaken for the lamina if the tube has been docked too laterally.

The microdiscectomy portion of the operation then proceeds in standard fashion after the microscope or endoscope is brought in. The base of the spinous process and inferior edge of the lamina are identified after dissection of the soft tissue. A matchstick drill is then used to drill a laminotomy down to the ligamentum flavum. The ligamentum is carefully removed with a combination of curettes and Kerrison rongeurs until the dura and nerve root are identified. The thecal sac and nerve root shoulder are then carefully retracted and the offending herniated disc is subsequently removed. Appropriate decompression is then confirmed by tactile feel with a curette or nerve hook.

Copious irrigation is used to clean out the wound. The fascia, dermis, and skin are subsequently closed in multiple layers with absorbable sutures.

1.7 Surgical Technique in Open Surgery

Following informed consent, the patient is brought to the operating room and endotracheal anesthesia is administered. Preoperative antibiotics are given, lower extremity pneumatic compression devices are placed, and the patient is positioned prone on either a Wilson frame, or longitudinal or transverse gel rolls, or Jackson frame, with the abdomen free and all bony prominences padded. After partitioning off the region of interest, we prefer to prepare the operative area with chlorhexidine scrub, followed by drying and then using C-arm fluoroscopy imaging in anteroposterior and lateral planes, to mark our site for incision. The patient is then sterilely prepped and draped, and following an intraoperative time-out and the injection of 0.25% Marcaine with epinephrine, an incision is made in the midline with dissection toward the side of the herniation. The incision is typically just over 2 cm, but may be larger in larger patients. In most cases, we prefer the use of an intraoperative microscope, both for teaching purposes and for visualization. Dissection ensues through subcutaneous tissue, lumbodorsal fascia, and then onto the spinous process of the affected area. A Cobb and Bovie are used to expose the bony anatomy along the spinous process and onto the lamina. This plane is developed to the facet joint capsule, which is identified and preserved. The pars is identified above and below the facet joint, which often lies at the level of, and just caudal to, the more ventrally located herniated disc. A McCullough retractor is generally preferred. C-arm fluoroscopy imaging is brought in to verify the correct level of surgery prior to significant dissection. A spinal needle can be placed in the interspinous process ligaments on a Penfield 4 just under the inferior edge of the superior lamina of the space prior to obtaining the image. A matchstick burr can be used to thin the lamina overlying the disc, if needed (thick, overhanging) and a curette used to develop a plane on the underside of the remaining superior lamina and ligamentum flavum. Bone and ligamentum flavum are removed or released with Kerrison rongeurs to develop the working window laminotomy for discectomy, working proximally and laterally to free tethered ligamentum as needed. Once the epidural fat/space is identified, bipolar cautery and gentle retraction are used to optimize hemostasis and identify the offending disc herniation. An annulotomy knife is used, if necessary, and the disc is removed using a pituitary or other micro-instruments. Closure is done following irrigation and obtaining hemostasis, with #1 Vicryl, 0-Vicryl, and 2-0 Vicryl, and then Monocryl in running fashion. Dermabond is applied, followed by a sterile dressing. Ropivacaine can be infiltrated prior to final closure to help with postoperative anesthesia and pain control.

1.8 Discussion of Minimally Invasive Surgery

Multiple advantages of the MIS approach over standard approaches have been shown, with the MIS tubular technique showing lower infection rates, lower cerebrospinal fluid (CSF) leak rates, and shorter hospital stays, with outcomes similar to open surgery (▶ Table 1.1).

1.8.1 Level I Evidence in Minimally Invasive Surgery

Arts et al performed a prospective, multicenter, double-blinded randomized trial comparing 8-week and 1-year outcomes in patients undergoing tubular discectomy versus conventional open microdiscectomy for treatment of disc herniation refractory to conservative measures.[26] In total, 167 patients were assigned to receive discectomy via endoscopic approach and 161 were assigned to a conventional microdiscectomy approach. At 1 year, patients in the open approach reported higher improvements in back and leg pain (visual analog scale [VAS]: –4.2 mm for open group vs. –3.5 mm for MIS group). Sixty-nine percent of patients in the MIS discectomy group reported good outcomes at 1 year, compared with 79% of patients in the conventional microdiscectomy group. However, when results were expanded to 2-year follow-up, no statistically significant differences were found in good clinical outcomes (71% of patients in MIS group vs. 77% of patients in open group) or reoperation rates (15% of patients in MIS group vs. 10% of patients in open group) between patients undergoing minimal invasive versus microdiscectomy. Of note, similar disc reherniation rates were seen between the two groups, with patients in the minimally invasive group having shorter hospital stays, earlier time to mobilization, and less progression of sensory and motor deficits postoperatively.

A Cochrane review by Rasouli et al compared the benefits and harms of MIS discectomy versus standard microdiscectomy or OD in symptomatic lumbar disc herniation.[27] They identified 11 randomized controlled trials (1,172 patients) which compared the two approaches for the treatment of adults with lumbar discectomy caused by discopathy. They found low-quality evidence that MIS approaches were associated with worse leg pain at follow-up from 6 months to 2 years, but differences were small (less than 0.5 points on a 0 to 10 scale) and did not meet thresholds for clinically meaningful significance. Low-quality evidence also suggested no significant differences in back pain comparing the two approaches out to 1 year of follow-up. The authors also found no differences on outcomes related to functional disability as measured by the Oswestry

Disability Index (ODI). With regard to secondary outcomes, MIS approaches were associated with a lower risk of surgical site infections and shorter hospital stay, although available evidence was inconsistent.

Gempt et al randomized 60 patients to receive either a traditional open approach or an MIS approach discectomy for single-level lumbar disc herniations.[28] Over a mean follow-up time of 33 months, patients were evaluated with physical health, mental health, and pain relief questionnaires using the ODI, Short Form Health Survey (SF-36), and the VAS for back and leg pain. Patients in both groups demonstrated significant improvements in leg and low back pain with good to excellent recoveries by ODI and SF-36 evaluations. There was no statistically significant difference observed between the two groups with regard to long-term VAS, ODI, or SF-36 outcomes.

1.8.2 Level II Evidence in Minimally Invasive Surgery

Kamper et al recently conducted a meta-analysis of 29 studies examining differences between minimally invasive and conventional microdiscectomy in 4,472 patients with sciatica from lumbar disc herniation.[29] They found low-quality evidence to support a shorter mean hospital stay in the MIS group, with a difference of 1.5 days. Although the analysis was in favor of the MIS group, the hospital times were variable and the source of the variability was unclear to the authors. There was moderate to low-quality evidence to suggest no differences in clinical outcomes, complications, or reoperations between MIS and open approaches for discectomy.

1.8.3 Level III and IV Evidence in Minimally Invasive Surgery

Harrington and French sought to compare operative times, length of hospital stay, and narcotic use in their retrospective review of single lumbar microdiscectomy patients performed by a single surgeon using a traditional open versus a minimally invasive approach.[30] There were 35 patients in the open group and 31 in the minimally invasive group. No differences were found with regard to intraoperative complications, surgical time, blood loss, or outcome. However, 45.2% of MIS approach patients were discharged on the same day versus 5.75% in the OD group ($p = 0.001$). The MIS group also used less intravenous morphine ($p = 0.04$) and less hydrocodone ($p = 0.03$), and did not use any oxycodone for pain control (vs. an average of 11.7-mg oxycodone in the open group).

Lau et al also compared differences in microdiscectomy performed via MIS techniques or open approaches by a single surgeon.[31] A retrospective analysis of 25 patients undergoing open microdiscectomy as compared with 20 patients receiving an MIS approach found no statistically significant differences in operative time, length of stay, outcome, or complication rates.

1.9 Complications in Minimally Invasive Surgery

Surgical site infections can be a source of significant morbidity that itself can lead to further major complications and worse

Table 1.1 Literature on minimally invasive versus open discectomy

Study	Level	Surgical technique	Number of patients	Follow-up	Significantly different outcome MIS/open	Nonsignificantly different outcome MIS/open
Arts et al	I	Tubular discectomy vs. conventional microdiscectomy	166 vs. 159	4, 8, 26, 52 wk	• Higher rate of recovery in open group at 1 year (79 vs. 69%) • Greater improvement in VAS leg and back pain scores in the open group • Longer operative time with tubular discectomy	No significant difference in complication rates, RDQ, SF-36, or hospital stay
Teli et al	I	Microendoscopic discectomy vs. microdiscectomy vs. open discectomy	70 vs.72 vs. 70	6, 12, 24 mo	• MED associated with more frequent severe complications (dural tear, nerve root injury, and recurrent herniation) compared to MD or OD • Higher cost per case for MED compared to MD or OD • Longer operative time with MED	No significant difference in VAS scores for leg and back pain, ODI, SF-36, or hospital stay
Righesso et al	I	Micro endoscopic discectomy vs. open discectomy	19 vs. 21	1, 3, 6, 12, 24 mo	• Less pain at 12 h postoperation with OD • Longer operative time with MED • 2-h shorter hospital stay with MED	No significant difference in ODI, change in motor/sensory deficits, or VAS for pain (except at 12 h after surgery)
Cochrane review	I	Minimally invasive discectomy vs. microdiscectomy or open discectomy	1,172	5 d to 56 mo	• Open: less leg pain at 6 mo to 2 y • Less back pain at 6 mo and 2 y • Higher quality-of-life scores on SF-36 subclasses (physical functioning, bodily pain, general health) after 6 mo • Lower risk of recurrent disc herniations requiring rehospitalization, but higher risk of surgical site/wound infections	No difference in ODI, persistence of neurological deficits, sciatica bothersome index, or sciatica frequency index
Garg et al	I	Microendoscopic discectomy vs. open discectomy	55 vs. 57	12–18 mo	• Longer operative time with MED, but less blood loss and shorter hospital stay	No difference in ODI, low back pain, or complications rate
Ruetten et al	I	Full endoscopic discectomy vs. microdiscectomy	91 vs. 87	1 d, 3, 6, 12, 24 mo	n/a	No difference in VAS for leg and back pain, ODI, recurrent disc herniations, or North American Spine Society (NASS) Instrument scores for pain and neurogenic symptoms
SPORT randomized trial	I	Open discectomy vs. nonoperative management	245 vs. 256	1.5, 3, 6, 12, 24 mo	• Due to significant crossover, OD improvements were less pronounced	
SPORT observational cohort	II	Open discectomy vs. nonoperative management	528 vs. 191	1.5, 3, 6, 12, 24 mo	• Improvements in ODI and SF-36 subclasses, sciatica bothersome index, self-reported improvements, and satisfaction in OD over nonoperative management	
Lau et al	III	Minimally invasive discectomy vs. open discectomy	20 vs. 25	8.2 mo	n/a	No difference in pain, complications, blood loss, operative time, length of hospital stay, and neurological function

Abbreviations: MD, microdiscectomy; MED, microendoscopic discectomy; MIS, minimally invasive surgery; OD, open discectomy; ODI, Oswestry Disability Index; SF-36, Short Form Health Survey; SPORT, Spine Patient Outcomes Research Trial; VAS, visual analog scale.

outcomes.[16,32,33,34,35,36,37] The treatment of these complications can require long-term antibiotic therapy, additional procedures or operations, and prolonged hospitalizations. Identifying risk factors to reduce infection is important toward developing a strategy of preventing this complication.

Ee et al conducted a retrospective review of 2,299 patients undergoing transforaminal lumbar interbody fusion, laminectomy, or discectomy and identified 27 cases of surgical site infections.[15] After matching with controls and stratifying by procedure, they found that patients undergoing open spinal surgery were 5.77 times more likely to develop infections compared with MIS approaches. Specifically in patients undergoing laminectomy or laminotomy with or without discectomy, there were seven cases of infection in the open group as compared to three in the MIS group. Although their statistical significance was borderline, they suggested that surgical approach was an independent risk factor for postoperative surgical site infections.

O'Toole et al sought to determine the rate of surgical site infections for MIS spinal surgeries.[16] They reviewed their experience of 1,338 MIS spinal surgeries and found an overall infection rate of only 0.22%. When looking specifically at MIS discectomy, foraminotomy, or decompression, the infection was lower at only 0.10% inclusive of both superficial and deep infections. This is in comparison to recent literature on open laminectomy reporting a surgical site infection of 1.0% among 6,365 patients.[38] Authors of other series have similarly reported rates of surgical site infections of 0.2 to 2% after simple open decompressive procedures, in particular microdiscectomy.[16,31,32,33,38,39,40,41,42,43] They also concluded that a reduction in postoperative wound infection is one possible advantage of MIS techniques for spinal surgery.

There are several mechanisms that may explain the lower published infection rates of MIS spinal approaches as compared to their open counterparts. The deep tissue area and potential dead space at risk for infection are reduced in MIS surgery with the use of the tubular retractor. This reduction may help prevent postoperative hematomas or seromas that may lead to infection.[44] The tubular retractor itself also physically blocks the local contamination of deep tissue by surface skin flora and only permits the use of surgical instruments rather than the surgeon's hands.

Another complication that may result from lumbar microdiscectomies is an unintentional durotomy leading to a CSF leak. This can further lead to postural headaches, pseudomeningocele, wound infection, meningitis, or remote intracranial complications of subdural or cerebellar hemorrhage.[13,45,46,47,48,49,50,51,52] Repair of these leaks involves the risks associated with prolonged bed rest, lumbar drain placement, blood patch injection, or revision surgery for repair. Long-term consequences of untreated CSF leaks may include worsening back pain, arachnoiditis, and an overall poor functional outcome.[53] Unrecognized durotomies can occur in 6.8% of cases.[54]

Recent literature shows that a potential benefit for MIS approaches for microdiscectomy is lower incidences of CSF leaks over open approaches. Shih et al reported a series of 49 patients who required one-level or two-level lumbar decompression for degenerative lumbar stenosis, with 23 patients receiving an MIS approach and 26 patients getting an open approach.[55] They found that the open lumbar decompression group was more than four times more likely to develop a CSF leak, with 19.2% in the open group as compared to 4.3% in the

MIS group. There was no significant difference in age or number of operative levels between the two groups.

Wong et al reviewed a series of 863 consecutive patients undergoing one- or two-level discectomy, foraminotomy, or laminectomy through either MIS or open approaches at their institution over a 5-year period.[53] They reported 15 CSF leaks (4.7%) in the MIS group as compared with 49 CSF leaks (9.0%) in the open group. Of the patients with CSF leak in the open group, 8 required lumbar drainage and 12 required reoperation for repair, as compared to zero patients in the MIS group for both interventions. They found that patients undergoing open surgery were twice as likely to have a CSF leak ($p = 0.01$) for these operations. Their group concluded that rates of durotomy and symptomatic CSF leak were more prevalent in open surgery than for MIS approaches to the lumbar spine.

Multiple studies have shown that MIS techniques have lower rates of postoperative symptomatic CSF leaks when compared with open approaches.[12,26,53,56,57,58,59,60,61] More common use of the operative microscope in MIS cases provides higher magnification with brighter lighting, which may improve visualization enough to reduce the occurrence of durotomy and CSF leak. Surgeons may also operate with slower and more controlled movements under the microscope because of their exaggerated motions under high magnification.[53] In the event of a durotomy during an MIS approach that requires treatment, the re-expansion of the paraspinal musculature after removal of the tubular retractors creates a physical barrier to the hydrostatic pressure of the intradural space. This likely guards against the development of a large pseudomeningocele or symptomatic CSF leak, especially those that may require intervention with a blood patch or lumbar drain.

While CSF leak repair typically requires the use of primary watertight closure with suture, there is evidence to argue that primary dural closure is not always necessary. One successful treatment algorithm involves the use of fibrin glue alone or in conjunction with blood-soaked Gelfoam, muscle graft, or collagen matrix.[53,60] This is especially important for MIS approaches where the narrow tubular corridor is particularly prohibitive for a direct repair of durotomy with suture. Likewise, there is no direct access to native tissue patches without removal of the retractor and loss of the surgical field. Experience has shown, however, that CSF leaks in MIS cases can be sufficiently treated with just a thin layer of fibrin sealant and Gelfoam.[53] Expansion of the muscle upon removal of the retractor system will then assist in closing off dead space and tamponading CSF egress. Subsequent inpatient management typically involves flat bed rest for 24 hours to reduce the intrathecal hydrostatic pressure at the durotomy site.[53,55]

1.10 Conclusion of Minimally Invasive Surgery

Careful patient selection and adequate nerve root decompression remain the mainstay of surgical principles to optimize outcomes for lumbar disc herniation.[62] With functional outcomes being comparable to open microdiscectomy, the argument for MIS approaches lies in the lower rates of surgical site infection, rates of durotomy and symptomatic CSF leak, and shorter hospital stays. Using the grading scale of Guyatt et al,[8] we suggest a Grade 1B recommendation that MIS and open approaches are generally equivalent in overall clinical outcome. There is level III and IV evidence to suggest that MIS approaches have reduced surgical site infections and symptomatic CSF leaks (Grade 2C).

1.11 Discussion of Open Surgery

1.11.1 Level I Evidence in Open Surgery

The Spine Patient Outcomes Research Trial[25] (SPORT) reported one of the largest series to date comparing OD to nonoperative management in a prospective multicenter randomized clinical trial of 501 patients with lumbar disc herniation with persistent symptoms for ≥ 6 weeks. Follow-up ranged from 6 weeks to 8 years. Although a significant crossover rate occurred between groups (50% of patients assigned to surgery and 30% to nonsurgical management), "as-treated" analyses of results demonstrated strong, statistically significant advantages for patients undergoing OD. Limitations of the study include the high degree of nonadherence to initial treatment, eligibility criteria for persistent symptoms lasting ≥ 6 weeks, and choice for nonoperative management being left to the discretion of the treating physician.

Open versus Minimally Invasive Surgery

A Cochrane review[27] was performed to compare outcomes in MID and microdiscectomy to open discectomy (MD/OD). Eleven high-level studies were identified, with a range of 22 to 325 patients in the studies, with a total of 1,172 patients, in all studies combined. Statistically significant differences were found *in favor* of MD/OD for leg pain, back pain, complications, and health-related quality of life measures. However, these findings were small and not considered clinically significant as determined by failing to exceed the threshold for minimum clinically important difference.[63,64] The comparable outcomes support the efficacy of both MD/OD and MID. The outcomes of surgical techniques are inherently based on a surgeon's comfort level with the procedure or approach. Nevertheless, patients who underwent MD/OD had lower VAS scores for leg pain measured at 6 months to 2 years, and back pain at 6 months and 2 years. MD/OD patients had higher quality-of-life scores on the SF-36 subclasses, including physical functioning, bodily pain, and general health. OD/MD was associated with a lower risk of recurrent disc herniations requiring rehospitalization, but higher risk of surgical site/wound infections. There was no statistically significant difference in Roland-Morris Disability Questionnaire (ODI/RDQ), persistence neurological deficits, sciatica bothersome index, or sciatica frequency index between the two groups. Weaknesses of the Cochrane review include small sample sizes for many of the studies and high risk of bias. Also, 5 of the 11 studies were not blinded.

Five randomized controlled studies from the Cochrane review in favor of open procedures were chosen, including the individual study with the largest series of patients comparing conventional OD with MID. MID studies included MED and tubular discectomy, for the treatment of lumbar disc herniation with radiculopathy in adults. All patients failed at least 6 weeks of conservative treatment and all studies had follow-up times ≥ 12 months. The conclusion of these studies are described below.

Arts et al[26] reported a prospective, multicenter, double-blinded randomized trial and compared recovery rates, pain scores, complication, and functional outcomes in tubular discectomy ($n = 166$) and conventional microdiscectomy ($n = 159$). All patients had a herniated lumbar disc with radiculopathy refractory to conservative treatment for ≥ 8 weeks with 1-year follow-up. More patients achieved full recovery from surgery in the OD group (79%) compared to the MID group (69%) at 6 months ($p < 0.03$) and 1-year ($p < 0.05$). Full recovery was defined as complete or nearly complete resolution of symptoms. VAS pain scores for leg and back improved significantly in both groups, and a statistically significant difference was found in favor of OD for both leg and back pain scores. Complication rates differences were not significantly significant, but a higher incidence was seen in the minimally invasive group with 8% dural tears, 2% nerve root injuries, and 7% recurrent herniations compared to 4, 2, and 5%, respectively, in the open group. The operative time was statistically longer in the minimally invasive group even though all participating surgeons fulfilled criteria to overcome the learning curve.[17,44,65] Functional outcomes measured by the Roland-Morris Disability Questionnaire and SF-36 form were not significantly different between the groups. A major limitation of the study included inadequate power to account for the heterogeneity between centers. Also, recovery times may be underestimated because they were based on fixed predefined follow-up time points.

Teli et al[66] reported a randomized controlled trial of 212 patients comparing outcomes and complications between MED ($n = 70$), microdiscectomy (MD, $n = 72$), and OD ($n = 70$). Complications such as dural tears, nerve root injuries, and recurrent herniations requiring reoperation were significantly more common in MED (9, 3, and 11.4%) compared to MD (3, 0, and 4%) or OD (3, 0, and 3%). One case (1.4%) of spondylodiscitis occurred with MED. Wound infections were only seen in the open groups. Mean operative time was statistically significantly longer in MED (56 min) compared to MD (43 min) and OD (36 min). Surgeons involved in the study had over 5 years of experience with MED and over 10 years with MD and OD. Average cost per case was significantly higher with MED ($p = 0.002$) at 3,010 euros compared to MD (2,450 euros) and OD (2,310 euros). No significant difference was found in VAS scores for back and leg, or in ODI or SF-36. Weaknesses of the study include inability to blind patients to treatment groups, but all treatments were presented as having equal validity. Nine percent of patients dropped out after treatment.

Righesso et al[67] reported a prospective, randomized controlled study of 40 patients who underwent MED ($n = 19$) or OD ($n = 21$). No significant difference was found in the main outcomes of ODI, changes in neurological status, including motor or sensory deficits and altered reflexes, and VAS for pain, except at 12 hours after surgery ($p < 0.01$) in favor of the open group. Mean operative time was significantly longer ($p < 0.01$) with MED (82.6 min) compared to OD (63.7 min). Length of stay was 2 hours longer with OD. The main study criticism of this, as with others, is its small sample size. The Cochrane review was unable to determine which technique had a significantly shorter LOS.

Garg et al[68] reported on a prospective randomized trial of 112 patients comparing MED to OD and found no significant difference in clinical outcomes based on ODI, low back pain,

Table 1.2 Complication rates comparing open versus MIS discectomy

Complications	MIS discectomy (%)	MD/open discectomy (%)
Infection[31,55,68,71,72]	0.27	2.7
Nerve root injury[68,71]	2.5	0.5
Dural tear[31,55,68,71,72]	7.3	4.2
Disc reherniation[31,55,68,71,72]	8.9	4.2

Abbreviations: MD, microdiscectomy; MIS, minimally invasive surgery.

and complication rates for up to 18 months postoperatively. MED was found to have longer operative times, but decreased blood loss and length of stay.

Ruetten et al[69] reported a prospective, randomized, controlled trial of 178 patients who underwent either endoscopic or conventional microdiscectomy, and found no significant difference in VAS for leg and back pain, ODI, recurrent disc herniations or North American Spine Society (NASS) Instrument scores.

1.11.2 Level II Evidence in Open Surgery

The SPORT[25] reported a prospective multicenter observational cohort of 743 patients with symptomatic lumbar disc herniation for ≥ 6 weeks who underwent OD or nonoperative management. Significant improvements were seen in bodily pain, physical functioning, ODI, and the sciatica bothersome index (▶ Table 1.2). Prior to OD, 89% of patients reported being very dissatisfied with symptoms, which improved after OD, with 71.5% of patients reporting being very or somewhat satisfied with symptoms. These significantly greater improvements were maintained at 4- and 8-year follow-ups.[20,24] Limitations of the study include the inherent lack of randomization and blinding, eligibility criteria for persistent symptoms lasting ≥ 6 weeks, nonstandardized nonoperative management, and missing data. Significantly improved results were similarly reported by Weber[21] in 1983 and by the Maine Lumbar Spine Society[18,19] in a large prospective study with over 500 patients.

1.11.3 Level III and IV Evidence in Open Surgery

Lau et al[31] reported a retrospective cohort of 45 patients with lumbar disc herniation who underwent MID or OD and found no significant difference in all primary and secondary outcomes measures including pain improvement, complication rate, blood loss, operative time, length of hospital stay, and neurological function according to the American Spinal Injury Association scale. Limitations of the study include its small sample size, retrospective nature, single institution, and single operating surgeon over a period of 3 years.

1.12 Complications in Open Surgery

Although MIS techniques were initially introduced to decrease morbidity, reported complication rates have not been significantly different,[26,67,68,69,70] with randomized trials showing an increase in severe complications.[27,66] In addition, all these

studies utilized experienced surgeons who have passed the learning curve,[44,65,71] suggesting a potentially increased risk of complications for the average spine surgeon with less experience in MIS techniques. Several reasons may be proposed to explain these results. The ubiquitous nature and long history of success of the open approach ensures that the average spine surgeon has performed multiple cases and is familiar with the technique. Also, MIS techniques may suffer from restricted visualization (i.e., from the tubular retractor) and poor depth perception from the orthogonal 2D image (i.e., from the endoscope), while the open approach allows for direction visualization of the dural sac and migrating disc fragments, thereby minimizing iatrogenic dural and nerve root injuries. The open approach allows the surgeon to utilize reliable tactile feedback, which can avoid difficulty interpreting fluoroscopic imaging used in MIS, particularly in cases of altered anatomy (i.e., scoliosis) or poor bone quality. Operative time is also clearly longer in MIS, thereby not only increasing radiation to the patient, surgeon, and operating room staff, but also increasing the risk for intraoperative and perioperative complications.

1.13 Conclusion of Open Surgery

The cumulative evidence argues that OD patients in all outcome measures are comparable to, if not better than, those undergoing MID. In some high-level studies, MD/OD patients do better than MID patients in VAS back pain and leg pain scores, SF-36 physical functioning, bodily pain, and general health, and have a lower risk of recurrent herniation. The studies are summarized in ▶ Table 1.1. In addition, patients undergoing MD/OD may have shorter operative times, do not incur costs of specialized MIS instruments, and typically will have less exposure to radiation/fluoroscopy. While complication rates such as durotomies may also be less in MD/OD, OD patients may have a slightly higher rate of infection. Although it is possible that the already short length of stay is slightly shorter in MED/MIS discectomy procedures, definitive data are lacking to make this a generalized statement. Using the Guyatt et al[8] grading scale, a Grade 1B recommendation can be assigned to the evidence, suggesting there is no significant difference in improvements in pain and functional outcomes in patients undergoing a minimally invasive versus open microdiscectomy. In addition, a Grade 1B recommendation can be given to evidence supporting longer operative times for minimally invasive discectomies, with slightly higher complication rates when compared to open approaches. The overall comparable outcomes of these techniques support the efficacy of both MD/OD and MID, and the notion that differences in outcomes between these surgical techniques are inherently based on a surgeon's comfort level with the approach/procedure for the specific pathology being addressed.

1.14 Editors' Commentary

1.14.1 Minimally Invasive Surgery

Open microdiscectomy is the most common operation performed in spine surgery and enjoys excellent outcomes. MIS discectomy achieves similar outcomes, and it is difficult to argue that it is a "better" technique for treating lumbar disc herniation based solely on outcome. However, there are several advantages that the MIS approach offers even in this comparison. First, infection rates are lower than those seen in the open approach. Second, as determined from serum stress hormones, tissue trauma is less in the MIS approach. Finally, in the unfortunate situation where a durotomy is obtained, 20 years of experience with the MIS technique have demonstrated that direct closure of the dural opening is not necessary, and the incidence of pseudomeningocele is lower than that seen with the open procedure. Thus, even though the overall long-term outcome may be similar, these advantages suggest that the MIS technique is still the preferred technique for treating lumbar disc herniation.

1.14.2 Open Surgery

Open microdiscectomy is one of the least invasive and most successful procedures in the spine surgeon's armamentarium. In this regard, it is difficult to substantially improve on, particularly in a manner dramatic enough to be statistically proven. Reductions in incision length measured in millimeters and length of stay measured in hours already have a minimal footprint with smaller open incision microdiscectomy techniques. It is precisely this scenario of minimal gain that calls into question the net patient benefit of adopting surgical techniques with steep learning curves. With all sides conceding long-term outcome equivalence, the open procedure is likely to be more cost-effective as well, given the current disposable-heavy financial strategy that companies that specialize in this area utilize.

There are few complications which routinely occur during microdiscectomy, and dural injuries with associated CSF leak are among the most common. The reported increase in dural injury in open surgery is difficult to reconcile to the contrary of many spine surgeons and may reflect increased rates of unrecognized dural injury in the MIS group due to poor visualization. In addition, few surgical technique descriptions for MIS discectomy actually advocate repair of dural injuries, instead proposing these injuries are best treated with patching techniques, surgical strategies akin to promoting establishment of a pseudomeningocele.

Given the similarities in perioperative measures as well as clinical outcome, MIS discectomy may never experience any meaningful advantage over open microdiscectomy techniques. Compared with the reliability, familiarity, minimal surgical footprint, and clinical success of open microdiscectomy, "MIS" discectomy does not provide enough potential for improvement to warrant widespread adoption.

References

[1] Mixter W, Barr J. Rupture of the intervertebral disc with involvement of the spinal canal. N Engl J Med. 1934; 211:210–215

[2] Love J. Removal of protruded intervertebral disc without laminectomy. Proc Staff Meet Mayo Clin. 1939; 14:800–805

[3] Love J, Walsh M. Protruded intervertebral disks. Report of one hundred cases in which operation was performed. JAMA. 1938; 111:396–400

[4] Yasargil MG. Microsurgical operation for herniated lumbar disc. Adv Neurosurg. 1977; 4:81

[5] Caspar W. A new surgical procedure for lumbar disk herniation causing less tissue damage through a microsurgical approach. Adv Neurosurg. 1977; 4: 74–80

[6] Arts MP, Peul WC, Koes BW, Thomeer RT, Leiden-The Hague Spine Intervention Prognostic Study (SIPS) Group. Management of sciatica due to lumbar disc herniation in the Netherlands: a survey among spine surgeons. J Neurosurg Spine. 2008; 9(1):32–39

[7] Gibson JNA, Waddell G. Surgical interventions for lumbar disc prolapse: updated Cochrane Review. Spine. 2007; 32(16):1735–1747

[8] Haines SJ, Jordan N, Boen JR, Nyman JA, Oldridge NB, Lindgren BR, LAPDOG/LEAPDOG Investigators. Discectomy strategies for lumbar disc herniation: results of the LAPDOG trial. J Clin Neurosci. 2002; 9(4):411–417

[9] Koebbe CJ, Maroon JC, Abla A, El-Kadi H, Bost J. Lumbar microdiscectomy: a historical perspective and current technical considerations. Neurosurg Focus. 2002; 13(2):E3

[10] Deen HG, Fenton DS, Lamer TJ. Minimally invasive procedures for disorders of the lumbar spine. Mayo Clin Proc. 2003; 78(10):1249–1256

[11] Foley KT, Smith MM. Microendoscopic discectomy. Tech Neurosurg. 1997; 3: 301–307

[12] Fourney DR, Dettori JR, Norvell DC, Dekutoski MB. Does minimal access tubular assisted spine surgery increase or decrease complications in spinal decompression or fusion? Spine. 2010; 35(9) Suppl:S57–S65

[13] Kawaguchi Y, Matsui H, Tsuji H. Back muscle injury after posterior lumbar spine surgery. A histologic and enzymatic analysis. Spine. 1996; 21(8):941–944

[14] Sihvonen T, Herno A, Paljärvi L, Airaksinen O, Partanen J, Tapaninaho A. Local denervation atrophy of paraspinal muscles in postoperative failed back syndrome. Spine. 1993; 18(5):575–581

[15] Ee WW, Lau WL, Yeo W, Von Bing Y, Yue WM. Does minimally invasive surgery have a lower risk of surgical site infections compared with open spinal surgery? Clin Orthop Relat Res. 2014; 472(6):1718–1724

[16] O'Toole JE, Eichholz KM, Fessler RG. Surgical site infection rates after minimally invasive spinal surgery. J Neurosurg Spine. 2009; 11(4):471–476

[17] Smith JS, Shaffrey CI, Sansur CA, et al. Scoliosis Research Society Morbidity and Mortality Committee. Rates of infection after spine surgery based on 108,419 procedures: a report from the Scoliosis Research Society Morbidity and Mortality Committee. Spine. 2011; 36(7):556–563

[18] Atlas SJ, Keller RB, Chang Y, Deyo RA, Singer DE. Surgical and nonsurgical management of sciatica secondary to a lumbar disc herniation: five-year outcomes from the Maine Lumbar Spine Study. Spine. 2001; 26(10):1179–1187

[19] Atlas SJ, Keller RB, Wu YA, Deyo RA, Singer DE. Long-term outcomes of surgical and nonsurgical management of sciatica secondary to a lumbar disc herniation: 10 year results from the maine lumbar spine study. Spine. 2005; 30(8):927–935

[20] Lurie JD, Tosteson TD, Tosteson A, et al. Long-term outcomes of lumbar spinal stenosis: eight-year results of the Spine Patient Outcomes Research Trial (SPORT). Spine. 2015; 40(2):63–76

[21] Weber H. Lumbar disc herniation. A controlled, prospective study with ten years of observation. Spine. 1983; 8(2):131–140

[22] Weinstein JN, Lurie JD, Tosteson TD, et al. Surgical vs nonoperative treatment for lumbar disk herniation: the Spine Patient Outcomes Research Trial (SPORT) observational cohort. JAMA. 2006; 296(20):2451–2459

[23] Weinstein JN, Tosteson TD, Lurie JD, et al. Surgical vs nonoperative treatment for lumbar disk herniation: the Spine Patient Outcomes Research Trial (SPORT): a randomized trial. JAMA. 2006; 296(20):2441–2450

[24] Weinstein JN, Tosteson TD, Lurie JD, et al. Surgical versus nonoperative treatment for lumbar spinal stenosis four-year results of the Spine Patient Outcomes Research Trial. Spine. 2010; 35(14):1329–1338

[25] Williams RW. Microlumbar discectomy: a conservative surgical approach to the virgin herniated lumbar disc. Spine. 1978; 3(2):175–182

[26] Arts MP, Brand R, van den Akker ME, Koes BW, Bartels RH, Peul WC, Leiden-The Hague Spine Intervention Prognostic Study Group (SIPS). Tubular diskectomy vs conventional microdiskectomy for sciatica: a randomized controlled trial. JAMA. 2009; 302(2):149–158

[27] Rasouli MR, Rahimi-Movaghar V, Shokraneh F, Moradi-Lakeh M, Chou R. Minimally invasive discectomy versus microdiscectomy/open discectomy for symptomatic lumbar disc herniation. Cochrane Database Syst Rev. 2014; 9(9): CD010328

[28] Gempt J, Jonek M, Ringel F, Preuss A, Wolf P, Ryang Y. Long-term follow-up of standard microdiscectomy versus minimal access surgery for lumbar disc herniations. Acta Neurochir (Wien). 2013; 155(12):2333–2338

[29] Kamper SJ, Ostelo RW, Rubinstein SM, et al. Minimally invasive surgery for lumbar disc herniation: a systematic review and meta-analysis. Eur Spine J. 2014; 23(5):1021–1043

[30] Harrington JF, French P. Open versus minimally invasive lumbar microdiscectomy: comparison of operative times, length of hospital stay, narcotic use and complications. Minim Invasive Neurosurg. 2008; 51(1):30–35

[31] Lau D, Han SJ, Lee JG, Lu DC, Chou D. Minimally invasive compared to open microdiscectomy for lumbar disc herniation. J Clin Neurosci. 2011 Jan;18 (1):81–84. doi: 10.1016/j.jocn.2010.04.040. Epub 2010 Sep 20.

[32] Beiner JM, Grauer J, Kwon BK, Vaccaro AR. Postoperative wound infections of the spine. Neurosurg Focus. 2003; 15(3):E14

[33] Chaudhary SB, Vives MJ, Basra SK, Reiter MF. Postoperative spinal wound infections and postprocedural diskitis. J Spinal Cord Med. 2007; 30(5):441–451

[34] Olsen MA, Mayfield J, Lauryssen C, et al. Risk factors for surgical site infection in spinal surgery. J Neurosurg. 2003; 98(2) Suppl:149–155

[35] Patel N, Bagan B, Vadera S, et al. Obesity and spine surgery: relation to perioperative complications. J Neurosurg Spine. 2007; 6(4):291–297

[36] Sasso RC, Garrido BJ. Postoperative spinal wound infections. J Am Acad Orthop Surg. 2008; 16(6):330–337

[37] Whitehouse JD, Friedman ND, Kirkland KB, Richardson WJ, Sexton DJ. The impact of surgical-site infections following orthopedic surgery at a community hospital and a university hospital: adverse quality of life, excess length of stay, and extra cost. Infect Control Hosp Epidemiol. 2002; 23(4):183–189

[38] Friedman ND, Sexton DJ, Connelly SM, Kaye KS. Risk factors for surgical site infection complicating laminectomy. Infect Control Hosp Epidemiol. 2007; 28 (9):1060–1065

[39] Boselie TF, Willems PC, van Mameren H, de Bie R, Benzel EC, van Santbrink H. Arthroplasty versus fusion in single-level cervical degenerative disc disease. Cochrane Database Syst Rev. 2012; 9(9):CD009173

[40] Brown EM, Pople IK, de Louvois J, et al. British Society for Antimicrobial Chemotherapy Working Party on Neurosurgical Infections. Spine update: prevention of postoperative infection in patients undergoing spinal surgery. Spine. 2004; 29(8):938–945

[41] Dobzyniak MA, Fischgrund JS, Hankins S, Herkowitz HN. Single versus multiple dose antibiotic prophylaxis in lumbar disc surgery. Spine. 2003; 28 (21):E453–E455

[42] Mastronardi L, Tatta C. Intraoperative antibiotic prophylaxis in clean spinal surgery: a retrospective analysis in a consecutive series of 973 cases. Surg Neurol. 2004; 61(2):129–135, discussion 135

[43] Schnöring M, Brock M. Prophylactic antibiotics in lumbar disc surgery: analysis of 1,030 procedures [in German]. Zentralbl Neurochir. 2003; 64(1):24–29

[44] Parikh K, Tomasino A, Knopman J, Boockvar J, Härtl R. Operative results and learning curve: microscope-assisted tubular microsurgery for 1- and 2-level discectomies and laminectomies. Neurosurg Focus. 2008; 25(2):E14

[45] Beier AD, Soo TM, Claybrooks R. Subdural hematoma after microdiscectomy: a case report and review of the literature. Spine J. 2009; 9(10):e9–e12

[46] Burkhard PR, Duff JM. Bilateral subdural hematomas following routine lumbar diskectomy. Headache. 2000; 40(6):480–482

[47] Friedman JA, Ecker RD, Piepgras DG, Duke DA. Cerebellar hemorrhage after spinal surgery: report of two cases and literature review. Neurosurgery. 2002; 50(6):1361–1363, discussion 1363–1364

[48] Khalatbari MR, Khalatbari I, Moharamzad Y. Intracranial hemorrhage following lumbar spine surgery. Eur Spine J. 2012; 21(10):2091–2096

[49] Konya D, Ozgen S, Pamir MN. Cerebellar hemorrhage after spinal surgery: case report and review of the literature. Eur Spine J. 2006; 15(1):95–99

[50] Kuhn J, Hofmann B, Knitelius HO, Coenen HH, Bewermeyer H. Bilateral subdural haematomata and lumbar pseudomeningocele due to a chronic leakage of liquor cerebrospinalis after a lumbar discectomy with the application of ADCON-L gel. J Neurol Neurosurg Psychiatry. 2005; 76(7):1031–1033

[51] Parpaley Y, Urbach H, Kovacs A, Klehr M, Kristof RA. Pseudohypoxic brain swelling (postoperative intracranial hypotension-associated venous congestion) after spinal surgery: report of 2 cases. Neurosurgery. 2011; 68 (1):E277–E283

[52] Thomas G, Jayaram H, Cudlip S, Powell M. Supratentorial and infratentorial intraparenchymal hemorrhage secondary to intracranial CSF hypotension following spinal surgery. Spine. 2002; 27(18):E410–E412

[53] Wong AP, Shih P, Smith TR, et al. Comparison of symptomatic cerebral spinal fluid leak between patients undergoing minimally invasive versus open lumbar foraminotomy, discectomy, or laminectomy. World Neurosurg. 2014; 81(3–4):634–640

[54] Cammisa FP, Jr, Girardi FP, Sangani PK, Parvataneni HK, Cadag S, Sandhu HS. Incidental durotomy in spine surgery. Spine. 2000; 25(20):2663–2667

[55] Shih P, Wong AP, Smith TR, Lee AI, Fessler RG. Complications of open compared to minimally invasive lumbar spine decompression. J Clin Neurosci. 2011; 18(10):1360–1364

[56] German JW, Adamo MA, Hoppenot RG, Blossom JH, Nagle HA. Perioperative results following lumbar discectomy: comparison of minimally invasive discectomy and standard microdiscectomy. Neurosurg Focus. 2008; 25(2):E20

[57] Khoo LT, Fessler RG. Microendoscopic decompressive laminotomy for the treatment of lumbar stenosis. Neurosurgery. 2002; 51(5) Suppl:S146–S154

[58] Lee P, Liu JC, Fessler RG. Perioperative results following open and minimally invasive single-level lumbar discectomy. J Clin Neurosci. 2011; 18(12):1667–1670

[59] Rahman M, Summers LE, Richter B, Mimran RI, Jacob RP. Comparison of techniques for decompressive lumbar laminectomy: the minimally invasive versus the "classic" open approach. Minim Invasive Neurosurg. 2008; 51(2):100–105

[60] Ruban D, O'Toole JE. Management of incidental durotomy in minimally invasive spine surgery. Neurosurg Focus. 2011; 31(4):E15

[61] van den Akker ME, Arts MP, van den Hout WB, Brand R, Koes BW, Peul WC. Tubular diskectomy vs conventional microdiskectomy for the treatment of lumbar disk-related sciatica: cost utility analysis alongside a double-blind randomized controlled trial. Neurosurgery. 2011; 69(4):829–835, discussion 835–836

[62] Evaniew N, Khan M, Drew B, Kwok D, Bhandari M, Ghert M. Minimally invasive versus open surgery for cervical and lumbar discectomy: a systematic review and meta-analysis. CMAJ Open. 2014; 2(4):E295–E305

[63] Copay AG, Glassman SD, Subach BR, Berven S, Schuler TC, Carreon LY. Minimum clinically important difference in lumbar spine surgery patients: a choice of methods using the Oswestry Disability Index, Medical Outcomes Study questionnaire Short Form 36, and pain scales. Spine J. 2008; 8(6):968–974

[64] Ostelo RW, Deyo RA, Stratford P, et al. Interpreting change scores for pain and functional status in low back pain: towards international consensus regarding minimal important change. Spine. 2008; 33(1):90–94

[65] McLoughlin GS, Fourney DR. The learning curve of minimally-invasive lumbar microdiscectomy. Can J Neurol Sci. 2008; 35(1):75–78

[66] Teli M, Lovi A, Brayda-Bruno M, et al. Higher risk of dural tears and recurrent herniation with lumbar micro-endoscopic discectomy. Eur Spine J. 2010; 19 (3):443–450

[67] Righesso O, Falavigna A, Avanzi O. Comparison of open discectomy with microendoscopic discectomy in lumbar disc herniations: results of a randomized controlled trial. Neurosurgery. 2007; 61(3):545–549, discussion 549

[68] Garg B, Nagraja UB, Jayaswal A. Microendoscopic versus open discectomy for lumbar disc herniation: a prospective randomised study. J Orthop Surg (Hong Kong). 2011; 19(1):30–34

[69] Ruetten S, Komp M, Merk H, Godolias G. Full-endoscopic interlaminar and transforaminal lumbar discectomy versus conventional microsurgical technique: a prospective, randomized, controlled study. Spine. 2008; 33(9):931–939

[70] Lau D, Han SJ, Lee JG, Lu DC, Chou D. Minimally invasive compared to open microdiscectomy for lumbar disc herniation. J Clin Neurosci. 2011; 18(1):81–84

[71] Wang B, Lü G, Patel AA, Ren P, Cheng I. An evaluation of the learning curve for a complex surgical technique: the full endoscopic interlaminar approach for lumbar disc herniations. Spine J. 2011; 11(2):122–130

[72] Arts M, Brand R, van der Kallen B, Lycklama à Nijeholt G, Peul W. Does minimally invasive lumbar disc surgery result in less muscle injury than conventional surgery? A randomized controlled trial. Eur Spine J. 2011; 20 (1):51–57

2 Is Lumbar Stenosis Best Treated with an Open Laminectomy?

MIS: Hasan R. Syed and Sylvain Palmer
Open: Jonathan M. Karnes and Scott D. Daffner

2.1 Introduction

Lumbar spinal stenosis is defined as any condition that leads to narrowing of the lumbar spinal canal and exiting nerve roots. It can be divided into congenital, acquired, iatrogenic, spondylotic, and posttraumatic stenosis, as defined by Arnoldi et al and modified by Katz and Harris.[1,2] Lumbar stenosis is a chronic debilitating condition that affects 5 out of 1,000 Americans older than 50 years. The most common pathophysiology results from degenerative arthritic changes in relatively mobile segments combined with axial loading. These changes include a combination of hypertrophied facet joints and ligaments, osteophyte overgrowth, disc herniation, and spondylolisthesis that can lead to decreased diameter of the spinal canal and subsequent symptoms as a result of neurologic compression and/or mechanical pain.[3] Prospective, randomized clinical trials have shown significantly greater improvements in patient's functional outcome and quality of life with surgical intervention compared to medical management.[4,5,6]

Surgical decompression of lumbar stenosis is the most common surgery for patients older than 65 years.[5] The initial description of the surgical treatment of spinal stenosis was by Sachs and Fraenkel in 1900.[7] Bailey and Casamajor in 1911 published work linking the findings of osteoarthritis of the lumbar spine with compression of the spinal cord and nerve roots.[8] Lumbar stenosis has traditionally been treated with an open, decompressive laminectomy, including partial facetectomy and foraminotomies with or without fusion.[5,9] While this is an effective treatment strategy, open decompression (OD) is associated with disruption of normal anatomic support structures and muscle atrophy that can theoretically lead to iatrogenic instability.[10,11]

Adams and Hutton showed that the tendency toward anterolisthesis is resisted by multiple spinal elements. The facet joints have been shown to resist 33% of shear forces, with the disc resisting 67%.[12] The supraspinous and interspinous ligaments resist 19% of flexion forces, with the facet capsular ligaments resisting 39% and the disc resisting 29%.[12,13] The force exerted on the spine in physiologic flexion by the trunk is more than double that required to injure the facet joints, and these articulating structures would fail if unaided by other supporting tissues.[12,13] The supraspinous/intraspinous ligamentous complex has the greatest mechanical advantage, being furthest from the axis of rotation. Cusick et al designed a biomechanical study of sequential sectioning of the posterior ligaments and facets using a two-motion segment model.[14] They found that the complex was stable until the supraspinous/interspinous ligaments and associated residual tendinous, midline muscle, and fascial attachments were violated.[12,13,14]

Subsequently, minimally invasive spine surgery was developed to address the diseased structures while minimizing the disruption of normal anatomic structures. Muscle-splitting serial tubular dilators and retractors were designed to access the spinal pathology without stripping, devascularizing, or denervating paraspinal musculature and preserving ligamentous and bony anatomy. Decompression can take place with the assistance of endoscopic or microscopic visualization. Interest in less invasive options has led to direct decompressions with bilateral laminotomies and foraminotomies[15,16,17] or unilateral approaches to bilateral decompression.[16,18,19,20,21] As with any new surgical technique, minimally invasive spine surgery is associated with an initial learning curve.

2.2 Indications for Minimally Invasive Surgery

Minimally invasive surgery (MIS) is generally indicated for the treatment of degenerative spinal stenosis involving any lumbar level as a result of bulging of the intervertebral discs, hypertrophy of the facet joints, and thickening or buckling of the ligamentum flavum. The clinical symptoms of this condition consist of mechanical back pain and radicular pain, as well as classic neurogenic claudication, leading to uni- or bilateral symptoms of the legs. Patients with spinal claudication complain of weakness or heaviness in the lower extremities, with variable sensory deficits or paresthesias when standing and walking. The pain commonly progresses from proximal to distal and is improved by spinal flexion with leaning forward or sitting. Spinal claudication can also be associated with radicular symptoms produced by direct nerve compression that is localized to a particular dermatomal level. A component of mechanical back pain is also commonly present.

There are no absolute contraindications for the use of MIS in the approach to lumbar decompression. Relative contraindications include multiple levels of spinal disease requiring treatment, though surgical time in multiple levels decreases with experience. In addition, exposures deeper than 9 cm (maximum standard retractor depth) and distorted anatomic landmarks, such as those found with reoperation or deformity, are challenging candidates for the minimally invasive approach and are best reserved for the seasoned MIS surgeon.

2.3 Advantages of Minimally Invasive Surgery

The MIS technique utilizes a tubular or bladed retractor system to provide a working corridor for decompression of the neural elements. This approach utilizes "muscle-splitting" dilators and retractors that are designed to minimize disruption of normal anatomy. This leads to decreased trauma to paravertebral musculature on the ipsilateral side and no trauma to the musculature on the contralateral side. In addition, decompression via MIS completely preserves the posterior tension band and spares bony elements, particularly the contralateral lamina and facet joint, as compared to open surgery (OS). Finally, bilateral decompression of the spinal canal can be performed through a unilateral approach by rotating the patient table and angling the approach to optimize the surgeon's line of sight.

The theoretical advantages of an MIS approach to lumbar decompression include a quicker recovery, short hospital stay, decreased blood loss, and preservation of midline structural elements.[22] While OS has demonstrated excellent clinical results, the risk of iatrogenic instability and poor outcome exists.[23,24] In those patients in whom instability is of concern or in those with preexisting spondylolisthesis, or scoliosis with primarily lower extremity symptom, MIS may be an attractive option and has the advantage of preserving posterior stabilizing structures. MIS has also shown advantages in the obese and elderly patient populations, owing to the minimally disruptive nature of the approach and the preservation of normal anatomy.[25,26]

2.4 Indications for Open Surgery

The indications for open surgical management of lumbar stenosis are to primarily relieve symptoms of neurogenic claudication or radiculopathy that are resistant to nonoperative therapy.[27] The patient-reported history and symptoms, clinical examination, and advanced imaging studies must be consistent with lumbar stenosis in order to expect good results from the surgery. Surgical intervention is indicated when the patient has failed an extended period of appropriate nonoperative treatment and continues to have severe, life-altering symptoms attributable to lumbar stenosis. Open surgical decompression using laminectomy with or without foramenotomy for lumbar stenosis has been the most commonly used operative strategy.

2.5 Advantages of Open Surgery

Lumbar stenosis is most commonly found in elderly patients who develop age-related constriction of the lumbar spinal canal from hypertrophy and distortion of the ligamentum flavum and facet joints as well as posterior displacement of the intervertebral disc. Less commonly, sagittal imbalance and segmental instability can create spinal canal constriction and create or amplify lumbar stenosis. OD provides several advantages. First, it utilizes a standard posterior lumbar approach, which is familiar to all spine surgeons. Consequently, it is less technically demanding. In addition, OD allows direct visualization of the neural elements while performing the decompression and provides more space for placement of surgical instruments. Lastly, in patients presenting with spinal stenosis with a component of vertebral instability or malalignment, OS may provide the additional benefit of facilitating more complex reconstructive techniques.

2.6 Case Illustration

The patient is a 68-year-old man with a long-standing history of intermittent back pain, which he has managed well with over-the-counter nonsteroidal anti-inflammatory drugs. Six months ago, he began developing pain radiating from his back to his right lower extremity, which is worse with standing or walking. His symptoms are relieved after sitting for a few minutes, and he notes he must lean on a shopping cart to make it through the market.

His past history is significant only for hypertension. Medications include baby aspirin, blood pressure medications, and diclofenac. He is a nonsmoker. Outcomes measures obtained at his initial visit include an Oswestry Disability Index (ODI) score of 42, with average visual analog scale (VAS) pain score for the past 24 hours of 6 for back pain and 9 for leg pain.

Physical examination is notable for limited lumbar range of motion on flexion, with some palpable back spasm. Motor strength is 5/5 in his bilateral lower extremities, sensation of light touch is intact, and deep tendon reflexes are 2 + symmetrically. Distal pulses are palpable.

Plain radiographs (▶ Fig. 2.1) demonstrate mild degenerative disc space loss of height and well-maintained overall alignment, with no evidence of spondylolisthesis on flexion/extension images. His MRI (▶ Fig. 2.2) demonstrates moderate to severe central and bilateral lateral recess stenosis at L4–L5 due to degenerative disc bulge, facet hypertrophy, and ligamentum flavum hypertrophy.

Since his symptoms became worse, he has been taking diclofenac twice daily. He has tried 6 weeks of physical therapy. An L4–L5 epidural injection provided 3 weeks of excellent relief before symptoms returned. He continues to have significant discomfort and is interested in surgical treatment.

2.7 Surgical Technique in Minimally Invasive Surgery

The patient is brought into the operating room, and most commonly general endotracheal anesthesia is obtained, although it can also be performed under spinal or local anesthesia. A Foley catheter can be placed at the discretion of the surgeon for longer cases, usually two or more levels. The procedure has been described previously[21] and is a modification of the microendoscopic discectomy detailed by Foley and Smith.[28] The patient is positioned prone, or lateral, and the level of interest is localized with fluoroscopy. The patient is prepped and draped and the skin is infiltrated with a local anesthetic. A paramedian incision is planned just lateral to the spinous process on the more symptomatic side. Fluoroscopy is utilized to localize the level of the disc space by placing a 22-G spinal needle. If there is a collapsed disc space, then the upper end plate of the lower vertebral body is the target because of the resulting low-lying lamina. Ideally, the inferior laminar edge is in the middle of the exposed field. The direction of approach can be modified in all directions by angling or "wanding" of the retractor to bring the intended structures into view.

When using a tubular system, a 20-mm incision is made, exposing the fascial layer above the paraspinal muscles. A scalpel or unipolar electrocautery is used to incise the fascial layer. The paraspinal muscles are sequentially dilated using tubular dilators, followed by placement of an 18-mm working channel of the shortest length that allows adequate depth of access (usually 50–70 mm). The level of interest and depth of the working channel is confirmed using fluoroscopy. The operative microscope is then moved into the field or an endoscope can be attached. Bovie electrocautery is used to expose and identify

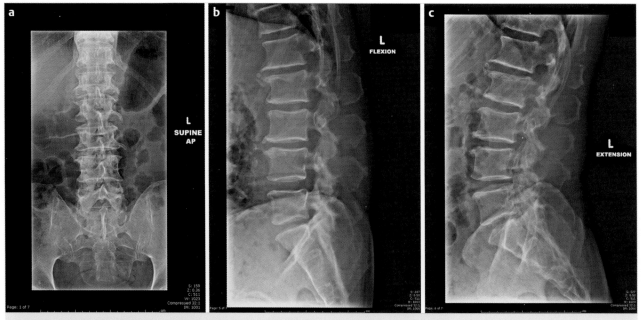

Fig. 2.1 (a) Anteroposterior, (b) lateral flexion, and (c) extension radiographs of a 68-year-old man with back and leg pain.

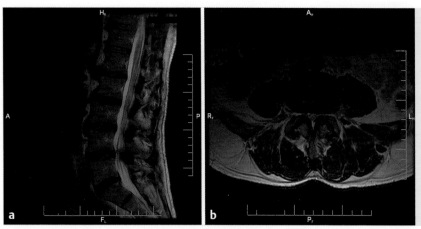

Fig. 2.2 (a) T2-weighted sagittal and (b) axial MRI images of the patient in ▶ Fig. 2.1 demonstrating moderate to severe central and bilateral lateral recess stenosis at L4–L5.

the laminar edge. A laminotomy is performed using a combination of diamond burr, Kerrison punches, and curettes. The laminotomy is extended cephalad to above the insertion of the ligamentum flavum on the inferior surface of the superior lamina (to ensure complete resection of ligamentous compressive elements) and caudally to include a smaller portion of the superior aspect of the inferior lamina exposing the pedicle. Partial resection of the medial facet complex is performed as necessary to adequately decompress the lateral recess and the neural foramina.

The working channel is then angled medially, exposing the anterior aspect of the spinous process, which is then removed utilizing a diamond burr. This exposes the lateral recess on the contralateral side where residual lamina, ligamentum flavum, and medial facet can be resected as needed for neural decompression. The angle of approach is the same as that commonly taken during an open laminectomy, making the anatomy familiar to most spine surgeons. Satisfactory decompression of the

lateral recess and foramina is achieved under direct vision. Palpation of the pedicle and foramina, with a blunt ball-tipped nerve hook, ensures correct orientation and complete decompression. If decompression is required at another level, the incision can be elongated and a separate dilation performed. The wound is copiously irrigated, and hemostasis is achieved using electrocautery as the working channel is slowly removed under direct vision. The wound is closed in layers with absorbable sutures and Steri-Strips or Dermabond can be used on the skin.

2.8 Surgical Technique in Open Surgery

For the open technique, a patient is placed under general anesthesia and positioned prone on a Jackson or Andrews frame, with all bony prominences well padded. It is important to ensure that the patient's abdomen hangs freely; this decreases intra-abdominal pressure, which in turn will help reduce the distension and bleeding from epidural veins. Alternately, the patient may be placed on a Wilson frame, which allows the spine to be flexed, opening the interspace and providing easier access to the epidural space. The authors, however, prefer a Jackson frame because it places the spine in a more anatomic position with lumbar lordosis, positioning the spine in the position of greatest symptomatic stenosis. Fluoroscopy or surface anatomic landmarks may be used to localize the incision. A midline incision is centered over the affected level(s). Dissection is carried down through the skin and subcutaneous tissue to the fascia. The fascia is incised in the midline and the underlying spinous processes and laminae are exposed in a subperiosteal fashion. Care must be taken to preserve the facet capsules. In addition, the pars interarticularis should be identified at each level. Deep self-retaining retractors are then placed, and exposure of the intended levels is confirmed radiographically.

The interspinous ligament is removed at the intended level(s) of decompression. Using a rongeur or bone cutter, the spinous processes are removed. A high-speed burr can be used to create a small trough medial to the facet joints on each side. The lamina is then thinned with the burr, and the laminectomy completed using a Kerrison rongeur. Alternately, an ultrasonic bone scalpel may be used to cut through the lamina on each side, after which the lamina can be elevated and removed en bloc. Once the midline laminectomy is performed, the remaining ligamentum flavum is also removed. The lateral recesses bilaterally are then decompressed by undercutting the lamina with a Kerrison rongeur. The decompression can be extended laterally to the medial third of the facet joint, and foraminotomies can be performed to decompress the exiting nerve roots through the neuroforamina. The midline laminectomy should extend just lateral to the lateral border of the thecal sac; however, care must be taken to leave at least 5 mm of pars interarticularis intact; thinning the pars too much from medial to lateral (or from ventral to dorsal while decompressing the lateral recess) can predispose to fracture. Palpation within the epidural space, following the nerve roots into the neuroforamina, confirms that the decompression is complete.

The wound is then copiously irrigated with saline solution and hemostasis is achieved. A Valsalva maneuver is performed to ensure there is no leakage of cerebrospinal fluid (CSF). The deep retractors are released, the muscle is allowed to fall back into the midline, and the wound is closed in layers.

2.9 Discussion for Minimally Invasive Surgery

Minimally invasive lumbar decompression is commonly performed for the treatment of degenerative spinal stenosis as a result of intervertebral disc bulge, ligamentum flavum hypertrophy and calcification, and facet joint hypertrophy. This technique provides excellent access for decompressing the neural elements and offers advantages over traditional open laminectomies. Furthermore, the MIS technique minimizes approach-related morbidity and disruption of normal anatomy incurred with OS. In this chapter's illustrative case, a minimally invasive approach for lumbar decompression via tubular retractors should allow for adequate direct decompression of the entire spinal canal using a unilateral approach. A critical review of published results should provide insight into the advantages of a minimally invasive approach compared to traditional open laminectomy (▶ Table 2.1).

2.9.1 Level I Evidence in Minimally Invasive Surgery

There are no level I studies available.

2.9.2 Level II Evidence in Minimally Invasive Surgery

Two prospective, randomized trials comparing MIS to open laminectomy have been published in the literature, albeit in small cohorts. Mobbs et al compared MIS to open laminectomy with respect to postoperative recovery and clinical outcomes by enrolling a total of 79 patients (data for analysis were available for only 54 patients) with symptomatic, radiographically confirmed lumbar spinal stenosis at a maximum of two levels between 2007 and 2009.[29] The patients were randomly assigned to either open decompressive laminectomy or MIS according to their sequence of presentation. The authors demonstrated statistically significant improvements in clinical outcome, that is, ODI and VAS scores for both open and minimally invasive interventions. However, patients treated with the MIS technique had a significantly better mean improvement in the VAS score but not the ODI scores compared with patients in the open laminectomy group. In addition, Mobbs et al noted shorter length of postoperative hospital stay (55.1 vs. 100.8 hours) and time to mobilization (15.6 vs. 33.3 hours) and reduced opioid use for postoperative pain (15.4 vs. 51.9%) in patients undergoing MIS compared to open laminectomy. This study provides level II evidence that MIS achieves similar functional outcomes when compared with open laminectomy (ODI score), with the additional benefits of a greater decrease in pain (VAS score), postoperative recovery time, time to mobilization, and opioid use.

Yagi et al performed a prospective, randomized trial comparing the traditional open laminectomy approach to MIS using endoscopy for bilateral decompression of lumbar stenosis in 41 patients.[30] The authors reported no significant clinical differences (JOA [Japanese Orthopaedic Association] scale) between the two groups but noted a statistically significant lower VAS score for back pain at 1-year follow-up, and less blood loss (37 vs. 71 mL) and damage to the paravertebral muscles as measured by creatine phosphokinase muscular type isoenzyme (CPK-MM). This study provides level II evidence that MIS is comparable to clinical outcomes achieved with open laminectomy, while reducing postoperative back pain, blood loss, and length of stay.

2.9.3 Level III and IV Evidence in Minimally Invasive Surgery

Several therapeutic cohort studies comparing MIS and OS with respect to clinical outcome and perioperative factors have been reported in the literature. Palmer et al and Khoo and Fessler were the first authors to describe the endoscopically assisted MIS technique in 2001 and published in 2002.[21,31] In Khoo and

Table 2.1 Literature on MIS versus OS and MIS alone

Authors (year)	Level	Study	Patients	ORT	EBL (mL)	LOS	Findings
Mobbs et al (2014)[29]	II	Prospective	27 MI 27 O	NR NR	110 40	56 h 101 h	VAS/ODI scores better and shorter time to mobilization in MILD; more likely to not use opioids in MILD
Yagi et al (2009)[30]	II	Prospective	20 MI 21 O	71.1 63.6	37 71	3 d 12 d	VAS scores better in MILD; lower CPK-MM and muscle atrophy in MILD; JOA similar
Khoo and Fessler (2002)[31]	III	Retrospective	25 MI 25 O	109 88	68 193	42 h 94 h	Clinical outcome similar; no delayed spinal instability in MILD; 3 patients required delayed fusion in OD
Ikuta et al (2005)[32]	III	Retrospective	47 MI 29 O	124 101	68 110	18d 24d	Clinical outcome similar; effective decompression demonstrated on MRI; complications slightly higher in MILD compared to OD
Asgarzadie and Khoo (2007)[33]	III	Retrospective	48 MI	55 NR	25 193	36 h 94 h	Patient satisfaction 78% at 4 years in MILD; clinical outcomes (ODI, SF-36) improved
Rahman et al (2008)[34]	III	Retrospective	38 MI 88 O	110 157	50 244	0.7 d 3.2 d	Complications: 16.1% of OD and 7.9% of MILD patients
Parker et al (2013)[35]	III	Retrospective	27 MI 27 O	NR	NR	NR	MILD ($23,109) vs. OD ($25,420) associated with similar costs, utility, and cumulative gain (QALY)
Palmer et al (2002)[20]	IV	Retrospective	17 MI	90	20	NR	Postoperative MRI showed improvement in stenosis; majority of cases performed on outpatient basis
Castro-Menendez (2009)[36]	IV	Prospective	50 MI	94.3	NR	3.2 d	Good or excellent results in 72% of patients; improvement in VAS and ODI statistically significant
Rosen et al (2007)[26]	IV	Prospective	57 MI	NR	NR	2.3 d	Average age: 80 y; VAS, ODI, SF-36 improved; no major complications or deaths
Pao (2009)[37]	IV	Prospective	53 MI	127	105	NR	Significant improvement in ODI (86% of patients); excellent or good results in 80% of patients based on JOA score; no postoperative instability at last follow-up
Sasai (2008)[38]	IV	Retrospective	48 MI	NR	NR	NR	23 degenerative spondylolisthesis with stenosis and 25 degenerative stenosis patients treated with MILD; clinical outcome similar; no patient in either group required additional fusion
Ikuta et al (2008)[39]	IV	Retrospective	37 MI	NR	NR	NR	MILD for degenerative spondylolisthesis with stenosis; 73% of patients with excellent or good results based on JOA, VAS, and RMDQ; 19% of patients had increase in sagittal motion after surgery
Mannion (2012)[40]	IV	Prospective	50 MI	NR	NR	NR	Significant improvement in ODI, SF-36; significant association between case number and change in ODI; operative time decreased based on surgeon's experience
Palmer (2012)[41]	IV	Retrospective	54 MI	78	37	NR	Improvement in VAS; 80% of patients pleased with outcome at 27 mo; 2% of patients required fusion for iatrogenic spondylolisthesis
Wada (2010)[42]	IV	Retrospective	15 MI	144	60	NR	Average age: 72; dural sac diameter increased by 408% postoperatively
Xu (2010)[43]	IV	Retrospective	32 MI	70	150	7	McNab scale: 65% of patients with excellent results; 35% of patients with good results
Minamide (2013)[44]	IV	Prospective	366 MI	NR	NR	NR	Clinical outcomes significantly improved (JOA, RMDQ, JOABPEQ, SF-36) over 2-year follow-up period

Abbreviations: CPK-MM, creatine phosphokinase muscular type isoenzyme; EBL, estimated blood loss; JOA, Japanese Orthopaedic Association; JOABPEQ, Japanese Orthopedic Association Back Pain Evaluation Questionnaire; LOS, length of stay; MI(S), minimal invasive (surgery); MILD, minimally invasive lumbar decompression; MRI, magnetic resonance imaging; NR, not recorded; O(S), open (surgery); OD, open discectomy; ODI, Oswestry Disability Index; ORT, operative time; QALY, quality-adjusted life year; RMDQ, RolandMorris Disability Questionnaire; SF-36, 36-Item Short Form Health Survey; VAS, visual analog scale.

Fessler's study, 25 consecutive patients with lumbar stenosis were treated with MIS and retrospectively compared to a historical control group of 25 patients treated with OS for lumbar decompression. The authors reported a similar short-term clinical outcome (i.e., resolution or relief of symptoms) after 1-year follow-up and a statistically significant decrease in operative blood loss (60 vs. 193 mL), postoperative narcotic requirement (31.8 vs. 73.7 eq), and length of stay (42 vs. 94 hours).

In Palmer et al's study, 54 patients underwent decompression at 77 levels. The average operative time was 78 minutes and the average blood loss was 37 mL per level. Twenty-seven patients had preoperative degenerative spondylolisthesis (Grade 1 = 26; Grade 2 = 1). Eight patients had discectomies and four had synovial cysts. Patient satisfaction was high. Use of pain medication for leg and back pain was low, and VAS scores improved by more than half. There were three dural tears. There were no deaths or infections. One patient with an unrecognized dural tear required re-exploration for repair of a pseudomeningocele and one patient required a lumbar fusion for pain associated with progression of her spondylolisthesis.[21]

In a retrospective cohort study comparing 47 patients undergoing endoscopically assisted MIS and 29 patients undergoing OS, Ikuta et al in 2005 demonstrated shorter hospital stay and reductions in duration of fever, use of postoperative analgesics, and estimated blood loss (EBL) in patients treated with MIS. Clinical outcomes (JOA score) were similar in both groups, and there was no evidence of postoperative instability on dynamic X-rays.[32] Asgarzadie and Khoo in 2007 compared 48 MIS patients to a historical control of 32 OS patients with a follow-up of 4 years.[33] The average EBL for the MIS group was 25 versus 193 mL for the OS group. The average length of hospital stay for MIS was 36 hours compared to 94 hours in the OS group. Rahman et al performed a comparative analysis in 2008 of 38 patients treated with MIS and 88 patients with OD.[34] Similar to previous reports, patients undergoing the minimally invasive approach experienced shorter operating times (37–47 minutes less than OD), less EBL (50 vs. 243 mL), shorter length of stay (0.75 vs. 3.2 days in patients with two-level surgery), and fewer complications.

In a study of 2-year cost–utility comparing MIS to OS in patients with multilevel degenerative lumbar spinal stenosis, Parker et al in 2013 assessed health state values via quality-adjusted life years (QALYs) after 2-year follow-up and comprehensive health care costs associated with each technique.[35] Fifty-four patients underwent treatment with MIS ($n = 27$) or OS ($n = 27$). The authors demonstrated similar cost over 2 years ($23,109 vs. $25,420), while providing equivalent improvement in QALYs, and concluded that MIS is a cost-equivalent technology for the treatment of lumbar stenosis. These studies provide level III evidence that MIS is equivalent to OS in improving clinical symptoms and functional outcome but leads to shortened operative time and length of hospital stay, less blood loss, and a trend toward benefit in cost-effectiveness technology.

2.10 Complications in Minimally Invasive Surgery

While many studies have demonstrated the benefit of MIS relative to OS, both approaches are associated with potential complications. In particular, there remains a high rate of initial complication in early case series owing to the steep learning curve of a new surgical technique.[45] The incidences of surgical complications have been reported to range from 0 to 19% for open lumbar decompression surgery and 0 to 25% for minimally invasive lumbar decompression,[46] with durotomies as high as 18% in OS.[4] In subsequent reports published in the literature, the authors have shown rapid improvement in their surgical skills and associated complications arising from a novel technique.[22]

In an early retrospective case series focusing on complications, Ikuta et al in 2007 examined 114 patients treated with MIS for lumbar stenosis and reported a 7.9% rate of intraoperative complications, including 6 dural tears and 3 fractures of the inferior facet.[46] The authors, however, noted that the rate of neurological complications in the first 34 patients was 18%, which decreased to 6.8% in the latest 80 patients. In the aforementioned retrospective cohort study comparing MIS to OS, Rahman et al reported more complications in OS (16.1%) versus MIS (7.9%) with the most common being a higher rate of dural tears, infection, and other medical complications.[34] Shih et al performed another retrospective cohort study in 2011 on 26 OS and 23 MIS patients and found no statistically significant difference in the rate of complications between the two groups.[47] With regard to CSF leak, the authors reported a rate of 19.2% in OS versus 4.3% in MIS patients. In addition, several studies have reported a decreased rate of infection in MIS compared to OS.[22,48] These studies provide level III evidence that the rate of complications is at least similar in both groups with a lower rate of infection.

Minimally invasive techniques may be particularly advantageous in elderly or medically frail patients, given that these techniques promote a less disruptive approach to spinal pathology. Previously published data reported a complication rate of 18% in OS for patients older than 75 years.[49] In contrast, Rosen et al reported their experience with MIS for lumbar stenosis in patients at least 75 years old.[26] The elderly population demonstrated improvements in VAS, ODI, and 36-Item Short Form Health Survey (SF-36) after surgery. In addition, the authors showed no major complications or perioperative deaths; minor complications included urinary retention and transient delirium.

Another subgroup of patients who may benefit from minimally invasive techniques are obese patients who tend to have longer operative times, increased blood loss, larger exposures requiring soft-tissue dissection, and increased complications.[50] By using a tubular retractor system, the spine may be accessed through the same incision in an obese patient as a nonobese patient. In theory, there would be minimal disruption of soft tissue, resulting in decreased tissue trauma and potential space for infection. Senker et al treated 72 patients with a minimally invasive approach for a transforaminal lumbar interbody fusion (TLIF) and decompression.[25] The authors reported no difference between normal, overweight, and obese patients based on BMI (body mass index) in terms of complication rates, operative time, EBL, or hospital stay. Similar results, including improvement in self-reported pain and quality-of-life measures, were documented by Rosen et al in overweight and obese patients undergoing minimally invasive TLIF.[51]

The use of tubular retractors for lumbar decompression may also be advantageous in maintaining normal spinal anatomy and reducing complications related to spinal instability. A minimally invasive approach may minimize postoperative progression to spinal instability by maintaining the posterior tension band and contralateral facet. Ikuta et al examined 37 patients surgically treated with MIS for spinal stenosis associated with degenerative spondylolisthesis and noted "percent slip" changed from 14.1 to 15.7%.[39] In addition, the authors documented 19% of patients developed spinal instability on postoperative imaging, including one that required fusion, after a mean follow-up of 38 months. However, Matsunaga et al reviewed the natural history of lumbar spondylolisthesis and reported 30% of patients eventually progressing to spinal instability.[52] This suggests that MIS in patients with lumbar stenosis associated with spondylolisthesis is no worse than the natural history of progression. Furthermore, MIS may actually minimize iatrogenic spinal instability compared to OS by reducing muscle dissection and maintaining the structural stability provided by the posterior tension band and contralateral facet.

2.11 Conclusion of Minimally Invasive Surgery

While there is a steep learning curve associated with minimally invasive approaches, these techniques may be beneficial for patients and may improve clinical outcomes. Although no level I randomized comparisons exist on MIS, several level II studies have demonstrated comparable clinical and functional outcomes, while also showing benefits of decreased blood loss, shorter hospital stay and time to mobilization, decreased narcotic use, and faster recovery. There are level III data that may indicate a slightly higher complication profile in MIS compared to OS due to the learning curve associated with a new technique; however, level III data suggest a lower infection rate and preservation of spinal stability in the minimally invasive treatment group. Finally, level III data exist showing comparable improvement in clinical symptoms and functional outcomes with a trend in the MIS group toward benefit in cost effectiveness compared to OS. Using the grading scale of Guyatt et al,[53] we suggest a Grade 2B recommendation that MIS and OS are equivalent in terms of clinical and functional outcomes. Also, we suggest a Grade 2B recommendation that MIS decreases blood loss and is associated with shorter hospital stay, faster recovery, and reduced narcotic use compared to OD. Finally, we suggest a Grade 2B recommendation that MIS decreases the risk of postoperative infection.

2.12 Discussion of Open Surgery

The decision to use either an open approach or MIS for laminectomy for surgical management of lumbar stenosis is primarily driven by surgeon preference, as both strategies have been shown to improve patient outcomes. Furthermore, as both procedures are attempting to achieve decompression of the affected levels, only the portal and its capacity to allow for the required work differ between the two approaches. It has been suggested that MIS can result in reduced blood loss, reduced risk of surgical infection, earlier discharge from the hospital, reduced narcotic administration, and reduced dependence on ancillary support services following discharge.[54] It is interesting to note that the majority of these outcome measures were not included in the original publications examining OD for lumbar stenosis and only became included in the literature in studies comparing MIS to open procedures. Despite these theoretical advantages, MIS procedures can expose patients to more radiation from intraoperative fluoroscopy, can make the repair of an iatrogenic dural tear more difficult, and have a significant learning curve.[54] Furthermore, using an open approach for laminectomy in cases of spinal stenosis is a less technically challenging procedure that still allows for consistent and satisfactory decompression of the central spinal canal, lateral recess, and neuroforamina under direct visualization. ▶ Table 2.2 summarizes the data for studies comparing OD and MIS procedures.

2.12.1 Level I Evidence in Open Surgery

There are no level I studies comparing open and minimally invasive approaches for laminectomy for the treatment of lumbar stenosis available.

2.12.2 Level II Evidence in Open Surgery

Two level II trials compare open and minimally invasive approaches for lumbar laminectomy. Mobbs et al[29] report on a matched cohort randomized trial with 79 patients. This group used the ODI, VAS, the SF-12, and a patient satisfaction index, and secondary outcome measures included postoperative opioid use, length of stay following surgery, and time to mobilization. The average follow-up was 44.3 months in the cohort undergoing OD and 36.9 months in the minimally invasive group. There are several attributes to appreciate in order to accurately interpret the results of this study. First, there was only a 68.4% follow-up rate because 13 from the open group and 12 from the minimally invasive group were not included in the final assessment. Also, the group receiving an OD had much more severe symptoms (66.7 vs. 40.7% for low back pain; 88.9 vs. 66.7% for radiculopathy), while the minimally invasive group had more classical symptoms of neurogenic claudication (66.7 vs. 59.3%). Therefore, given the OD cohort had almost a 50% higher incidence of back pain and radiculopathy, one would anticipate that the OS cohort likely had more severe pathology. Furthermore, the higher incidence of back pain, which does not respond well to decompression, likely influences the postoperative outcome assessments. Therefore, one must exercise caution when interpreting the finding that the VAS scores were better in the minimally invasive group, which is further emphasized by the observation that there was no difference in the ODI or SF-12 scores between the two groups at the final follow-up. Furthermore, the documentation of the time to mobility, postoperative opioid consumption, and time to discharge are susceptible to bias given these outcomes are heavily influenced by the surgeon and may reflect care decisions rather than patient experience. Lastly, all MIS procedures were performed by an experienced surgeon, who had already progressed through the learning curve associated with MIS, and may not reflect the results of an average spine surgeon.

Yagi et al[30] reported a prospective trial with 21 OD and 20 MIS patients with single-level stenosis receiving decompression. All subjects were followed for 1 year, and outcomes were assessed with the JOA and VAS scores, and secondary outcomes

Table 2.2 Comparison of outcomes, open versus MIS decompression

Authors (year)	Level	Study	Type	Patients	ORT	EBL (mL)	LOS	Findings
Mobbs et al (2014)[29]	II	Prospective	OD vs. MIS	OD 27 / MIS 27	NR	OD 110 / MIS 40	OD 101 h / MIS 56 h	MIS group had earlier mobility, shorter surgery, less EBL, and less postoperative opioid requirements. There was no significant difference in ODI or SF-12 scores despite the nearly 50% higher incidence of back pain and radicular symptoms on the OD group
Yagi et al (2009)[30]	II	Prospective	OD vs. MIS	OD 21 / MIS 20	OD 63.6 / MIS 71.1	OD 71 / MIS 37	OD 3 d / MIS 12 h	There was no significant clinical differences between either group with the exception of a lower VAS score in the MIS group
Khoo and Fessler (2002)[31]	III	Retrospective	OD vs. MIS	OD 25 / MIS 25	OD 88 / MIS 109	OD 193 / MIS 68	OD 94 h / MIS 42 h	No clinical outcome score used; 64% had disease at one level and 36% had disease at two levels; more dural tears in MIS vs. OD (16 vs. 8%)
Asgarzadie and Khoo (2007)[33]	III	Retrospective	OD vs. MIS	OD 32 / MIS 48	OD NR / MIS 55 min	OD 193 / MIS 25	OD 94 h / MIS 36 h	No comparison of clinical outcomes between OD and MIS approaches; perioperative parameters of EBL and LOS super or
Ikuta et al (2005)[32]	III	Prospective with retrospective control	OD vs. MIS	OD 29 / MIS 47	OD 101 / MIS 124	OD 110 / MIS 68	OD 24 d / MIS 18 d	No difference in clinical outcome scores between OD and MIS; there were more complications in the MIS group, 14 vs. 25%, and including several dural tears and a case of cauda equina
Parker et al (2013)[35]	III	Retrospective	OD vs. MIS	OD 27 / MIS 27	NR	NR	NR	Concluded that the 2-year costs associated with OD and MIS was equivalent without significantly different quality-adjusted life years (QALYs)
Shih et al (2011)[47]	IV	Retrospective	OD vs. MIS	OD 26 / MIS 23	OD 112 / MIS 141	OD 139.8 / MIS 62.0	OD 2.92 d / MIS 2.04 d	Not patient outcomes reported, only compared perioperative parameters
Rahman et al (2008)[34]	IV	Retrospective	OD vs. MIS	OD 88 / MIS 38	OD 136.9 / MIS 109	"OD lost 194 mL more on average"	"OD had an average 2.52 day longer stay"	MIS patients had less EBL, shorter hospitalization, and shorter operating time. No clinical outcomes measures reported
Weinstein et al (2008)[55]	I	RCT	OD	OD 394 / Non-op 240	Median 120	Mean 314	NR	Open decompression produces more improvement in patient outcomes at 2-year follow-up
Weinstein et al (2010)[6]	I	RCT	OD	OD 423 / Non-op 221	Median 129	Mean 311	NR	Spinal stenosis patients undergoing open decompression still had superior results at 4 years compared to nonoperative patients
Malmivaara et al (2007)[56]	I	RCT	OD	OD 50 / Non-op 44	NR	NR	NR	Patients undergoing decompressive surgery had greater relief of leg and back pain at 2 years
Amundsen et al (2000)[59]	II	RCT	OD	OD 32 / Non-op 68	NR	NR	NR	Results favored surgery over nonoperative management at 10-year follow-up
Athiviraham and Yen (2007)[57]	II	Prospective	OD	88 (49 w/o fusion; 39 w/ fusion)	NR	NR	NR	Surgical cohort had significantly better Roland-Morris scores compared to nonoperative cohort; however, only 63.3% in the decompression only and 61.5% in the decompression with fusion had improvement
Javid and Hadar (1998)[64]	III	Prospective	OD	170	NR	NR	NR	Found that approximately two-thirds of patients had improvement following open laminectomy and that there was no significant difference between patients with stenosis, stenosis with a herniated disc, and lateral recess stenosis

Table 2.2 (continued)

Authors (year)	Level	Study	Type	Patients	ORT	EBL (mL)	LOS	Findings
Atlas et al (2005)[65]	III	Prospective	OD	148	NR	NR	NR	Patients undergoing surgery had similar results when compared to patients undergoing conservative treatment at 8 to 10 y
Arinzon et al (2003)[66]	IV	Retrospective	OD	283	54.5 min for 65- to 74-year-olds 53.1 min for >75-year-olds	NR	NR	Compared surgical outcomes in patients older than 75 years and patients between 65 and 74 years and found significant improvement in pain while performing daily activities in both cohorts at a mean of 42 mo
Arinzon et al (2004)[67]	IV	Retrospective	OD	257	NR	NR	NR	Found that surgical management of lumbar stenosis in diabetic patients was effective, but had poorer outcomes than in nondiabetics
Airaksinen et al (1997)[60]	IV	Retrospective	OD	438	NR	NR	NR	Evidence suggested that prior lumbar surgery, diabetes, hip arthritis, previous spine trauma were associated with inferior outcomes of OD for lumbar stenosis
Gelalis et al (2006)[68]	IV	Retrospective	OD	54	NR	NR	NR	Found that patients with a longer duration of preoperative symptoms have less satisfaction with surgery at an average 11.6-year follow-up
Jolles et al (2001)[61]	IV	Retrospective	OD	155	NR	NR	NR	Excellent or good outcome noted in 79% of patients and Roland-Morris scores were significantly improved at mean 6.5-year follow-up

Abbreviations: EBL, estimated blood loss; LOS, length of stay; MIS, minimally invasive surgery; NR, not recorded; OD, open decompression; ODI, Oswestry Disability Index; ORT, operative time; RCT, randomized controlled trial; SF-12, 12-Item Short Form Health Survey; VAS, visual analog scale.

included EBL, operative time, length of stay, CPK-MM, and CT/MRI assessment of paraspinal muscle atrophy. At 1 year, there was no difference in JOA score, but the MIS cohort had a significantly lower VAS score. The operative time was higher in the MIS cohort (71.1 vs. 63.6 minutes), EBL was lower in the MIS cohort (37 vs. 71 mL), the length stay was lower in the MIS cohort (42 vs. 94 hours), and there were lower CPK-MM levels and less paraspinal muscle atrophy in the MIS cohort. All of these associations were statistically significant. Although the perioperative benefits presented in that report are promising, they are achieved in a patient cohort with single-level stenosis and minimal spondylolisthesis. This, however, represents the minority of lumbar stenosis patients, as previous reports have suggested that approximately 60 to 75% of patients present with two or more levels affected.[6,55,56,57]

2.12.3 Level III and IV Evidence in Open Surgery

Khoo and Fessler[31] compared the results of 25 patients undergoing MIS for spinal stenosis to a historical cohort of 25 patients treated with an OD. Of the 25 patients treated with MIS, 16 had disease at one level and 9 had disease at two levels. Primary outcomes were the SF-36 and the VAS; however, the authors did not include these in the article due to "the lack of validity in our brief [MIS] group follow-up period." Instead, the authors report that 30% of patients had almost complete symptom resolution, 68% report improved symptoms, and 10% remained unchanged at 12-month follow-up. Similarly, the authors report that back pain was resolved in 16%, improved in 68%, and unchanged in 16% of patients at 12 months. MIS surgery had longer OR times (109 vs. 88 minutes), but less blood loss (68 vs. 193 mL) and shorter hospitalizations (42 vs. 94 hours). Overall, the ability to compare outcomes between the OD and MIS cohorts is severely limited by the authors' omission of the results of validated outcome measure, despite having collected the data. The reasoning that the VAS and ODI are not validated at 12-month follow-up does not provide a clear explanation and suggests that follow-up should have been longer prior to publication or a different outcome score should have been implemented in order to facilitate objective comparison. The 4-year results from this cohort were later published,[33] but no comparison between the OD and MIS patient outcomes was made.

Ikuta et al[32] performed a prospective study of 47 patients undergoing MIS with a historical control of 25 patients treated with an OD. Of the MIS group, 35 patients had single-level disease, 11 had two-level disease, and one had three-level disease, and there was no description of the control group. The MIS cohort was followed for a mean of 22 months and the open cohort was followed for a mean of 23 months. Primary outcome scores were the JOA and VAS scores, and there was no difference at 3 months or final follow-up between the control and MIS groups. The MIS cohort had a longer mean operative time (124 vs. 101 minutes), less blood loss (61 vs. 100 mL), and a shorter length of stay (18 vs. 24 days). However, the MIS group had a significantly higher incidence of complications (25 vs. 14%) and included serious occurrences such as an 8.5% incidence of dural tears and a 14.9% incidence of transient neurological symptoms. Overall, this study suggests that equivalent clinical outcomes can be achieved between OD and MIS

approaches, but that MIS surgery carries a potentially higher complication rate—specifically increased risk of neural injury and dural tears.

Shih et al[47] performed a retrospective chart review of 26 open and 23 MIS patients with one- or two-level uncomplicated stenosis. No patient outcomes were assessed or reported but the perioperative parameters operative time, EBL, complications, and length of stay were assessed. The duration of surgery was greater in the MIS cohort (141 vs. 112 minutes), but there was less blood loss (140 vs. 62 mL) and the postoperative length of stay was shorter (2.04 vs. 2.92 days). Although not statistically significant, there was a higher number of postoperative complications (34.7 vs. 30.1%) in the MIS group, although the OD group had a higher risk of CSF leak (19.2 vs. 4.3%). Overall, the study suggests that there is a nonsignificant increase in complication rate for MIS procedures and a longer duration of surgery, but patients in the MIS cohort had an average 68 mL less blood loss and 1 day earlier discharge. However, the lack of patient outcome measures limits the ability to assess relative value each surgery provides to patients.

Parker et al[35] performed retrospective study comparing the total costs associated with open or MIS approaches in patients with multilevel disease at 2 years. For these cohorts, the OD costs slightly more ($25,420 vs. $23,109), but the difference was not statistically significant. Furthermore, the benefit of the surgeries, as measured by QALYs, was not statistically different. Overall, the theoretical benefits of reduced ancillary dependence following discharge and the shorter duration of hospitalization associated with an MIS did not affect the cost differential between the two procedures.

Rahman et al[34] performed a retrospective review of 88 patients receiving OD and 38 patients undergoing MIS for lumbar stenosis. No patient outcomes were reported but operative times were longer in the OD cohort (136.9 vs. 109 minutes); the OD cohort had a 194 mL greater blood loss and a 2.5 day greater length of stay following surgery. Although statistically significant, the clinical significance of these improved parameters is unclear as there are no patient outcomes reported.

2.13 Complications in Open Surgery

One of the central criticisms of OD for lumbar stenosis is the theory that this approach significantly traumatizes the paraspinal muscles, resulting in inferior clinical outcomes, which is thought to occur from prolonged retraction causing ischemia and denervation in open cases.[10,58] This seems to be supported by the observation that MIS procedures have lower perioperative CPK-MM values and less postoperative paraspinal muscle atrophy.[30] However, critical analysis of the eight investigations comparing open and MIS cohorts fails to support the clinical relevance of these findings, as short-term patient outcomes are equivalent.

Another complication associated with OD is increased blood loss compared to MIS. Critically examining the evidence suggests that there is a significant difference between the two procedures, but the largest average blood loss reported for the OD cohorts was 193 mL and the largest difference between the OD and MIS groups was 168 mL.[33] Although blood loss is to

Table 2.3 Comparison of complication between open and MIS decompression

Complication	Open	MIS
Dural tear	2%[34]; 9%[55]; 15%[56]; 3.7%[29]; 6.8%[57]; 8%[31]; 8%[32]; 1%[64]; 3%[60]; 1%[61]	3% (required conversion to open procedure)[34]; 3.7%[29]; 16%[31]; 8.5% (1 required conversion to open)[32]; 4%[33]
Wound infection/ postoperative drainage	3%[34]; 2%[55]; 3.4%[57]; 1%[64]; 3.4%,[60] 1%[61]	Not investigated[32]; 3%[34]
Cerebrospinal fluid leak	3%[34]	3%[34]
Synovial cyst	1%[34]	3%[34]
Hematoma	2%[55]; 3.7%[29]	
Misplaced pedicle screw	2%[56]	
Foot drop or other nerve complications	3.7%[29]; 4%[32]; 12%,[61]	14.9%[32]
Fracture of inferior articular process	4%[32]	6.3%[32]
Cauda equina syndrome	NR	2.1%[32]
Other	6%[55]; 4.3%[60]	NR

be avoided during surgery, the clinical significance of the difference between OD and MIS approaches in unclear—especially when EBL is subject to reporting bias.

The rate of complications in OD ranges from 0 to 14%,[30,32,55,59,60,61] and the rate of revision surgery in OD has been reported to be 8% at 2 years[55] and 13% at 4 years.[6] A systematic review of OD, with or without spinal fusion, for lumbar stenosis found that 5.4 to 14% of patients sustained operative complications and 8.2 to 18% of patients had a postoperative event, but nearly 90% of patients experienced an uncomplicated surgery.[62] Revision procedures were reported to occur in 1.3 to 2% at 1 year, 6 to 11% at 2 years, and 15% at 4 years.[62] Complications are summarized in ▶ Table 2.3.

2.14 Conclusion of Open Surgery

The literature reviewed, with the levels of evidence, is summarized in ▶ Table 2.1 and ▶ Table 2.2. There are no level I studies. There is level II evidence to suggest that MIS procedures create less blood loss, have shorter hospitalizations following surgery, and also have longer operative times. There is level II evidence suggesting that there is no difference in clinical outcomes between OD and MIS procedures. With the exception of a single study, there is an absence of level III and level IV evidence comparing clinical outcomes between MIS and OD. The single level III study demonstrated no significant difference in clinical outcomes between the two groups. There is level III and IV evidence that MIS surgery has shorter hospitalizations and less EBL than OD, and there is mixed evidence over duration of operative time to complete each surgery, with the majority of reports suggesting that MIS procedures have longer OR times. Using the grading scale of Guyatt et al,[63] we agree with our coauthors with a Grade 2B recommendation that MIS and OD have equivalent clinical and functional outcomes as well as the Grade 2B recommendation that MIS is associated with

decreased blood loss and shorter hospital stay, faster recovery, and reduced postoperative narcotic use compared to OD.

Overall, the quality of published studies comparing both approaches is insufficient to support clinical superiority of one approach over the other, as the majority of these reports omit or have equivalent outcome scores. The reports directly comparing open and MIS approaches potentially introduce a bias as the lead authors are experienced MIS surgeons and the reported outcomes may not be generalizable to all surgeons. Furthermore, the majority of patients in MIS versus OD studies have single-level disease, limiting the extrapolation of the benefits for MIS surgery to patients with more involved pathology. OD remains a reliable and effective procedure. MIS may be an option in certain patients, but the surgeon must weigh the theoretical perioperative benefits against a steep learning curve and a higher risk of complications.

2.15 Editors' Commentary

2.15.1 Minimally Invasive Surgery

The published benefits of minimally invasive decompression of stenosis are now so overwhelming that it is approaching the time when OD will have to be considered an antiquated treatment modality. Published literature now shows that MIS decompression of stenosis is associated with less blood loss, less pain and requirement for pain medication, shorter hospital stay, faster return to normal activities, fewer infections, lower complications overall, less paraspinal muscle destruction, less need for rehabilitation, equivalent dural decompression in even the most extreme stenotic canals, maintenance of normal spinal biomechanics, and less risk of iatrogenic instability and therefore no need for fusion.

Just as endoscopic cholecystectomy replaced open cholecystectomy as a result of the obvious and substantial benefits, it is time for MIS decompression of stenosis to replace open laminectomy. Reliance on antiquated data and/or lack of the necessary skill set to perform MIS decompression are not acceptable excuses to ignore the accumulating, overwhelming data supporting the advantages of MIS technique for this pathology.

2.15.2 Open Surgery

Open laminectomy is one of the most successful surgeries performed by spinal surgeons with respect to restoration of function and resolution of pain and has a relatively easy, short postoperative recovery period. For this reason, attempts to improve on this operation through MIS techniques are often an uphill battle. This uphill battle is best exemplified by the attempted management of a dural tear, a common intraoperative complication, which is difficult to address through an MIS incision. While a dural tear is easily addressed when using an OD technique, this common problem is difficult for all but the most experienced MIS surgeon to repair through a tubular retractor. Indeed, many MIS technique guides recommend the use of sealants instead of primary repair.

While a population of patients with minimal spondylosis would be ideal candidates for MIS decompression, patients belonging to such a spinal stenosis cohort are rare. The typical elderly patient with spinal stenosis in the absence of spinal instability has advanced spondylosis, distorted landmarks, thin dura, and atrophic paraspinal muscles, mitigating many of the proposed advantages of MIS techniques. In addition, most patients present with more than one level of spinal stenosis, making an MIS decompression more tedious and less surgeon-friendly as more levels are included. Patients with spinal stenosis and neurogenic claudication should be treated with the most effective and least complicated surgery available, which is open laminectomy in the vast majority of cases.

References

[1] Arnoldi CC, Brodsky AE, Cauchoix J, et al. Lumbar spinal stenosis and nerve root entrapment syndromes. Definition and classification. Clin Orthop Relat Res. 1976(115):4–5

[2] Katz JN, Harris MB. Clinical practice. Lumbar spinal stenosis. N Engl J Med. 2008; 358(8):818–825

[3] Osenbach R. Lumbar laminectomy. In: Sekhar L, Fessler R, eds. Atlas of Neurosurgical Techniques: Spine and Peripheral Nerves. 1st ed. New York, NY: Thieme; 2006

[4] Turner JA, Ersek M, Herron L, Deyo R. Surgery for lumbar spinal stenosis. Attempted meta-analysis of the literature. Spine. 1992; 17(1):1–8

[5] Gibson JNA, Waddell G. Surgery for degenerative lumbar spondylosis: updated Cochrane Review. Spine. 2005; 30(20):2312–2320

[6] Weinstein JN, Tosteson TD, Lurie JD, et al. Surgical versus nonoperative treatment for lumbar spinal stenosis four-year results of the Spine Patient Outcomes Research Trial. Spine. 2010; 35(14):1329–1338

[7] Sachs B, Fraenkel J. Progressive ankylotic rigidity of the spine (spondylose rhizomelique). J Nerv Ment Dis. 1900; 27:1–15

[8] Bailey P, Casamajor L. Osteoarthritis of the spine as a cause of compression of the spinal cord and its roots. J Nerv Ment Dis. 1911; 38:588–609

[9] Verbiest H. Results of surgical treatment of idiopathic developmental stenosis of the lumbar vertebral canal. A review of twenty-seven years' experience. J Bone Joint Surg Br. 1977; 59(2) 59B:181–188

[10] Gejo R, Matsui H, Kawaguchi Y, Ishihara H, Tsuji H. Serial changes in trunk muscle performance after posterior lumbar surgery. Spine. 1999; 24(10):1023–1028

[11] Sengupta DK, Herkowitz HN. Degenerative spondylolisthesis: review of current trends and controversies. Spine. 2005; 30(6) Suppl:S71–S81

[12] Adams MA, Hutton WC. The mechanical function of the lumbar apophyseal joints. Spine. 1983; 8(3):327–330

[13] Adams MA, Hutton WC, Stott JR. The resistance to flexion of the lumbar intervertebral joint. Spine. 1980; 5(3):245–253

[14] Cusick JF, Yoganandan N, Pintar FA, Reinartz JM. Biomechanics of sequential posterior lumbar surgical alterations. J Neurosurg. 1992; 76(5):805–811

[15] Young S, Veerapen R, O'Laoire SA. Relief of lumbar canal stenosis using multilevel subarticular fenestrations as an alternative to wide laminectomy: preliminary report. Neurosurgery. 1988; 23(5):628–633

[16] Aryanpur J, Ducker T. Multilevel lumbar laminotomies: an alternative to laminectomy in the treatment of lumbar stenosis. Neurosurgery. 1990; 26 (3):429–432, discussion 433

[17] Thomas NW, Rea GL, Pikul BK, Mervis LJ, Irsik R, McGregor JM. Quantitative outcome and radiographic comparisons between laminectomy and laminotomy in the treatment of acquired lumbar stenosis. Neurosurgery. 1997; 41(3):567–574, discussion 574–575

[18] Herkowitz HN, Kurz LT. Degenerative lumbar spondylolisthesis with spinal stenosis. A prospective study comparing decompression with decompression and intertransverse process arthrodesis. J Bone Joint Surg Am. 1991; 73(6): 802–808

[19] Dirksmeier P, Parson I, Kang J. Microendoscopic and open laminotomy and discectomy in lumbar disc disease. Semin Spine Surg. 1999; 11:138–146

[20] Palmer S, Turner R, Palmer R. Bilateral decompression of lumbar spinal stenosis involving a unilateral approach with microscope and tubular retractor system. J Neurosurg. 2002; 97(2) Suppl:213–217

[21] Palmer S, Turner R, Palmer R. Bilateral decompressive surgery in lumbar spinal stenosis associated with spondylolisthesis: unilateral approach and use of a microscope and tubular retractor system. Neurosurg Focus. 2002; 13 (1):E4

[22] Wong AP, Smith ZA, Lall RR, Bresnahan LE, Fessler RG. The microendoscopic decompression of lumbar stenosis: a review of the current literature and clinical results. Minim Invasive Surg. 2012; 2012(2012):325095

[23] Herkowitz HN, Kurz LT. Degenerative lumbar spondylolisthesis with spinal stenosis. A prospective study comparing decompression with decompression and intertransverse process arthrodesis. J Bone Joint Surg Am. 1991; 73(6): 802–808

[24] Bridwell KH, Sedgewick TA, O'Brien MF, Lenke LG, Baldus C. The role of fusion and instrumentation in the treatment of degenerative spondylolisthesis with spinal stenosis. J Spinal Disord. 1993; 6(6):461–472

[25] Senker W, Meznik C, Avian A, Berghold A. Perioperative morbidity and complications in minimal access surgery techniques in obese patients with degenerative lumbar disease. Eur Spine J. 2011; 20(7):1182–1187

[26] Rosen DS, O'Toole JE, Eichholz KM, et al. Minimally invasive lumbar spinal decompression in the elderly: outcomes of 50 patients aged 75 years and older. Neurosurgery. 2007; 60(3):503–509, discussion 509–510

[27] Sengupta DK, Herkowitz HN. Lumbar spinal stenosis. Treatment strategies and indications for surgery. Orthop Clin North Am. 2003; 34(2):281–295

[28] Foley K, Smith M. Microendoscopic discectomy. Tech Neurosurg. 1997; 3(4): 301–307

[29] Mobbs RJ, Li J, Sivabalan P, Raley D, Rao PJ. Outcomes after decompressive laminectomy for lumbar spinal stenosis: comparison between minimally invasive unilateral laminectomy for bilateral decompression and open laminectomy: clinical article. J Neurosurg Spine. 2014; 21(2):179–186

[30] Yagi M, Okada E, Ninomiya K, Kihara M. Postoperative outcome after modified unilateral-approach microendoscopic midline decompression for degenerative spinal stenosis. J Neurosurg Spine. 2009; 10(4):293–299

[31] Khoo LT, Fessler RG. Microendoscopic decompressive laminotomy for the treatment of lumbar stenosis. Neurosurgery. 2002; 51(5) Suppl:S146–S154

[32] Ikuta K, Arima J, Tanaka T, et al. Short-term results of microendoscopic posterior decompression for lumbar spinal stenosis. Technical note. J Neurosurg Spine. 2005; 2(5):624–633

[33] Asgarzadie F, Khoo LT. Minimally invasive operative management for lumbar spinal stenosis: overview of early and long-term outcomes. Orthop Clin North Am. 2007; 38(3):387–399, abstract vi–vii

[34] Rahman M, Summers LE, Richter B, Mimran RI, Jacob RP. Comparison of techniques for decompressive lumbar laminectomy: the minimally invasive versus the "classic" open approach. Minim Invasive Neurosurg. 2008; 51(2):100–105

[35] Parker SL, Adogwa O, Davis BJ, et al. Cost-utility analysis of minimally invasive versus open multilevel hemilaminectomy for lumbar stenosis. J Spinal Disord Tech. 2013; 26(1):42–47

[36] Castro-Menendez M, Bravo-Ricoy JA, Casal-Moro R, Hernandez-Blanco M, Jorge-Barreiro FJ. Midterm outcome after microendoscopic decompressive laminotomy for lumbar spinal stenosis: 4-year prospective study. Neurosurgery 2009;1(1):100–110

[37] Pao JL, Chen WC, Chen PQ. Clinical outcomes of microendoscopic decompressive laminotomy for degenerative lumbar spinal stenosis. European Spine Journal 2009;18:672

[38] Sasai K, Umeda M, Maruyama T, Wakabayashi E, Iida H. Microsurgical bilateral decompression via a unilateral approach for lumbar spinal canal stenosis including degenerative spondylolisthesis. J Neurosurg Spine 2008;9 (6):554–9

[39] Ikuta K, Tono O, Oga M. Clinical outcome of microendoscopic posterior decompression for spinal stenosis associated with degenerative spondylolisthesisminimum 2-year outcome of 37 patients. Minim Invasive Neurosurg 2008;51(5):267–271

[40] Mannion RJ, Guilfoyle MR, Efendy J, Nowitzke AM, Laing RJ, Wood MJ. Minimally invasive lumbar decompression: long-term outcome, morbidity, and the learning curve from the first 50 cases. J Spinal Disord Tech 2012;25 (1):47–51

[41] Palmer S, Davison L. Minimally invasive surgical treatment of lumbar spinal stenosis: Two-year follow-up in 54 patients. Surg Neurol Int 2012;3:41

[42] Wada K, Sairyo K, Sakai T, Yasui N. Minimally invasive endoscopic bilateral decompression with a unilateral approach (endo-BiDUA) for elderly patients with lumbar spinal canal stenosis. Minim Invasive Neurosurg 2010;53(2):65–8

[43] Xu BS, Tan QS, Xia Q, Ji N, Hu YC. Bilateral decompression via unilateral fenestration using mobile microendoscopic discectomy technique for lumbar spinal stenosis. Orthopedic Surgery 2010;2(2):106–110

[44] Minamide A, Yoshida M, Yamada H, Nakagawa Y, Kawai M, Maio K, et al. Endoscope-assisted spinal decompression surgery for lumbar spinal stenosis. J Neurosurg Spine 2013;19(6):664–71

[45] Perez-Cruet MJ, Fessler RG, Perin NI. Review: complications of minimally invasive spinal surgery. Neurosurgery. 2002; 51(5) Suppl:S26–S36

[46] Ikuta K, Tono O, Tanaka T, et al. Surgical complications of microendoscopic procedures for lumbar spinal stenosis. Minim Invasive Neurosurg. 2007; 50 (3):145–149

[47] Shih P, Wong AP, Smith TR, Lee AI, Fessler RG. Complications of open compared to minimally invasive lumbar spine decompression. J Clin Neurosci. 2011; 18(10):1360–1364

[48] O'Toole JE, Eichholz KM, Fessler RG. Surgical site infection rates after minimally invasive spinal surgery. J Neurosurg Spine. 2009; 11(4):471–476

[49] Deyo RA, Cherkin DC, Loeser JD, Bigos SJ, Ciol MA. Morbidity and mortality in association with operations on the lumbar spine. The influence of age, diagnosis, and procedure. J Bone Joint Surg Am. 1992; 74(4):536–543

[50] Patel N, Bagan B, Vadera S, et al. Obesity and spine surgery: relation to perioperative complications. J Neurosurg Spine. 2007; 6(4):291–297

[51] Rosen DS, Ferguson SD, Ogden AT, Huo D, Fessler RG. Obesity and self-reported outcome after minimally invasive lumbar spinal fusion surgery. Neurosurgery. 2008; 63(5):956–960, discussion 960

[52] Matsunaga S, Sakou T, Morizono Y, Masuda A, Demirtas AM. Natural history of degenerative spondylolisthesis. Pathogenesis and natural course of the slippage. Spine. 1990; 15(11):1204–1210

[53] Guyatt G, Schunëmann H, Cook D, Jaeschke R, Pauker S, Bucher H, American College of Chest Physicians. Grades of recommendation for antithrombotic agents. Chest. 2001; 119(1) Suppl:3S–7S

[54] Reitman CA, Anderson DG, Fischgrund J. Surgery for degenerative spondylolisthesis: open versus minimally invasive surgery. Clin Orthop Relat Res. 2013; 471(10):3082–3087

[55] Weinstein JN, Tosteson TD, Lurie JD, et al. SPORT Investigators. Surgical versus nonsurgical therapy for lumbar spinal stenosis. N Engl J Med. 2008; 358(8):794–810

[56] Malmivaara A, Slätis P, Heliövaara M, et al. Finnish Lumbar Spinal Research Group. Surgical or nonoperative treatment for lumbar spinal stenosis? A randomized controlled trial. Spine. 2007; 32(1):1–8

[57] Athiviraham A, Yen D. Is spinal stenosis better treated surgically or nonsurgically? Clin Orthop Relat Res. 2007; 458(458):90–93

[58] Weiner BK, Fraser RD, Peterson M. Spinous process osteotomies to facilitate lumbar decompressive surgery. Spine. 1999; 24(1):62–66

[59] Amundsen T, Weber H, Nordal HJ, Magnaes B, Abdelnoor M, Lilleâs F. Lumbar spinal stenosis: conservative or surgical management?: A prospective 10-year study. Spine. 2000; 25(11):1424–1435, discussion 1435–1436

[60] Airaksinen O, Herno A, Turunen V, Saari T, Suomlainen O. Surgical outcome of 438 patients treated surgically for lumbar spinal stenosis. Spine. 1997; 22(19):2278–2282

[61] Jolles BM, Porchet F, Theumann N. Surgical treatment of lumbar spinal stenosis. Five-year follow-up. J Bone Joint Surg Br. 2001; 83(7):949–953

[62] Kovacs FM, Urrútia G, Alarcón JD. Surgery versus conservative treatment for symptomatic lumbar spinal stenosis: a systematic review of randomized controlled trials. Spine. 2011; 36(20):E1335–E1351

[63] Guyatt GH, Cook DJ, Jaeschke R, et al. Grades of recommendation for antithrombotic agents: American College of Chest Physicians Evidence-Based Clinical Practice Guidelines (8th Edition). Chest. 2008; 133(6)(Suppl):123S–131S

[64] Javid MJ, Hadar EJ. Long-term follow-up review of patients who underwent laminectomy for lumbar stenosis: a prospective study. J Neurosurg. 1998; 89(1):1–7

[65] Atlas SJ, Keller RB, Wu YA, Deyo RA, Singer DE. Long-term outcomes of surgical and nonsurgical management of lumbar spinal stenosis: 8 to 10 year results from the maine lumbar spine study. Spine. 2005; 30(8):936–943

[66] Arinzon ZH, Fredman B, Zohar E, et al. Surgical management of spinal stenosis: a comparison of immediate and long term outcome in two geriatric patient populations. Arch Gerontol Geriatr. 2003; 36(3):273–279

[67] Arinzon Z, Adunsky A, Fidelman Z, Gepstein R. Outcomes of decompression surgery for lumbar spinal stenosis in elderly diabetic patients. Eur Spine J. 2004; 13(1):32–37

[68] Gelalis ID, Stafilas KS, Korompilias AV, Zacharis KC, Beris AE, Xenakis TA. Decompressive surgery for degenerative lumbar spinal stenosis: long-term results. Int Orthop. 2006; 30(1):59–63

3 Facet Cysts: Is There an Advantage to Treating Synovial Cysts with Minimally Invasive Techniques?

MIS: Jose M. Torres-Campa, Marjan Alimi, and Roger Härtl
Open: Brian W. Su

3.1 Introduction

Synovial cysts are well-known (although relatively uncommon) pathologies in the spine involving the synovium of the facet joints. Synovial cysts were first described in the knee in 1885,[1] and in the spine in 1950.[2] Their relationship to the facet joint, however, was not clearly described until 2010 by Spinner et al.[3] Synovial cysts of the spine usually originate from degenerative facet joints, although occasional cases arising from microtraumatized joints have also been reported.[4]

Synovial cysts can be found throughout the spinal axis, but most commonly occur within the lumbar spine. Among all patients with synovial cysts on the magnetic resonance imaging (MRI), 0.5 to 2.3% are found to be symptomatic.[5] Wilby et al demonstrated that osteoarthritis of the facet joints can result in the release of cartilage and bone fragments into the synovial fluid of the joint, which can then provoke granulation tissue and cyst formation.[6] Synovial cysts of the lumbar spine typically cause nerve compression in the lateral recess adjacent to the joint. The traversing nerve root is more commonly affected (e.g., L5 nerve is affected by an L4/L5 cyst), although extension of the cysts into the foramen may also happen, resulting in compression of the exiting nerve root as well (e.g., L4 nerve becomes affected by an L4/L5 cyst). Symptomatic facet cysts present with pain and paresthesias within the distribution of the compressed nerve root. Although exceedingly rare, lumbar facet cysts have also been reported to present as cauda equina syndrome.[7,8,9]

Since instability alters the biomechanics of the facet joint, lumbar synovial cysts may be associated with degenerative spondylolisthesis. Lumbar synovial cysts are more commonly seen at the L4/L5 level.[10,11] For evaluation of patients with synovial cysts, it is critical to obtain dynamic flexion/extension X-rays in order to rule out concomitant spondylolisthesis and instability. While the majority of facet cysts are fluid filled, chronic cysts may occasionally be calcified following percutaneous aspiration.[12] In such cases, computed tomography (CT) scans need to be done for evaluation and surgical planning.

3.2 Indications for Surgical Treatment of a Synovial Cyst

Initial treatment of synovial cyst is nonoperative, which includes oral medication, cyst injection or aspiration, and selective nerve root injections. Slipman et al reported 33% long-term improvement of symptoms with corticosteroid use.[13] Martha et al proposed that fluoroscopy-guided injection results in concurrent rupture of the cyst and introduction of the corticosteroids into the synovial cyst space.[14] They successfully treated 46% of their patients by injection, and the other 54% surgically. Cyst aspiration, however, may appear to be challenging, due to gelatinous consistency of the cyst fluid or presence of a calcified component within the cyst.[15,16]

Surgical intervention should be considered after failure of nonoperative management and/or where the extremity pain interferes with the patient's functionality and quality of life. While facet cysts can also cause axial back pain, surgical intervention should generally be reserved for patients with radiculopathy and/or weakness secondary to nerve compression.

Surgical treatment of the lumbar facet cyst involves resection of the cyst. Fusion is indicated only if concomitant dynamic instability of the spinal segment is detected or when over 30% of the facet joint is resected during surgery.

3.3 Advantages of Minimally Invasive Surgery

There are several advantages of using the techniques of minimally invasive surgery (MIS). MIS procedures allow for reduced retraction of muscles and result in less soft-tissue damage compared to open procedures. It has been shown that they allow earlier ambulation and shorten the hospital stay.[17,18,19,20] MIS treatment of the herniated lumbar discs and MIS fusion, in particular, result in reduced muscle atrophy, as shown on the postoperative MRI.[21]

Treatment of synovial cysts using MIS technique has similar advantages. It is associated with reduced blood loss (MIS: 74–158 mL; vs. open: 460–930 mL).[22,23] In this instability-prone pathology, a tubular approach can avoid fusion in patients without mechanical back pain and/or movement on the flexion/extension films.[24] The tubular approach preserves the majority of the posterior elements, thereby minimizing instability.[25,26,27] Moreover, a contralateral approach (contrary to an ipsilateral approach) allows for resection of the cyst through normal anatomy; the normal dura is identified first, therefore minimizing the risk of cerebrospinal fluid (CSF) leak. A contralateral approach also reduces the extent of the facet joint that needs to be removed.[24]

CSF leaks, if they occur, can be treated with CSF sealants such as Tissucol (Baxter Healthcare SA Inc.; Zurich, Switzerland) or Duraseal (Confluent Surgical Inc.; Waltham, MA). Direct mechanical repair in our experience is rarely necessary and can be accomplished with endoscopic tools through tubular retractors.

3.4 Advantages of Open Surgery

Resection of facet cysts through an open ipsilateral microdiscectomy/microdecompression approach has several advantages. The open technique allows for avoidance of the demanding learning curve associated with minimally invasive approaches, particularly the contralateral approach. Facet cysts often require widespread resection of laminae and/or facet joints, to ensure complete removal of the facet cyst and decompression of the affected nerve root. The broader field of view in an ipsilateral

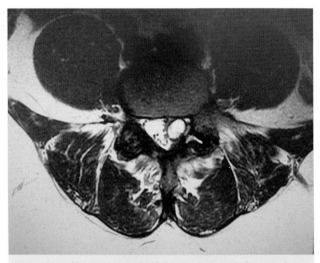

Fig. 3.1 A case example of a patient with a synovial cyst on the left at L4–L5: the T2-weighted MRI.

open technique permits better visualization of the surgical region during resection. An incidental durotomy due to removal of an adherent cyst can easily be repaired through an ipsilateral open technique, as opposed to a contralateral minimally invasive approach. In addition, when fusion becomes necessary during the surgery, an open technique can rapidly be converted to a fusion procedure.[16,28,29]

3.5 Case Illustration

A 64-year-old woman presented with a 5-month history of severe left leg pain along L5 dermatome. There was no relief of the symptoms with the use of oral medications, physical therapy, and epidural steroid injections.

MRI and flexion/extension X-rays were obtained, showing a large left synovial cyst at L4–L5 level, without spondylolisthesis and no instability (▶ Fig. 3.1).

A minimally invasive tubular surgical resection and decompression via a contralateral approach was performed. The operative technique has been fully described following the current case example (under "The MIS Surgical Technique"). Briefly, under the microscope and through a 19-mm-diameter tubular retractor, the inferior edge of the lamina contralateral to the cyst was removed; the retractor was angled medially, and the spinous process and the contralateral lamina were undercut. The ligamentum flavum was exposed bilaterally, and the cyst was exposed from the contralateral, normal anatomy. The cyst was then carefully resected. The patient ambulated within a few hours after surgery and was discharged home within 24 hours.

At 4 years' follow-up, the sciatic pain and neurological claudication remained resolved. No worsening of the spondylolisthesis was detected in any of the postoperative studies.

3.6 Surgical Technique in Minimally Invasive Surgery

The microendoscopic tubular approach was first described by Foley and Smith in 1997.[30] We have been using a modification of this approach since 2004, by replacing the endoscope with an operating microscope.[23] In the operating room, patients under general anesthesia are placed prone on a Wilson frame. Fluoroscopy is used for localization of the correct level. A skin incision is made approximately 1.5 cm lateral to the midline on the side opposite to the juxtafacet cyst. A tubular retractor is placed over serial dilators and is fixed in place using a table-mounted arm; an 18- or 19-mm-diameter tubular retractor is used for this procedure. The correct level is confirmed. An operating microscope is brought in. The base of the spinous process and the inferior edge of the lamina contralateral to the cyst are identified and removed using a high-speed drill with a curved 3-mm matchstick attachment (Anspach; Palm Beach Gardens, FL). The yellow ligamentum flavum is identified and exposed bilaterally. Subsequently, the retractor is angled toward the midline, and the lamina and facet joint contralaterally are undercut. In the cases where lumbar spinal stenosis coexists with the cyst, a bilateral MIS laminectomy is performed. The operating table is then rotated away from the surgeon, which provides a wide access to the ligamentum flavum, which needs to be carefully resected for exposure of the facet cyst. The dura is then carefully dissected off the cyst wall.

During this maneuver, the dura is depressed using the suction device. After adequate exposure, the medial edge of the juxtafacet cyst is meticulously identified and carefully dissected off the dural attachment along the cranial, caudal, and medial aspect of the cyst. It is then typically possible to remove the juxtafacet cyst in a piecemeal manner using Kerrison rongeurs and other microsurgical instruments. Occasionally, when clearance cannot be achieved due to the large size of the cyst, in order to prevent excessive retraction of the dura, the cyst is deliberately ruptured and decompressed, which allows complete removal of the cyst. Resection of the facet joint is not required. If a dural tear is observed, it is covered at the end of the procedure by Tissucol or Duraseal, and the patient is kept flat after surgery. At the end of the procedure, the operative field is irrigated by antibiotic solution, the tubular retractor is removed, and every attempt is made to close the fascia before skin closure is obtained.

3.7 Surgical Technique in Open Surgery

Preoperative planning of the location and extent of the cyst is critical. The surgery should be performed under a microscope or 3.5 × loupe magnification. The patient is placed in a prone position on a Wilson or Andrews frame. This position allows for opening of the interlaminar space, which eases the access to the spinal canal. The patient's knees are positioned at 90 degrees to allow for the nerve to be manipulated while avoiding a stretch injury. A small longitudinal midline skin incision is made at the level of the cyst and dissection is taken down to the thoracolumbar fascia. The muscles are then elevated in a subperiosteal manner on the ipsilateral side to expose the interlaminar space. The correct level of surgery is verified with X-ray guidance. A self-retaining Taylor or McCullough-type retractor is then placed over the facet joint. A laminoforaminotomy is then made with an AM-8 matchstick burr at the inferior aspect of the superior lamina until the ligamentum flavum is identified.

The ligamentum flavum inserts approximately at the level of the inferior pedicle of the superior vertebrae and protects the burr from damaging the dura. The lamina is then resected with a 4–0 Kerrison rongeur up until the insertion of the flavum. The flavum is then separated from the lamina with a 0 curved curette and removed either en-bloc or piecemeal with a Kerrison rongeur in order to expose the dura. The lateral recess is then completely decompressed with removal of the superior articular process up until the medial aspect of the pedicle. At that point, the cyst is typically seen originating from the facet joint and adherent to the traversing nerve root. Caution should be used as the capsule of the facet can mimic the appearance of dura. Once the entire extent of the cyst is identified, the capsule of the cyst is gently peeled off the dura with the use of a Woodsen and Penfield 4. This is best accomplished by starting on normal dura and developing a plane between normal dura and the cyst capsule. An assistant can provide tension on the cyst with a pituitary roungeur to aid in peeling the cyst off the dura. It is important to resect enough lamina and facet to ensure that the entire extent of the cyst has been excised. At the conclusion of the decompression, the traversing nerve should be completely decompressed and easily mobilized from the medial pedicle of the interior vertebrae. A Valsalva maneuver should be performed to carefully check for a durotomy. The wound is then irrigated and bleeding is stopped with liquid Gelfoam and bipolar cautery. Closure is completed with interrupted sutures and deep fascia and a running absorbable skin suture. Patients are typically sent home on the day of surgery and permitted to ambulate with a soft corset for comfort.

3.8 Discussion of Minimally Invasive Surgery

Since the original description of a microendoscopic tubular approach by Foley and Smith in 1997,[30] it has been gaining more popularity and its indications have constantly been expanding. Within the last decade, synovial cysts have also been added to the indications of tubular approach,[24,31,32,33] and more recently a contralateral approach has been used to perform this procedure.[24,32] Initially, an ipsilateral approach was used, requiring at minimum a partial removal of the facet joint for complete resection of the cyst. James et al and Rhee et al, however, recently reported a contralateral approach.[24,32] The contralateral approach allows for resection of the cyst from a normal anatomy, and identification of normal dura prior to cyst resection. It also minimizes the extent of facet that needs to be removed. The studies on MIS treatment of synovial cyst have been summarized in ▶ Table 3.1 (54 patients).

Up until now, no studies have compared open and MIS techniques for synovial cyst removal. However, comparisons of MIS and open technique for fusion and discectomies have shown MIS to be superior to open technique in terms of earlier ambulation, less blood loss, reduced postoperative opioid medication, and shorter hospital stay. Similar favorable results were found on MIS technique for treatment of synovial cysts.[19,20]

The primary advantage of treating synovial cyst with an MIS contralateral approach through tubular retractors is minimization of segmental instability through preservation of most of the posterior elements and the facet joints. Another advantage

Table 3.1 Literature on minimally invasive treatment of synovial cysts

	Number of cases	Age (y)	Presence of radicular pain	L4/L5 level of surgery	Presence of listhesis	Follow-up time (mo)	Outcome (excellent/good) (%)	Time of surgery (min)	Length of hospital stay	Blood loss (mL)	Complications
Sehati et al (2006)[33]	19	69 (43–80)	16/19	16/19	2/19	16	95	158 (75–770)	13→0 d; 2→1 d; 1→2 d	31 (10–100)	2 dural tears
Sandhu et al (2004)[31]	17	64 (46–82)	17/17	14/17	8/17 (47%)	12	94	97 (50–180)	7→0 d; 7→1 d; 3→2–3 d	35 (5–100)	1 dural tear
James et al (2012)[24]	16	66.5 ± 10.7 48–83	72%	9/16	9/16 (56%)	18	87.5	105 ± 37	8→1 d; 2→2 d; 6→>3 d	<40	2 dural tear; 1 transient L5 weakness
Rhee et al (2012)[32]	2	70	2/2	2/2	0/2	12	100%	74	2→0 d	27	–

of MIS treatment of synovial cyst is its avoidance of fusion in most cases, unless there is clear evidence of instability such as severe mechanical back pain and/or movement on flexion/extension films. According to North American Spine Society guidelines, fusion is recommended in the presence of degenerative spondylolisthesis, a pathology which is likely to occur after resection of synovial cyst.[34] In contrast, Khan et al argue for fusion in all open cases.[23] However, even after open resection, there is no evidence in the literature that supports fusion in all cases. Most publications do not provide a criteria for determination of a need for fusion.[12,26] In Bydon et al's meta-analysis, the recurrence rate after cyst excision without fusion was 1.8%, and the reoperation rate requiring fusion was 5.8%.[35] In the same study, the recurrence rate after excision and fusion was found to be 0%, and the overall reoperation rate was 6.2%. Lyons et al found similar results; in their study of 194 patients with symptomatic synovial cysts, half of the patients were found to have concomitant spondylolisthesis; among all, only 18 patients required fusion, while the clinical outcome was reported as good pain relief in 91% of the patients, demonstrating favorable results.[36] Due to the complications and increased cost of surgery associated with instrumentation, fusion may not be cost effective.[22] MIS treatment for synovial cysts minimizes the need for fusion because it preserves stability of the spine.

3.8.1 Level I Evidence in Minimally Invasive Surgery

There is no level I study available.

3.8.2 Level II Evidence in Minimally Invasive Surgery

There is no level II study available.

3.8.3 Level III and IV Evidence in Minimally Invasive Surgery

Only four papers have been published on MIS treatment for synovial cyst.[24,31,32,33] All are prospective or retrospective cohort studies with no control groups for comparison. Pain relief and rates of intraoperative and postoperative complications are comparable in all four studies.

3.9 Complications in Minimally Invasive Surgery

A number of complications have been described. Five dural tears (9% of MIS patients) were reported, compared to 3.4% in open surgery. However, no CSF leakage occurred in MIS operations, whereas 1% of open surgeries resulted in CSF leakages requiring a second surgery.[35] The advantage of MIS surgery over open approaches in this regard could be explained by the absence of dead space after removal of the tubular retractor. There were no cases of reoperation for new cyst resection and no reports of instability. Partial neurological deterioration (transient weakness at L5) was detected in one case, but no permanent neurological deficit was reported.

3.10 Conclusion of Minimally Invasive Surgery

MIS treatment for synovial cyst and spondylolisthesis has several advantages over open surgery. MIS surgery is less invasive, resulting in reduced blood loss, shorter hospital stay, and less muscle damage. Minimal facet joint is resected, minimizing the progression of spondylolisthesis. Reoperation rates are lower, and the need for fusion or repair of CSF leakage is low. Modifications to the initial MIS treatment of synovial cyst by a contralateral approach allow for no or almost no resection of the facet joint and a better view of the interface between the dura and the cyst.[24] Additional data with higher number of patients are needed for further evaluation of long-term follow-up.

3.11 Discussion of Open Surgery

Although, no studies have specifically compared MIS to mini-open approaches for resection of lumbar synovial cysts, it seems that differences in postoperative pain, incision size, and blood loss are likely to be negligible between the two techniques. The purported benefits of MIS techniques are more significant in larger surgeries such as multilevel laminectomies, pedicle screw placement, and fusion. Facet joint resection, however, may be considered as analogous to MIS microdiscectomy which has been shown to have no differences in the outcome, in postoperative back or leg pain.[20,29] A review study on clinical papers on the facet cyst resection, in which majority of the cases were treated by resection without fusion, demonstrated the efficacy of cyst excision and partial facetectomy without fusion with an open approach.

3.11.1 Level I Evidence in Open Surgery

There are no level I studies on the open treatment of lumbar synovial facet cysts.

3.11.2 Level II Evidence in Open Surgery

There are no level II studies on the open treatment of lumbar synovial facet cysts.

3.11.3 Level III and IV Evidence in Open Surgery

All studies on the open treatment of lumbar facet cysts are case–controlled, retrospective cohorts or case series, and are summarized in ▶ Table 3.2. Two series involve treatment with an open laminectomy and cyst resection. It should be noted that these studies did not employ a microdecompressive approach as described in this chapter.[36,37] Nonetheless, in Lyons et al's study, only 4 out of 176 patients undergoing laminectomy and cyst excision required subsequent fusion for symptomatic spondylolisthesis, and overall 91% of patients reported good pain relief.[36] Other studies employing a microdecompressive-type approach have shown similar results, with outcome scores ranging from 80 to 100%.[16,22,23,28,38,39,40,41] Two studies included patients with a preexisting spondylolisthesis, and both reported an approximate 80% of good outcome, with few cases of progression of instability.[38,40]

Table 3.2 Literature on open treatment of synovial cysts

	Number of cases	Surgical treatment	Follow-up time (mo)	Progression of listhesis	Outcome (excellent/ good)
Epstein (2004)[37]	45 (cyst) 35 (cyst and spondylolisthesis)	Open laminectomy and cyst excision	24	11% in patients w/o listhesis 31% in patients w/ listhesis	58% (cyst) 63% (cyst and spondylolisthesis)
Lyons et al (2000)[36]	147 patients with at least 6-month follow-up (50% with spondylolisthesis)	Open laminectomy and cyst excision (partial hemilaminectomy or total hemi- or bilateral laminectomy)	26	2% developed symptomatic spondylolisthesis	91%
Banning et al (2001)[38]	29 (41% with spondylolisthesis)	Mini-open decompression	24	Not specified (7% had concurrent fusion)	90% with similar grading ("completely improved" or "better—still some problems")
Boviatsis et al (2008)[39]	7	Mini-open decompression	6	0%	100%
Deinsberger et al (2006)[40]	31 (41% with spondylolisthesis)	27 mini-open decompression 4 laminectomy and cyst excision	12–30	0%	81%
El Shazly and Khattab (2011)[16]	13	10 partial hemilaminectomy 3 bilateral decompressive laminectomies	50	7% required subsequent fusion	92%
Ganau et al (2013)[22]	15	Mini-open decompression	28	0%	100%
Hsu et al (1995)[41]	8	Mini-open decompression	Not precisely noted (a 10 years' experience)	Not specified	87.5%
Landi et al (2012)[28]	15 (without instability)	Mini-open decompression	24	0%	100%

3.12 Complications in Open Surgery

When performing an open decompression, care should be taken to minimize damage to the lateral facet capsule. It is important to expose the midlateral pars of the superior vertebrae to avoid overresection of the pars. Every effort should be made to preserve at least 7 mm of the midlateral pars and 30% of the facet joint. Over-resection of the pars can lead to iatrogenic pars fracture and overresection of the facet joint can lead to instability. Another complication is cyst recurrence. In that setting, management is identical to that of a primary cyst, with the exception of having a lower threshold to perform a fusion to permanently treat the pathology. If the cyst is very adherent, it may be necessary to puncture the cyst and remove as much of the dorsal portion of the cyst as possible, while leaving a portion of the back wall of the cyst on the nerve. Since a generous decompression has been performed, the nerve is decompressed even if the wall of the cyst is left adherent to the nerve. Adherence of the cyst to the nerve can lead to an incidental durotomy. Incidental durotomy is the most common surgical complication and occurs 9% of the times.[38] When possible, a dural tear should undergo a primary watertight closure with 6–0 Gore-Tex suture and then bolstered with Duragen and Duraseal.

3.13 Conclusion of Open Surgery

The purpose of a new technology or different surgical approach is to improve the outcome and minimize the complications. MIS approaches to facet cyst have not demonstrated superiority to the mini-open approach due to relative less invasive nature of mini-open surgeries. Benefits of MIS techniques are not outweighed by the learning curve associated with a contralateral decompression and its potential for intraoperative complications. In addition, good outcomes following treatment of facet cysts through a mini-open technique is well described by multiple studies and have stood the test of time.[16,28,29] The most important factor in choosing a surgical technique for treating facet cysts is the surgeon's comfort; the surgeon must be certain enough that the cyst is completely excised and that the nerve is thoroughly decompressed.

3.14 Editors' Commentary

3.14.1 Minimally Invasive Surgery

MIS treatment of synovial cysts represents one of the "no-brainer" applications of this technique. By essentially performing an MIS foraminotomy, it enables removal of the cyst with minimal disruption of the adjacent anatomy, thus reducing the incidence of delayed spondylolisthesis while maintaining all the other known advantages of MIS surgery (e.g., less blood loss, less pain, faster recovery). In doing so, the necessity for fusion is also eliminated, unless there is also preexisting instability.

3.14.2 Open Surgery

The surgical excision of facet cysts is a minimally invasive technique regardless of the method used; a 1.25-inch incision can be used even when an "open" technique is utilized. While this is an uncommonly performed surgery, patients who undergo isolated cyst resection without fusion would be expected to go home on the day of surgery regardless of technique. Excising a facet cyst carries a higher rate of dural injury due to frequent adhesions between the cyst and the dura when compared to other decompression procedures. Given the relative equivalence in the incision length and a superior ability to repair dural injuries with an open technique, there is little benefit to performing this surgery through a tubular retractor. The MIS technique detailed above suggests that dural repair should not be attempted and that surgeons encountering a dural injury should simply put Duraseal or another sealant over the defect. This strategy has a high failure rate, particularly given the acknowledged difficulty obtaining a watertight fascial closure through a tubular retractor. This MIS shortcoming should discourage surgeons from applying MIS techniques in the setting of facet cyst excision.

A frequent underlying cause of facet cysts is spinal instability. As the degree of instability may be underrepresented on preoperative radiographs due to patient effort or lack of flexion/extension views, surgeons must approach the resection of facet cysts with an awareness that unanticipated segmental instability may present itself; in these cases, the patient may benefit from fusion surgery to prevent cyst recurrence. Assessment of instability is easier through an open approach, and conversion to a fusion surgery when necessary can be done without the need for additional incisions.

References

[1] Baker WM. Formation of synovial cyst in connection with joints. St Bartholomews Hosp Rep. 1885; 21:177–199

[2] Vossschulte K, Borger G. Anatomische und funktionelle Untersuchungen über den Bandscheibenprolaps. Langenbecks Arch Klin Chir Ver Dtsch Z Chir. 1950; 265(3–4):329–355

[3] Spinner RJ, Hébert-Blouin MN, Maus TP, Atkinson JL, Desy NM, Amrami KK. Evidence that atypical juxtafacet cysts are joint derived. J Neurosurg Spine. 2010; 12(1):96–102

[4] Ramieri A, Domenicucci M, Seferi A, Paolini S, Petrozza V, Delfini R. Lumbar hemorrhagic synovial cysts: diagnosis, pathogenesis, and treatment. Report of 3 cases. Surg Neurol. 2006; 65(4):385–390, discussion 390

[5] Doyle AJ, Merrilees M. Synovial cysts of the lumbar facet joints in a symptomatic population: prevalence on magnetic resonance imaging. Spine. 2004; 29(8):874–878

[6] Wilby MJ, Fraser RD, Vernon-Roberts B, Moore RJ. The prevalence and pathogenesis of synovial cysts within the ligamentum flavum in patients with lumbar spinal stenosis and radiculopathy. Spine. 2009; 34(23):2518–2524

[7] Tatter SB, Cosgrove GR. Hemorrhage into a lumbar synovial cyst causing an acute cauda equina syndrome. Case report. J Neurosurg. 1994; 81(3):449–452

[8] Muir JJ, Pingree MJ, Moeschler SM. Acute cauda equina syndrome secondary to a lumbar synovial cyst. Pain Physician. 2012; 15(5):435–440

[9] Machino M, Yukawa Y, Ito K, Kanbara S, Kato F. Spontaneous hemorrhage in an upper lumbar synovial cyst causing subacute cauda equina syndrome. Orthopedics. 2012; 35(9):e1457–e1460

[10] Mavrogenis AF, Papagelopoulos PJ, Sapkas GS, Korres DS, Pneumaticos SG. Lumbar synovial cysts. J Surg Orthop Adv. 2012; 21(4):232–236

[11] Chaput C, Padon D, Rush J, Lenehan E, Rahm M. The significance of increased fluid signal on magnetic resonance imaging in lumbar facets in relationship to degenerative spondylolisthesis. Spine. 2007; 32(17):1883–1887

[12] Boissière L, Valour F, Rigal J, Soderlund C. Lumbar synovial cyst calcification after facet joint steroid injection. BMJ Case Rep. 2013:; 2013:2013

[13] Slipman CW, Lipetz JS, Wakeshima Y, Jackson HB. Nonsurgical treatment of zygapophyseal joint cyst-induced radicular pain. Arch Phys Med Rehabil. 2000; 81(7):973–977

[14] Martha JF, Swaim B, Wang DA, et al. Outcome of percutaneous rupture of lumbar synovial cysts: a case series of 101 patients. Spine J. 2009; 9(11):899–904

[15] Epstein NE, Baisden J. The diagnosis and management of synovial cysts: Efficacy of surgery versus cyst aspiration. Surg Neurol Int. 2012; 3 Suppl 3: S157–S166

[16] El Shazly AA, Khattab MF. Surgical excision of a Juxtafacet cyst in the lumbar spine: a report of thirteen cases with long-term follow up. Asian J Neurosurg. 2011; 6(2):78–82

[17] Datta G, Gnanalingham KK, Peterson D, et al. Back pain and disability after lumbar laminectomy: is there a relationship to muscle retraction? Neurosurgery. 2004; 54(6):1413–1420, discussion 1420

[18] Kawaguchi Y, Yabuki S, Styf J, et al. Back muscle injury after posterior lumbar spine surgery. Topographic evaluation of intramuscular pressure and blood flow in the porcine back muscle during surgery. Spine. 1996; 21(22):2683–2688

[19] Podichetty VK, Spears J, Isaacs RE, Booher J, Biscup RS. Complications associated with minimally invasive decompression for lumbar spinal stenosis. J Spinal Disord Tech. 2006; 19(3):161–166

[20] Parikh K, Tomasino A, Knopman J, Boockvar J, Härtl R. Operative results and learning curve: microscope-assisted tubular microsurgery for 1- and 2-level discectomies and laminectomies. Neurosurg Focus. 2008; 25(2):E14

[21] Bresnahan LE, Smith JS, Ogden AT, et al. Assessment of paraspinal muscle cross-sectional area following lumbar decompression: minimally invasive versus open approaches. Clin Spine Surg. 2017; 30(3):E162–168

[22] Ganau M, Ennas F, Bellisano G, et al. Synovial cysts of the lumbar spine–pathological considerations and surgical strategy. Neurol Med Chir (Tokyo). 2013; 53(2):95–102

[23] Khan AM, Synnot K, Cammisa FP, Girardi FP. Lumbar synovial cysts of the spine: an evaluation of surgical outcome. J Spinal Disord Tech. 2005; 18(2):127–131

[24] James A, Laufer I, Parikh K, Nagineni VV, Saleh TO, Härtl R. Lumbar juxtafacet cyst resection: the facet sparing contralateral minimally invasive surgical approach. J Spinal Disord Tech. 2012; 25(2):E13–E17

[25] Müslüman AM, Cansever T, Yılmaz A, Çavuşoğlu H, Yüce İ, Aydın Y. Midterm outcome after a microsurgical unilateral approach for bilateral decompression of lumbar degenerative spondylolisthesis. J Neurosurg Spine. 2012; 16(1):68–76

[26] Palmer S, Turner R, Palmer R. Bilateral decompressive surgery in lumbar spinal stenosis associated with spondylolisthesis: unilateral approach and use of a microscope and tubular retractor system. Neurosurg Focus. 2002; 13 (1):E4

[27] Pao JL, Chen WC, Chen PQ. Clinical outcomes of microendoscopic decompressive laminotomy for degenerative lumbar spinal stenosis. Eur Spine J. 2009; 18(5):672–678

[28] Landi A, Marotta N, Tarantino R, et al. Microsurgical excision without fusion as a safe option for resection of synovial cyst of the lumbar spine: long-term follow-up in mono-institutional experience. Neurosurg Rev. 2012; 35(2):245–253, discussion 253

[29] Arts MP, Brand R, van den Akker ME, et al. Tubular diskectomy vs conventional microdiskectomy for the treatment of lumbar disk herniation: 2-year results of a double-blind randomized controlled trial. Neurosurgery. 2011; 69(1):135–144, discussion 144

[30] Foley KT, Smith MM. Microendoscopic discectomy. Tech Neurosurg. 1997; 3: 301–307

[31] Sandhu FA, Santiago P, Fessler RG, Palmer S. Minimally invasive surgical treatment of lumbar synovial cysts. Neurosurgery. 2004; 54(1):107–111, discussion 111–112

[32] Rhee J, Anaizi AN, Sandhu FA, Voyadzis JM. Minimally invasive resection of lumbar synovial cysts from a contralateral approach. J Neurosurg Spine. 2012; 17(5):453–458

[33] Sehati N, Khoo LT, Holly LT. Treatment of lumbar synovial cysts using minimally invasive surgical techniques. Neurosurg Focus. 2006; 20(3):E2

[34] Baisden J, Easa J, Fernand R, et al. North American Spine Society Evidence-Based Clinical Guidelines for Multidisciplinary Spine Care. Burr Ridge, IL: North American Spine Society; 2008

[35] Bydon A, Xu R, Parker SL, et al. Recurrent back and leg pain and cyst reformation after surgical resection of spinal synovial cysts: systematic review of reported postoperative outcomes. Spine J. 2010; 10(9):820–826

[36] Lyons MK, Atkinson JL, Wharen RE, Deen HG, Zimmerman RS, Lemens SM. Surgical evaluation and management of lumbar synovial cysts: the Mayo Clinic experience. J Neurosurg. 2000; 93(1) Suppl:53–57

[37] Epstein NE. Lumbar laminectomy for the resection of synovial cysts and coexisting lumbar spinal stenosis or degenerative spondylolisthesis: an outcome study. Spine. 2004; 29(9):1049–1055, discussion 1056

[38] Banning CS, Thorell WE, Leibrock LG. Patient outcome after resection of lumbar juxtafacet cysts. Spine. 2001; 26(8):969–972

[39] Boviatsis EJ, Stavrinou LC, Kouyialis AT, et al. Spinal synovial cysts: pathogenesis, diagnosis and surgical treatment in a series of seven cases and literature review. Eur Spine J. 2008; 17(6):831–837

[40] Deinsberger R, Kinn E, Ungersböck K. Microsurgical treatment of juxta facet cysts of the lumbar spine. J Spinal Disord Tech. 2006; 19(3):155–160

[41] Hsu KY, Zucherman JF, Shea WJ, Jeffrey RA. Lumbar intraspinal synovial and ganglion cysts (facet cysts). Ten-year experience in evaluation and treatment. Spine. 1995; 20(1):80–89

4 Transforaminal Lumbar Interbody Fusion: Minimally Invasive versus Open

MIS: Rory J. Petteys, Anthony Conte, and Faheem A. Sandhu
Open: Jason C. Eck

4.1 Introduction

Lumbar interbody fusion was first described by Cloward[1,2] in 1952 via a posterior approach (posterior lumbar interbody fusion [PLIF]), which proved effective in achieving interbody fusion, but required significant nerve root and thecal sac retraction.[3] Subsequently, Harms and Rolinger described a less invasive approach in 1982 via transforaminal route (transforaminal lumbar interbody fusion [TLIF]).[4] This approach provides a more lateral point of access to the disc space, thus limiting retraction of the neural elements. While clinical outcomes have been favorable with both of these approaches, the amount of muscle dissection and retraction required to expose the spine was thought to adversely affect patient recovery.[5,6,7,8,9,10,11] As an alternative to these standard open techniques and with technological advancements in illumination, retractors, and magnification, Foley et al introduced the minimally invasive TLIF (MIS TLIF) in an attempt to reduce muscle damage associated with the subperiosteal exposure.[12,13] MIS TLIF has subsequently become a commonly used and effective technique for achieving lumbar interbody fusion.

4.2 Indications of Transforaminal Lumbar Interbody Fusion

Lumbar arthrodesis is generally employed in the treatment of degenerative diseases of the spine including facet arthropathy, spondylolisthesis, degenerative disc disease, and mechanical instability. While lumbar arthrodesis has been shown to be beneficial in degenerative conditions, the benefits of posterolateral versus interbody fusion are less clear. Many advocate interbody fusion because it permits deformity reduction, indirect decompression, foraminal distraction, and placement of the graft under compression, and is associated with a higher fusion rate among other benefits.[12,13,14,15,16,17,18] Therefore, interbody fusion via TLIF or PLIF is indicated when patients present with grade I or II spondylolisthesis with instability and/or foraminal stenosis with radiculopathy, severe degenerative disc disease with back pain, multiple recurrent disc herniation with back pain or radiculopathy, and postlaminectomy kyphosis.[19,20] Indications for MIS TLIF do not differ substantially from standard open TLIF, but advantages of MIS TLIF will be discussed below. Higher grades of spondylolisthesis can be treated via an MIS approach, but are associated with technical difficulties. Two-level TLIF is indicated in patients who present with the above conditions at consecutive spinal levels. Contraindications to TLIF include poor bone quality that would make graft subsidence likely, severe spondylolisthesis and scoliosis, and anatomic variations of the foraminal contents, such as conjoined nerve roots or the presence of a foraminal mass.

4.3 Advantages of Minimally Invasive Surgery

Minimally invasive or minimal access techniques offer several advantages over their traditional open counterparts. As mentioned above, the amount of muscle dissection and retraction necessary to expose the spine leads to significant muscle damage and atrophy.[5,6,7,8,10,11] MIS techniques do not require the same degree of muscle, fascia, and soft-tissue disruption. In addition, several authors report other advantages, including less intraoperative blood loss, less postoperative pain and narcotic use, earlier ambulation, and decreased length of hospital stay (▶ Table 4.1).[12,13,14,15,16,17,18] As the MIS TLIF procedure becomes more popularized and widespread, numerous studies comparing it to traditional open approaches have been published, most notably over the last several years.

4.4 Surgical Technique in Minimally Invasive Surgery

The patient is brought to the operating room where general endotracheal anesthesia is administered. A Foley catheter is inserted, pneumatic compression devices and neurophysiological monitoring leads placed, and an arterial line may be used if indicated. The patient is then positioned prone on a Jackson flat top table with chest roll(s) to maintain lumbar lordosis. Preoperative antibiotics are then administered. The fluoroscopic arm is then positioned such that the base of the device is on the side opposite the surgeon. The surgeon should stand on the side of the most significant pathology or symptoms.

Using anteroposterior fluoroscopy, the midline is marked on the skin and a parallel line is drawn 4 to 4.5 cm away on the side nearest the surgeon. Then, using lateral fluoroscopy, the correct levels are identified and marked. For two-level TLIF, the incision should span the intervening vertebral body from one disc space to the next along the paramedian line that was previously marked with the incision centered over the pedicle of the middle lumbar level. The patient is then draped after antiseptic is applied and the skin is infiltrated with local anesthetic. The level with the worst pathology or referable symptoms should be addressed first. A small puncture is made with a number 11 blade over the disc space and a Kirschner wire or Steinmann pin is inserted along a slight medial trajectory under fluoroscopic guidance. The goal is to "dock" the wire on the ipsilateral facet joint of the level in question. Once "docked" at the appropriate level, the incision is lengthened to accommodate a 25-mm tubular retractor. Serial dilators are then inserted followed by the tubular retractor, which is secured by a table-mounted arm. Final placement is then confirmed by fluoroscopy.

With the working channel in place, it is important to confirm placement under direct visualization. Ideally, the laminofacet

Table 4.1 Literature on MIS versus open TLIF and MIS TLIF alone

Authors (year)	Level	Study	Type	Patients	OR time	EBL (mL)	LOS	Fusion	Findings
Peng et al (2009)[23]	II	Prospective	MIS vs. open	29 MI 29 O	216 h 170 h	150 681	4 d 6.7 d	80% 86.7%	Pain scores similar, though increase morphine in open
Schizas et al (2009)[24]	II	Prospective	MIS vs. open	18 MI 18 O	5.8 h 5.2 h	456 961	6.1 d 8.2 d	15/18 18/18	Narcotic use same, VAS/ODI similar
Ghahreman et al (2010)[22]	II	Prospective	MIS vs. open	23 MI 24 O					Both had decreased leg/back pain; shorter LOS and earlier to mobilize in MIS
Shunwu et al (2010)[25]	II	Prospective	MIS vs. open	32 MI 30 O	159 h 142 h	400 517	9.3 d 12.5 d	100% both	VAS/ODI scores better in MIS
Wang et al (2010)[26]	II	Prospective	MIS vs. open	42 MI 43 O	156 h 145 h	264 673	10.6 d 14.6 d	41/42 42/43	VAS better in MIS, ODI same
Lee et al (2012)[21]	II	Prospective	MIS vs. open	72 MI 72 O	166 h 181 h	50 447	3.2 d 6.8 d	97% 98.5%	VAS/ODI similar, 10-fold less narcotic use in MIS
Isaacs et al (2005)[15]	III	Retrosective	MES vs. open	20 ME 24 O	5 h 4.6 h	226 1,147	3.4 d 5.1 d		Half post-op morphine use in MIS
Scheufler et al (2007)[33]	III	Retrospective	MIS vs. mini-open	43 MI 51 O	104 h 132 h	55 125			VAS decreased after POD #2
Bagan et al (2008)[60]	III	Retrospective	MIS vs. open	28 MI 19 O					Complications 18% MI 37% O
Dhall et al (2008)[34]	III	Retrospective	MIS vs. open	21 MI 21 O	223 h 215 h	194 505	3 d 5.5 d	20/21 100%	Pain scores similar
Wu et al (2010)[35]	III	Meta-analysis	MIS vs. open	312 MI 716 O	–	–	–	94.8% 90.9%	
Villavicencio et al (2010)[40]	III	Retrospective	MIS vs. open	76 MI 63 O	223 h 215 h	163 367	3 d 4.2 d	–	VAS/ODI similar, 10% neuro injury in MIS
Adogwa et al (2011)[61]	III	Retrospective	MIS vs. open	15 MI 15 O	–	–	3 d 5.5 d	–	Less narcotics in MIS, VAS/ODI similar
McGirt et al (2011)[36]	III	Retrospective	MIS vs. open	5,170	–	–	–	SSI less in MI (2)	Less infections in MIS
Beringer and Mobasser (2006)[65]	III	Prospective	MIS	8				100%	Pain better in MIS
Deutsch and Musacchio (2006)[62]	III	Prospective	MIS	20	4.1 h	100	2.5 d		Pain better in MIS
Jang and Lee (2005)[56]	III	Prospective	MIS	23	150 h	310		22/24	Pain better in MIS
Foley et al (2003)[12]	IV	Retrospective	MIS	39				–	38/39 good to excellent results
Kim et al (2012)[58]	IV	Retrospective	MIS	44				97.7% (6 mo)	VAS/ODI better in MIS
Lee et al (2008)[49]	IV	Retrospective	MIS elders	27	172 h	338		77.8%	VAS/ODI better in MIS
Park et al (2011)[66]	IV	Retrospective	MIS	66	–	–	–	51/66	Pain and narcotic use decreased
Park and Foley (2008)[67]	IV	Retrospective	MI	40				–	Pain improved in MIS, 76% reduction in spondylolisthesis
Rouben et al (2011)[63]	IV	Retrospective	MIS	169	183 h	–	15 d	96%	Pain improved, narcotic use decreased
Schwender et al (2005)[18]	IV	Retrospective	MIS	49	240 h	140	1.9 d	100%	Narcotics use decreased, VAS improved
Tsahtsalis and Wood (2012)[64]	IV	Prospective	MIS	34	173 h		4 d	97% (6 mo)	ODI decreased 27 points

Abbreviations: EBL, estimated blood loss; LOS, length of stay; MIS, minimally invasive surgery; ODI, Oswestry Disability Index; OR, operative; POD, postoperative day #; SSI, surgical site infection; VAS, visual analog scale.

junction should be in the lateral half of the working field and the lateral half of the lamina in the medial field. Electrocautery is then used to clear the field of remaining muscle and soft tissue until the facet and lamina are exposed. The sublaminar plane is defined with curettes and the ligamentum flavum elevated from the underside of the lamina. This will help ensure the ligamentum remains intact during bone removal, thus minimizing the risk of dural injury. A generous hemilaminotomy and facetectomy is then performed with curettes, rongeurs, and high-speed drill, and should extend from the rostral to the caudal pedicle. Bone fragments can be harvested to use later as autograft.

Once bone removal is completed, the remaining ligamentum flavum is removed with curettes and rongeurs. The disc space, traversing nerve root, and thecal sac are now in view and should be carefully identified before proceeding. The thecal sac is gently retracted medially and all epidural veins coagulated so as to further expose the disc space. The disc space is then incised and a thorough discectomy is performed with curettes and rongeurs. The end plates are then prepared with scrapers and rotating rasps to remove all cartilaginous and disc material. Dilators are then employed to distract the disc space, increasing overall disc space height in preparation for the interbody grafting material. The graft may consist of polyether-ether ketone (PEEK), autograft, cadaver allograft, titanium or carbon-fiber cages, or absorbable materials. Graft placement can also be supplemented with recombinant human bone morphogenetic protein.

Once the discectomy is completed, pedicle screws can then be placed under direct visualization. If a two-level TLIF is planned, the retractor is then removed and a Steinmann pin or Kirschner wire is advanced through the skin incision under fluoroscopic guidance toward the facet of the next level to be addressed. Typically, this will require more rostrocaudal angulation than is used for a single-level TLIF. Serial dilators are advanced and the retractor is "docked" at the laminofacet junction in the manner described above. The removal of bone and ligament and discectomy proceeds as described above. A second interbody graft is placed once the discectomy and end-plate preparation is completed. Pedicle screws are then placed at the remaining two levels under direct visualization and a rod is placed. The disc spaces can then be compressed prior to securing the rod. The lumbodorsal fascia and skin are then closed in layers. Percutaneous pedicle screw fixation is then performed on the contralateral side.

4.5 Surgical Technique in Open Surgery

The patient is brought to the operating room and undergoes general anesthesia with endotracheal intubation. The patient is then turned to the prone position on the Jackson table with standard precautions to avoid decubitus ulcers and minimized upper extremity neuropraxia. The patient should be positioned to maintain the normal lordotic lumbar spine curvature. Positioning should allow for intraoperative radiographic imaging to confirm spinal alignment and implant position.

A lateral fluoroscopic image can be obtained to verify the location of the operative levels. A midline posterior incision is made over the operative levels, and the erector spinous muscles subperiosteally elevated to expose the posterior elements of the spine bilaterally. The spinous processes, laminae, facet joints, pars interarticularis, and transverse processes are visible. Self-retaining retractors are placed to maintain exposure and should be released and repositioned at least each hour to maintain adequate soft-tissue perfusion. A lateral image can then be obtained to verify operative levels.

Exposure for the TLIF is achieved by removing the superior and inferior articulating processes of the facet joint and performing a hemilaminotomy and partial resection of the pars interarticularis. This provides a rectangular window through which you can visualize the underlying disc space, lateral edge of the dura, and the exiting nerve root.

The disc space can then be exposed by removing the overlying ligamentum flavum and fatty tissues. With careful nerve root protection, a 15-blade scalpel can then be used to incise the posterolateral annulus. The annulotomy should be large enough to pass the interbody implant after the disc space is final prepared. A lamina spreader can be utilized if needed for further distraction to facilitate passage of instruments into the disc space. A series of curettes and pituitary rongeurs can be used for removal of the disc material. The end plates can be prepared with a variety of curettes and shavers. Meticulous discectomy and end-plate preparation are essential for facilitating interbody fusion. Once the disc space is prepared, trial interbody spacers are placed to determine the optimal implant size. Implants are available in a wide variety of sizes, shapes, and materials based on surgeon preference. The implant should be selected to maximize the contact of the implant and the prepared end plates. Morselized bone graft is then placed into the periphery of the disc space, followed by placement of the implant. Any previously placed distraction should be removed, and the implant should be assessed for adequate tightness in the interbody space. Any remaining voids in the interbody space can be filled with additional morselized bone graft.

Pedicle screws are then placed bilaterally in the vertebrae above and below the disc to be fused. Placement of the pedicles screws can be performed through a variety of techniques including anatomic placement, fluoroscopically guided placement, or computer navigation–assisted placement. After placement of the pedicles screws, connecting rods are placed, set caps applied, and final tightened to the rods. Anteroposterior and lateral images should be obtained to verify proper placement of the interbody implant and pedicle screws. Decortication of the transverse processes and remaining lamina and placement of additional bone graft allow for a 360° fusion. A standard layered closure is then performed after achieving meticulous hemostasis.

4.6 Discussion of Minimally Invasive Surgery

Low back pain is a common complaint among adults in the United States, and many of these patients require surgical treatment. Lumbar fusion, via TLIF or other techniques, is utilized to treat a variety of conditions, including degenerative disc disease, facet arthropathy, spondylolisthesis, scoliosis, tumors, and fractures. The TLIF approach is a well-established method for achieving circumferential arthrodesis through a single posterior approach, and recent advancements have allowed the procedure to be performed with minimally invasive techniques. However, considerable questions remain as to whether MIS TLIF is superior to standard open TLIF or *vice versa*.

4.6.1 Level I Evidence in Minimally Invasive Surgery

There are no level I studies available.

4.6.2 Level II Evidence in Minimally Invasive Surgery

Several authors have performed prospective cohort studies comparing MIS and open TLIF, albeit in relatively small cohorts. The largest of these studies by Lee et al[21] compared 72 consecutive MIS and 72 consecutive open TLIF patients at a single institution. The authors demonstrated significantly lower blood loss, length of hospital stay, and postoperative narcotic use in patients undergoing MIS TLIF, while operative time and fusion rates were similar. Ghahreman et al,[22] Peng et al,[23] and Schizas et al[24] also demonstrated decreased blood loss and shorter hospital stay in MIS patients, also with similar clinical and radiographic outcomes compared with patients treated with standard open techniques. Ghahreman et al also reported earlier independent ambulation in patients who had MIS TLIF than in patients who had open fusion.[22] Shunwu et al[25] and Wang et al[26] both demonstrated modest improvements in short-term clinical outcomes, that is, visual analog scale (VAS) scores and Oswestry Disability Index (ODI) scores, in patients treated with MIS TLIF over open TLIF. Early experience appeared to show some modest benefits for MIS TLIF in the short term, but overall clinical outcome was essentially unchanged.

More recent studies point to equivalent, with even potential trends toward benefits in long-term clinical outcomes when compared to traditional open TLIF. In the only randomized, nonblinded, control study investigating MIS versus open TLIFs, Wang et al[27] showed less sacrospinalis muscle injury with significantly better 3- to 6-month ODI scores in patients undergoing MIS TLIF. Gu et al[28] compared 44 patients treated with two-level MIS TLIF versus 38 patients treated with an open two-level procedure, observing similar back and leg VAS scores and ODI scores at an average of 20-month follow-up. Parker et al[29] examined a cohort of 100 patients undergoing TLIF, half via a minimally invasive approach. Results at 2 years showed similar pain and quality-of-life scores, with shorter hospital stays and earlier return-to-work periods for patients in the MIS cohort. A prospective study by Rodríguez-Vela et al,[30] comparing 3- to 4-year postoperative results of MIS versus open TLIF patients, showed similar North American Spine Society (NASS) lumbar spine and VAS back pain scores, with a trend toward lower ODI scores in the MIS group. Wong et al[31] compared 4-year postoperative results in 144 patients undergoing MIS TLIF versus 54 patients undergoing open TLIF. Both groups showed similar fusion rates, with the MIS group exhibiting improvements in estimated blood loss (EBL), shorter operative times, and lower infection and complication rates. The MIS group showed a significant improvement in VAS back pain scores at the 4-year mark when compared to the open group, with a 15% better ODI score at that time. In a meta-analysis by Khan et al[32] comparing surgical outcomes for MIS versus open TLIF procedures, the authors found improvements in length of hospital stay, average blood loss, complication rates, and long-term VAS back scores (minimum > 1 year postoperatively).

4.6.3 Level III and IV Evidence in Minimally Invasive Surgery

To date, there has been no level I study comparing MIS and open TLIF, although a number of level III/IV retrospective studies have been performed. Several studies since the initial report by Foley et al have also demonstrated benefits of MIS TLIF over standard open techniques in head-to-head comparison.

Several retrospective cohort studies appear in the literature comparing MIS and standard open TLIF. Scheufler et al[33] compared percutaneous TLIF in 43 patients with mini-open TLIF in 51 patients. They demonstrated similar operative times and fusion rates, but statistically significant reductions in blood loss and postoperative pain in patients who had MIS TLIF procedures.[33] There were no differences in clinical outcomes at 8 and 16 months as measured by standard questionnaires.

In a study of mini-open TLIF versus open TLIF with 21 patients in each group, Dhall et al[34] also showed significantly less blood loss and hospital stay in mini-open patients, while fusion rates and overall clinical outcomes were similar. However, there were two cases of neurologic injury and two cases of instrumentation malpositioning requiring revision in the mini-open group. Isaacs et al[15] performed a comparative analysis of 20 patients treated with endoscopically assisted MIS TLIF and 24 with standard open techniques. The authors demonstrated significant reductions in operative blood loss (226 vs. 1,147 mL), postoperative blood transfusion, length of hospital stay (3.4 vs. 5.1 days), and postoperative analgesia use in patients treated with MIS TLIF; clinical and radiographic outcomes were similar. In a 2010 meta-analysis, Wu et al[35] reviewed fusion rates of MIS versus open TLIF patients and found comparable results (MIS: 94.8%; open: 90.9%). Furthermore, a multicenter retrospective study by McGirt et al[36] of 5,170 patients treated with either MIS or open TLIF showed that surgical site infections were less common in patients treated with MIS techniques, especially for multilevel procedures. A recent review by Habib et al,[37] which included seven articles directly comparing MIS and open TLIF, found operative time to be 220 minutes for MIS TLIF and 218 minutes for open TLIF. Furthermore, blood loss was found to be 282 and 693 mL, and hospital stay 5.6 and 8.1 days, for MIS TLIF and open TLIF, respectively.

Several retrospective cohort studies have displayed the improvement in pain reduction and functional status in the short-term postoperative period for patients undergoing MIS TLIF. Cheng et al[38] showed significant decreases in operative length and EBL in MIS TLIF patients, with improvements in immediate postoperative mobility when compared with patients undergoing open TLIF. MIS TLIF patients used only one-third of the daily around-the-clock pain medication postoperatively when compared with patients in the open cohort, indicating a lower overall baseline pain level.

Seng et al[39] compared 5-year clinical outcomes between 40 patients undergoing MIS TLIF versus 40 patients undergoing open surgery. The authors found similar fusion rates between the two groups, with lower operative blood loss and shorter hospitalizations in the MIS group. Patients in the MIS cohort used less morphine postoperatively; however, self-reported pain scores and functional status was similar for both groups between 6 months and 5 years postoperatively.

4.7 Complications in Minimally Invasive Surgery

While many studies have demonstrated the benefit of MIS TLIF relative to open TLIF, both approaches are associated with potential complications (▶ Table 4.2). Complications common to both procedures include interbody graft malpositioning, graft subsidence, pedicle screw malposition, and infection.[40] Other less frequent complications found in both procedures include hematoma, anemia, and cerebrospinal fluid leak.[40] Several studies have reported higher rates of infectious complications including surgical site infections and urinary tract infection in open TLIF than in MIS TLIF.[37] In addition, the need for blood transfusion is higher in open TLIF.[37] There are level III data showing decreased infection rate and need for blood transfusion in MIS TLIF.

Although infectious and bleeding complications are less frequent with MIS TLIF, hardware-related complications were more common than in open TLIF.[37] These included screw malpositioning, cage misplacement or dislodgement, and cage subsidence. Many authors attribute these complications to the learning curve associated with MIS techniques and the relative inexperience of many surgeons with MIS compared to open techniques.[24] The limited visualization provided by tubular and independent blade retractors combined with the reliance on two-dimensional radiographic images to place instrumentation makes MIS techniques a unique skill set that are not easily acquired. In addition to instrumentation-related complications, neurological complications were also more common in MIS TLIF.[37] This may also be related to technical limitations of visualization and exposure that can limit decompression and increase likelihood of nerve root injury. However, a previously aforementioned systemic review by Khan et al[32] showed a lower complication rate in patients undergoing MIS TLIF. The authors attributed these findings to a trend in recently published studies with lower complication rates in MIS patients, implying progression of spine surgeons along the learning curve for this challenging procedure.

Several authors have commented on the amount of radiation exposure associated with MIS techniques. Studies that reported fluoroscopy time for MIS versus open techniques found that radiation exposure was greater in MIS TLIF.[23,24,26] This presents a possible concern for the well-being not only of the patient, but also of the surgeon and the operating room personnel. However, the long-term effects of this increased radiation exposure are not yet known. Recent technological advances in intraoperative image guidance systems via multidimensional fluoroscopy or computed tomography (CT) may help reduce this radiation exposure and are a promising development. Furthermore, increased surgeon experience with MIS techniques may decrease the fluoroscopy time, although this was not reflected in one study that examined this variable.[24]

Minimally invasive techniques (including MIS TLIF) may be particularly advantageous in obese patients. These patients are particularly prone to wound and surgical site complications in open lumbar surgery because of the larger incision required and larger cavity created to expose the deep spine.[41,42,43,44] By using a tubular retractor, the spine may be accessed through the same-size incision in an obese patient as in a nonobese patient. Obese patients do present some challenges, including poor fluoroscopic visualization of anatomical landmarks and limitations of the length of tubular retractors. However, obese patients have been evidenced to show numerous benefits afforded by MIS—decreased blood loss and narcotic use—and one study found that BMI (body mass index) had no significant relationship with self-reported outcome measures, operative time, hospital stay, and complications.[45] In a prospective study directly comparing MIS versus open TLIF in overweight and obese patients, Wang et al[46] showed similar fusion rates and pain scores at 1 to 2 years after surgery, with the MIS cohort experiencing shorter operative times, less blood loss, lower immediate postoperative VAS scores, and a significant decrease in operative complications and postoperative infections. Terman et al[47] and Adogwa et al[48] reviewed obese or morbidly obese patients undergoing MIS or open TLIF, ultimately arriving at similar results with regard to postoperative pain relief and functional disability.

Elderly patients may also benefit from MIS procedures, especially with the possibility of less blood loss. Lee et al[49] found a low complication rate in a retrospective review of 27 consecutive patients older than 65 years treated with MIS TLIF. Fusion rates were 80% at 3 years, comparable with studies of open fusion in elderly patients. These are level III data that MIS procedures provide some advantage over open techniques in the obese and elderly population.

MIS TLIF is relatively contraindicated in some situations, including lumbar arthrodesis of greater than two levels, severe osteoporosis, high-grade spondylolisthesis, some fractures, and severe scoliosis where localization under fluoroscopy can be difficult due to anatomical irregularities. In addition, very thin patients with little subcutaneous fat may not benefit from MIS procedures because the amount of muscle dissection required may actually be greater than standard open subperiosteal exposure. However, in most cases, MIS TLIF is an option for achieving lumbar fusion.

Table 4.2 Breakdown of complications by TLIF approach

Complications	MI (%)	Open (%)
Infection	6.9	23.5
UTI	3.4	11.8
Neurologic deficits	20.7	11.8
Screw/cage complications	44.8	11.8
CSF leak	10.3	5.9
Blood transfusion/coagulation	3.4	11.8
Other	10.5	23.4

Abbreviations: CSF, cerebrospinal fluid; MI, minimally invasive; TLIF, transforaminal lumbar interbody fusion; UTI, urinary tract infection.

4.8 Conclusion of Minimally Invasive Surgery

While there is a steep learning curve associated with MIS techniques, these techniques may be beneficial for patients and improve clinical outcomes. Although no level I randomized comparisons exist, multiple level II studies have demonstrated comparable clinical outcomes and fusion rates while also demonstrating benefits including decreased blood loss, decreased postoperative pain and narcotic use, and shorter hospital stays. The decreased postoperative pain could lead to earlier ambulation, return to function, and return to work, which may reduce direct (hospital) and indirect (lost work days) costs. In addition, a decrease in total operative and anesthesia time with MIS TLIF approach may lead to total decreased hospital costs when compared to open TLIF.[50] Level II data suggest a slightly higher complication rate with MIS TLIF, but there are level III data showing decreased infection rates and need for blood transfusion among the MIS group. Using the grading scale of Guyatt et al, we suggest a Grade 1C recommendation that MIS TLIF and open TLIF are generally equivalent in terms of clinical outcomes, fusion results, and cost-effectiveness.[21] Also, we suggest a Grade 2A recommendation that the MIS TLIF decreases the risk of postoperative infection and need for blood transfusions.

4.9 Discussion of Open Surgery

The purported advantages of these minimally invasive techniques include decreased blood loss, decreased muscle damage from dissection, shorter hospital stay, and faster return to activities. However, as with all new technology, the surgeon must carefully examine the published results to determine the actual risks and benefits of using these new techniques.

4.9.1 Level I Evidence in Open Surgery

There are no level I studies available.

4.9.2 Level II Evidence in Open Surgery

A frequent criticism of utilizing a new technique is the associated learning curve. During this period of time, the surgeon might experience longer operative times and more complications than with the traditional technique. In some cases, after the surgeon becomes more proficient with the new technique, these differences begin to normalize. There are several studies that have reported on the effects of the learning curve associated with MIS TLIF. Lee et al reported on a prospective consecutive case series of patients undergoing MIS TLIF.[51] In this study, it was determined that surgeons reached the end of their learning curve with this procedure after 30 cases, which was longer than the surgeons believed they had achieved technical proficiency. When comparing patient data of the initial 30 patients with those performed after the learning curve, there were statistically significant improvements in terms of operative time, EBL, and time to ambulation. This study provides level II evidence that a learning curve is achieved after 30 cases of MIS TLIF, and initial cases have worse operative times, blood loss, and time to ambulation. This curve, although expected with any new technical procedure, poses an ethical challenge for the novice embarking on a technique that is destined to commit the initial 30 patients to a suboptimal outcome. This dilemma must be addressed through other means of learning that can mitigate such a reality.

In addition, not all studies have reported improved results with MIS TLIF techniques. Peng et al[23] reported on a prospective comparison between MIS TLIF versus open TLIF and found no statistically significant difference in outcomes based on ODI, NASS, and VAS at either 6 months or 2 years postoperatively. However, there was a statistically higher fluoroscopy time for the minimally invasive group (105.5 seconds) as compared to the open group (35.2 seconds) ($p < 0.05$). In a randomized control trial of 41 patients undergoing MIS TLIF versus 38 patients undergoing the open procedure, Wong et al[31] did not find any difference in VAS scores between groups at 3, 6, 12, and 24 months after surgery. A similar prospective cohort study by Gu et al[28] showed no difference in back or leg VAS scores or ODI scores at a mean follow-up of 20 months, with a significantly longer amount of fluoroscopy time for patients undergoing MIS TLIF. In a study by Adogwa et al,[52] comparison of creatinine phosphokinase levels in patients undergoing MIS versus open TLIF showed a higher level of muscle trauma in the MIS group, without any difference between the groups at 2 years with regard to pain scores, functional disability, or SF-36 patient satisfaction scores. These studies provided level II evidence that there was no difference in clinical outcomes between the two groups, and there was significantly higher radiation exposure in the minimally invasive group.

One method to determine the utility of a given surgical procedure is to calculate the cost-effectiveness. Adogwa et al performed a cost-effectiveness analysis of open TLIF for the treatment of grade I degenerative spondylolisthesis.[53] They reported on statistically significant improvements in back pain VAS score, leg pain VAS score, and ODI at 2 years postoperatively with the TLIF procedure. In addition, they found that TLIF had a mean 2-year cost per quality-adjusted life year (QALY) gain of $42,845, which is within the accepted limit of $50,000. This study provides level II evidence that the traditional open TLIF procedure is cost-effective for the treatment of degenerative spondylolisthesis.

In another cost-effectiveness study from the same institution, Parker et al compared the cost-effectiveness of the MIS TLIF versus the traditional open TLIF.[29] While there were some benefits of the minimally invasive approach, there was no statistical significance between the two approaches in terms of cost-effectiveness. This study again provides level II evidence that there is no difference in cost-effectiveness between the two techniques.

4.9.3 Level III Evidence in Open Surgery

In a recent review article, Habib et al reported that, based on a comprehensive review of the literature, high-class data comparing the two groups are lacking, and the current evidence supports the use of the MIS TLIF as having comparable results to the traditional open technique.[37] In a retrospective review, Sulaiman and Singh[54] did not find any significant differences in postoperative VAS scores in MIS versus open TLIF patients at 6 weeks, 6 months, or 1 year. Cheng et al,[38] in their retrospective review of 50 patients undergoing MIS TLIF versus 25 patients undergoing open surgery, found no difference in VAS scores or change in VAS score from preoperative score at 3- to 6-year follow-up. These results were similar to a review by Zairi et al,[55] where a comparison between 40 patients undergoing MIS TLIF and 60 patients undergoing open TLIF did not yield any difference in 2-year postoperative VAS scores, ODI scores, or fusion rates. These studies provide level III evidence that the two techniques produce equivalent long-term clinical outcomes.

The other common method utilized to compare the outcomes of different surgical techniques that have numerous previously published studies is a meta-analysis of the literature. Wu et al performed a meta-analysis comparing MIS TLIF with the traditional open technique and reported no statistically significant differences between the two techniques in terms of fusion rates or complications.[35] This study again provides level III evidence that there is no difference between the two techniques in terms of fusion rates or complications.

4.10 Complications in Open Surgery

One of the most commonly reported benefits of the minimally invasive approach is the limited need for muscle dissection and subsequent muscle damage. Previous studies have documented that there are MRI changes in the cross-sectional area of the erector spinae muscles following open lumbar fusion.[4,19] However, other studies have suggested that this change is temporary, and there are no significant differences in muscle atrophy at 1 year following surgery.[15] In addition, the use of either a posterior spinous process–splitting approach or a far lateral Wiltse approach is an alternative method for performing a TLIF through an open approach but without the high learning curve and radiation exposure associated with the minimally invasive techniques.[7,8,56]

One of the most significant criticisms of the MIS TLIF approach is the reliance on intraoperative imaging and the associated radiation exposure to the patient and operating room staff. In a prospective study, Bindal et al investigated the radiation dose to the surgeon and the patient during a series of 24 consecutive MIS TLIF procedures using fluoroscopic guidance.[57] The mean fluoroscopy time per case was 1.69 minutes (range, 0.82–3.73 minutes). The highest radiation exposure to the surgeon was localized to the dominant hand with a mean of 76 mRem, with 27 mRem at the waist. The mean exposure to the patient's skin was 59.5 mGy (range, 8.3–252 mGy) in the posteroanterior plane and 78.8 mGy (range, 6.3–29.5 mGy) in the lateral plane. The maximum allowed annual radiation exposure is 5 Rem to the body.[58]

More recent advances have combined intraoperative CT with navigation systems for the placement of percutaneous pedicle screws. This eliminates the need for fluoroscopic imaging during placement of percutaneous pedicle screws and decreases the associated radiation exposure to the surgical team. However, even if the operative team is able to leave the room or remain behind a shield during the intraoperative CT scan, there is still a large amount of radiation imparted to the patient. Lange et al investigated the radiation dose imparted to patients through an intraoperative cone-beam CT scan used with a navigation system to insert percutaneous pedicle screws.[59]

They reported that the mean effective dose of radiation imparted during a single scan for a "small patient" setting was 3.24 mSv (range, 2.37–4.12 mSv), and for a "large patient" setting it was 8.09 mSv (range, 5.91–10.27 mSv). In each case, the scan has to be performed twice, once for the initial registration and another after placement of instrumentation. These values remain within the previously reported values associated with an abdominal CT scan, which range from 1 to 31 mSv.

While there are various studies that have reported on improved benefits of MIS TLIF over the traditional open technique, this new technique is not without risk or the potential for complications. Villavicencio et al retrospectively investigated the safety and efficacy of MIS TLIF versus open TLIF with a 37.5-month follow-up.[40] While there were improvements in blood loss and duration of stay, they came at the cost of significantly higher rates of neurologic injury in the minimally invasive group (10.2%) versus the open group (1.6%) ($p = 0.02$). This study provides level III evidence of higher rates of neurologic injury related to the minimally invasive approach as compared to the open TLIF.

4.11 Conclusion of Open Surgery

Based on the review of the literature presented above, there are multiple level II studies reporting no significant difference in clinical outcomes between the MIS TLIF and open TLIF techniques. There is level II evidence supporting a higher risk of radiation exposure in the minimally invasive technique compared to the open TLIF. There is level II evidence that both open TLIF and MIS TLIF are cost-effective, but there is no difference in cost-effectiveness between the two techniques. There is level II evidence that operative time, blood loss, and time to ambulation are worse in the learning curve compared to MIS TLIF cases performed by more experienced surgeons. There is conflicting level III evidence regarding the risk of neurologic injury when comparing the two techniques. Based on the grading scale of Guyatt et al, these data provide a Grade 1C recommendation that traditional open and MIS TLIF are equivalent in terms of clinical outcomes, fusion results, and cost-effectiveness.[34] They also provide a Grade 2B recommendation that the MIS TLIF carries a higher risk of radiation exposure than the traditional open technique.

4.12 Editors' Commentary
4.12.1 Minimally Invasive Surgery

TLIF was among the earliest operations converted to MIS technique, and has become one of the most frequently performed MIS procedures in spine surgery. The reasons for this are multiple. First, the advantages of MIS are evident in this procedure. Incision is smaller, muscle destruction is minimized, pain is decreased, hospitalization is decreased, rehabilitation is faster, blood loss is decreased, and infection is decreased. Perhaps, most important to its widespread adoption is the fact that, because the "tube" utilized for the procedure is larger, the learning curve is much easier for most surgeons. Thus, it is an improved procedure that requires minimal investment to adopt and become proficient. Long-term results appear equivalent to open TLIF, but the short-term benefits listed above are significant. Although this advantage is often disregarded in outcome studies, one might consider this advantage in the context of this analogy. Imagine that you are standing at a point "A" and that you are starving. You need to get to point "B," which is where lunch is located and happens to be 20 feet away. You are given the option of two pathways. One is to walk directly to point B and have lunch. The other is to walk a 2.5-mile circuit uphill to arrive at point B, and then have lunch. Which are you going to choose? The point is, even though the end result may be the same, the "price" you pay to get there is important!

4.12.2 Open Surgery

When considering adoption of a new surgical technique, it is incumbent on surgeons to carefully weigh whether the new technique accomplishes the same surgical goals and additionally provides other advantages to motivate a change in practice. Although proponents of MIS TLIF may point eagerly to slight decreases in length of stay and postoperative narcotic use and clinically insignificant reductions in blood loss, the reality is that such arguments for the use of MIS TLIF are trivial compared to the increased rate of neurologic injury and malpositioned instrumentation. A higher risk of an iatrogenic postoperative neurologic deficit is not worth an extra day recovering at home or a small reduction in the need for blood transfusion, to either the patient or the surgeon. Similarly, short advantages in length of stay are quickly eliminated by a single return to the operation room to address malpositioned or migrated instrumentation.

More than most other MIS procedures, the MIS TLIF is a complicated surgery with a steep learning curve. Surgical steps such as disc preparation, facetectomy, and cage placement are difficult to perform through a tubular retractor and may be poorly performed by inexperienced surgeons. The fact that many important outcomes (fusion rate, validated clinical outcome measures, cost-effectiveness) are equivalent between open and MIS TLIF patients in most series suggests that patients treated early in the learning curve will have inferior results. Results from patients treated with MIS TLIF must be better than those from patients treated using open techniques to justify the increased risk of neurological injury and radiation exposure and to compensate for the cohort of patients treated during the learning curve who are only rarely described in the literature.

References

[1] Cloward RB. The treatment of ruptured lumbar intervertebral disc by vertebral body fusion. III. Method of use of banked bone. Ann Surg. 1952; 136 (6):987–992

[2] Cloward RB. The treatment of ruptured lumbar intervertebral discs by vertebral body fusion. I. Indications, operative technique, after care. J Neurosurg. 1953; 10(2):154–168

[3] Ray CD. Threaded titanium cages for lumbar interbody fusions. Spine. 1997; 22(6):667–679, discussion 679–680

[4] Harms J, Rolinger H. A one-stager procedure in operative treatment of spondylolistheses: dorsal traction-reposition and anterior fusion (author's transl) [in German]. Z Orthop Ihre Grenzgeb. 1982; 120(3):343–347

[5] Datta G, Gnanalingham KK, Peterson D, et al. Back pain and disability after lumbar laminectomy: is there a relationship to muscle retraction? Neurosurgery. 2004; 54(6):1413–1420, discussion 1420

[6] Gejo R, Matsui H, Kawaguchi Y, Ishihara H, Tsuji H. Serial changes in trunk muscle performance after posterior lumbar surgery. Spine. 1999; 24(10): 1023–1028

[7] Kawaguchi Y, Matsui H, Tsuji H. Back muscle injury after posterior lumbar spine surgery. Part 1: Histologic and histochemical analyses in rats. Spine. 1994; 19(22):2590–2597

[8] Kawaguchi Y, Matsui H, Tsuji H. Back muscle injury after posterior lumbar spine surgery. Part 2: Histologic and histochemical analyses in humans. Spine. 1994; 19(22):2598–2602

[9] Mayer TG, Vanharanta H, Gatchel RJ, et al. Comparison of CT scan muscle measurements and isokinetic trunk strength in postoperative patients. Spine. 1989; 14(1):33–36

[10] Sihvonen T, Herno A, Paljärvi L, Airaksinen O, Partanen J, Tapaninaho A. Local denervation atrophy of paraspinal muscles in postoperative failed back syndrome. Spine. 1993; 18(5):575–581

[11] Styf JR, Willén J. The effects of external compression by three different retractors on pressure in the erector spine muscles during and after posterior lumbar spine surgery in humans. Spine. 1998; 23(3):354–358

[12] Foley KT, Holly LT, Schwender JD. Minimally invasive lumbar fusion. Spine. 2003; 28(15) Suppl:S26–S35

[13] Foley KT, Lefkowitz MA. Advances in minimally invasive spine surgery. Clin Neurosurg. 2002; 49:499–517

[14] German JW, Foley KT. Minimal access surgical techniques in the management of the painful lumbar motion segment. Spine. 2005; 30(16) Suppl:S52–S59

[15] Isaacs RE, Podichetty VK, Santiago P, et al. Minimally invasive microendoscopy-assisted transforaminal lumbar interbody fusion with instrumentation. J Neurosurg Spine. 2005; 3(2):98–105

[16] Khoo LT, Palmer S, Laich DT, Fessler RG. Minimally invasive percutaneous posterior lumbar interbody fusion. Neurosurgery. 2002; 51(5) Suppl:S166–S181

[17] Kim KT, Lee SH, Suk KS, Bae SC. The quantitative analysis of tissue injury markers after mini-open lumbar fusion. Spine. 2006; 31(6):712–716

[18] Schwender JD, Holly LT, Rouben DP, Foley KT. Minimally invasive transforaminal lumbar interbody fusion (TLIF): technical feasibility and initial results. J Spinal Disord Tech. 2005; 18 Suppl:S1–S6

[19] Holly LT, Schwender JD, Rouben DP, Foley KT. Minimally invasive transforaminal lumbar interbody fusion: indications, technique, and complications. Neurosurg Focus. 2006; 20(3):E6

[20] Selznick LA, Shamji MF, Isaacs RE. Minimally invasive interbody fusion for revision lumbar surgery: technical feasibility and safety. J Spinal Disord Tech. 2009; 22(3):207–213

[21] Lee KH, Yue WM, Yeo W, Soeharno H, Tan SB. Clinical and radiological outcomes of open versus minimally invasive transforaminal lumbar interbody fusion. Eur Spine J. 2012; 21(11):2265–2270

[22] Ghahreman A, Ferch RD, Rao PJ, Bogduk N. Minimal access versus open posterior lumbar interbody fusion in the treatment of spondylolisthesis. Neurosurgery. 2010; 66(2):296–304, discussion 304

[23] Peng CW, Yue WM, Poh SY, Yeo W, Tan SB. Clinical and radiological outcomes of minimally invasive versus open transforaminal lumbar interbody fusion. Spine. 2009; 34(13):1385–1389

[24] Schizas C, Tzinieris N, Tsiridis E, Kosmopoulos V. Minimally invasive versus open transforaminal lumbar interbody fusion: evaluating initial experience. Int Orthop. 2009; 33(6):1683–1688

[25] Shunwu F, Xing Z, Fengdong Z, Xiangqian F. Minimally invasive transforaminal lumbar interbody fusion for the treatment of degenerative lumbar diseases. Spine. 2010; 35(17):1615–1620

[26] Wang J, Zhou Y, Zhang ZF, Li CQ, Zheng WJ, Liu J. Comparison of one-level minimally invasive and open transforaminal lumbar interbody fusion in degenerative and isthmic spondylolisthesis grades 1 and 2. Eur Spine J. 2010; 19(10):1780–1784

[27] Wang HL, Lü FZ, Jiang JY, Ma X, Xia XL, Wang LX. Minimally invasive lumbar interbody fusion via MAST Quadrant retractor versus open surgery: a prospective randomized clinical trial. Chin Med J (Engl). 2011; 124(23): 3868–3874

[28] Gu G, Zhang H, Fan G, et al. Comparison of minimally invasive versus open transforaminal lumbar interbody fusion in two-level degenerative lumbar disease. Int Orthop. 2014; 38(4):817–824

[29] Parker SL, Mendenhall SK, Shau DN, et al. Minimally invasive versus open transforaminal lumbar interbody fusion for degenerative spondylolisthesis: comparative effectiveness and cost-utility analysis. World Neurosurg. 2014; 82(1-2):230238

[30] Rodríguez-Vela J, Lobo-Escolar A, Joven E, Muñoz-Marín J, Herrera A, Velilla J. Clinical outcomes of minimally invasive versus open approach for one-level transforaminal lumbar interbody fusion at the 3- to 4-year follow-up. Eur Spine J. 2013; 22(12):2857–2863

[31] Wong AP, Smith ZA, Stadler JA, III, et al. Minimally invasive transforaminal lumbar interbody fusion (MI-TLIF): surgical technique, long-term 4-year

prospective outcomes, and complications compared with an open TLIF cohort. Neurosurg Clin N Am 2014;25(2):279304

[32] Khan NR, Clark AJ, Lee SL, Venable GT, Rossi NB, Foley KT. Surgical outcomes for minimally invasive vs open transforaminal lumbar interbody fusion: an updated systematic review and meta-analysis. Neurosurgery 2015;77(6):847874, discussion 874

[33] Scheufler KM, Dohmen H, Vougioukas VI. Percutaneous transforaminal lumbar interbody fusion for the treatment of degenerative lumbar instability. Neurosurgery. 2007; 60(4) Suppl 2:203–212, discussion 212–213

[34] Dhall SS, Wang MY, Mummaneni PV. Clinical and radiographic comparison of mini-open transforaminal lumbar interbody fusion with open transforaminal lumbar interbody fusion in 42 patients with long-term follow-up. J Neurosurg Spine. 2008; 9(6):560–565

[35] Wu RH, Fraser JF, Härtl R. Minimal access versus open transforaminal lumbar interbody fusion: meta-analysis of fusion rates. Spine. 2010; 35(26):2273–2281

[36] McGirt MJ, Parker SL, Lerner J, Engelhart L, Knight T, Wang MY. Comparative analysis of perioperative surgical site infection after minimally invasive versus open posterior/transforaminal lumbar interbody fusion: analysis of hospital billing and discharge data from 5170 patients. J Neurosurg Spine. 2011; 14(6):771–778

[37] Habib A, Smith ZA, Lawton CD, Fessler RG. Minimally invasive transforaminal lumbar interbody fusion: a perspective on current evidence and clinical knowledge. Minim Invasive Surg. 2012; 2012:657342

[38] Cheng JS, Park P, Le H, Reisner L, Chou D, Mummaneni PV. Short-term and long-term outcomes of minimally invasive and open transforaminal lumbar interbody fusions: is there a difference? Neurosurg Focus. 2013; 35(2):E6

[39] Seng C, Siddiqui MA, Wong KP, et al. Five-year outcomes of minimally invasive versus open transforaminal lumbar interbody fusion: a matched-pair comparison study. Spine. 2013; 38(23):2049–2055

[40] Villavicencio AT, Burneikiene S, Roeca CM, Nelson EL, Mason A. Minimally invasive versus open transforaminal lumbar interbody fusion. Surg Neurol Int. 2010; 1:12

[41] Olsen MA, Mayfield J, Lauryssen C, et al. Risk factors for surgical site infection in spinal surgery. J Neurosurg. 2003; 98(2) Suppl:149–155

[42] Patel N, Bagan B, Vadera S, et al. Obesity and spine surgery: relation to perioperative complications. J Neurosurg Spine. 2007; 6(4):291–297

[43] Telfeian AE, Reiter GT, Durham SR, Marcotte P. Spine surgery in morbidly obese patients. J Neurosurg. 2002; 97(1) Suppl:20–24

[44] Wimmer C, Gluch H, Franzreb M, Ogon M. Predisposing factors for infection in spine surgery: a survey of 850 spinal procedures. J Spinal Disord. 1998; 11(2):124–128

[45] Rosen DS, Ferguson SD, Ogden AT, Huo D, Fessler RG. Obesity and self-reported outcome after minimally invasive lumbar spinal fusion surgery. Neurosurgery. 2008; 63(5):956–960, discussion 960

[46] Wang J, Zhou Y, Feng Zhang Z, Qing Li C, Jie Zheng W, Liu J. Comparison of the clinical outcome in overweight or obese patients after minimally invasive versus open transforaminal lumbar interbody fusion. J Spinal Disord Tech. 2014; 27(4):202–206

[47] Terman SW, Yee TJ, Lau D, Khan AA, La Marca F, Park P. Minimally invasive versus open transforaminal lumbar interbody fusion: comparison of clinical outcomes among obese patients. J Neurosurg Spine. 2014; 20(6):644–652

[48] Adogwa O, Carr K, Thompson P, et al. A prospective, multi-institutional comparative effectiveness study of lumbar spine surgery in morbidly obese patients: does minimally invasive transforaminal lumbar interbody fusion result in superior outcomes? World Neurosurg. 2015; 83(5):860–866

[49] Lee DY, Jung TG, Lee SH. Single-level instrumented mini-open transforaminal lumbar interbody fusion in elderly patients. J Neurosurg Spine 2008;9(2):137144

[50] Singh K, Nandyala SV, Marquez-Lara A, et al. A perioperative cost analysis comparing single-level minimally invasive and open transforaminal lumbar interbody fusion. Spine J. 2014; 14(8):1694–1701

[51] Lee, JC, Jang HD, Shin BJ. Learning Curve and Clinical Outcomes of Minimally-Invasive Transforaminal Lumbar Interbody Fusion: Our Experience in 86 Consecutive Cases. Spine 2012. 37(18):1548-1557

[52] Adogwa O, Johnson K, Min ET, et al. Extent of intraoperative muscle dissection does not affect long-term outcomes after minimally invasive surgery versus open-transforaminal lumbar interbody fusion surgery: a prospective longitudinal cohort study. Surg Neurol Int. 2012; 3 Suppl 5: S355–S361

[53] Adogwa O, Parker S, Davis B, Aaronson O, Devin C, Cheng J, McGirt M. Cost-effectiveness of transforaminal lumbar interbody gusion for grade I fegenerative spondylolisthesis. J Neurosurg Spine 2011;15:138-143

[54] Sulaiman WA, Singh M. Minimally invasive versus open transforaminal lumbar interbody fusion for degenerative spondylolisthesis grades 1–2: patient-reported clinical outcomes and cost-utility analysis. Ochsner J. 2014; 14(1):32–37

[55] Zairi F, Arikat A, Allaoui M, Assaker R. Transforaminal lumbar interbody fusion: comparison between open and mini-open approaches with two years follow-up. J Neurol Surg A Cent Eur Neurosurg. 2013; 74(3):131–135

[56] Jang JS, Lee SH. Minimally invasive transforaminal lumbar interbody fusion with ipsilateral pedicle screw and contralateral facet screw fixation. J Neurosurg Spine 2005;3(3):218223

[57] Bindal R, Glaze S, Ognoskie M, Tunner V, Malone R, Ghosh S. Surgeon and patient radiation exposure in minimally-invasive transforaminal lumbar interbody fusion. J Neurosurg Spine 2008;9:570-573

[58] Kim JS, Jung B, Lee SH. Instrumented minimally invasive spinal-transforaminal lumbar interbody fusion (MIS-TLIF); minimum 5-years follow-up with clinical and radiologic outcomes. J Spinal Disord Tech 2012 [Epub ahead of print]

[59] Lange J, Karellas A, Street J, Eck J, Lapinsky A, Connolly P, DiPaola C. Estimating the effective radiation dose imparted to patients by intraoperative cone-beam computed tomography in thoracolumbar spinal surgery. Spine 2013;38(5):206-312

[60] Bagan B, Patel N, Deutsch H, et al. Perioperative complications of minimally invasive surgery (MIS): comparison of MIS and open interbody fusion techniques. Surg Technol Int. 2008; 17:281–286

[61] Adogwa O, Parker SL, Bydon A, Cheng J, McGirt MJ. Comparative effectiveness of minimally invasive versus open transforaminal lumbar interbody fusion: 2-year assessment of narcotic use, return to work, disability, and quality of life. J Spinal Disord Tech. 2011; 24(8):479–484

[62] Deutsch H, Musacchio MJ, Jr. Minimally invasive transforaminal lumbar interbody fusion with unilateral pedicle screw fixation. Neurosurg Focus 2006;20(3):E10

[63] Rouben D, Casnellie M, Ferguson M. Long-term durability of minimal invasive posterior transforaminal lumbar interbody fusion: a clinical and radiographic follow-up. J Spinal Disord Tech 2011;24(5):288296

[64] Tsahtsarlis A, Wood M. Minimally invasive transforaminal lumber interbody fusion and degenerative lumbar spine disease. Eur Spine J 2012;21(11):23002305

[65] Beringer WF, Mobasser JP. Unilateral pedicle screw instrumentation for minimally invasive transforaminal lumbar interbody fusion. Neurosurg Focus 2006;20(3):E4

[66] Park Y, Ha JW, Lee YT, Oh HC, Yoo JH, Kim HB. Surgical outcomes of minimally invasive transforaminal lumbar interbody fusion for the treatment of spondylolisthesis and degenerative segmental instability. Asian Spine J 2011;5(4):228236

[67] Park P, Foley KT. Minimally invasive transforaminal lumbar interbody fusion with reduction of spondylolisthesis: technique and outcomes after a minimum of 2 years' follow-up. Neurosurg Focus 2008;25(2):E16

[68] Archavlis E, Carvi y Nievas M. Comparison of minimally invasive fusion and instrumentation versus open surgery for severe stenotic spondylolisthesis with high-grade facet joint osteoarthritis. Eur Spine J 2013;22(8):17311740

5 The Lateral Transpsoas Approach versus ALIF: Do the Risks of Lateral Interbody Fusion Outweigh the Benefits Compared to Anterior Lumbar Interbody Fusion?

MIS: Steven M. Spitz, Hasan R. Syed, and Jean-Marc Voyadzis
Open: David L. Scott and Peter G. Whang

5.1 Introduction

Lumbar interbody fusion has been successfully used for decades to manage degenerative, neoplastic, developmental, and traumatic conditions of the lumbar spine. Potential advantages of interbody fusion over posterolateral arthrodesis include the ability to place a large graft under compressive forces to enhance fusion, restoration of disc height, foraminal distraction and indirect decompression, and deformity correction.[1,2] Lumbar interbody fusion utilizing a posterior approach (posterior lumbar interbody fusion [PLIF]) was first described in 1952 by Cloward. This technique proved effective in achieving interbody fusion but required extensive nerve root and thecal sac retraction to allow for adequate disc excision for placement of the interbody graft.[3] In an attempt to minimize the risk of nerve root retraction and injury, Harms and Jeszensky popularized a technique that utilized a transforaminal corridor (transforaminal lumbar interbody fusion [TLIF]) for interbody graft placement. This approach provides greater lateral access with enhanced visualization of the intervertebral disc.[4] These traditional posterior procedures have proven to be relatively safe and effective in achieving spinal fusion with favorable clinical outcomes; however, they require significant soft-tissue dissection, muscle retraction, and the removal of osteoligamentous structures, all of which can adversely affect patient recovery.[3,5]

The anterior transabdominal approach for interbody fusion (anterior lumbar interbody fusion [ALIF]), first described in 1932 by Capener for the treatment of spondylolisthesis and later modified to a retroperitoneal approach in 1960 by Harmon, provides wide anterior access to the lumbar disc space without disruption of the posterior spinal elements, with the advantage of placing a larger interbody graft than afforded by the posterior approaches.[6,7] Mayer in 1997 modified the retroperitoneal approach utilizing a smaller incision combined with a muscle-splitting exposure.[8] There remains, however, an increased approach-related risk of vascular and visceral injury, along with sympathetic dysfunction in males.[9,10,11,12] Recently, technological advancements in spinal instrumentation along with an improved understanding of surgical anatomy have led to minimally invasive techniques to mitigate muscle damage and blood loss and to reduce patient recovery time incurred by traditional open spinal fusions. The lateral transpsoas approach to the lumbar spine (lateral lumbar interbody fusion [LLIF]) was first introduced in 2006 by Pimenta and colleagues as the extreme lateral interbody fusion (XLIF).[13] Unlike ALIF, this approach does not require mobilization of the bowel, great vessels, or autonomic plexus. It involves the use of tubular retractors through a small incision that allows for a wide discectomy while maintaining the competence of the anterior and posterior longitudinal ligaments, and as such represents a true minimally

disruptive technique. Only a few clinical studies directly comparing LLIF and ALIF have been published (▶ Table 5.1).

5.2 Indications of Lateral Lumbar Interbody Fusion

LLIF is generally indicated for the treatment of degenerative conditions of the spine, including degenerative disc disease, spondylolisthesis, degenerative scoliosis, mechanical instability, and facet arthropathy involving all lumbar levels with the exception of L5–S1. The ability to place a large interbody graft makes it ideal for the restoration of disc height and indirect decompression of severe foraminal stenosis and moderate canal stenosis in the setting of degenerative disc disease with radiculopathy[14,15] LLIF has also been used successfully for the treatment of Grade 1 to 2 spondylolisthesis (▶ Table 5.2). Lateral positioning, disc space preparation, and height expansion can allow for reduction, particularly in cases of overt instability. Multilevel LLIF has also been shown to be a powerful procedure for the correction of coronal deformities (▶ Table 5.3).[16,17] Other indications include nonunion, discitis and osteomyelitis, and trauma.[2,13,16] Instrumentation options following LLIF include lateral plating, pedicle or transfacet screws, or the use of an interspinous device.[18,19,20,21,22] Recent biomechanical studies have shown that lateral plating is not as robust when compared to posterior fixation in resisting flexion and extension forces.[18,23] Posterior fixation typically requires prone repositioning, although posterior percutaneous screw insertion has been described in the lateral decubitus position.[22] Several studies have shown that stand-alone LLIF, particularly with larger grafts, is safe and effective owing to the minimal disruption of osteoligamentous structures afforded by this approach (▶ Table 5.4).[15,24]

Relative contraindications to LLIF include previous retroperitoneal surgery or fibrosis, vascular abnormalities, Grade 3 and above spondylolisthesis, severe disc space collapse with osteophyte formation, and L5–S1 pathology due to the anatomic constraints of the iliac crest. Patients with concomitant severe canal stenosis require a decompressive laminectomy because indirect decompression will be ineffective. This can be performed through a tubular retractor in the prone position after LLIF. Alternatively, a posterior approach for fusion with decompression should be considered. A standard preoperative anteroposterior (AP) X-ray is essential when considering an L4–L5 approach, given the presence of a "high-riding" crest at the L4 pedicle or above may complicate the approach. A "rising psoas sign" on axial magnetic imaging at L4–L5 manifested by a more ventral and lateral position of the psoas muscle with respect to the vertebral body may portend difficulty during the initial docking phase due to the proximity of the lumbar plexus.[25]

Table 5.1 Clinical studies directly comparing ALIF with LLIF

Authors (year)	Type	Patients	FUP (mo)	EBL (mL)	LOS (d)	Study parameters	No. (%) of patients	Conclusion(s)
Smith et al[36] (2012) III-R (2004–2008)[a]	ALIF vs. XLIF	87 115	24 24	242 354 79.1 95.6	3[b] 4[c] 1.5[b] 1.8[c]	Infection, MI, pneumonia, DVT	16 (16.7) 9 (8.2)	VAS and ODI comparable, XLIF has lower complications and costs
Hrabalek et al[10] (2014) III-R (1996–2011)[a]	ALIF vs. XLIF	120 88	>6	—	—	Sympathetic dysfunction Vascular injury Nerve injury Sexual dysfunction Left groin pain Left groin numb Infection	(16/5) (0/0) (5/1.1) (0/0) (0/12.5) (0/10.2) (0/0)	No statistical difference in complications (26.6% ALIF vs. 25.0% XLIF)
Hrabalek et al (2013) *Biomed Pap Med Fac Univ Palacky Olomouc Czech Repub* III-R (1996–2012)[a]	ALIF (L5/S1) vs. ALIF (T12–L5) vs. XLIF	210 120 101	>6	—	—	Post-op sympathetic dysfunction	1 (0.5) 18 (15) 4 (4)	Risk of injury to sympathetics highest for ALIF above L5; clinical impact generally modest
Watkins et al[58] (2013) III-R (2007–2010)[a]	ALIF vs. LLIF vs. TLIF (360)	184 86 39 220 patients/309 discs	19.2	—	—	Lordosis improve Disc height improve Slip correction	4.5° 2.2° 0.8° 2.2 mm 2.0 mm 0.5 mm 3.3 mm 3.5 mm 2.6 mm	For lordosis improvement: ALIF > LLIF = TLIF For disc height improvement: ALIF = LLIF > TLIF For slip: ALIF = LLIF = TLIF

Abbreviations: ALIF, anterior lumbar interbody fusion; DVT, deep vein thrombosis; EBL, estimated blood loss; FUP, follow-up; LLIF, lateral lumbar interbody fusion; LOS, length of stay; MI, minimally invasive; ODI, Oswestry Disability Index; VAS, visual analog scale; XLIF, extreme lateral interbody fusion.

[a]Time interval during which surgeries were performed.

[b]One surgical level.

[c]Two surgical levels.

Table 5.2 Recent ALIF or LLIF studies for spondylolisthesis (2005–2013)

Authors (year)	Type	Patients	FUP (mo)	EBL (mL)	LOS (d)	Fusion (%)	Conclusion(s)
Ohtori et al (2011) *J Orthop Sci* 16(4):352 II-P	ALIF vs. PLIF	22 24	42 29	200 321	26 19	91 88–92	All L4/L5; low back pain more improved in ALIF; low back/leg pain, patient satisfaction equal
Min et al (2007) *J Neurosurg Spine* 7(1):21 III-R	ALIF vs. PLIF	25 23	42.8 46.4	–	–	100 100	Success rates similar; complication rate higher for ALIF
Kim et al (2010) *World Neurosurg* 73(5):565 III-R	ALIF + Perc vs. ALIF + PLIF	43 32	41.1 32.9	300 379	7.4 15.2	97.7 100	No significant difference in VAS and ODI scores; ALIF + Perc = improved operative data
Shim et al (2011) *J Neurosurg Spine* 15(3):311 III-R	ALIF + Perc vs. ALIF + PLIF	26 23	30.3 30.3	163 305	7.2 10.3	76.9 91.3	Age of all patients >65 y; L5–S1 only; results favor ALIF with PLIF
Kanamori et al (2012) *Asian Spine J* 6(2):105 IV-R	ALIF	20	197	–	–	–	Adjacent level disease worsened long-term results
Riouallon et al (2013) *Orthop Trauma Surg Res* 99(2):155 IV-R	ALIF	65	79.2	–	–	91	ALIF comparable to other techniques
Ahmadian et al (2013) *J Neurosurg Spine* 19 (3):314 IV-P	XLIF L4–L5	31	18.2	94	3.5	100	Safe and effective technique
Rodgers et al (2012) *Sci World J* 2012 356712 IV-R	XLIF L4–L5 Grade 2	63	12	–	1.21	100	Safe and effective technique for Grade 2 spondylolisthesis

Abbreviations: ALIF, anterior lumbar interbody fusion; EBL, estimated blood loss; FUP, follow-up; LLIF, lateral lumbar interbody fusion; LOS, length of stay; ODI, Oswestry Disability Index; Perc, percutaneous; PLIF, posterior lumbar interbody fusion; VAS, visual analog scale; XLIF, extreme lateral interbody fusion

Table 5.3 Recent ALIF or LLIF studies for scoliosis (2005–2013)

Authors (year)	Type	Patients	FUP (mo)	EBL (mL)	LOS (d)	Fusion (%)	Conclusion(s)
Dorward et al[65] (2013) III-R	ALIF vs. TLIF	42 42	24 24	1.3 l 2.0 l	12.3 7.9	98 100	No difference in complication rates
Phillips et al[37] (2013) III-P	XLIF	107	178	100	3.8	97	Mean 4.4 levels treated per patient
Anand et al (2008) *J Spinal Disorder Tech* 21:459 IV-P	XLIF DLIF AxiaLIF	12	240	164	8.6	–	Pain improved; deformity correction excellent
Anand and Baron[55] (2013) IV-R	XLIF DLIF AxiaLIF	28	232	241	20	100	All patients had PS instrumentation; VAS, ODI, SF-36 improved
Dakwar et al[16] (2010) IV-R	XLIF	25	108	53	6.2	100	Pain and functional outcome better
Wang et al (2010) *Neurosurg Focus* 28: E9 IV-R	XLIF DLIF	23	401	477	–	–	Average pre-op Cobb's angle 31.4° corrected to 11.5°
Caputo et al (2013) *Clin Neurosci* 20:1558 IV-R	XLIF	30	–	–	–	88.2	Cobb's angle corrected 72.3%; disc height increased 116.7%

Abbreviations: ALIF, anterior lumbar interbody fusion; DLIF, direct lateral interbody fusion; EBL, estimated blood loss; FUP, follow-up; LLIF, lateral lumbar interbody fusion; LOS, length of stay; ODI, Oswestry Disability Index; PS, posterior spinal; SF-36, 36-Item Short Form Health Survey; TLIF, transforaminal lumbar interbody fusion; VAS, visual analog scale; XLIF, extreme lateral interbody fusion.

Table 5.4 Representative LLIF studies (2005–2013)

Authors (year)	Patients	ORT (min)	EBL (mL)	LOS (d)	Fusion (%)	Conclusions
Rodgers et al[2] (2007) IV-R	100	–	–	1.5	–	Pain improved
Knight et al[38] (2009) IV-R	58	161	136	5	–	No clinical outcomes reported
Rodgers et al (2009) *Internet J Minim Invasive Spine Technol* IV-R	100	–	–	1.13	–	Pain improved
Rodgers et al[28] (2010) IV-R	313 (156 obese)	–	–	1.24	–	Pain improved; lower complications in obese
Ozgur et al[13] (2006) IV-R	62	240	183	3.9	91	VAS and ODI improved; 73% posterior fixation; 71% clinical success
Oliveira et al[15] (2010) IV-R	15	67.3	50	1	100	VAS and ODI improved
Youssef et al (2010) *Spine* 35:S302 IV-R	84	199	155	2.6	81	XLIF/PSF group had longer ORT; VAS and ODI improve
Sharma et al (2011) *J Spinal Disord Tech* 24:242 IV-R	43	–	–	3.4	–	Significant improvement in VAS, ODI, and SF-12
Rodgers et al[24] (2011) IV-P	600	–	–	1.2	–	Pain improved; 87% patient satisfaction
Karikari et al (2011) *Neurosurg* 68:897 IV-R	41 (aged)	–	46–175	3.5	–	Average age 74.9; complication rate 7.4%
Elowitz et al[14] (2011) IV-R	25	–	–	–	–	VAS and ODI improved; dural sac area increased 143%
Berjano et al (2012) *Eur Spine J* 21 S1:S37 IV-R	93	–	–	–	–	92% clinical success; 8/93 failed to improve
Malham et al (2012) *Sci World J* 2012:246989 IV-P	30	60	50	–	85	VAS, ODI, and SF-36 improved; 1 bowel injury

Abbreviations: EBL, estimated blood loss; LLIF, lateral lumbar interbody fusion; LOS, length of stay; ODI, Oswestry Disability Index; ORT, operative time; PSF, posterior spinal fusion; SF-12, 12-Item Short Form Health Survey; SF-36, 36-Item Short Form Health Survey; VAS, visual analog scale; XLIF, extreme lateral interbody fusion.

5.3 Advantages of Lateral Lumbar Interbody Fusion

The LLIF technique utilizes a lateral retroperitoneal approach to access the psoas major muscle that is subsequently traversed to expose the lateral intervertebral disc space. This approach, as with the ALIF, provides a wide working corridor for intervertebral disc excision and end plate preparation, leading to a larger surface area available for fusion. Furthermore, this approach, as with ALIF, allows for the insertion of a larger interbody graft that engages the cortical ring apophysis, which may lessen the risk of subsidence and hence maintain disc height, indirect foraminal decompression, and/or deformity correction.[20,26] The lateral transpsoas approach, in contradistinction to ALIF, does not require an approach surgeon and minimizes dissection or manipulation of the great vessels, viscera, and sympathetic chain, thus potentially mitigating the attendant risks associated with injury to these structures. In addition, LLIF maintains the structural integrity of the anterior and posterior longitudinal ligaments, reducing the potential for iatrogenic destabilization.[15,18] LLIF can be utilized to treat all lumbar levels with the exception of L5–S1.

The use of tubular retractors with LLIF reduces incision size and tissue dissection, thus minimizing blood loss, infection rates, and postoperative pain. This has translated into shortening hospital stays and faster return to work.[2,5,16,24,27,28]

5.4 Indications for Anterior Lumbar Interbody Fusion

Despite ALIF's long-standing use and popularity, evidence-based indications continue to evolve.[29,30] Improved instrumentation, better graft materials, and a reduction in associated complications have expanded its clinical application. ALIF, in comparison to traditional posterior approaches, is associated with reduced operative times, results in less blood loss, and yields comparable outcomes. The anterior approach provides direct, unobstructed, and unmatched access to the disc space, allowing complete removal of disc material, meticulous preparation of the vertebral end plates, and the insertion of a large graft or implant. The technique may prove particularly useful for patients who have one or more risk factors for poor bone healing. The ALIF technique permits restoration of disc space height, correction of sagittal and coronal balance, and the reduction of spondylolisthesis. Posterior elements, including facet joints and pars, must be carefully scrutinized preoperatively to determine the need for ancillary stabilization.

Operative indications are often subjective (severe back pain), and surgery should be restricted to patients who have failed a reasonable trial of nonoperative care. Clinical research supports the use of ALIF for the following: grade I or II isthmic or degenerative spondylolisthesis (72–94% success); degenerative disc disease with disabling central or discogenic low back pain (71–100% success); degenerative lumbar scoliosis; pseudoarthrosis after posterior procedures; recurrent disc herniation; and the revision or retrieval of failed XLIF grafts. Contraindications to ALIF include osteoporosis severe enough to compromise graft stability, a Grade 3 or higher spondylolisthesis, prior retroperitoneal surgery, severe peripheral vascular disease, active disc space infection, an infrarenal aortic aneurysm, an anomalous genitourinary system with only a single ureter, obesity, and men still desiring to father children. All patients should undergo a preoperative bone density testing and males with a history of sexual dysfunction referred for evaluation. Although posterior surgical approaches and techniques are generally indicated for patients with severe nerve compression, ALIF, either alone or with supplemental foraminal decompression, may be sufficient to improve modest radicular symptoms.

5.5 Advantages of Anterior Lumbar Interbody Fusion

The anterior approach to the spine has become popular, in part due to its relative ease and its potential for application to all lumbar segments. Degenerative disc disease most commonly affects the L4–L5 and L5–S1 disc levels. Lateral approaches are unable to provide access to the L5–S1 disc space due to the constraints of the bony pelvis. Surgery at the L4–L5 level may also prove impossible or difficult if the patient has relatively high-riding iliac crests. Access to more rostral levels (e.g., L2–L3) may be limited by the rib cage. Although orthopaedic and neurological surgeons who are uncomfortable with the anterior approach should rely on the assistance of a general or vascular access surgeon, well-trained spine surgeons can achieve safe and comparable outcomes.[31]

The anterior column of the spine bears 80% of the forces associated with axial physiological loads. ALIF reconstructs the anterior load-bearing column of the spine, places the graft under compression, thereby increasing the likelihood of fusion, and improves sagittal and coronal alignment. The ideal position for fused lumbar segments is in lordosis, and ALIF restores this through resection of the anterior longitudinal ligament, through discectomy and annular release, by allowing the insertion of large lordotic grafts and by retaining the posterior tension band. Lateral interbody techniques also preserve the posterior tension band but fail to provide an anterior release and often cannot accommodate comparably sized grafts or implants. Obtaining autograft, particularly from the iliac crests, is much easier with the supine positioning of ALIF and may not require a separate incision. Both anterior and lateral approaches leave the paravertebral muscles and facet joints untouched, and the spinal canal inviolate, and may reduce the potential for iatrogenic adjacent level disease.[32]

The anterior approach provides an unobstructed view of the entire disc space, permitting complete removal of the disc and a thorough anterior decompression. Lateral interbody techniques, in contrast, provide a more limited view of the disc space and nociceptive disc remnants may be retained. Disc space elevation during ALIF graft or cage placement can increase spinal volume and neural foramen cross-sectional area by 20 and 30%, respectively. Additional anterior techniques such as microscopic anterior foraminal decompression have been developed to supplement this indirect nerve decompression.

Although resection of the anterior longitudinal ligament and the anterior annulus fibrosus during ALIF has been determined to be destabilizing, particularly in extension and axial rotation, the relevance of this biomechanical finding to fusion success and clinical outcome is unclear. Anterior fusion with structural grafting, threaded cages, or stand-alone anterior cages is often augmented with posterior pedicle screws (open or percutaneous), low-profile anterior plates, translaminar facet screws, and spinous process anchors. The posterior procedures significantly increase both operative time and costs but the increased stability appears to improve outcomes, particularly for patients with preoperative spondylolistheses or instability. Newer anterior devices constructed of PEEK (polyetheretherketone) with integrated locking screws offer more secure stand-alone fixation.

5.6 Case Illustration

A 50-year-old woman developed worsening low back and right leg pain that failed to respond to conservative measures, including physical therapy and epidural injections over the course of 1 year. Imaging studies demonstrate a Grade 1 spondylolisthesis at L4–L5 with a broad disc protrusion causing significant foraminal stenosis without significant canal stenosis (▶ Fig. 5.1). Flexion and extension radiographs showed 5 mm of anterolisthesis on flexion without reduction on extension.

5.7 Surgical Technique (Lateral Lumbar Interbody Fusion)

After starting intravenous lines and the administration of preoperative antibiotics, general endotracheal anesthesia is obtained. A Foley can be placed at the surgeon's discretion. The side of the approach should be chosen based on a careful assessment of preoperative X-ray and magnetic resonance imaging (MRI). The patient is placed in a true lateral decubitus position with the table break at the midpoint of the iliac crest and greater trochanter. All pressure points are padded, and the leg is flexed to relax the psoas muscle. The patient's chest and hip are secured to the table with elastic tape. The table is then flexed in such a way as to increase the distance between the

iliac crest and the rib cage. Once in position, a proper fluoroscopic AP view is obtained demonstrating parallel end plates, with the spinous processes being equidistant to the pedicles. Proper lateral imaging is also confirmed, eliminating parallax of the end plates and pedicles with adjustments of the table. A Kirschner wire (K-wire) is used to identify the intervertebral disc of interest at its midpoint with fluoroscopy. A mark is made on the flank overlying the center of the affected disc space. The patient is then draped after antiseptic is applied and the skin is infiltrated with a local anesthetic.

A 3- to 4-cm transverse incision is made along Langer's line. The incision is then carried down to the aponeurosis of the external oblique. Access to the retroperitoneal space is performed by blunt dissection in parallel to the orientation of the muscle fibers of the external oblique, followed by the internal oblique, and finally the transversus abdominis. Blunt dissection is of paramount importance so as not to injure the superficial sensory nerves (subcostal, iliohypogastric, ilioinguinal, and lateral femoral cutaneous) and motor fibers of the abdominal wall musculature.[1,33] At this point, the retroperitoneal fat will be in view, and blunt dissection is continued using sweeping movements to mobilize the peritoneum and its contents anteriorly to visualize the psoas major muscle with the aid of hand-held retractors. Once the psoas major is in view, the surgeon's index finger is then used to guide the first dilator through the abdominal musculature to the surface of the psoas major overlying the center of the disc space. A lateral fluoroscopic image is obtained to ensure that the first dilator is coaxial with the center of the disc space of interest.

Given the intrapsoas location of the lumbar contribution to the lumbosacral plexus, it is extremely important to have real-time electrophysiologic monitoring to aid in safe passage through the psoas muscle.[1,3,3,34,35] Each dilator is equipped with an isolated electrode at its distal tip. Prior to traversing the psoas muscle, a stimulation clip is applied to the proximal end of the dilator for intraoperative continuous electromyographic (EMG) monitoring. With this system, safe passage is most likely

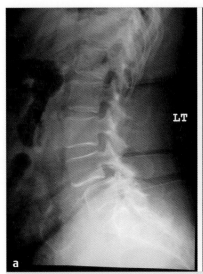
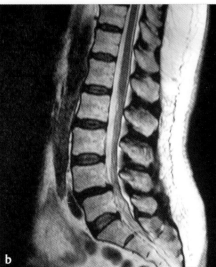
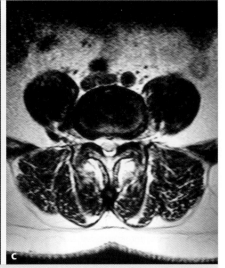

Fig. 5.1 Imaging studies of a 50-year-old woman with low back and right leg pain that failed to improve with conservative measures. **(a)** Standing lateral X-ray and **(b)** sagittal and **(c)** axial MRI showing a Grade 1 L4–L5 spondylolisthesis and a broad disc protrusion causing significant foraminal stenosis without canal stenosis.

if the EMG threshold is greater than 8 mA, thus demonstrating that the nerve is a safe distance from the dilator. The dilator is passed through the psoas muscle and docked on the center of the disc space. At this point, a K-wire is advanced through the dilator to the middle of the disc space. Successively larger dilators are then placed over the K-wire, followed by the retractor system, which in turn is affixed to the table-mounted flexible arm. All these steps are performed with stimulation and EMG. Lateral fluoroscopy is obtained to confirm placement over the center of the index disc space. A blunt-tip nerve probe is then used to confirm the location of lumbar nerves outside the confines of the retractor system, and the working channel is secured to the disc space or vertebral body and expanded. If the dilation was effective, only scant muscular fibers are identified and easily swept away exposing the disc space. A discectomy is performed in standard fashion using a combination of pituitary rongeurs, end plate shavers, rasps, and curettes. A Cobb elevator is used to release the contralateral annulus with AP fluoroscopy to allow for distraction and disc height expansion. All cartilaginous material is meticulously removed from the end plates. A series of trials are then inserted to determine the appropriate dimensions of the spacer. The graft is filled with bone graft extenders and is then tapped into place as confirmed with AP and lateral fluoroscopy. The wound is copiously irrigated and hemostasis deemed appropriate with bipolar electrocautery and the application of commercially available hemostatic agents. The retractor is slowly removed and any bleeding cauterized under direct visualization to insure meticulous hemostasis. The fascia of the external oblique is closed when possible, and the wound is closed in layers with absorbable sutures.

5.8 Surgical Technique (Anterior Lumbar Interbody Fusion)

The patient should undergo a thorough bowel clean-out the night prior to surgery. Prophylactic intravenous antibiotics are infused approximately 1 hour before the planned incision. The patient is positioned supine on the cystoscopy table with legs abducted (French position), allowing direct caudal access to the lower abdomen. Both arms are positioned at 90° to the plane of the operating table to permit unfettered lateral access to the abdomen by the surgeon and by the fluoroscopic unit. Vulnerable sites, including elbows and heels, are carefully padded to reduce the incidence of peripheral nerve injury. Additional lumbar lordosis, if needed, can be obtained either by reverse flexing of the table or by positioning a lumbar bump. Endotracheal intubation is performed, general anesthesia provided, and a Foley catheter placed. Ureteral stents may be advisable for women or for individuals with complex abdominal anatomy. Oxygenation probes and pulse oximeters are placed on toes and neuromonitoring considered. Patients should be typed and cross-matched. The abdomen is prepped, with inclusion of the anterior iliac crest if bone grafting is planned.

A left paramedian vertical incision is marked below the umbilicus with fluoroscopic guidance. The incision is carried through the subcutaneous tissues using electrocautery to expose the anterior rectus sheath. The sheath is divided longitudinally in the direction of its fibers with preservation of a tissue cuff to permit tight closure. The rectus muscle is retracted medially and the posterior rectus sheath/transversalis fascia divided as required. The ureters are identified and protected. Great care is also taken to prevent damage to the iliohypogastric and ilioinguinal nerves between the layers of the internal and transverse abdominal muscles.

The peritoneum and its contents are retracted medially by blunt dissection to expose the iliopsoas muscles and the anterior longitudinal ligament. Even small rents in the peritoneum are immediately repaired to reduce the possibility of herniation. A circular frame (e.g., Synthes SynFrame) is attached to the operating table and the abdominal contents gently retracted behind padded blades. The left common iliac artery and vein are traced to their bifurcations, and the iliolumbar vein (for L4–L5), middle sacral vessels (for L5–S1), and segmental vessels (for proximal exposure) are ligated and divided as necessary. The great vessels, including the aorta, inferior vena cava, and iliac, are mobilized to the right with hand-held retractors. Pressure on the vessels is ideally released at least hourly.

The appropriate disc level is confirmed by AP and lateral fluoroscopy. The annulus fibrosus is vertically incised at its midline and the two halves retracted laterally. The disc is incised and then completely removed. End plates are curetted, removing cartilaginous remnants while avoiding deep penetration. The disc space is distracted and the cage/graft size determined by an intraoperative assessment of annular tension with temporary trials.

Tricortical structural graft or cancellous graft for packing for the interior of titanium or PEEK spacers is harvested from the anterior iliac crest. For ALIF at the L4–L5 level, a separate incision is not needed. The graft or cage is impacted under lateral fluoroscopic guidance. The interbody can now be further stabilized, if indicated, with either anterior screws or a plate. The final construct is evaluated critically on both AP and lateral fluoroscopic views and the wound thoroughly lavaged. A suction drain is placed retroperitoneally, and the fascia, subcutaneous tissue, and skin closed meticulously.

Although this patient's spondylolisthesis appears stable on flexion–extension views (▶ Fig. 5.1), she would still likely benefit from posterior stabilization. The degree of foraminal compromise, the radiological improvement seen with the ALIF, and the patient's tolerance of the anterior procedure would be important variables in determining whether the patient undergoes a subsequent foraminotomy/open fusion or a percutaneous posterior procedure. In addition to the usual postoperative neural checks, lower extremity pulses, particularly the dorsalis pedis artery, must be carefully evaluated.

5.9 Discussion (Lateral Lumbar Interbody Fusion)

LLIF is commonly performed for the treatment of degenerative disc disease with associated radiculopathy due to foraminal stenosis, spondylolisthesis, and scoliosis. This technique provides excellent access for anterior interbody fusion and offers the same advantages of an ALIF. Furthermore, the lateral approach minimizes approach-related morbidity incurred with ALIF, notably the risk of injury to the great vessels, abdominal viscera, and hypogastric plexus, while eliminating the need for an approach surgeon. However, the greatest potential risk associated with LLIF is injury to the lumbar plexus, particularly at L4–L5. In this chapter's illustrative case, a lateral approach for lumbar interbody fusion should restore disc height, reduce the spondylolisthesis, and allow for an indirect decompression of foraminal stenosis and relief of her radiculopathy. Posterior stabilization can be achieved using percutaneous pedicle or transfacet screws in either the lateral or prone position.[22] A critical review of published results should provide insight into whether the potential risks of a lateral approach outweigh the benefits compared to ALIF (▶ Table 5.1).

5.9.1 Level I Evidence in Lateral Lumbar Interbody Fusion

There are no level I studies available.

5.9.2 Level II Evidence in Lateral Lumbar Interbody Fusion

There are no level II studies available.

5.9.3 Level III Evidence in Lateral Lumbar Interbody Fusion

One retrospective cohort study comparing LLIF and ALIF with respect to clinical outcome and costs has been reported in the literature. Smith et al compared 87 ALIF and 115 XLIF patients at a single institution between 2004 and 2008.[36] The authors demonstrated a statistically significant lower mean operative time (94.4 vs. 150.6 min), estimated blood loss (79.1 vs. 241.7 mL), length of hospital stay (36.3 vs. 71.9 hours), and mean charges ($91,995 vs. $102,146) in patients undergoing single-level XLIF compared to ALIF. These treatment differences were noted for two-level procedures as well. Smith et al also reported similar improvements in functional outcomes, that is, visual analog scale (VAS) and Oswestry Disability Index (ODI) scores, at 2 years for both cohorts. This study provides level III evidence that LLIF is more cost-effective and achieves similar clinical and functional outcomes when compared with ALIF, while reducing operative times, blood loss, and length of stay. In a prospective, nonrandomized, multicenter, single-arm study of 107 patients with degenerative scoliosis who underwent the XLIF procedure, Phillips et al showed significant improvement in all clinical outcome measures at 24 months, including ODI, VAS for back and leg pain, and 36-Item Short Form Health Survey mental and physical component summaries (SF-36).[37] The authors reported an overall correction of coronal deformity as measured by Cobb's angle from 20.9 to 15.2° and a significant increase in disc height from 5.2 mm preoperatively to 7.5 mm at 24-month follow-up. This study provides level III data that LLIF is comparable to clinical outcomes achieved with ALIF that are reported in the literature.

5.9.4 Level IV Evidence for Lateral Lumbar Interbody Fusion

Numerous retrospective cohort reviews exist that report the benefits of the lateral approach over historical controls or traditional interbody techniques. These studies describe improvements in clinical and functional outcome of patients with radiographic confirmation while emphasizing the minimally disruptive nature of the LLIF technique.

One of the earlier reports with clinical outcomes was presented by Rodgers et al in 2007, who described the results of 100 patients undergoing XLIF for multiple degenerative conditions.[2] The authors reported a low complication rate (2%), short length of hospital stay (1.5 days), and improvements in clinical outcomes, including a significant reduction in VAS pain scores by 68.7% and restoration of disc height at 6-month follow-up. Knight et al reported in 2009 on the results of 58 patients undergoing lateral approach surgeries, including XLIF and direct lateral interbody fusion (DLIF), by four different surgeons.[38] Mean operative time, estimated blood loss, and hospital stay was 161 minutes, 131 mL, and 5 days, respectively. The overall complication rate reported was 22.4%. These relatively longer operative times and hospital stays, higher blood loss, and an increased rate of complications were attributed to the associated learning curve. During the same year, Rodgers et al reported on 100 patients with adjacent segment degeneration after a prior history of lumbar fusion and again noted fast recovery with an average hospital stay of 1.13 days and significant reduction in VAS pain score by 67.4% in the 6-month follow-up period (▶ Table 5.4).

Since then, many reports in the literature have corroborated these initial results of LLIF with respect to clinical and radiographic outcomes. Ozgur et al,[13] Oliveira et al,[15] and Youssef et al described short operative times, minimal blood loss, and brief hospital stays (▶ Table 5.4). In addition, patients were able to ambulate early, and the authors noted an improvement in both clinical and functional outcomes measured by VAS pain score and ODI along with radiographic success in the follow-up period. In the larger of these studies, Youssef et al reported on 84 XLIF patients with a mean follow-up time of 15.7 months for treatment of degenerative disc disease, spinal stenosis, spondylolisthesis, and scoliosis, and found operative time, estimated blood loss, and length of hospital stay to be 199 minutes, 155 mL, and 2.6 days, respectively. Average pain (77% reduction in VAS) and function scores (56% reduction in ODI) significantly improved, and solid arthrodesis was obtained in 81% of patients. The authors reported that these results were similar or superior to conventional approaches.

Rodgers et al further assessed patient outcome and fusion rates in 66 patients undergoing XLIF 1 year after surgery and found 96.6% of levels fused on computed tomography (CT) scan with nearly 90% of patients "satisfied or very satisfied."[40] Finally, Ozgur et al reported a series of 62 patients who had 2-year follow-up after XLIF and reported a 91% fusion rate and 75% frequency of "clinical success," as measured by ODI-change definition.[41]

More recently, Berjano et al conducted in 2012 a retrospective cohort review of 97 consecutive patients across three centers with a mean follow-up of 12 months (▶ Table 5.4). Clinical success, defined by improvement in ODI and VAS, was demonstrated in 92% of cases at time of last follow-up. Transient neurological symptoms presented in 7% of cases postoperatively, but all resolved within 1 month from surgery. Malham et al reported on clinical and radiographic outcomes in their initial 30 patients treated with XLIF by a single surgeon with an average follow-up of 11.5 months (▶ Table 5.4). Operative time averaged 60 minutes per level with a mean blood loss of 50 mL. Furthermore, VAS back and leg pain decreased 63 and 56%, respectively, and complete fusion was observed in 85%. Ahmadian et al reported in 2013 the clinical outcome and efficacy of 31 LLIF patients with Grade 1 or 2 spondylolisthesis at L4–L5 over a period of 18.2 months (▶ Table 5.2). The total blood loss and length of hospital stay were found to be 94 mL and 3.5 days, respectively. Clinical outcomes, as measured by VAS, ODI, and SF-36, were all significantly improved. The benefits of the lateral transpsoas approach for lumbar interbody fusion have also been reported in patients of older age in addition to the obese population.[28,44] These studies provide level IV evidence that LLIF leads to shortened operative time and length of hospital stay, less blood loss, a significant reduction in VAS pain scores, and improvement in functional outcome.

5.10 Complications (Lateral Lumbar Interbody Fusion)

Complications associated with LLIF have been reported by many authors over the past several years as the popularity of the technique has increased (▶ Table 5.5). These largely comprise various nerve-related syndromes given the lumbar contribution to the lumbosacral plexus lies within the substance of the psoas major muscle. Quadriceps weakness and leg dysesthesias can occur from stretch injury to the femoral nerve during the insertion of the tubular dilators and placement and use of the retractor.[13,24] Motor injuries during lateral approaches may manifest as hip flexor and/or knee extensor weakness. These injuries are more apt to occur at the L4–L5 junction because of the more ventral presence of the lumbar plexus at this level.[33,34,45,46] Postoperative sensory symptoms are difficult to accurately

quantify due to the varying definitions reported in the literature. The incidence of transient sensory deficits in intermediate- and large-sized case series ranges between 1.6 and 22.5%,[47,48] the majority of which resolved by the end of the postoperative follow-up period.

In the largest prospective observational study on the lateral transpsoas approach to date, Rodgers et al specifically evaluated complications after XLIF in 600 patients.[24] In this series, 641 levels were treated, with 59.3% including the L4–L5 level. The overall complication rate was reported to be 6.2%, with 2.5% directly related to the surgical procedure; the inclusion of the L4–L5 level was a significant factor in the incidence of complications. With respect to neural complications, 0.7% of patients experienced either quadriceps or anterior tibialis weakness that resolved by 3 months postoperatively. This reported complication rate is significantly lower than most other published studies, which have documented motor weakness due to lumbar plexus injury occurring between 1.7 and 6.8%, the majority of which resolved during the postoperative follow-up period.[49,50] In comparison, permanent motor deficits have also been reported following ALIF, occurring in up to 6.5% of endoscopic ALIFs[51] and 1.5% of open ALIFs.[52]

In the aforementioned retrospective cohort study comparing XLIF to ALIF, Smith et al reported significantly more complications in ALIF (16.7%) versus XLIF (8.2%), with the most common being a higher rate of infection.[36] Hrabalek et al performed a comparative analysis on 120 ALIF and 88 XLIF patients and found no statistically significant difference in the rate of complications between the two groups.[10] With regard to neurologic complications, they reported a lumbar postsympathectomy syndrome in 15.8% of ALIF patients and partial and transient injury to the L5 nerve root in 1.1% of XLIF patients. These studies provide level III data that the rate of complications is *at least* similar in both groups or lower in the LLIF population of patients.

The most severe complications associated with ALIF have been visceral and vascular injuries. Visceral injuries in ALIF have ranged from 0.0 to 3.3% in intermediate-sized series[12] and have only been reported in two LLIF cases in the literature (▶ Table 5.5). Larger series have discussed vascular injuries in ALIF with rates ranging from 1.9 to 6.2%.[16,52,53] While there have been no published reports of vascular injuries associated with the lateral transpsoas technique to our knowledge, one such injury occurred in our hands.[54]

The use of tubular retractors in spine surgery is associated with reduced rates of infection. There were no infections in Rodgers et al's series of 600 XLIF patients,[24] with an overall infection rate of 0.4% following LLIF based on a review of published reports.[17,24,36,41,50] Postoperative hernias, ureteral injury, and psoas muscle hematoma, while uncommon, have also been documented complications in the LLIF literature.[41,49,55] The incidence of retrograde ejaculation, which has ranged from 0.6 to 45% in ALIF patients,[11,12,56] has not been reported in the LLIF population.

5.11 Conclusion (Lateral Lumbar Interbody Fusion)

No level I randomized comparisons or level II studies exist on LLIF. Level III studies have demonstrated comparable clinical

Table 5.5 Literature review of complications associated with LLIF and ALIF (aggregate data)

Complication type	LLIF[47] % (n)	ALIF[55] % (n)
Infection	0.4 (9)	2.2 (32)
Vascular injury	0 (0)	4.1 (74)
Visceral injury	0.01 (2)	0.3 (4)
Hernia	0.4 (8)	0.3 (5)
Neurological deficits	–	–
Motor	4.5 (99)	0.2 (5)
Sensory	5.6 (123)	0.6 (9)
Sympathetic	–	2.8 (41)
Vertebral body fracture	0.9 (19)	0.1 (2)
Hardware	0.6 (13)	0 (0)
Sexual dysfunction	–	1.2 (19)
Ileus	–	1.2 (22)
Urinary retention	–	0.5 (10)
DVT	–	0.7 (13)
Medical-related	3.6 (79)	0.6 (9)
Other	1.5 (34)	3.7 (54)
Total	17.5 (386)	15.4 (298)

Abbreviations: ALIF, anterior lumbar interbody fusion; DVT, deep vein thrombosis; LLIF, lateral lumbar interbody fusion.

and functional outcomes, while also showing benefits of decreased blood loss, operative time, shorter hospital stay, and lower cost. There are level III data indicating a comparable complication profile between the two groups. Finally, level IV data exist showing a significant reduction of major visceral and vascular injury but a higher rate of transient postoperative neurologic symptoms compared to ALIF. Using the grading scale of Guyatt et al,[57] we suggest a Grade 2B recommendation that LLIF and ALIF are generally equivalent in terms of clinical and functional outcome and fusion rates. Also, we suggest a Grade 2B recommendation that LLIF decreases blood loss and is associated with shorter operative time and hospital stay compared to ALIF. Finally, we suggest a Grade 2C recommendation that LLIF decreases the risk of infection, as well as the risk of visceral, vascular, and hypogastric plexus injuries when compared to ALIF.

5.12 Discussion (Anterior Lumbar Interbody Fusion)

Anterior approaches to the spine, originally developed for the surgical treatment of tuberculosis, offer a time-tested and effective means for lumbar fusion. The retroperitoneal approach was first reported by Iwahara in 1944 and refined by Southwick and Robinson. Subsequent variations on the anterior approach include mini-open, laparoscopic, and AxiaLIF.[11] The ALIF literature is extensive with interpretation of aggregate data confounded by variations in technique, the choice of interbody (e.g., auto- or allograft, titanium or PEEK cages), and the type of ancillary stabilization (stand-alone devices with integrated screws, anterior or lateral plates, posterior fusion and/or instrumentation).

More recently, the less invasive lateral (LLIF, XLIF, DLIF) approach to the lumbar spine has been popularized by reports of comparable biomechanical and clinical results to ALIF with a favorable complication profile. In the absence of well-controlled randomized studies directly comparing the two methods, however, it is difficult to determine which method is most suitable for a particular patient.

We used the terms ALIF/anterior lumbar interbody fusion, XLIF (lateral interbody fusion), and spondylolisthesis as key words to search the databases of the U.S. National Library of Medicine and the National Institutes of Health (www.pubmed. gov). All English language articles were reviewed for inclusion, with particular emphasis on papers reporting clinical outcomes.

5.12.1 Level I Evidence in Anterior Lumbar Interbody Fusion

There are no level I published studies that compare ALIF with LLIF.

5.12.2 Level II Evidence in Anterior Lumbar Interbody Fusion

There are no level II published studies that compare ALIF with LLIF.

5.12.3 Level III Evidence in Anterior Lumbar Interbody Fusion

There are only four published level III clinical studies that directly compare ALIF and LLIF techniques (▸ Table 5.1). Watkins et al compared ALIF, LLIF, and TLIF with regard to postoperative radiological parameters including lordosis, disc height, and spondylolisthesis correction.[58] Although ALIF restored lumbar lordosis to a greater degree than LLIF, the two approaches were otherwise comparable and the clinical relevance of the lordosis difference is unclear. Hrabalek et al published two level III papers focusing specifically on ALIF and XLIF complications (▸ Table 5.1).[10] No significant difference was found for overall complication rates (ALIF 26.6% vs. XLIF 25.0%); however, the types of complications differed markedly. The more comprehensive study of Smith et al associated XLIF surgery with reduced hospital length of stay and costs, a lower mean operative time, and reduced blood loss.[36] The overall complication rate was higher for the ALIF group (16.7 vs. 8.2%) but the paper provides insufficient data to draw specific conclusions as to cause (e.g., why 5.7% of the ALIF patients but only 0.9% of the XLIF recipients would develop infections of the posterior instrumentation). The higher overall complication rate for ALIF determined by Smith et al[36] is not supported by either the data of Hrabalek et al[10] or calculations made from aggregate data (▸ Table 5.5). Outcomes (VAS and ODI) measured by Smith et al were comparable for ALIF and XLIF at the 2-year follow-up.

5.12.4 Level IV Evidence for Anterior Lumbar Interbody Fusion

There are no published level IV studies that directly compare ALIF with LLIF.

5.13 Complications (Anterior Lumbar Interbody Fusion)

Complications specific to ALIF arise from the surgical approach, the discectomy and cage/graft insertion, and/or from the autograft donor site.[52] Most immediate or short-term complications are related to difficulties encountered with prevertebral structures. Dissection into the retropsoas space can result in thirdspacing of fluids and injury to the genitofemoral and/or ilioinguinal nerves. Perforation of the bowel necessitates immediate repair and case cancellation. Even small, inadequately repaired, violations of the peritoneum may result in postoperative hernias or bowel incarceration.

Vascular complications are not infrequent regardless of whether the approach is transperitoneal or retroperitoneal.[12,59,60] Despite a drop in the reported risk of injury after the mid-1990s to < 5% of cases, concerns regarding vascular injury continue to limit the popularity of ALIF. The abdominal aorta and the inferior vena cava bifurcate at the level of the L4 and the L5 vertebral bodies, respectively. Venous injuries are more frequent than arterial and are associated primarily with surgery at the L4–L5 disc space. The most commonly compromised vessels are the dorsally located left common iliac vein, the inferior vena cava, and the left iliolumbar vein. Although the ascending lumbar veins run vertically along the course of the inferior vena cava, the iliolumbar vein and its tributaries create a horizontal drainage system with known anatomic variations.[61] These tethering vessels may be easily injured by overzealous retraction. The left-sided retroperitoneal approach takes advantage of the relatively long and more pliable left common iliac vein and associated venules. Early identification and ligation of the left iliolumbar vein avoids later, potentially catastrophic, avulsion of the vein off of the vena cava. Risk factors for injury to the major vascular structures include osteomyelitis, discitis, previous anterior spinal surgery, spondylolisthesis, large osteophytes, transitional lumbosacral vertebrae, and the anterior migration of an interbody device. Although most surgeons approach the anterior spine from the left, a right-sided midline anterior retroperitoneal approach appears to be a safe alternative with a relatively low rate of venous injury and retrograde ejaculation.[62]

The most common arterial injury is left iliac artery thrombosis, presumably caused by prolonged retraction of the common iliac arteries to the right. Brau et al observed that 57% of patients undergoing ALIF at L4–L5 were subject to transient leg ischemia due to compression of the left iliac arteries, and recommended that continuous retraction of the iliac artery should be no longer than 1 hour.[53] Other factors predisposing to arterial thrombosis include traumatic dissections/previous surgeries, obesity, prolonged surgical time, hypotensive anesthesia, smoking, previous thrombosis, age, and anatomic variations in vascular tortuosity and bifurcation.

Urological complications related to the approach include urinary retention (5–27%) that is usually temporary. More problematic is retrograde ejaculation from iatrogenic injury to the sympathetic fibers of the hypogastric plexus that are adherent to the posterior surface of the peritoneum at the level of L5–S1 (0.42–22.5%).[9] The hypogastric plexus is a continuation of the preaortic sympathetic chain in the retroperitoneal space, and damage to these nerves may result in abnormal relaxation of the internal bladder sphincter with retrograde flow of ejaculate into the bladder. This problem is managed nonoperatively and resolves in 25 to 33% of patients by the end of the second postoperative year. Postoperative retrograde ejaculation has been reported to be almost 10-fold more common with the transperitoneal approach.

Although the use of synthetic bone growth factors remains controversial, the harvest of autograft is not without complications.[63] Medial placement of the incision for iliac crest grafting may injure the lateral femoral cutaneous nerve with potentially permanent anesthesia of the ventrolateral skin of the thigh. Poor hemostasis and closure of the graft site can result in a substantial hematoma or herniation of bowel through the transversalis fascia. Graft site discomfort can be substantial and persistent, although it may not affect overall clinical patient satisfaction. For cage implants, harvesting cancellous bone from the vertebral body itself and replacing the void by a tricalcium phosphate plug has been proposed as a safe and effective alternative.[51]

Enthusiasm for the use of autograft substitutes, particularly recombinant human bone morphogenetic protein-2 (rhBMP-2), has been tempered by recent data (▶ Table 5.6).[64] Although prospective randomized clinical studies comparing BMP-2 with that of iliac crest bone graft (ICBG) fail to show a statistical difference with regard to overall patient-based outcomes (ODI and SF-36), complications associated with BMP-2 use include postoperative leg pain without MRI evidence of root compression in 17%, and urinary retention and retrograde ejaculation in 9% of males. RhBMP appears to be directly toxic to neural tissue and its use has been associated with migration of interbody implants, delayed pseudoarthrosis, unwarranted bony outgrowths, pseudocyst formation, and osteolysis/subsidence of allograft cages.

Adynamic postoperative ileus is frequently observed in extraperitoneal operations including ALIF and results in delayed hospital discharge and increased health care costs. Acute colonic pseudo-obstruction, or Ogilvie's syndrome, may be related to mechanical disruption of parasympathetic innervation to the colon and can result from direct manipulation, retroperitoneal hematoma, or ischemic insult to the sacral plexus. Colonic distension can usually be successfully treated conservatively with nasogastric suction, bowel rest, and correction of underlying medical issues but may benefit from the use of methylnaltrexone bromide (for opiate-induced constipation), parasympathomimetics (neostigmine), and colonic decompression. The numerous lymphatic vessels and nodes located lateral to the left common iliac artery can also be injured during dissection of the left ascending lumbar vein at the L3–L4 or L4–L5 disc space. The clear fluid oozing from the lymphatic system in the lower lumbar region distal to the cisterna chili can be easily overlooked. Persistent leakage can result in lymphedema, lymphoceles, chyloretroperitoneum, nutritional deficiencies, and immune suppression. If necessary, drainage via a peritoneal window is generally curative.

Neurologic complications include dural tears and partial sympathectomy. During discectomy, aggressive decompression may violate the posterior annulus and permit inadvertent entrance into the epidural space. Even small dural tears generally cannot be adequately visualized, and treatment consists of bed rest and a lumbar subarachnoid drain. The lumbar sympathetic chain is located on the anterolateral aspect of the vertebral body, and partial sympathectomy may induce vasodilation of vessels in the ipsilateral leg with clinical complaints of a cold contralateral foot. Fortunately, this complication often resolves 3 to 6 months postoperatively.

Postoperative complications include deep vein thrombosis (DVT), cage subsidence, and pseudoarthrosis. Cage subsidence is, at least partially, correlated with cage size and reaming depth, and is inversely related to bone quality. Multiple patient and surgical variables contribute to the risk for pseudoarthrosis, with reported fusion rates ranging from 47 to 100%.

5.14 Conclusion (Anterior Lumbar Interbody Fusion)

Evidence-based comparison of ALIF and LLIF outcomes and complications suffers from the absence of suitable well-controlled studies. Selected intraoperative and outcome data directly comparing the two techniques are available primarily from a single study at a single institution with a relatively small patient panel.[36] Indirect comparison of ALIF and LLIF is possible by analyzing the data from studies that compare either ALIF or LLIF to the same "gold standard" surgical technique (e.g., PLIF or TLIF) or clinical application (e.g., spondylolisthesis or scoliosis

Table 5.6 Representative ALIF studies (2005–2013)

Authors (year)	Type	Patients	FUP (mo)	EBL (mL)	Fusion (%)	Conclusion(s)
Hsieh et al (2007) J Neurosurg Spine 7(4):379 III-R	ALIF vs. TLIF	32 (46 l) 25 (34 l)	45.7 44.1	–	–	ALIF is superior to TLIF for restoring foraminal height, local disc angle, and lordosis. 2-year clinical outcomes equivalent (VAS)
Kurtz et al (2012) J Neurosurg Spine 17(4):342 III-R	ALIF 360 P/TLF TLF PLF	544 492 5,851 917 7,840	120	–	–	Approach had no effect on deep (subfascial) infection rate; modest effect on superficial
Sasso et al[63] (2005) II-P	ALIF + iliac crest bone graft	208	24	–	–	Donor-site pain remains a significant postoperative management problem
Arlet et al[51] (2006) II-P	ALIF + vertebral body graft	21	28	250	100%	Local harvest of autograft core from adjacent vertebral body with a β-TCP plug is safe and effective
Whang et al (2013) J Spinal Disord Tech 26(8)437 III-R (2002–2010)	ALIF vs. AxiaLIF (all at L5–S1)	48 48	>24	–	79% 85%	AxiaLIF appears to provide similar radiographic results and complications as ALIF
Aghayev et al (2012) Eur Spine J 21(8):1640 III-R (2005–2010)	ALIF vs. TDA	50 534	12	–	–	Pain alleviation after ALIF and TDA was similar
Behrbalk et al (2013) Eur Spine J 22(12):2869 IV-R	ALIF + PEEK/BMP	25 (32 levels)	17	–	90.6%	SynFix-LR System. No BMP-related complication at 6-mg dose level
Quraishi et al (2013) Eur Spine J 22 (Supp 1):S16 III-R (2001–2010)	ALIF or TDR	304	–	–	–	With adequate training, spine surgeons can safely perform anterior approaches to the lumbar spine
Jarrett et al[31] (2009) III-R (2003–2005)	Spine Surgery Vascular Surgery	63 202	–	–	–	With adequate training, spine surgeons can safely perform anterior approaches to the lumbar spine
Garg et al[60] (2010) III-R (2004–2009)	ALIF L4/5 and/or L5/S1	212	–	143	–	Increased vascular injury in two-level exposures and in males, no effect of aorta-iliac calcification
Kalb et al[68] (2016) IV-R (2004–2010)	ALIF	242	11	–	99%	No correlation among patients' demographics, comorbidities and previous lumbar surgical interventions with complications
Choi et al (2011) Acta Neurochir 153(3):567 IV-R (2007–2008)	ALIF	200	18.4	–	98%	Unfavorable outcome associated with obese patients at L5/S1, high-grade slip, or severe facet arthropathy
Lindley et al (2012) Spine 37(20):1785 III-R (2004–2011)	ALIF + BMP vs. ADR (All at L5/S1)	54 41	–	–	–	No significant difference in incidence of RE
Carragee et al (2011) Spine J 11(6):511 III-R (2002–2004)	ALIF vs. rhBMP-2	–	69 174	–	–	Use of rhBMP-2 during ALIF appears to increase risk of RE
Snyder et al (2013) J Spinal Disord Tech III-R (2004–2010)	ALIF + anterior plate vs. ALIF – plate	146 85	11.2 13.7	–	–	Anterior plating results in no statistical difference in Prolo or ODI scores
Sasso et al[52] (2005) III-R (1992–2002)	ALIF (–) vs. (+) TIB	243 228	–	–	–	Threaded interbodies associated with more complications (8.3%) than nonthreaded (2.1%)
Lubelski et al (2013) J Neurosurg Spine 18(2):126 III-R	ALIF ± rhBMP-2	59 51	17.5 30.8	–	–	No significant difference in urological complications with (22%) or without (19.6%) rhBMP-2

Abbreviations: ALIF, anterior lumbar interbody fusion; Beta-TCP, beta-tricalcium phosphate; EBL, estimated blood loss; FUP, follow-up; PEEK, polyetheretherketone; RE, retrograde ejaculation; rhBMP-2, recombinant human bone morphogenetic protein-2; TDA, total disc arthroplasty; TLIF, transforaminal lumbar interbody fusion; VAS, visual analog scale.
Note: LLIF patients = 2,207 (Ahmadian et al 2013, Anand et al 2008, Berjano et al 2012, Caputo et al 2013, Malhan et al 2012, Rodgers et al 2009, Rodgers et al 2012, Sharma et al 2011, Tormenti et al 2010, Wang et al 2010, Youssef et al 2010).[10,16,17,24,36,38,41,44,48,49,50]
ALIF patients = 1,938 (Asha et al 2012, Hrabaek et al 2012, Hsieh et al 2007, Quraishi et al 2013).[10,12,31,36,52,60,68]
The overall complication rates for ALIF and LLIF do not significantly differ at the 95% confidence level (p-value = 0.06724).

correction[65]) (► Table 5.2 and ► Table 5.3). These comparisons are weakened by the inclusion of the L5–S1 level in many of the ALIF studies, a level anatomically inaccessible to current LLIF technology. The cumulative level II, III, and IV data (► Table 5.1, ► Table 5.2, ► Table 5.3, ► Table 5.4, ► Table 5.5 and ► Table 5.6) strongly suggest, but do not prove, that the two approaches generate comparable biomechanical results,[66] clinical outcomes, and overall complication rates.[30]

The prominent complications associated with these two approaches are either vascular and urologic (ALIF) or neurologic (LLIF). Complications that are subgroup specific (e.g., retrograde ejaculation in males undergoing ALIF) may provide additional impetus for the choice of one approach over the other. Retrograde ejaculation, often cited as a major drawback for choosing an ALIF, is simply not relevant to the female patient described in ► Fig. 5.1. Various strategies have been cited to reduce the incidence of ALIF-related complications, and published complication rates vary widely.[67]

Using the grading scale of Guyatt et al,[57] we suggest a Grade 2B recommendation that LLIF and ALIF are generally equivalent in terms of biomechanical stability, clinical outcome, and fusion rates. Although the overall complications rates for the two techniques appear similar, ALIF carries a higher risk of vascular damage, sexual dysfunction, and sympathetic dysregulation, whereas LLIF surgery is more likely to result in motor and sensory nerve damage (Grade 1C). There is substantial level III and IV evidence supporting the use of both ALIF and LLIF for the treatment of Grade I or II lumbar spondylolisthesis (Grade 1C). ALIF appears to be superior to LLIF in restoring lumbar lordosis (Grade 2C).

5.15 Editors' Commentary

5.15.1 Minimally Invasive Surgery

LLIF and ALIF are procedures with widely different indications. It is quite true that LLIF cannot be easily and safely performed at L5–S1. There is little question that ALIF is the preferred approach to this level. That being said, the incidence of retrograde ejaculation, iliolumbar vein avulsion, lower extremity DVT, and ileus associated with this approach cannot be ignored. Furthermore, the incidence of complications increases dramatically when the ALIF approach is performed at L4–L5 or higher levels. These levels, then, are where the LLIF is the preferred approach.

It is hard to accept the argument that a 3-cm incision on the lateral abdominal wall, enabling approach to, and fusion of, three or more disc levels, is not less invasive than the equivalent approach using the ALIF technique. In the LLIF approach, no abdominal muscles are cut, the iliopsoas muscle can be safely dilated to access the disc space using neuromonitoring techniques, with minimal risk to the femoral nerve, no bowel or vascular mobilization or retraction is necessary, and all abdominal structures are safely protected by "360°" retractors. When used for correction of adult degenerative scoliosis, the recent development of hyperlordotic cages and advanced posterior instrumentation techniques have made sagittal plane correction nearly equivalent to open correction.

In summary, ALIF and LLIF have very different surgical indications in lumbar spine surgery. When used appropriately, each yields excellent results. When pushed beyond their appropriate indication, the complication profile can escalate dramatically.

5.15.2 Open Surgery

It is difficult to defend the lateral anterior interbody surgical approach as a "less invasive" technique or as an alternative to ALIF given the lateral approach complication profile and the inability of this technique to address the L5–S1 disc space, the most likely to require discectomy and reconstruction.

Lumbar lateral approach surgery passes through the psoas muscle, potentially contributing to ipsilateral lower extremity weakness through injury to the psoas muscle belly or via a lumbar plexus injury. In ► Table 5.6, the two complications with the highest rates are presumably related to lumbar plexus injury during the surgical exposure. Depending on the level, this injury can be benign or, as seen in upper lumbar levels, a more serious injury resulting in quadriceps deficiency, a limitation that makes walking difficult without an assistive device. Given the typically benign nature of the anterior retroperitoneal approach with rare iliac or iliolumbar vein injuries as the predominant vascular complication, an argument could be made that ALIF is the less invasive, less morbid procedure. Limitations of LLIF in accessing the L5–S1 level further narrow the indications for use of this procedure. Finally, segmental sagittal plane correction may be limited when LLIF is performed properly by failure to release the anterior longitudinal ligament, often a contracted structure in adult scoliosis with flatback deformity or spondylolisthesis. In summary, LLIF is essentially a procedure that should be used in limited spinal conditions and cannot keep pace with open ALIF in terms of patient safety profile, surgical levels, or reconstructive potential.

References

[1] Dakwar E, Vale FL, Uribe JS. Trajectory of the main sensory and motor branches of the lumbar plexus outside the psoas muscle related to the lateral retroperitoneal transpsoas approach. J Neurosurg Spine. 2011; 14(2):290–295

[2] Rodgers WB, Cox C, Gerber EJ. Experience and early results with a minimally invasive technique for anterior column support through extreme lateral interbody fusion (XLIF). US Musculoskelet Rev. 2007; 1:28–32

[3] Cloward RB. The treatment of ruptured lumbar intervertebral disc by vertebral body fusion. III. Method of use of banked bone. Ann Surg. 1952; 136(6):987–992

[4] Harms J, Jeszensky D. The unilateral, transforaminal approach for posterior lumbar interbody fusion. Orthop Traumatol. 1998; 6:88–99

[5] Foley KT, Holly LT, Schwender JD. Minimally invasive lumbar fusion. Spine. 2003; 28(15) Suppl:S26–S35

[6] Meyerding HW. Spondylolisthesis. Surg Gynecol Obstet . 1932; 54:371–377

[7] Harmon P. Anterior extraperitoneal lumbar disc excision and vertebral body fusion. Clin Orthop. 1960; 18:168–173

[8] Mayer HM. A new microsurgical technique for minimally invasive anterior lumbar interbody fusion. Spine. 1997; 22(6):691–699, discussion 700

[9] Flynn JC, Price CT. Sexual complications of anterior fusion of the lumbar spine. Spine. 1984; 9(5):489–492

[10] Hrabalek L, Adamus M, Gryga A, Wanek T, Tucek P. A comparison of complication rate between anterior and lateral approaches to the lumbar spine. Biomed Pap Med Fac Univ Palacky Olomouc Czech Repub. 2014; 158(1):127–132

[11] Kaiser MG, Haid RW, Jr, Subach BR, Miller JS, Smith CD, Rodts GE, Jr. Comparison of the mini-open versus laparoscopic approach for anterior

lumbar interbody fusion: a retrospective review. Neurosurgery. 2002; 51(1): 97–103, discussion 103–105

[12] Rajaraman V, Vingan R, Roth P, Heary RF, Conklin L, Jacobs GB. Visceral and vascular complications resulting from anterior lumbar interbody fusion. J Neurosurg. 1999; 91(1) Suppl:60–64

[13] Ozgur BM, Aryan HE, Pimenta L, Taylor WR. Extreme lateral interbody fusion (XLIF): a novel surgical technique for anterior lumbar interbody fusion. Spine J. 2006; 6(4):435–443

[14] Elowitz EH, Yanni DS, Chwajol M, Starke RM, Perin NI. Evaluation of indirect decompression of the lumbar spinal canal following minimally invasive lateral transpsoas interbody fusion: radiographic and outcome analysis. Minim Invasive Neurosurg. 2011; 54(5)(−)(6):201–206

[15] Oliveira L, Marchi L, Coutinho E, Pimenta L. A radiographic assessment of the ability of the extreme lateral interbody fusion procedure to indirectly decompress the neural elements. Spine. 2010; 35(26) Suppl:S331–S337

[16] Dakwar E, Cardona RF, Smith DA, Uribe JS. Early outcomes and safety of the minimally invasive, lateral retroperitoneal transpsoas approach for adult degenerative scoliosis. Neurosurg Focus. 2010; 28(3):E8

[17] Isaacs RE, Hyde J, Goodrich JA, Rodgers WB, Phillips FM. A prospective, nonrandomized, multicenter evaluation of extreme lateral interbody fusion for the treatment of adult degenerative scoliosis: perioperative outcomes and complications. Spine. 2010; 35(26) Suppl:S322–S330

[18] Cappuccino A, Cornwall GB, Turner AWL, et al. Biomechanical analysis and review of lateral lumbar fusion constructs. Spine. 2010; 35(26) Suppl:S361–S367

[19] Le TV, Smith DA, Greenberg MS, Dakwar E, Baaj AA, Uribe JS. Complications of lateral plating in the minimally invasive lateral transpsoas approach. J Neurosurg Spine. 2012; 16(3):302–307

[20] Oliveira L, Marchi L, Coutinho E, Pimenta L. The subsidence rate in XLIF osteoporotic patients in standalone procedures. Spine. 1976; 2010(10):S51–S52

[21] Park SH, Park WM, Park CW, Kang KS, Lee YK, Lim SR. Minimally invasive anterior lumbar interbody fusion followed by percutaneous translaminar facet screw fixation in elderly patients. J Neurosurg Spine. 2009; 10(6):610–616

[22] Voyadzis JM, Anaizi AN. Minimally invasive lumbar transfacet screw fixation in the lateral decubitus position after extreme lateral interbody fusion: a technique and feasibility study. J Spinal Disord Tech. 2013; 26(2):98–106

[23] Kim SM, Lim TJ, Paterno J, Park J, Kim DH. Biomechanical comparison: stability of lateral-approach anterior lumbar interbody fusion and lateral fixation compared with anterior-approach anterior lumbar interbody fusion and posterior fixation in the lower lumbar spine. J Neurosurg Spine. 2005; 2(1):62–68

[24] Rodgers WB, Gerber EJ, Patterson J. Intraoperative and early postoperative complications in extreme lateral interbody fusion: an analysis of 600 cases. Spine. 2011; 36(1):26–32

[25] Voyadzis JM, Felbaum D, Rhee J. The rising psoas sign: an analysis of preoperative imaging characteristics of aborted minimally invasive lateral interbody fusions at L4–5. J Neurosurg Spine. 2014; 20(5):531–537

[26] Lowe TG, Hashim S, Wilson LA, et al. A biomechanical study of regional endplate strength and cage morphology as it relates to structural interbody support. Spine. 2004; 29(21):2389–2394

[27] Perez-Cruet MJ, Fessler RG, Perin NI. Review: complications of minimally invasive spinal surgery. Neurosurgery. 2002; 51(5) Suppl:S26–S36

[28] Rodgers WB, Cox CS, Gerber EJ. Early complications of extreme lateral interbody fusion in the obese. J Spinal Disord Tech. 2010; 23(6):393–397

[29] Heary RF, Yanni DS, Benzel EC. Anterior lumbar interbody fusion. In: Benzel EC, ed. Spine Surgery. Philadelphia, PA: Saunders; 2012:523–534

[30] Mobbs RJ, Loganathan A, Yeung V, Rao PJ. Indications for anterior lumbar interbody fusion. Orthop Surg. 2013; 5(3):153–163

[31] Jarrett CD, Heller JG, Tsai L. Anterior exposure of the lumbar spine with and without an "access surgeon": morbidity analysis of 265 consecutive cases. J Spinal Disord Tech. 2009; 22(8):559–564

[32] Tang S. Does TLIF aggravate adjacent segmental degeneration more adversely than ALIF? A finite element study. Turk Neurosurg. 2012; 22(3):324–328

[33] Uribe JS, Arredondo N, Dakwar E, Vale FL. Defining the safe working zones using the minimally invasive lateral retroperitoneal transpsoas approach: an anatomical study. J Neurosurg Spine. 2010; 13(2):260–266

[34] Benglis DM, Vanni S, Levi AD. An anatomical study of the lumbosacral plexus as related to the minimally invasive transpsoas approach to the lumbar spine. J Neurosurg Spine. 2009; 10(2):139–144

[35] Tohmeh AG, Rodgers WB, Peterson MD. Dynamically evoked, discrete-threshold electromyography in the extreme lateral interbody fusion approach. J Neurosurg Spine. 2011; 14(1):31–37

[36] Smith WD, Christian G, Serrano S, Malone KT. A comparison of perioperative charges and outcome between open and mini-open approaches for anterior lumbar discectomy and fusion. J Clin Neurosci. 2012; 19(5):673–680

[37] Phillips FM, Isaacs RE, Rodgers WB, et al. Adult degenerative scoliosis treated with XLIF: clinical and radiographical results of a prospective multicenter study with 24-month follow-up. Spine. 2013; 38(21):1853–1861

[38] Knight RQ, Schwaegler P, Hanscom D, Roh J. Direct lateral lumbar interbody fusion for degenerative conditions: early complication profile. J Spinal Disord Tech. 2009; 22(1):34–37

[39] Youssef JA, McAfee PC, Patty CA, Raley E, DeBauche S, Shucosky E, Chotikul L. Minimally invasive surgery: lateral approach interbody fusion: results and review. Spine (Phila PA 1976) 2010;35(26):S302-11

[40] Rodgers WB, Gerber EJ, Patterson JR. Fusion after minimally disruptive anterior lumbar interbody fusion: Analysis of extreme lateral interbody fusion by computed tomography. SAS J. 2010; 4(2):63–66

[41] Ozgur BM, Agarwal V, Nail E, Pimenta L. Two-year clinical and radiographic success of minimally invasive lateral transpsoas approach for the treatment of degenerative lumbar conditions. SAS J. 2010; 4(2):41–46

[42] Berjano P, Balsano M, Buric J, Petruzzi M, Lamartina C. Direct lateral access lumbar and thoracolumbar fusion: preliminary results. Eur Spine J 2012;21:S37-42

[43] Malham GM, Ellis NJ, Parker RM, Seex KA. Clinical outcome and fusion rates after the first 30 extreme lateral interbody fusions. ScientificWorldJournal 2012;2012:246989

[44] Rodgers WB, Gerber EJ, Rodgers JA. Lumbar fusion in octogenarians: the promise of minimally invasive surgery. Spine. 2010; 35(26) Suppl:S355–S360

[45] Kepler CK, Bogner EA, Herzog RJ, Huang RC. Anatomy of the psoas muscle and lumbar plexus with respect to the surgical approach for lateral transpsoas interbody fusion. Eur Spine J. 2011; 20(4):550–556

[46] Park DK, Lee MJ, Lin EL, Singh K, An HS, Phillips FM. The relationship of intrapsoas nerves during a transpsoas approach to the lumbar spine: anatomic study. J Spinal Disord Tech. 2010; 23(4):223–228

[47] Ahmadian A, Deukmedjian AR, Abel N, Dakwar E, Uribe JS. Analysis of lumbar plexopathies and nerve injury after lateral retroperitoneal transpsoas approach: diagnostic standardization. J Neurosurg Spine. 2013; 18(3):289–297

[48] Le TV, Burkett CJ, Deukmedjian AR, Uribe JS. Postoperative lumbar plexus injury after lumbar retroperitoneal transpsoas minimally invasive lateral interbody fusion. Spine. 2013; 38(1):E13–E20

[49] Cahill KS, Martinez JL, Wang MY, Vanni S, Levi AD. Motor nerve injuries following the minimally invasive lateral transpsoas approach. J Neurosurg Spine. 2012; 17(3):227–231

[50] Cummock MD, Vanni S, Levi AD, Yu Y, Wang MY. An analysis of postoperative thigh symptoms after minimally invasive transpsoas lumbar interbody fusion. J Neurosurg Spine. 2011; 15(1):11–18

[51] Arlet V, Jiang L, Steffen T, Ouellet J, Reindl R, Aebi M. Harvesting local cylinder autograft from adjacent vertebral body for anterior lumbar interbody fusion: surgical technique, operative feasibility and preliminary clinical results. Eur Spine J. 2006; 15(9):1352–1359

[52] Sasso RC, Best NM, Mummaneni PV, Reilly TM, Hussain SM. Analysis of operative complications in a series of 471 anterior lumbar interbody fusion procedures. Spine. 2005; 30(6):670–674

[53] Brau SA, Delamarter RB, Schiffman ML, Williams LA, Watkins RG. Vascular injury during anterior lumbar surgery. Spine J. 2004; 4(4):409–412

[54] Syed HR, Spitz SM, Voyadzis JM, Sandhu FA. Complications associated with minimally invasive extreme lateral interbody fusion (XLIF): an analysis of 300 cases. Paper presented at: Congress of Neurological Surgeons Poster Presentation; 2013; San Francisco, CA

[55] Anand N, Baron EM. Urological injury as a complication of the transpsoas approach for discectomy and interbody fusion. J Neurosurg Spine. 2013; 18(1):18–23

[56] Villavicencio AT, Burneikiene S, Bulsara KR, Thramann JJ. Perioperative complications in transforaminal lumbar interbody fusion versus anterior-posterior reconstruction for lumbar disc degeneration and instability. J Spinal Disord Tech. 2006; 19(2):92–97

[57] Guyatt G, Schünemann H, Cook D, Jaeschke R, Pauker S, Bucher H, American College of Chest Physicians. Grades of recommendation for antithrombotic agents. Chest. 2001; 119(1) Suppl:3S–7S

[58] Watkins RG, IV, Hanna R, Chang D, Watkins RG, III. Sagittal alignment after lumbar interbody fusion: comparing anterior, lateral, and transforaminal approaches. J Spinal Disord Tech. 2014; 27(5):253–256

[59] Fantini GA, Pawar AY. Access related complications during anterior exposure of the lumbar spine. World J Orthop. 2013; 4(1):19–23

[60] Garg J, Woo K, Hirsch J, Bruffey JD, Dilley RB. Vascular complications of exposure for anterior lumbar interbody fusion. J Vasc Surg. 2010; 51(4):946–950, discussion 950

[61] Kunakornsawat S, Prasartritha T, Korbsook P, Vannaprasert N, Tungsiripat R, Tansatit T. Variations of the iliolumbar and ascending lumbar veins. J Spinal Disord Tech. 2012; 25(8):433–436

[62] Edgard-Rosa G, Geneste G, Nègre G, Marnay T. Midline anterior approach from the right side to the lumbar spine for interbody fusion and total disc replacement: a new mobilization technique of the vena cava. Spine. 2012; 37(9):E562–E569

[63] Sasso RC, LeHuec JC, Shaffrey C, Spine Interbody Research Group. Iliac crest bone graft donor site pain after anterior lumbar interbody fusion: a prospective patient satisfaction outcome assessment. J Spinal Disord Tech. 2005; 18 Suppl:S77–S81

[64] Comer GC, Smith MW, Hurwitz EL, Mitsunaga KA, Kessler R, Carragee EJ. Retrograde ejaculation after anterior lumbar interbody fusion with and without bone morphogenetic protein-2 augmentation: a 10-year cohort controlled study. Spine J. 2012; 12(10):881–890

[65] Dorward IG, Lenke LG, Bridwell KH, et al. Transforaminal versus anterior lumbar interbody fusion in long deformity constructs: a matched cohort analysis. Spine. 2013; 38(12):E755–E762

[66] Laws CJ, Coughlin DG, Lotz JC, Serhan HA, Hu SS. Direct lateral approach to lumbar fusion is a biomechanically equivalent alternative to the anterior approach: an in vitro study. Spine. 2012; 37(10):819–825

[67] Than KD, Wang AC, Rahman SU, et al. Complication avoidance and management in anterior lumbar interbody fusion. Neurosurg Focus. 2011; 31(4):E6

[68] Kalb S, Perez-Orribo L, Kalani MY, et al. The influence of common medical conditions on the outcome of anterior lumbar interbody fusion. Clin Spine Surg. 2016; 29(7):285–290

6 Is AxiaLIF Comparable to Open Fusion with ALIF and Posterolateral 360° Fusion at L5–S1?

MIS: Venu M. Nemani and Oheneba Boachie-Adjei
Open: John D. Koerner and Todd J. Albert

6.1 Introduction

Arthrodesis at the lumbosacral junction is the treatment of choice for a wide variety of spinal diseases, including but not limited to trauma, instability, tumor, deformity, and degenerative conditions. While spinal fusion can be performed via a variety of approaches and techniques, obtaining an interbody fusion is often desirable due to the favorable biomechanical environment and the ability to achieve indirect foraminal decompression and restoration of sagittal alignment via restoration of intervertebral height. Interbody fusions can be performed via several different approaches, all with their own unique advantages and disadvantages. The traditional open approaches include anterior lumbar interbody fusion (ALIF), posterior lumbar interbody fusion, and transforaminal interbody fusion.

The ALIF technique was first described by Lane and Moore in 1948, using a transperitoneal approach and autograft for degenerative disorders of the spine.[1] Compared to the transperitoneal approach, the retroperitoneal approach is associated with lower rates of retrograde ejaculation,[2] and is more commonly used today. Circumferential fusion with combined anterior/posterior (AP) procedures became popular for the treatment of iatrogenic flat-back syndrome[3,4] as well as high-grade spondylolisthesis.[5,6] In addition to autograft and allograft, numerous implants made of metal and other materials have been developed for implantation within the disc space from an anterior approach. While the ALIF procedure can be used in isolation, it is often combined with a posterior fusion procedure and/or decompression for various indications. More recently, "minimally invasive" lateral and presacral approaches to obtain interbody fusion have been described. While a lateral approach to the L5–S1 disc space is typically not possible due to anatomical constraints, the presacral approach takes advantage of a naturally occurring tissue plane between the anterior sacrum and the peritoneal contents to allow access to the lumbosacral junction.

6.2 Indications for Circumferential Fusion at L5–S1

The indications for combined interbody and posterolateral fusion include painful disc degeneration after the failure of nonoperative treatment, low- or high-grade spondylolisthesis, and revision surgery for failed posterior fusion. Interbody support is also important at the lumbosacral junction below long fusion constructs for adult idiopathic or degenerative scoliosis. Degenerative disc disease (DDD) is usually confirmed radiographically by decreased disc height and signal changes within the disc.

6.3 Advantages of Minimally Invasive Surgery

The benefits of the presacral approach versus ALIF include avoidance of a traditional transperitoneal or retroperitoneal dissection, which can be complicated by vessel injury, retrograde ejaculation, and postoperative ileus. The presacral approach also preserves the anterior longitudinal ligament and the anterior annulus, both of which are critical to the stability of the motion segment. Furthermore, the approach involves minimal dissection and is muscle-sparing, which theoretically can minimize postoperative pain. Lastly, the AxiaLIF implant (Baxano Surgical; Raleigh, NC) is unique in that it resists the shear stresses that predominate at the lumbosacral junction in cases of spondylolisthesis. The AxiaLIF rod thus resists anterior translation at L5–S1 and protects the posterior pedicle screw fixation, while an ALIF cage or graft alone does not.

6.4 Advantages of Open Surgery

An open anterior procedure allows for direct visualization of the disc space and complete preparation of the end plates, which provides a larger surface area to promote fusion. This approach also allows a more thorough removal of the disc, including part of the annulus fibrosis (AF) if necessary, which is not removed in the AxiaLIF procedure. Increased nerve ingrowth in the AF has been demonstrated in painful degenerative discs[7] and could continue to be a pain generator if not completely removed. Placement of a lordotic graft in the disc space can also help improve sagittal alignment—a benefit not possible with the AxiaLIF procedure, which only maintains preexisting sagittal alignment. These gains in intersegmental sagittal correction are not as successful with any posterior technique other than osteotomies. The indications for open AP fusion also include higher grades of spondylolisthesis, which cannot be done with the minimally invasive technique. Finally, as with most techniques of minimally invasive surgery (MIS), there is a steep learning curve and increased radiation exposure compared to the traditional open approach.

6.5 Case Illustration

The patient is a 51-year-old man with severe back pain and grade II isthmic spondylolisthesis with disc degeneration at L5–S1. The patient failed conservative treatment. Preoperative lateral radiograph is seen in ▶ Fig. 6.1.

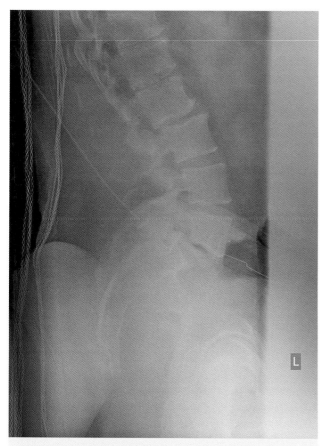

Fig. 6.1 Preoperative lateral radiograph showing a degenerative grade II spondylolisthesis.

6.6 Surgical Technique in Minimally Invasive Surgery

Before considering presacral interbody fusion, patients receive a magnetic resonance imaging (MRI) of the pelvis to ensure there is a safe fat plane devoid of vascular structures separating the visceral peritoneum from the anterior sacral wall, to allow for an appropriate corridor to pass the implant. This percutaneous procedure is contraindicated in patients with extensive vasculature in this plane or those who have retroperitoneal scarring from previous procedures.

Patients undergo a standard bowel prep using GoLYTELY. Patients are positioned prone on a flat Jackson table with all bony prominences well padded. In this case, we would begin with a standard midline posterior approach to the spine for reduction and instrumentation of L5 and S1 with pedicle screws. Reduction of the spondylolisthesis is achieved by bringing the spine to bilateral rods fixed distally. The facet joints and transverse processes are decorticated, and local bone graft and graft extenders are placed to encourage a posterolateral fusion. The posterior procedure could also be performed in a minimally invasive fashion using percutaneous screws.

Presacral interbody fusion can proceed using the same prone patient positioning without a separate prep and drape; however, in practice, we usually close and dress the posterior wound and reposition the patient with an additional pillow underneath the hips to maximize hip flexion. Two C-arms are needed to obtain simultaneous AP and lateral views. We also usually exclude the previous wound from the surgical field to minimize risk of contamination.

A 3-cm transverse incision is made on the right buttock next to the coccygeal area. We utilize a transverse incision because it reduces the risk of wound dehiscence with sitting. The ligamentous fascia is exposed bluntly to the presacral region using a curved Kelly clamp turned toward the anterior surface of the sacrum. Next, under fluoroscopy, a blunt dissecting tool is then advanced along the midline of the sacrum to the S1–S2 level. Then, the inner blunt stylet is exchanged for a guide pin that is tapped into the S1 vertebral body, across the L5–S1 disc space, and 1 to 2 mm into the L5 vertebral body under fluoroscopic visualization. A series of dilators are then passed over the guide pin to dilate the sacral implant tract. A working cannula is then secured into place to allow for drilling of an osseous path from the anterior sacrum through S1 into the L5–S1 disc space. The discectomy is then performed using radial and down-cutting blades. The disc space is then typically packed using local bone and a graft extender, with our preference being cancellous allograft chips. If the disc space is felt to be relatively large, then 2-mg bone morphogenetic protein (BMP; without a collagen sponge) mixed with demineralized bone matrix and local bone is used to pack the disc space. The discectomy is followed by insertion of exchange cannulas to allow passage of the threaded AxiaLIF rod. A nondistracting rod is used when posterior fixation is performed as the first stage and no further distraction is needed. Closure is performed in layers as per routine.

6.7 Surgical Technique in Open Surgery

The patient is placed in the supine position. After induction of general anesthesia and placement of an endotracheal tube, the abdomen is prepped and draped. A low transverse incision is made through the skin and subcutaneous tissue, the fascia is divided, and rectus muscles are split in the midline. The preperitoneal and left-sided retroperitoneal space is entered. The L5–S1 disc space is approached at the confluence of the iliac veins. At this level, mobilization of the vascular structures may not be necessary, other than the middle sacral vessels. An X-ray marker is placed and confirms the appropriate level. After incising and removing the disc, a curette is used to gently remove the cartilaginous end plates of the vertebral bodies above and below the interspace. After squaring off the end plates, a rasp is used to further refine and smooth the end plates and to expose bleeding bone across both surfaces. In addition to allograft, a variety of interbody implants are available today, including threaded interbody devices, lumbar tapered devices, PEEK (polyetheretherketone) cages, and titanium mesh cages. Regardless of the device chosen, appropriate sizing and placement is key, ideally countersunk a few millimeters, without protruding posteriorly. Imaging is obtained to confirm appropriate positioning within the disc space. The rectus is then reapproximated with Vicryl sutures, and the fascia is closed with running #1 PDS suture. Subcutaneous tissue is reapproximated with 3-0 Vicryl suture, and the skin is closed with a running subcuticular closure.

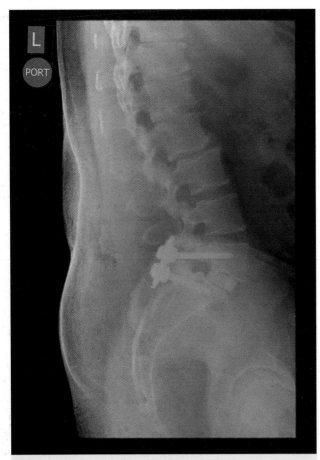

Fig. 6.2 Postoperative lateral radiograph. The lumbar fascia is then closed, followed by the subcutaneous tissue and skin.

The patient is then transferred to the prone position. A midline incision is centered over the surgical levels, and continues through the fascia. Subperiosteal dissection is performed to expose the spinous processes, lamina, and facet joints, and continued laterally to the transverse processes. If indicated, decompression can be performed before or after pedicle screw placement, if instrumentation is necessary. The bone over the lateral pars, facet joints, and transverse processes is then decorticated with a high-speed burr. The lamina and spinous processes can also be decorticated if a decompression was not done. Bone graft is then placed across the fusion bed and lateral gutters. The lumbar fascia is then closed, followed by the subcutaneous tissue and skin. Postoperative lateral radiograph is seen in ▶ Fig. 6.2.

6.8 Discussion of Minimally Invasive Surgery

6.8.1 Level I Evidence in Minimally Invasive Surgery

There is no level I study available.

6.8.2 Level II Evidence in Minimally Invasive Surgery

There is no level II study available.

6.8.3 Level III and IV Evidence in Minimally Invasive Surgery

Only one recently published level III study has directly compared ALIF with AxiaLIF for fusion across the lumbosacral junction. Whang and colleagues retrospectively examined 96 patients (48 patients in each group) who underwent circumferential fusion at L5–S1 with either ALIF or AxiaLIF for interbody fixation as well as supplemental posterior fixation.[8] Of note, 5 out of 48 of the ALIF cohort had stand-alone procedures without supplemental posterior fixation. In the ALIF cohort, 21 patients underwent placement of a femoral ring allograft, while 27 patients had placement of a PEEK cage for interbody support. All patients had 2 years of clinical and radiographic (X-rays and computed tomography [CT] scan) follow-up. The primary end point was fusion status on both X-rays and CT at 24 months postoperatively. At 2-year follow-up, 79% of patients in the ALIF cohort had solid fusions compared to 85% of patients in the AxiaLIF cohort ($p > 0.05$). There were 16 adverse events in 10 patients in the ALIF group, which included one left common iliac artery injury and one peritoneal laceration. There were 10 adverse events in 6 patients in the AxiaLIF group, including 3 patients with local infections, 2 of which required irrigation and debridement. There were no instances of bowel perforation or other visceral or vascular injury in the AxiaLIF group.

There have been several level III and IV studies examining presacral interbody fusion for various diagnoses. Gerszten and colleagues examined 26 patients with symptomatic L5–S1 isthmic spondylolisthesis treated with AxiaLIF combined with percutaneous posterior fixation.[9] All patients showed solid fusion at 2-year follow-up, with 81% of patients having an excellent or good result. Members of the same group also examined AxiaLIF without and without the use of rhBMP-2 at L5–S1, and found no significant difference in clinical outcomes or in complication rate between the two groups ($p = 0.27$). Fusion rates were 96% with rhBMP-2 and 93% without rhBMP-2 at 2-year follow-up.[10] Issack and Boachie-Adjei retrospectively evaluated nine patients who underwent presacral interbody fusion at the end of a long fusion construct for spinal deformity. The patients had no major complications, and the authors did not find any evidence of implant subsidence at 1-year follow-up, although two patients had pseudarthroses: one at L4–L5 and the other at L5–S1. There was a significant improvement in Scoliosis Research Society (SRS-22) scores at 1-year follow-up.[11] In a larger series, Tobler and colleagues examined the 2-year outcomes in a multicenter study including 156 patients who underwent AxiaLIF at L5–S1.[10] The vast majority of patients had preoperative diagnoses of DDD (62%) and spondylolisthesis (22%). They found a 63% overall improvement in pain score and a 54% improvement in Oswestry Disability Index (ODI) at 2 years and reported a fusion rate of 94%.

6.9 Complications in Minimally Invasive Surgery

Although presacral interbody fusion provides a relatively atraumatic, minimally invasive way to fuse the L5–S1 level, this approach is not without risks. As mentioned previously, it is very important to obtain preoperative imaging studies that ensure that there is a well-developed and safe plane between the abdominal and pelvic viscera and the anterior sacrum. There have been multiple reports of bowel injury during this approach,[12,13] which can have a delayed presentation.[14] Lindley and colleagues reported the overall complication rate in their series of 68 patients who underwent AxiaLIF with an average follow-up of 34 months.[15] They had 16 patients (23.5%) who had a total of 18 complications (26.5%). The complications included pseudarthrosis (8.8%), superficial infection (5.9%), sacral fracture (2.9%), pelvic hematoma (2.9%), failure of wound closure (1.5%), transient nerve root irritation (1.5%), and rectal perforation (2.9%) (▶ Table 6.2).

6.10 Conclusion in Minimally Invasive Surgery

Overall, the data show that presacral interbody fusion is a promising technique for obtaining interbody arthrodesis at the lumbosacral junction. There is, however, a notable lack of high-quality evidence examining the results of this technique and critically comparing it to other, more traditional methods of obtaining interbody fusion at L5–S1. With proper patient selection and the appropriate preoperative imaging and workup, AxiaLIF can generally be used with good results, a high fusion rate, and an acceptable complication rate compared to open techniques for L5–S1 fusion. This has been reported in multiple level III and IV studies. We therefore give a grade IC recommendation for AxiaLIF as a safe and efficacious procedure used in conjunction with posterior fixation to obtain a circumferential arthrodesis at L5–S1.

6.11 Discussion of Open Surgery

In theory, the minimally invasive presacral procedure for interbody fusion of L5–S1 avoids disruption of the anterior longitudinal ligament and annulus and the need for posterior fixation that is frequently needed with ALIF procedures. However, in the published studies of the AxiaLIF, most patients are supplemented with posterior fixation,[10,16] so it is difficult to isolate data for patients with stand-alone AxiaLIF. The indications for AxiaLIF include pseudoarthrosis, spondylolisthesis (grade I or II), or discogenic back pain.[16] Because there is only one study directly comparing AxiaLIF and ALIF with posterolateral fusion at L5–S1, data will be extracted from high-quality studies in which one of the treatment groups was ALIF with posterolateral fusion, and results will be compared to studies describing AxiaLIF. Higher quality studies that directly compare the AxiaLIF with open 360° fusion need to be performed to allow better comparison.

6.11.1 Level I Evidence in Open Surgery

There are several level I studies in which circumferential fusion is used as a control group to compare to new technology, such as lumbar disc arthroplasty. Results from the prospective, randomized, multicenter studies of the ProDisc-L disc replacement versus circumferential fusion have been published with up to 5-year clinical results.[17,18] The inclusion criteria for this study included a diagnosis of single-level DDD, as defined by back and/or leg pain, radiographic confirmation, an ODI of greater than or equal to 40, and failed conservative treatment of at least 6 months. The mean operative time for the 75 patients who underwent circumferential fusion was 229 minutes (SD, 75.9) with estimated blood loss (EBL) of 465 mL (SD, 440.0) and a mean length of hospital stay of 4.4 days (SD, 1.54). All procedures were one level, with 50/75 (66.7%) at L5–S1. There were no major complications (major vessel injury, neurologic damage, nerve root injury, or death), with 2/75 patients experiencing clinically significant blood loss (> 1,500 mL) and 2/75 patients developing an infection. There were no cases of retrograde ejaculation. At 2-year follow-up, 97% of patients were considered fused radiographically, and ODI had decreased from 62.7 (±10.3) at baseline to 39.8 (±24.3). Visual analog scale (VAS) pain assessment decreased from a mean of 75 preoperatively to 43 (±31.6) at 2-year follow-up.

The multicenter, prospective, randomized, controlled IDE study of the Flexicore artificial disc replacement (Stryker Spine; Allendale, NJ) also used circumferential fusion as their control group. The circumferential fusion group consisted of 23 patients, 17 of whom had the procedure at L5–S1. Mean operative time was 179 minutes, with EBL of 179 mL and mean hospital stay of 3 days. Baseline ODI was 58, which decreased to 25 at 6 months, 25 at 1 year, and 12 at 2 years. VAS pain assessment decreased from 82 preoperatively to 20 at 2-year follow-up. There were eight patients who had an adverse event requiring surgical intervention (three for wound infection, five for removal of instrumentation).[19]

6.11.2 Level II Evidence in Open Surgery

In addition to studies that compare circumferential fusion to disc arthroplasty, data can be extracted from studies comparing circumferential fusion to posterior-only fusion. In a prospective cohort study of posterior versus circumferential fusion for low back pain and grade I or II isthmic spondylolisthesis, 47 patients were treated with circumferential fusion. The mean operative time was 244 minutes (range, 195–330 minutes), with EBL of 355 mL (range, 200–1,100 mL) and mean hospital stay of 4.6 days (range, 3–7 days). Mean ODI at baseline was 53 (±16), and improved to 22.4 (±9.3) at 6 months, 16.7 (±7.2) at 12 months, and 14.6 (±9.6) at 24 months. The mean VAS for back pain was 6.7 preoperatively and 2.9 (±1.7) at 6 months, 2.6 (±1.7) at 12 months, and 2.2 (±1.6) at 24 months. There were nine reported major complications (one case each of deep vein thrombosis, iliac vein laceration requiring transfusion, transient retrograde ejaculation, postoperative new-onset clinical depression, transient L5 paresis, urinary tract infection with bacteremia, nonunion, hardware removal, and laminectomy/screw exploration).[20]

Table 6.1 Literature on ALIF with posterolateral fusion versus AxialIF

Author(s) (year)	Level	Study	Type	Pts	Operation time (min)	EBL (mL)	LOS (d)	Fusion rate	ODI baseline	ODI 2 year	ODI 5 year
Zigler et al (2007)	I	Prospective, randomized, multicenter	ProDisc-L vs. AP fusion	75 (50 at L5–S1)	229 (75.9)	465 (440.0)	4.4 (1.54)	97%	62.7 (10.3)	39.8 (24.3)	NA
Sasso et al (2008)	I	Prospective, randomized, multicenter	Flexicore arthroplasty vs. AP fusion	23 (17 at L5–S1)	179	179	3	NA	58	12	NA
Zigler and Delamarter (2012)	II	Prospective, randomized, multicenter	ProDisc-L vs. AP fusion	56 (out of original 75)	a	a	a	95.8%	a	a	36.2 (25.7)
Swan et al (2006)	II	Prospective cohort	Posterior fusion vs. AP fusion	47	244 (295–330)	355 (200–1,100)	4.6 (3–7)	97.9%	53	14.6 (9.6)	NA
Kwon et al (2005)	III	Systematic review	Approach for low-grade spondylolisthesis	170, 125	NA	NA	NA	98.2%	NA	NA	NA
Whang et al (2013)	III	Retrospective multicenter cohort	AxialIF vs. ALIF	96	NA	NA	NA	79% (ALIF) vs. 85% (AxiaLIF)	NA	NA	NA
Gerszten et al (2011)	III	Retrospective cohort	AxiaLIF ± rhBMP-2	45 (BMP) vs. 54 (no BMP)	60	87 (BMP) vs. <50 (no BMP)	NA	96% (BMP) vs. 93% (no BMP)	54.4 (BMP group only)	23.7 (BMP group only)	NA
Gerszten et al (2012)	IV	Retrospective cohort	AxiaLIF + PSF for spondylolisthesis	26	70 (AxiaLIF) + 75 (PSF)	Range 20–150 mL	1 (range <1–2)	100%	NA	NA	NA
Issack and Boachie-Adjei (2012)	IV	Retrospective case series	AxiaLIF for spinal deformity	9	94 (range 60–120 min)	NA	NA	78%	43	NA	NA
Tobler et al (2011)	IV	Retrospective multicenter case series	AxiaLIF at L5–S1	156	NA	NA	NA	94%	36.6	19.0	NA

Abbreviations: ALIF, anterior lumbar interbody fusion; AP, anterior/posterior; BMP, bone morphogenetic protein; EBL, estimated blood loss; LOS, length of stay; ODI, Oswestry Disability Index; PSF, posterolateral spinal fusion.

Note: Some ALIF data extracted from studies evaluating other techniques.

aData from same group of patients as Zigler et al (2007) study.

Table 6.2 Complications reported on ALIF with posterolateral fusion versus AxiaLIF

Authors (year)	Level	Study	Patients	Type	Major complications	Comments
Zigler et al (2007)	I	Prospective, randomized, multicenter	75 (50 at L5–S1)	ProDisc-L vs. AP fusion	0	
Sasso et al (2008)	I	Prospective, randomized, multicenter	23 (17 at L5–S1)	Flexicore arthroplasty vs. AP fusion	Eight patients required repeat surgical intervention (AP fusion group)	
Swan et al (2006)	II	Prospective cohort	47	Posterior fusion vs. AP fusion	4 (8%)	Three iliac vein lacerations, one retrograde ejaculation (resolved)
Whang et al (2013)	III	Retrospective multicenter cohort	96	AxiaLIF vs. ALIF	16 (ALIF) vs. 10 (AxiaLIF)	Iliac artery injury and peritoneal laceration (ALIF); no vessel or bowel injury (AxiaLIF)
Gerszten et al (2011)	III	Retrospective cohort	45 (BMP) vs. 54 (no BMP)	AxiaLIF ± rhBMP-2	None	
Gerszten et al (2012)	IV	Retrospective cohort	26	AxiaLIF + PSF for spondylolisthesis	None	
Issack and Boachie-Adjei (2012)	IV	Retrospective case series	9	AxiaLIF for spinal deformity	None	Two pseudarthroses
Tobler et al (2011)	IV	Retrospective multicenter case series	156	AxiaLIF at L5–S1	None	

Abbreviations: ALIF, anterior lumbar interbody fusion; AP, anterior/posterior; BMP, bone morphogenetic protein; PSF, posterolateral spinal fusion.
Note: some ALIF data extracted from studies evaluating other techniques

Five-year follow-up data are also available for the prospective, randomized, multicenter ProDisc-L trial using AP fusion as the control group, which was previously described in the "Level I Evidence" section. The lower follow-up rate of 74.7% at 5 years makes this level II evidence. Nonetheless, the AP fusion group had a 95.8% fusion rate at 5 years and an ODI of 36.2 (±25.7), down from 62.7 (±10.3) at baseline.

6.11.3 Level III and IV Evidence in Open Surgery

In a systematic review looking at the surgical approach and outcome for adult low-grade isthmic spondylolisthesis, the fusion rates and clinical outcomes were 98.2 and 86.4%, respectively, for combined AP procedures.[21] The data from these studies are summarized in ▶ Table 6.1.

6.12 Complications in Open Surgery

The anterior approach to the lumbar spine places major vascular structures as well as the hypogastric nerve plexus at risk. The L5–S1 disc space lies between the bifurcation of the great vessels, and the hypogastric plexus overlies the disc spaces. A vascular or general surgeon usually exposes the anterior lumbar spine; however, not all surgeons have the same level of comfort or experience with this approach. The incidence of vascular injury has been reported to be up to 15% in some series[22,23];

however, in two randomized prospective studies, there were no vascular injuries in a total of 101 patients during ALIF as part of a circumferential fusion.[17,19] Another review of a mini-open anterior approach in 686 patients by one surgeon demonstrated six arterial injuries (0.8%) and six venous injuries (0.8%).[24] There is a steep learning curve for this approach, and the experience of the approach surgeon can contribute to important operative outcomes, including blood loss and operative time.

Potential for damage to the hypogastric plexus is also concerning during the anterior approach, and can lead to retrograde ejaculation. The incidence of this complication can range from 0.42 to 5.9% of cases.[25,26] Utilizing a retroperitoneal approach, rather than a transperitoneal approach can minimize this risk.[2] In the prospective, randomized ProDisc L-trials, 0/75 patients in the circumferential fusion group experienced retrograde ejaculation,[17] and in a large review of one surgeon, the rate was 0.1%.[24] Damage to the sympathetic chain from excessive retraction on the psoas muscle can result in the patient feeling a sensation of relative coldness in the right leg, but this usually resolves (▶ Table 6.2).

6.13 Conclusion of Open Surgery

Open ALIF with posterior fusion has been validated by multiple level I studies as having a high fusion rate and low complication rate, with long-term follow-up available. Complete removal of the disc and a large surface area for fusion is obtained from the open anterior approach. The complications associated with the anterior approach can be minimal with an experienced approach surgeon. The data provide grade IA recommendation that ALIF with posterior fusion is a safe and efficacious procedure. There is only one level III study directly comparing open ALIF and posterior fusion to AxiaLIF, which provides a grade IIC recommendation that the two procedures are equivalent in clinical outcomes and fusion rates, as well as complication rates.

6.14 Editors' Commentary

6.14.1 Minimally Invasive Surgery

From its very inception, the likelihood of AxiaLIF successfully stabilizing the lumbosacral junction and achieving a high rate of fusion was marginal. This lesson had been learned at least a decade before from a minimally invasive procedure called the "transsacral L5/S1 fusion and instrumentation." In this procedure, tubular access to the L5/S1 disc space was achieved through bilateral transgluteal and transiliac wing approach. The significant advantage of this approach over the AxiaLIF approach was that it achieved bilateral, oblique purchase across the disc space, thus stabilizing across the instantaneous axis of rotation. Just as with the AxiaLIF procedure, however, adequate discectomy was difficult. Even with the superior biomechanics of this technique, however, it was found that without posterior instrumentation supplementation, fusion rates were only 60 to 65%. AxiaLIF, with its stabilization screw directly in line with the instantaneous axis of rotation (IAR), has had similarly low fusion success.

ALIF of L5/S1, on the other hand, has an excellent fusion profile, with relatively low complication rates. Complete discectomy can be reliably performed and verified under direct visualization. A large graft/cage can be inserted to cover the majority of the end plate surface area, and fixation/stabilization to the vertebral bodies can be performed anteriorly, thus eliminating the need for posterior instrumentation in many cases.

It has been argued that the "minimally invasive" benefit of AxiaLIF has significant advantages for patients. However, this advantage must be weighed against the success rate of the procedure itself. So far, AxiaLIF has not proven to be an improvement over ALIF.

6.14.2 Open Surgery

The limited biomechanical axial support alone eliminates AxiaLIF from being considered as a serious alternative to ALIF. Compared to ALIF, which creates two solid platforms for structural support following a thorough discectomy, AxiaLIF utilizes a suspect discectomy strategy. After removing whatever disc can be excavated blindly using curettes and shavers, the cage must be placed through a path drilled through the vertebrae, a process which removes much of the cage's structural support. A cage placed through this technique is less useful for resisting axial compression and serves more as a barrier to shearing forces across the disc space. Although anterior-based fusion strategies are typically thought of as providing the best opportunity for fusion to occur because of the advantageous biomechanical factors including compressive forces and large surface area, these advantages are largely forfeited in AxiaLIF because of the small volume of disc that is removed and the associated small surface area for bone grafting.

Innovative approaches often lead to better surgical techniques and hopefully to improved patient outcomes. A discriminating surgeon must gather evidence about the relative success of a novel technique and formulate a judgment about whether the technique is worth adopting to improve outcomes for their patients. ALIF has a long track record with well-described complication rates but recognized advantages over AxiaLIF in terms of the biomechanical environment for fusion and the likelihood of successful healing. The surgical technique, complication profile, familiarity of approach, and likelihood of clinical advantage are all unlikely to favor adoption of AxiaLIF over continued use of ALIF when anterior interbody support is needed.

References

[1] Lane JD, Jr, Moore ES, Jr. Transperitoneal approach to the intervertebral disc in the lumbar area. Ann Surg. 1948; 127(3):537–551

[2] Sasso RC, Kenneth Burkus J, LeHuec JC. Retrograde ejaculation after anterior lumbar interbody fusion: transperitoneal versus retroperitoneal exposure. Spine. 2003; 28(10):1023–1026

[3] Kostuik JP, Maurais GR, Richardson WJ, Okajima Y. Combined single stage anterior and posterior osteotomy for correction of iatrogenic lumbar kyphosis. Spine. 1988; 13(3):257–266

[4] Lagrone MO, Bradford DS, Moe JH, Lonstein JE, Winter RB, Ogilvie JW. Treatment of symptomatic flatback after spinal fusion. J Bone Joint Surg Am. 1988; 70(4):569–580

[5] Bradford DS. Treatment of severe spondylolisthesis. A combined approach for reduction and stabilization. Spine. 1979; 4(5):423–429

[6] McPhee IB, O'Brien JP. Reduction of severe spondylolisthesis. A preliminary report. Spine. 1979; 4(5):430–434

[7] Freemont AJ, Peacock TE, Goupille P, Hoyland JA, O'Brien J, Jayson MI. Nerve ingrowth into diseased intervertebral disc in chronic back pain. Lancet. 1997; 350(9072):178–181

[8] Whang PG, Sasso RC, Patel VV, Ali RM, Fischgrund JS. Comparison of axial and anterior interbody fusions of the L5-S1 segment: a retrospective cohort analysis. J Spinal Disord Tech. 2013; 26(8):437–443

[9] Gerszten PC, Tobler W, Raley TJ, Miller LE, Block JE, Nasca RJ. Axial presacral lumbar interbody fusion and percutaneous posterior fixation for stabilization of lumbosacral isthmic spondylolisthesis. J Spinal Disord Tech. 2012; 25(2):E36–E40

[10] Gerszten PC, Tobler WD, Nasca RJ. Retrospective analysis of L5-S1 axial lumbar interbody fusion (AxiaLIF): a comparison with and without the use of recombinant human bone morphogenetic protein-2. Spine J. 2011; 11(11):1027–1032

[11] Issack PS, Boachie-Adjei O. Axial lumbosacral interbody fusion appears safe as a method to obtain lumbosacral arthrodesis distal to long fusion constructs. HSS J. 2012; 8(2):116–121

[12] Botolin S, Agudelo J, Dwyer A, Patel V, Burger E. High rectal injury during trans-1 axial lumbar interbody fusion L5-S1 fixation: a case report. Spine. 2010; 35(4):E144–E148

[13] Siegel G, Patel N, Ramakrishnan R. Rectocutaneous fistula and nonunion after TranS1 axial lumbar interbody fusion L5-S1 fixation: case report. J Neurosurg Spine. 2013; 19(2):197–200

[14] Mazur MD, Duhon BS, Schmidt MH, Dailey AT. Rectal perforation after AxiaLIF instrumentation: case report and review of the literature. Spine J. 2013; 13(11):e29–e34

[15] Lindley EM, McCullough MA, Burger EL, Brown CW, Patel VV. Complications of axial lumbar interbody fusion. J Neurosurg Spine. 2011; 15(3):273–279

[16] Tobler WD, Gerszten PC, Bradley WD, Raley TJ, Nasca RJ, Block JE. Minimally invasive axial presacral L5-S1 interbody fusion: two-year clinical and radiographic outcomes. Spine. 2011; 36(20):E1296–E1301

[17] Zigler J, Delamarter R, Spivak JM, et al. Results of the prospective, randomized, multicenter Food and Drug Administration investigational device exemption study of the ProDisc-L total disc replacement versus circumferential fusion for the treatment of 1-level degenerative disc disease. Spine. 2007; 32(11):1155–1162, discussion 1163

[18] Zigler JE, Delamarter RB. Five-year results of the prospective, randomized, multicenter, Food and Drug Administration investigational device exemption study of the ProDisc-L total disc replacement versus circumferential arthrodesis for the treatment of single-level degenerative disc disease. J Neurosurg Spine. 2012; 17(6):493–501

[19] Sasso RC, Foulk DM, Hahn M. Prospective, randomized trial of metal-on-metal artificial lumbar disc replacement: initial results for treatment of discogenic pain. Spine. 2008; 33(2):123–131

[20] Swan J, Hurwitz E, Malek F, et al. Surgical treatment for unstable low-grade isthmic spondylolisthesis in adults: a prospective controlled study of posterior instrumented fusion compared with combined anterior-posterior fusion. Spine J. 2006; 6(6):606–614

[21] Kwon BK, Hilibrand AS, Malloy K, et al. A critical analysis of the literature regarding surgical approach and outcome for adult low-grade isthmic spondylolisthesis. J Spinal Disord Tech. 2005; 18 Suppl:S30–S40

[22] Rajaraman V, Vingan R, Roth P, Heary RF, Conklin L, Jacobs GB. Visceral and vascular complications resulting from anterior lumbar interbody fusion. J Neurosurg. 1999; 91(1) Suppl:60–64

[23] Baker JK, Reardon PR, Reardon MJ, Heggeness MH. Vascular injury in anterior lumbar surgery. Spine. 1993; 18(15):2227–2230

[24] Brau SA. Mini-open approach to the spine for anterior lumbar interbody fusion: description of the procedure, results and complications. Spine J. 2002; 2(3):216–223

[25] Flynn JC, Price CT. Sexual complications of anterior fusion of the lumbar spine. Spine. 1984; 9(5):489–492

[26] Tiusanen H, Seitsalo S, Osterman K, Soini J. Retrograde ejaculation after anterior interbody lumbar fusion. Eur Spine J. 1995; 4(6):339–342

7 Multiple-Level Interbody Fusion: How Do Two-Level Fusion Techniques Compare between Open and Minimally Invasive Surgery?

MIS: Christopher Clayton Hills and Robert E. Isaacs
Open: P. Justin Tortolani

7.1 Introduction

Lumbar interbody fusion, whether performed via the PLIF (posterior lumbar interbody fusion) technique as originally described by Cloward[1] in 1952 or via the TLIF (transforaminal lumbar interbody fusion) method as described by Harms,[2] is a technically demanding surgical technique which has a long learning curve. Epidural bleeding can be extensive, and numerous passes into the disc space are required in order to prepare the end plates appropriately. In addition, regardless of the technique employed (PLIF or TLIF, open or minimally invasive surgery [MIS]), some degree of nerve root retraction is required. While PLIF and TLIF techniques have been shown to enhance fusion rates when compared to posterolateral intertransverse fusion (PLF),[3,4,5] the risk of nerve root injury, dural tear, and the so-called battered root syndrome is higher.[6] Furthermore, Rampersaud et al[7] have elegantly demonstrated that the lifetime incremental cost-utility ratio (ICUR) for traditional PLF for focal stenosis due to grade I degenerative spondylolisthesis is $7,153 per quality-adjusted life year (QALY),[8] whereas the ICUR for total hip arthroplasty is $5,321 per QALY and the ICUR for total knee arthroplasty is $11,275 per QALY.[7,9] As the traditional benchmark for cost-effective treatment is $50,000 per QALY, lumbar decompression and PLF without interbody fusion is a justified treatment for spinal stenosis in the setting of spondylolisthesis. Considering these data as well as the additional costs associated with interbody implants, it strongly suggests that interbody fusions (whether single or multilevel) are not cost-effective for routine grade I degenerative spondylolisthesis cases[10] and, therefore, should be reserved for more complex surgical scenarios in which our current PLF methods will not predictably achieve the desired surgical outcomes. The focus of this chapter will be to compare and contrast the effectiveness of open vs MIS for two-level lumbar interbody fusion in appropriately selected individuals.

7.2 Indications of Two-Level Interbody Fusion

Evidence-based guidelines regarding the indications for single-level or multiple-level lumbar interbody versus standard posterolateral intertransverse (PL) arthrodesis have not been clearly defined. In general, lumbar arthrodesis following decompression for spinal stenosis is advocated for patients with gross instability (i.e., grade I spondylolisthesis with greater than 3 mm of translation on lateral flexion/extension radiographs or grade II or higher spondylolisthesis) or scoliosis. Lumbar arthrodesis has also been indicated in patients at risk for iatrogenic instability as may occur when more than 50% of the facet joint complex has been resected during the decompression.[4]

Severe mechanical back pain, due to facet arthritis and/or degenerative disc disease, is another potential indication for posterior spinal fusion. Nondegenerative conditions such as pyogenic vertebral osteomyelitis or pathologic (or impending) fracture due to infiltrative tumors represent additional indications for posterior spinal fusion.[11,12]

Interbody fusions, which employ the interbody application of structural bone graft or synthetic devices, have the added benefit of distracting the interbody space, which increases foraminal volume and facilitates sagittal and coronal plane deformity correction. By accessing the subchondral interbody region, open PLIF/TLIF procedures have been shown to increase fusion rates via increased surface area for bone healing, compression-loading of the graft, and exposure of the graft to greater numbers of osteoprogenitor cells.[13] Two-level interbody fusions are therefore indicated in degenerative conditions when restoration of foraminal height is needed to alleviate neurologic compression over two continuous levels.[14] Such clinical scenarios are often associated with some combination of spondylolisthesis, severe disc degeneration or herniation, lumbar flatback (as can occur with degenerative scoliosis, degenerative disc disease, postlaminectomy kyphosis, or spondylolisthesis), and scoliosis. Two-level (or greater) interbody device placement is also a powerful tool in restoring lumbar lordosis as a primary indication in association with posterior column osteotomies in patients with fixed sagittal plane imbalance.

7.3 Advantages of Minimally Invasive Surgery

McAfee et al in a summary statement defined MI spine surgery as "one that by virtue of the extent and means of surgical technique results in less collateral tissue damage, resulting in measurable decrease in morbidity and more rapid functional recovery than traditional exposures, without differentiation in the intended surgical goal."[15] Conventional open lumbar fusion techniques are associated with significant muscle stripping and retraction that can adversely affect both short- and long-term patient outcomes.[16,17,18,19,20,21,22,23] Recognizing the need for minimizing approach-related morbidities associated with open TLIF, Foley and colleagues introduced the MITLIF procedure, which utilizes a muscle-dilating approach and significantly diminishes the amount of soft-tissue disruption.[24,25] Since its introduction, a growing body of evidence has been reported on the advantages that include, but are not limited to, less intraoperative blood loss, less postoperative pain, decreased postoperative narcotic usage, early ambulation, and decreased length of stay in hospital.[24,25,26,27,28,29,30,31]

A steep learning curve, including the complexity of the MITLIF decompression via a unilateral approach, is argued as a disadvantage compared to the open procedure. There is no question that an open midline approach affords the surgeon a virtually limitless exposure for decompression utilizing familiar techniques and instrumentation. However, this advantage for the surgeon becomes a disadvantage to the patient, given that iatrogenic soft-tissue injury incurred from subperiosteal dissection and retraction leads to subsequent denervation and atrophy of back muscles, which has objectively been shown to adversely affect clinical outcomes.[16,18,19,20,22,23,28] The learning curve can be significantly shortened by combining the techniques utilized in open interbody fusion (OIF), percutaneous pedicle screw fixation, and MI microdiscectomy at hands-on didactic courses that are readily available, thus ensuring that patients are not subjects in the learning curve as inexperienced surgeons adopt this new technology. In addition, by utilizing this approach to gain experience with this MI technique, other factors debated as disadvantages such as operative time and radiation exposure will be improved upon. Furthermore, the risk of additional radiation exposure to the surgeon and operating room (OR) staff can be mitigated with the incorporation of image-guidance technology.

It was previously stated that MI screws are approximately 20% more expensive than traditional open screws, thus resulting in increasing implant costs for MI multiple-level fusion. Although this is a slight disadvantage of newer technology, implant cost difference is easily offset by the cost savings accrued by decreased length of hospital stay by MITLIF patients compared to open patients. In fact, a financial analysis performed by Singh et al evaluating single-level open versus MITLIF found lower total hospital direct costs over a 60-day perioperative period in the MIS versus the open group ($19,512 vs. $23,550).[32] In addition, McGirt and colleagues showed direct costs were greater in the OIF cases when compared to two-level minimally invasive interbody fusion (MIIF) due to increased prevalence of SSI in the open group ▶ Table 7.1).

7.4 Advantages of Open Surgery

According to Ockham's razor or "the principle of parsimony," the simplest solution to any given problem is the best solution.[33] At the most basic level, the main advantage of two-level OIF versus MIIF lies in its relative simplicity. OIF requires far less radiation exposure for the patient, provides better exposure and visualization of the relevant anatomy, is more versatile, and has a shorter learning curve. Extrapolating from single-level data, the radiation exposure for two-level OIF versus MIIF is less than 20 seconds versus 3 to 4 minutes.[34] Whether this 10× increase in exposure translates into greater risk for the patient or surgical staff in MIS cases has yet to be determined.

Open surgery enables the surgeon to decompress both sides of the spinal canal with similar techniques and instruments. MIIF generally incorporates a unilateral exposure in which the surgeon removes bone toward himself/herself for ipsilateral decompression and away from himself/herself for the contralateral decompression. This requires greater time to learn and increases the complexity of the procedure. Furthermore, in open techniques, the surgeon can employ virtually limitless lines of view for decompression and instrumentation, whereas lines of vision are constrained by the tubular retractor system in MIIF procedures. While this may not translate directly into

greater complications for MIIF, it increases the time to learn and the complexity of the technique. In addition, open surgery provides greater flexibility especially in cases with added complexity. In revision cases, for example, the epidural space is often scarred, making access to the interbody space difficult or impossible. In unilateral MIIF, the surgeon would have to abandon the technique on one side and make a separate contralateral exposure in such circumstances. Especially in two-level cases, this will add additional time and radiation exposure. This same rationale applies to cases of aberrant anatomy such as a conjoined nerve root or extensive epidural venous plexuses, which cannot be predicted preoperatively. Open surgery allows the surgeon to easily move to the opposite side for transforaminal disc space access without adding complexity (additional incision/incisions, radiation exposure, surgical time). In some cases, intraoperative circumstances such as ossification of the posterior annulus, rigid disc degeneration, and massive durotomy, the surgeon may elect to abort interbody graft placement. In open surgery, the intertransverse region can be easily accessed bilaterally, thereby salvaging many of the surgical goals, whereas MIIF exposure suboptimally exposes the ipsilateral intertransverse region and requires an additional incision and radiation exposure to expose the contralateral intertransverse region. Another advantage of OIF occurs in the treatment of deformity, in which the soft-tissue releases, which are routine components of the exposure, in addition to transfacet osteotomies, improve the potential for sagittal and coronal plane correction.

Another major advantage of open versus MIIF relates to implant costs. MI screws cost on average 20% more than open screws from the same manufacturer (personal communication). While cost-effectiveness studies have not been performed comparing two-level OIF versus MIIF, with increasing numbers of levels fused the direct implant costs become increasingly greater for MI cases.

Finally, in revision surgery, a midline incision as performed with an open approach provides unlimited access for handling numerous complications. Thorough lumbar wound irrigation and debridement for surgical-site infection (SSI), for example, cannot be adequately performed through an MIS portal.

7.5 Case Illustration

A 66-year-old man presents with 1-year history of progressive neurogenic claudication and weakness in the left quadriceps, left anterior tibialis, and left extensor hallucis longus refractory to multiple nonoperative treatment methods including physical therapy and epidural injections. Ten years prior, he underwent a successful L5/S1 microdiscectomy for severe sciatica. Currently, his walking tolerance was 50 yards and standing tolerance was 5 minutes before he felt as though he needed to sit down in order alleviate his leg symptoms. He rates leg pain to back pain as 80:20. After thorough discussion about the risks and benefits of continued nonoperative versus operative treatment methods, informed consent was obtained and the patient was consented for L3–L5 lumbar decompression with instrumentation and interbody fusion. Anteroposterior (AP) and lateral plain radiographs demonstrated multilevel lumbar degenerative disc disease with a lateral listhesis at L3/L4 and right-sided disc collapse at L4/L5 in the setting of a mild

Table 7.1 Two-level open TLIF versus two-level MITLIF and open TLIF alone

	Level	Study	Type	No. of patients	OR time (min)	EBL (mL)	Transfusion amount (mL)	X-ray exposure (s)	LOS (d)	Fusion	Outcome scores	Complications
Gu et al[14]	II	Prospective	MI vs. O	44 MI vs. 38 O	MI: 195 ±28; O: 186.6 ±23.4	MI: 248.4 ±94.3; O: 576.3 ±176.2	MI: 0; O: 94.7 ±165.9	MI: 45.3 ±11.7; O: 28.9 ±8.2	MI: 9.3 ±3.7; O: 12.1 ±3.6	MI 41/44; O 35/38	VAS-BP: MI, pre-op 7.3±1.2, 3 days post-op 2.2±0.6, at least 16 months post-op 1.7 ±0.6; O, pre-op 7.4±1.0, 3 days post-op 2.5±0.6, at least 16 months post-op 1.8 ±0.7 / VAS-LP: MI, pre-op 7.6±0.9, 3 days post-op 2.0±0.5, at least 16 months post-op 1.8 ±0.7	MI, 6: dura tear 2, superficial 2, overlong screws 2; O, 4: dura tear 1, superficial 3, overlong screws 0
Hackenberg et al[42]	III	Prospective	Single- vs. multilevel open TLIF	39 one-level, 11 two-level, 2 three-level	One-level: 173; multilevel: 238	One-level: 485; multilevel: 560				Overall 89%	VAS: one-level pre-op 7.8, 6 months 3.9, 24 months 4.3, 3 years 5.3; multilevel pre-op 8.2, 6 months 4, 24 months 4.8, 3 years 5.5	4: 1 deep infection, 1 L5 radiculopathy, 1 disc herniation, 1 pseudoarthrosis
Hee et al[43]	IV	Prospective	Open TLIF vs. open TLIF + AGF	Open TLIF: 111 total (50 one-level, 61 two-level) vs. open TLIF + AGF: 23 total (13 one-level, 10 two-level)	Open TLIF only: 172±46.6; open TLIF + AGF: 155 ±21.5	Open TLIF only: 808±686.6; open TLIF + AGF: 609 ±406.2				One-level 100%, two-level 90%		
Hioki et al[44]	IV	Retrospective series	Double PLIF	19	301 ±101.5	1,277.6 ±411.5 g					JOA score: pre-op 12.9±3.5, 6 months post-op 18.5±5.3, 2 years post-op 21.3±4.9	5 complications: 2 dural tear, 1 L3 radiculopathy, 1 PE, 1 spacer displacement
McGirt et al[38]	IV	Retrospective	Surgical-site infections; Single-level/multilevel open vs. MI PLIF/TLIF	5,170 total; single-level (848 MI PLIF/TLIF vs. 1,595 open PLIF/TLIF); two-level (588 MI PLIF/TLIF vs. 2,139 open PLIF/TLIF)								Surgical-site infections/surgical-site infections requiring surgical management; single-level (38 [4.5%]/16 [42.1%] MI PLIF/TLIF vs. 77 [4.8%]/31 [40.3%] open PLIF/TLIF); two-level (27 [4.6%]/10 [37.0%] MI PLIF/TLIF vs. 150 [7%]/61 [40.7%] open PLIF/TLIF)
Potter et al[45]	IV	Retrospective	Single-Level vs Multi-Level	100 patients: 64 single-level, 33 two-level, 2 three-level, and 1 four-level						Overall 94%	71% of patients narcotic-free at follow-up, 81% with back pain relief, 29% entirely pain free	22 complications: 5 wound infections, 4 GI complications, 7 transient radiculopathy, 6 dural tears
Salehi et al[46]	IV	Retrospective	Single level vs. double level	24 patients total: 13 patients single-level, 11 double level								

Table 7.1 (continued)

Study	Type	Level	No. of patients	OR time (min)	EBL (mL)	Transfusion amount (mL)	X-ray exposure (s)	LOS (d)	Fusion	Outcome scores	Complications
											Pseudarthrosis 10, instrumentation failure 2, deep surgical-site infection 1, dural injury w/ transient meningitis 1, hematoma 1, pneumonia 1, instrumentation failure 2 (2.3), deep surgical-site infection 1 (1.2), dural injury w/ transient meningitis 1 (1.2), hematoma 1 (1.2), pneumonia 1 (1.2)
Taneichi et al[47]	TLIF and b/l anterior column fixation	IV	38 one-level, 40 two-level, 8 three-level	Single-level, 202; two-level, 279; three-level, 337	Single-level 545; two-level 802; three-level 1,168					Overall population JOA: pre-op 10.6, post-op 24.9	Elderly: 3 wound problems, 1 CVA, 2 MI, 1 CSM, 3 lumbar compression fx, 1 knee joint dz, SI joint pain, reoperation for migrant implant 2 or additional lumbar decompression 2. Younger: 1 minor root injury, 2 wound problems, 1 dural tear, 1 lumbar compression fx, hip joint dz, 1 SI joint pain, reoperation for migrant implant 2 or additional lumbar decompression 1
Takahashi et al[48]	Open one- or two-level TLIF in older vs. younger patients	III	35 patients with age >65 y; 43 patients with age <65 y	237 ±67 in elderly; 230 ±63 in younger patients	173±92 in elderly patients; 1983±105 in younger patients			25.6 ±19 in elderly patients; 23.6 ±14 in younger patients	34/36 (94%) for elderly group, 44/45 (98%) for younger group		
Villavicencio et al[39]	MI vs. O (with BMP)	III	MI: 29 one-level, 14 two-level; O: 18 one-level, 10 two-level, 3 three-level or more	MI: one-level 192.5 ±51.0, two-level 297.7 ±43.4; O: one-level 219.2 ±74.0, two-level 360.6 ±101.4, three-level or more 429.0 ±166.9	MI: one-level 143.5 ±90.5, two-level 353.6 ±366.6; O: one-level 379.2 ±172.0, two-level 800.0 ±248.6, three-level or more 600.0 ±424.3			MI: one-level 2.8 ±1.8, two-level 3.8 ±2.2; O: one-level 4.4 ±2.1, two-level 6.2±2.9, three-level or more 3.0±2.0			MI, one-level: 1 CSF leak, 1 hematoma, 5 neural injury; two-level: 2 screw malposition, 1 infection, 1 neural injury; O, one-level: 2 CSF leak, 3 screw malposition, 1 graft malposition, 1 hematoma, 1 neural injury; two-level: 6 screw malposition; three-level or more: 1 screw malposition, 1 infection

Abbreviations: AGF, autologous growth factors; b/l, bilateral; BMP, bone morphogenetic protein 2; CSF, cerebrospinal fluid; CSM, cervical spondylotic myelopathy; CVA, cerebrovascular accident; EBL, estimated blood loss; GI, gastrointestinal; JOA, Japanese Orthopedic Association; LOS, length of stay; MI, minimally invasive; O, open; PE, physical exam; PLIF, posterior lumbar interbody fusion; SI, sacroiliac; TLIF, transforaminal lumbar interbody fusion; VAS-BP, visual analog scale for back pain; VAS-LP, visual analog scale for leg pain.

degenerative scoliosis (▶ Fig. 7.1). T2-weighted sagittal images in the midsagittal (▶ Fig. 7.2**a**) and left foraminal plane (▶ Fig. 7.2**b**) demonstrate severe central and lateral recess stenosis at L3/L4 and moderate stenosis at L4/L5, with severe narrowing in left L3 and L4 neuroforamina. T2-weighted axial image at L3/L4 (▶ Fig. 7.3**a**) demonstrates severe circumferential stenosis. T2-weighted axial image at L4/L5 (▶ Fig. 7.3**b**) demonstrates moderate circumferential stenosis.

7.6 Surgical Technique in Minimally Invasive Surgery

Positioning of the patient is no different than for an open procedure. Prior to prepping and draping the patient, fluoroscopy is brought in to obtain Ferguson's angles and marked these upon the Fluoro machine for later use in the procedure. We also mark the projection of the upper end plates of each level upon the patient's skin, and after obtaining 15-degree off-angle oblique images, we draw vertical lines on the skin corresponding to the

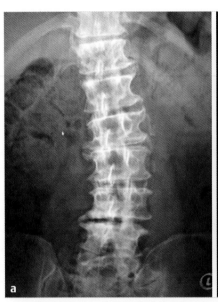
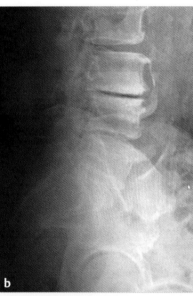

Fig. 7.1 (a) Anteroposterior and **(b)** lateral plain radiographs demonstrated multilevel lumbar degenerative disc disease with a lateral listhesis at L3/L4 and right-sided disc collapse at L4/L5 in the setting of a mild degenerative scoliosis.

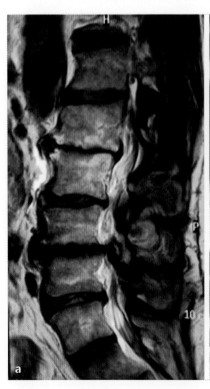
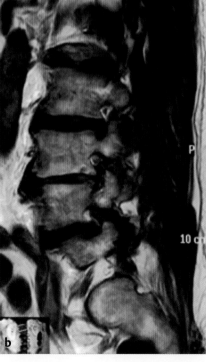

Fig. 7.2 (a) T2-weighted sagittal image in the midsagittal plane. **(b)** T2-weighted sagittal image at the level of the left foraminal plane.

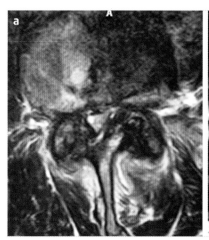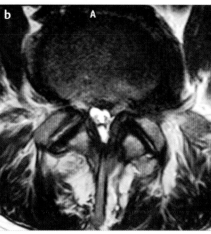

Fig. 7.3 (a) T2-weighted axial image at L3/L4 disc level. (b) T2-weighted axial image at L4/L5 disc level.

midpedicle line. These lines can help gauge the correct location of the incisions for the procedure, as they correspond to the correct trajectory for the screws and a TLIF approach. At this point, we prep and drape the patient.

Initially, we begin the procedure by serially, in turn, reobtaining each off-angle oblique Ferguson's angle so that we have in-line views down the pedicles bilaterally. We work by initially obtaining these images, determining the location of the pedicle, and placing a Jamshidi needle at the central portion of the pedicle radiographically. On the basis of these images, using the owl's-eye technique, we place the Jamshidi in line with the X-ray beam and then place a K-wire through the Jamshidi needle at approximately 1.5 cm. Once we confirm the location of the K-wire, we then shift our attention to the next off-angle oblique Ferguson's view and repeat the process, working to obtain all in-line views and place all K-wires prior to shifting to the lateral X-ray.

Under lateral fluoroscopy, once all are confirmed under the AP and off-angle oblique images, we advance the K-wires to midvertebral body. Then, we perform the following technique for each screw. We perform serial dilation, place a working channel, and follow this with a cannulated tap-awl through the pedicle. Care is taken not to advance the K-wire during this process. In this fashion, each screw pathway is prepared at the end of the procedure to simply place the screw in as soon as we reach that point in the procedure. The K-wires are secured to the drape.

At this point, we begin our decompression at each level, typically approaching from the side of the worst pathology. Specifically, the initial dilator is introduced through the aforementioned incision down to the facet complex. We serially dilate to a total of 21 mm, at which point a 21-mm working channel is placed in followed by a light source. The remainder of the case takes place through this.

Any soft tissue is removed and then we perform a unilateral laminotomy, drilling out the lamina out to the pars, with care taken to save as much bone as possible for locally harvested autograft. We use the yellow ligament as our guide. Once we had worked our way out fully laterally, we incise the capsular ligaments and remove en bloc the inferior facet. The yellow ligament is kept as our guide. We take a few small bites toward

both pedicles and use an osteotome to skeletonize down to the clean edge of the pedicles. In that fashion, we can fully decompress from a dorsal aspect of the exiting root. Only at this point we remove the yellow ligament and were able to visualize the traversing and exiting nerve roots. Care is taken not to place any undue pressure upon the exiting nerve root during this or any other portion of the procedure.

We eventually will do identical exposures at both levels. If we need to decompress across the canal to resolve stenosis, we will perform this next. When required, this begins by angling the working channel toward the contralateral side to decompress across the canal. We use the yellow ligament as our guide, drilling out the undersurface of the spinous process and lamina on the contralateral side. We drill the bone above the lateral recess contralaterally and then begin to elevate the yellow ligament circumferentially around the laminotomy. We palpate along the contralateral side, throughout the lateral recess, and out the foramen, ensuring adequate contralateral decompression as well. At this point, we work toward the ipsilateral side for the interbody fusion.

At this point, we incise the disc spaces and begin our interbody decompression. Specifically, after incising the disc space we take a combination of pituitary rongeurs, Kerrison rongeurs, Sypert impactors, and curettes to remove a majority of the disc material. We also work to prepare the end plates for accepting the interbody fusion. We remove the cartilaginous plate, preserving the cortical end plate if possible during this procedure. We serially dilate up in order to increase the size of the disc space, while protecting the traversing and exiting nerve roots, until we size up to a trial. Conversely, an expandable cage can be used. At this point, with the trial in position, when possible, we secure the screws from a contralateral side to maintain distraction in order to facilitate placement of the interbody fusion graft. Again, this is performed at both levels.

At this point, we begin packing the disc spaces with the graft material. Once we pack the disc spaces, we place a cage into the disc space while protecting the traversing and exiting nerve roots. It is confirmed radiographically and by direct palpation. Once in position and confirmed radiographically, we compress on the contralateral screws, and removed the extensions and began to work on the ipsilateral screws. Closure follows.

7.7 Surgical Technique in Open Surgery

Once informed consent is obtained, the patient is transported to the OR. Endotracheal general anesthesia is administered, a Foley catheter is inserted, and the patient is placed in prone position on the radiolucent Axis Jackson (Mizuho OSI; Union City, CA) table. The patient's hips can be flexed by bending the table, thereby reducing lumbar lordosis and facilitating access to the interlaminar space for the decompression. Proper space is preserved for C-arm entry and maneuvering in the operative field. Standard precautions are undertaken to avoid decubitus ulcers, venous engorgement from compression of the vena cava, and upper and lower extremity neuropraxias.

A midline posterior skin incision is made over the operative levels using anatomic landmarks for localization. The lumbodorsal fascia is incised in line with the skin incision and the paravertebral muscles are then subperiosteally dissected elevated from the posterior elements by detaching the tendinous attachments to the spinous processes (supraspinous ligaments). Care is taken to avoid muscle tearing or cutting and exposure beyond the lateral edge of the facet. A single, lateral fluoroscopic image or lateral plain radiograph is then obtained with a radioopaque marker affixed to the spine in order to confirm the appropriate spinal level. Self-retaining cerebellar or Gelpi retractors are inserted to maintain visibility of the three levels of interest (e.g., lamina and facet region of L3, L4, and L5 in case L3/L4 and L4/L5 two-level). A full, bilateral laminectomy and facetectomy is performed in patients with bilateral radicular symptoms; however, in patients with unilateral symptoms, a unilateral facetectomy and hemilaminectomy can be performed on only the symptomatic side. Establishing a rectangular work zone at the level of the disc lateral to the lateral edge of the traversing nerve root and caudal to the exiting nerve root is essential. Skeletonization of the caudal pedicle ensures maximum visibility of the superomedial aspect of the pedicle and is critical for protecting the traversing nerve root and preparing the disc space. Epidural bleeding is controlled with bipolar cautery and/or thrombin-soaked Gelfoam.

With Gelfoam in place in the transforaminal space, bilateral pedicle screws are inserted using anatomic landmarks into the vertebrae above and below. Once hemostasis is achieved, the Gelfoam is removed and the traversing nerve root and the thecal sac are protected with a nerve root retractor. A 15-blade is then used to create a box annulotomy, which should be sized according to the width of the desired implant to be inserted. A combination of disc space shavers, straight and angled curettes, and pituitary rongeurs is used to remove the intervertebral disc and cartilaginous end plate. A 3- or 4-mm Kerrison punch can be helpful in enlarging the annulotomy portal. Care is taken to not violate the end plates or the anterior annulus or longitudinal ligament. Depth markers etchings help to ensure that the interbody instruments (curettes, shavers, pituitary rongeurs) remain within the confines of the interbody space. Distraction of the interbody space via the pedicle screws or lamina spreader may facilitate disc space preparation and subsequent implant insertion.

After disc space preparation, trial interbody spacers are placed to determine implant height and depth that will maximize surface area of contact between implant and the prepared end plates. Once the implant is sized and the bone graft material is selected, the final implant can be tightly packed with morselized graft and carefully inserted into position. Additional morselized bone graft can then be placed around the interbody implant. Distraction (if utilized) is removed and the implant is assessed for adequate tightness in the interbody space. The procedure is then repeated at the second level. The bed is then brought into slight extension and the adequacy of the decompression is double checked by placing nerve probes through the foramen. Longitudinal rods are then connected to the pedicle screws under gentle compression. As long as access to the disc space is not impeded by excessive scar tissue, copious epidural veins, or a conjoined nerve root, our preference is to perform the TLIF on the patient's most symptomatic side. Satisfactory implant positions (pedicle screws and interbody devices) are then confirmed with single AP and lateral fluoroscopy or plain radiographs. Generally, three images are required for the entire procedure. Copious irrigation followed by standard layered closure is performed after hemostasis has been achieved.

7.8 Discussion of Minimally Invasive Surgery

The need for minimizing approach-related morbidity associated with open TLIF served as a catalyst for the introduction of MITLIF. McAfee and colleagues stated the justification of a procedure as "MIS" includes (1) reduced surgically induced tissue damage; (2) measureable clinical benefits such as lower blood loss, reduced surgical morbidity, reduced postoperative analgesic requirements, reduced length of hospitalization, and early resumption of activities; (3) clinical effectiveness; and (4) a favorable socioeconomic effect.[15] Although there currently is no level 1 evidence suggesting superiority of open multilevel TLIF, the available literature reveals potential advantages of MITLIF, including intraoperative blood loss, reduced need for blood transfusions, shorter length of hospital stay, decreased postoperative pain, and narcotic usage with at least comparable outcomes compared to open TLIF (▶ Table 7.1). Given these findings, the development of TLIF as an MI procedure is not only justified—it is a compelling technique in the armamentarium of a spine surgeon in achieving circumferential lumbar fusion.

7.9 Complications in Minimally Invasive Surgery

The MIS procedure is subject to the same complications as the open procedure. When performing an interbody fusion, there is a known risk to hardware malposition, infection, medical complications, and the like. Thankfully, the rate of nearly every complication is reduced with the MIS procedure relative to the open procedure.[28] What is clear from the Karikari compilation review of the MIS versus open TLIF literature is that medical complications and certain surgical complications (such as infections) are clearly diminished across the board in MIS TLIF series.[28] However, as is evident in both the Villavicencio and Silva reports, there is clearly a learning curve to performing their techniques well.[39,40]

7.10 Conclusion of Minimally Invasive Surgery

Although good prospective controlled studies had not been performed to clearly rest this debate, in general the data with respect to MIS surgery versus open surgery tend to favor MIS. While we would agree that any new technique has an associated learning curve, and during that learning curve there is an increased risk for complications, it appears that, once mastered, MIS surgery, and in particular MIIF, lowers the overall risk of perioperative complications. This comes with an overall lowering of the "costs" associated with surgery, including hospital direct costs, societal economic benefits, and direct patient benefits. Given this, it appears that the time and effort it takes to learn this technique is well justified. Having said that, MIIF is a viable technique with a long track record of success. Until controlled studies are performed, this debate will continue to rage on. A Grade 2C recommendation can be made for performing a two-level MITLIF.

7.11 Discussion of Open Surgery

Achieving the best outcomes in the safest fashion, at the lowest cost, with least trauma to normal and healthy tissue should be the goal of all surgical procedures. As summarized in the previous chapter, single-level MITLIF has not demonstrated long-term clinical superiority over open TLIF, and much needed prospective, randomized trials have not been performed comparing open versus MITLIF for single-level operations.[35,36,37] Evidence published to date suggests that single-level MITLIF in experienced hands may result in shorter hospitalization time and faster return to work, at the expense of a longer learning curve and increased radiation exposure for the patient and staff. The data comparing OIF versus MIIF in two-level cases are more limited, as summarized in ▶ Table 7.1.

7.11.1 Level I Evidence in Open Surgery

There are no level I studies available.

7.11.2 Level II Evidence in Open Surgery

Gu et al have published the only level II comparative study evaluating open versus MITLIFs.[14] They conducted a prospective cohort study of 82 patients comparing the clinical and radiographic results of open versus MITLIF for two-level degenerative lumbar disease.[14] Patients were randomized to undergo open versus MIS based on even versus odd numbered dates, respectively. At mean 20-month follow-up, they observed no statistically significant differences in leg pain, back pain, or Oswestry Disability Index (ODI) between the two groups. Intraoperative blood loss and length of hospital stay, however, were statistically significantly reduced in the MI cohort ($n = 44$) compared to the open group ($n = 38$). The fusion rates (93.2 and 92.1%) and complications (11 and 10.5%) between the two

groups were similar; however, the fluoroscopy time was greater in the MI cohort (mean: 45.3 seconds for MI vs. 28.9 seconds for open cases). These authors did not record the relative differences of radiation doses exposed to the surgical staff and patient or the implications of such.

7.11.3 Level III and IV Evidence in Open Surgery

As part of two larger comparative studies, patients undergoing two-level open TLIF versus two-level MITLIF have been evaluated.[38,39] In a retrospective study of 74 consecutive patients aimed at evaluating the safety of BMP-2 (bone morphogenetic protein 2) in open versus MITLIF, Villavicencio et al showed no differences in clinical or radiographic outcomes in 10 open versus 14 MI two-level cases. Importantly, preference was given to the open procedure in patients who had previous surgery or had bilateral disease and/or spondylolisthesis. Nonetheless, there were 2/14 neural injuries in the two-level MI group compared to the 0/10 in two-level open group.[39] Patient satisfaction, as analyzed by postoperative survey at most recent follow-up, was found to be statistically significantly better for the two-level MITLIF patients versus the open two-level patients.[39] To date, this is one of the only papers published to show fewer complications with open surgery.

In a retrospective study analyzing hospital billing and discharge data from 5,170 patients undergoing open interbody or MIIF, McGirt et al demonstrated statistically significantly greater prevalence of SSIs in 150/2,139 (7%) patients undergoing two-level open interbody versus 27/588 (4.6%) in the MI interbody group.[38] Although the two-level open and MI patients were not statistically significantly different based on the Charleston comorbidity index (CCI), the two-level open patients were statistically significantly older and more likely to have diabetes.[38] Importantly, in the single-level cases, there was no difference in age, diabetes, or CCI between open and MI groups and, perhaps not surprisingly, there were no differences in prevalence of SSI.[38] Due to the increased prevalence of SSI in the open two-level interbody cases, the direct costs were greater in the open group ($1,140/case) when compared to two-level MIIF ($756/case) group.[38] The authors did not provide a comparison of direct implant costs or indirect costs in their analysis.

7.12 Complications in Open Surgery

The most common complications of OIF include subsidence, osteolysis, postoperative radiculitis or radiculopathy, heterotopic ossification, dural tears, implant migration, and intraoperative neurologic injury. The overall complication rate varies from 8 to 80%, with an average of 36%.[10] Perhaps, the most disabling of all of the complications are the so-called battered root syndrome and severe postoperative radiculopathy, which has been recorded in 7% of cases.[10] These complications are not unique to open techniques and may occur with more prevalence in MI procedures, especially during the learning curve. In a review of open versus MITLIF cases, Habib et al report a nonstatistically significant increased rate of neurologic injuries and malpositioned instrumentation in predominantly single-level MI versus open cases.[35] In a retrospective study, however, Villavicencio et al have reported a statistically significant increased risk of neurologic injury in the MI group when compared to open in single-level TLIF cases.[39] In a recent study of 150 consecutive single-level MITLIF cases, Silva et al reported a 33% complication rate early in the learning curve, with dural tear being the most common.[40] Using surgery time for a single surgeon as the primary outcome, these authors estimate that overcoming the learning curve approximates 40 cases. In another consecutive series of single-level MITLIF cases, Lee et al estimated that overcoming the learning curve requires 30 cases, and during the learning curve, operative time, blood loss, and time to ambulation were statistically significantly inferior in comparison to postlearning curve cases.[41] Although these outcomes are not complications per se, they may expose the patient to additional risks for complications.

Given the greater amounts of soft-tissue exposure and retraction required to perform an OIF versus MIIF, one would expect to see greater rates of SSIs following open versus MI cases. Of the numerous articles published to date comparing open to MI single-level TLIF, a trend toward increased risk for infection has been suggested[35,36,37]; however, a statistically significant increased risk for infection has been demonstrated for two-level OIFs versus MIIF (see above section).[38]

7.13 Conclusion of Open Surgery

Whether interbody fusions, performed via open or MI methods, provide improved outcomes versus standard posterolateral fusion with instrumentation remains controversial. Furthermore, much needed prospective randomized trials have not been conducted comparing open to MI one- or two-level interbody fusions and interbody fusions to posterolateral fusions. Given the increased direct costs of MI implants, the long learning curve, increased radiation exposure, and lack of improved clinical outcomes, making the decision to embark on two-level MI interbody fusions remains an ethical consideration. Two-level OIF, however, remains time-consuming, can have extensive blood loss, and seems to require longer hospitalization time. Because of this, two-level OIF should be done in select cases in which the benefits of the interbody fusions clearly justify the increased risks. While the general indications for two-level OIF and MIIF are currently the same, identifying the best candidate for each procedure has not been elucidated, and patient selection criteria will likely evolve substantially as more information becomes available. A Grade 2B recommendation can be made for performing a two-level open TLIF procedure.

7.14 Editors' Commentary
7.14.1 Minimally Invasive Surgery

Using MITLIF technique to perform two-level fusions offers several advantages. First, particularly at L5/S1, both levels can be fused through the same size incision as a one-level fusion.

Thus, compared to the very large soft-tissue dissection required for a two-level open fusion, the advantages of minimizing soft-tissue destruction are even greater than when performing single-level fusions. Along with this, the known advantages of MIS surgery (e.g., less blood loss, less pain, less pain medication, less hospitalization) are even more evident.

The second advantage relates to time of surgery. One of the criticisms of MIS technique for multilevel fusions is that two-level surgery takes significantly longer than the equivalent open procedure. If a single surgeon is performing the procedure, this tends to be true. However, if the assistant surgeon is experienced in MIS technique, then each surgeon can work independently on opposite sides of the patient. In that case, a two-level MIS fusion can be performed in the same amount of time as required for a single-level MIS fusion.

Finally, one of the major advantages of MIS surgery is particularly important for two-level procedures. Unlike open surgery, MIS approaches do not devascularize or denervate the adjacent levels. This leads to a significantly lower incidence of adjacent level degeneration and the necessity of subsequent extensions of the fusion. These three factors combined make MITLIF for two-level fusions a very attractive alternative to open technique.

7.14.2 Open Surgery

Interbody fusion procedures present substantially greater technical challenges to the surgeon than posterolateral fusion techniques, which is reflected in operative times and learning curve. This difference is magnified in multilevel procedures and magnified to an even greater degree by utilizing an MIS technique. With only a very narrow set of indications to perform a posterior interbody fusion at two levels and the reluctance of MIS surgeons to perform isolated posterolateral fusion out of fear of nonunion, discussion of this procedure highlights the dependence of MIS surgery on interbody techniques. For many patients undergoing a two-level MIS interbody fusion, the most appropriate comparison group would be patients undergoing open posterolateral fusion, a procedure with lower complication rates. Nevertheless, even for this somewhat artificial comparison, there are several reasons to promote open procedures over MIS procedures.

The best available evidence as outlined above suggests no difference in outcome or complications for experienced surgeons performing open and MIS procedures. Such studies understate the influence of the increasing complexity of interbody and multilevel procedures on the learning curve. Eventual equivalence of outcome suggests that the average outcomes across a surgeon's entire experience would be lower for MIS techniques, although it is impossible to predict whether this would lead to a statistically significant difference.

MIS procedures are more challenged from a technical perspective than open procedures when encountering such anatomic variations or events as dural scarring, conjoined nerve roots, calcified disc spaces, or dural injury. Whether this leads to abandonment of interbody cage placement or unplanned contralateral exposure and instrumentation through a separate incision, this uncertainty can be disruptive for surgical scheduling and OR efficiency and forfeit many of the purported advantages of MIS surgery as well as being disconcerting to the patient and their family.

References

[1] Cloward RB. The treatment of ruptured lumbar intervertebral discs by vertebral body fusion. I. Indications, operative technique, after care. J Neurosurg. 1953; 10(2):154–168

[2] Harms J, Rolinger H. A one-stager procedure in operative treatment of spondylolistheses: dorsal traction-reposition and anterior fusion [author's transl; in German]. Orthop Ihre Grenzgeb. 1982; 120:343–347

[3] Audat Z, Moutasem O, Yousef K, Mohammad B. Comparison of clinical and radiological results of posterolateral fusion, posterior lumbar interbody fusion and transforaminal lumbar interbody fusion techniques in the treatment of degenerative lumbar spine. Singapore Med J. 2012; 53(3):183–187

[4] Herkowitz HN, Sidhu KS. Lumbar spine fusion in the treatment of degenerative conditions: current indications and recommendations. J Am Acad Orthop Surg. 1995; 3(3):123–135

[5] Kim KT, Lee SH, Lee YH, Bae SC, Suk KS. Clinical outcomes of 3 fusion methods through the posterior approach in the lumbar spine. Spine. 2006; 31 (12):1351–1357, discussion 1358

[6] Chrastil J, Patel AA. Complications associated with posterior and transforaminal lumbar interbody fusion. J Am Acad Orthop Surg. 2012; 20(5):283–291

[7] Rampersaud YR, Tso P, Walker K, et al. Comparative outcomes and cost-utility following surgical treatment of focal lumbar spinal stenosis compared with osteoarthritis of the hip or knee: part 2–estimated lifetime incremental cost-utility ratios. Spine J. 2014; 14(2):244–254

[8] La Puma J, Lawlor EF. Quality-adjusted life-years. Ethical implications for physicians and policymakers. JAMA. 1990; 263(21):2917–2921

[9] Tso P, Walker K, Mahomed N, Coyte PC, Rampersaud YR. Comparison of lifetime incremental cost:utility ratios of surgery relative to failed medical management for the treatment of hip, knee and spine osteoarthritis modelled using 2-year postsurgical values. Can J Surg. 2012; 55(3):181–190

[10] Moatz B, Tortolani PJ. Transforaminal lumbar interbody fusion and posterior lumbar interbody fusion utilizing BMP-2 in treatment of degenerative spondylolisthesis: neither safe nor cost effective. Surg Neurol Int. 2013; 4 Suppl 2:S67–S73

[11] Chen WH, Jiang LS, Dai LY. Surgical treatment of pyogenic vertebral osteomyelitis with spinal instrumentation. Eur Spine J. 2007; 16(9):1307–1316

[12] Kostuik JP, Errico TJ, Gleason TF, Errico CC. Spinal stabilization of vertebral column tumors. Spine. 1988; 13(3):250–256

[13] Cole CD, McCall TD, Schmidt MH, Dailey AT. Comparison of low back fusion techniques: transforaminal lumbar interbody fusion (TLIF) or posterior lumbar interbody fusion (PLIF) approaches. Curr Rev Musculoskelet Med. 2009; 2(2):118–126

[14] Gu G, Zhang H, Fan G, et al. Comparison of minimally invasive versus open transforaminal lumbar interbody fusion in two-level degenerative lumbar disease. Int Orthop. 2014; 38(4):817–824

[15] McAfee PC, Phillips FM, Andersson G, et al. Minimally invasive spine surgery. Spine. 2010; 35(26) Suppl:S271–S273

[16] Gejo R, Matsui H, Kawaguchi Y, Ishihara H, Tsuji H. Serial changes in trunk muscle performance after posterior lumbar surgery. Spine. 1999; 24(10):1023–1028

[17] Holly LT, Schwender JD, Rouben DP, Foley KT. Minimally invasive transforaminal lumbar interbody fusion: indications, technique, and complications. Neurosurg Focus. 2006; 20(3):E6

[18] Kawaguchi Y, Matsui H, Tsuji H. Back muscle injury after posterior lumbar spine surgery. A histologic and enzymatic analysis. Spine. 1996; 21(8):941–944

[19] Kawaguchi Y, Matsui H, Tsuji H. Back muscle injury after posterior lumbar spine surgery. Part 2: Histologic and histochemical analyses in humans. Spine. 1994; 19(22):2598–2602

[20] Mayer TG, Vanharanta H, Gatchel RJ, et al. Comparison of CT scan muscle measurements and isokinetic trunk strength in postoperative patients. Spine. 1989; 14(1):33–36

[21] Rantanen J, Hurme M, Falck B, et al. The lumbar multifidus muscle five years after surgery for a lumbar intervertebral disc herniation. Spine. 1993; 18(5):568–574

[22] Sihvonen T, Herno A, Paljärvi L, Airaksinen O, Partanen J, Tapaninaho A. Local denervation atrophy of paraspinal muscles in postoperative failed back syndrome. Spine. 1993; 18(5):575–581

[23] Styf JR, Willén J. The effects of external compression by three different retractors on pressure in the erector spine muscles during and after posterior lumbar spine surgery in humans. Spine. 1998; 23(3):354–358

[24] Foley KT, Lefkowitz MA. Advances in minimally invasive spine surgery. Clin Neurosurg. 2002; 49:499–517

[25] Foley KT, Holly LT, Schwender JD. Minimally invasive lumbar fusion. Spine. 2003; 28(15) Suppl:S26–S35

[26] German JW, Foley KT. Minimal access surgical techniques in the management of the painful lumbar motion segment. Spine. 2005; 30(16) Suppl:S52–S59

[27] Isaacs RE, Podichetty VK, Santiago P, et al. Minimally invasive microendoscopy-assisted transforaminal lumbar interbody fusion with instrumentation. J Neurosurg Spine. 2005; 3(2):98–105

[28] Karikari IO, Isaacs RE. Minimally invasive transforaminal lumbar interbody fusion: a review of techniques and outcomes. Spine. 2010; 35(26) Suppl:S294–S301

[29] Khoo LT, Palmer S, Laich DT, Fessler RG. Minimally invasive percutaneous posterior lumbar interbody fusion. Neurosurgery. 2002; 51(5) Suppl:S166–S181

[30] Kim KT, Lee SH, Suk KS, Bae SC. The quantitative analysis of tissue injury markers after mini-open lumbar fusion. Spine. 2006; 31(6):712–716

[31] Schwender JD, Holly LT, Rouben DP, Foley KT. Minimally invasive transforaminal lumbar interbody fusion (TLIF): technical feasibility and initial results. J Spinal Disord Tech. 2005; 18 Suppl:S1–S6

[32] Singh K, Nandyala SV, Marquez-Lara A, et al. A perioperative cost analysis comparing single-level minimally invasive and open transforaminal lumbar interbody fusion. Spine J. 2013; 14:S1529–S9430

[33] Carey TV. Parsimony, in as few words as possible. Philos Now. 2010; 81:6–8

[34] Bindal RK, Glaze S, Ognoskie M, Tunner V, Malone R, Ghosh S. Surgeon and patient radiation exposure in minimally invasive transforaminal lumbar interbody fusion. J Neurosurg Spine. 2008; 9(6):570–573

[35] Habib A, Smith ZA, Lawton CD, Fessler RG. Minimally invasive transforaminal lumbar interbody fusion: a perspective on current evidence and clinical knowledge. Minim Invasive Surg. 2012; 2012:657342

[36] Peng CW, Yue WM, Poh SY, Yeo W, Tan SB. Clinical and radiological outcomes of minimally invasive versus open transforaminal lumbar interbody fusion. Spine. 2009; 34(13):1385–1389

[37] Wu RH, Fraser JF, Härtl R. Minimal access versus open transforaminal lumbar interbody fusion: meta-analysis of fusion rates. Spine. 2010; 35(26):2273–2281

[38] McGirt MJ, Parker SL, Lerner J, Engelhart L, Knight T, Wang MY. Comparative analysis of perioperative surgical site infection after minimally invasive versus open posterior/transforaminal lumbar interbody fusion: analysis of hospital billing and discharge data from 5170 patients. J Neurosurg Spine. 2011; 14(6):771–778

[39] Villavicencio AT, Burneikiene S, Nelson EL, Bulsara KR, Favors M, Thramann J. Safety of transforaminal lumbar interbody fusion and intervertebral recombinant human bone morphogenetic protein-2. J Neurosurg Spine. 2005; 3(6):436–443

[40] Silva PS, Pereira P, Monteiro P, Silva PA, Vaz R. Learning curve and complications of minimally invasive transforaminal lumbar interbody fusion. Neurosurg Focus. 2013; 35(2):E7

[41] Lee JC, Jang HD, Shin BJ. Learning curve and clinical outcomes of minimally invasive transforaminal lumbar interbody fusion: our experience in 86 consecutive cases. Spine. 2012; 37(18):1548–1557

[42] Hackenberg L, Halm H, Bullmann V, Vieth V, Schneider M, Liljenqvist U. Transforaminal lumbar interbody fusion: a safe technique with satisfactory three to five year results. Eur Spine J. 2005; 14(6):551–558

[43] Hee HT, Majd ME, Holt RT, Myers L. Do autologous growth factors enhance transforaminal lumbar interbody fusion? Eur Spine J. 2003; 12(4):400–407

[44] Hioki A, Miyamoto K, Kodama H, et al. Two-level posterior lumbar interbody fusion for degenerative disc disease: improved clinical outcome with restoration of lumbar lordosis. Spine J. 2005; 5(6):600–607

[45] Potter BK, Freedman BA, Verwiebe EG, Hall JM, Polly DW, Jr, Kuklo TR. Transforaminal lumbar interbody fusion: clinical and radiographic results and complications in 100 consecutive patients. J Spinal Disord Tech. 2005; 18 (4):337–346

[46] Salehi SA, Tawk R, Ganju A, LaMarca F, Liu JC, Ondra SL. Transforaminal lumbar interbody fusion: surgical technique and results in 24 patients. Neurosurgery. 2004; 54(2):368–374, discussion 374

[47] Taneichi H, Suda K, Kajino T, Matsumura A, Moridaira H, Kaneda K. Unilateral transforaminal lumbar interbody fusion and bilateral anterior-column fixation with two Brantigan I/F cages per level: clinical outcomes during a minimum 2-year follow-up period. J Neurosurg Spine. 2006; 4(3):198–205

[48] Takahashi T, Hanakita J, Minami M, et al. Clinical outcomes and adverse events following transforaminal interbody fusion for lumbar degenerative spondylolisthesis in elderly patients. Neurol Med Chir (Tokyo). 2011; 51(12): 829–835

8 Is Lumbar Adjacent Segment Degeneration Best Treated Using Minimally Invasive Surgery over Open Fusion Techniques?

MIS: Luiz Pimenta, Luis Marchi, and Leonardo Oliveira
Open: Christopher M. Bono

8.1 Introduction

Lumbar fusion has been demonstrated to be a safe and effective surgical option for the treatment of a variety of degenerative conditions such as spondylolisthesis, dynamic instability, discogenic low back pain, and scoliosis.[1] However, fusion is not without its complications, both short and long term. One long-term complication that has received increasing attention in recent years is adjacent level degeneration.[2] Despite a large body of literature concerning this topic, full understanding of its risk factors, prevention, and treatment remains incomplete.[3]

Fueling this lack of clarity is variation of the definition and features of adjacent level degeneration among studies. These have included loss of disc height more than 2 mm, decreased lordosis or increased kyphosis of more than 5 degrees, disc herniation, acquired spondylosis, segmental instability, spinal stenosis, disc desiccation, dynamic translation more than 2 mm, spondylolisthesis, retrolisthesis, sclerosis of the adjacent end plate, and facet joint arthrosis.[4,5,6] These findings can be detected by combinations of plain radiographs, computed tomography (CT) scans, and magnetic resonance imaging (MRI). An important distinction should be made between adjacent level degeneration (ASDeg), which is characterized by radiographic findings, and adjacent level disease (ASDis), which is clinically symptomatic degeneration.[7,8,9,10] Likewise, the clinical criteria for ASDis have also been variably defined in the literature. Perhaps, the most controversial issue surrounding ASDeg/ASDis is its etiology, with some data suggesting that it is simply a result of natural degeneration progression and other studies making strong arguments that it is markedly accelerated (if not caused) by lumbar fusion.

Fortunately, the above controversies are beyond the scope of this chapter. This is not to disappoint the reader, of course, as what will be presented is a cordial debate about what is the "best" treatment of ASDis—minimally invasive or open surgery (▶ Table 8.1).

8.2 Indications of Minimally Invasive Lateral Interbody Fusion

Once ASDis has occurred, different surgical approaches and techniques can be performed to stabilize the adjacent level. One of these surgical options is lateral lumbar interbody fusion (LLIF) that was first indicated to treat degenerative disc disease above L5 level without severe central canal stenosis.[11] The development of this technique and its related instruments allowed the advancement of indications, which now includes indirect neural decompression by disc height restoration[12] and vertebral body derotation and coronal realignment obtained by ligamentotaxis.[13] Other indications for LLIF, with or without

pedicle screw supplementation, are pseudoarthrosis, discogenic low back pain, trauma, infection, sagittal alignment, spondylolisthesis, and especially adjacent level disease.[14]

The opportunity to access the operated site from a different approach avoids the manipulation of scar tissue and adhesions, making the procedure safer and more effective.[15] The advent of minimal invasive spine surgery enabled the achievement of good clinical and radiological results while minimizing collateral muscle and bone damage, with decreased risks and complications when compared to open techniques.[16]

8.3 Advantages of Minimally Invasive Surgery

One of the biggest advantages of the lateral approach is the opportunity to insert larger implants into the densest area of the vertebral end plate, reaching both sides of the ring apophysis that enhances primary fusion. The transpsoas approach for patients with scoliosis has been proven to be very effective.[13] Despite its minimally invasive features, the maintenance of the longitudinal ligaments, particularly the anterior longitudinal ligament, associated with the implantation of a large device results in the correction of the rotational deformity in addition to the coronal and sagittal deformities, without the risks, comorbidities, and complications related to standard open surgeries. In spondylolisthesis, a through discectomy itself partially reduces vertebral slippage. The maintenance of the anterior and posterior portions of the disc, keeping intact the longitudinal ligaments, allows ligamentotaxis, which is partly responsible for slippage reduction.[17] Disc height restoration has been proven to indirectly decompress the neural structures,[12] without the need of posterior laminectomy or pedicle screw supplementation, minimizing muscle splitting, blood loss, hospital stay, and operative time, and improving patient's recovery and satisfaction with the procedure.[14] Moreover, several clinical reports have emerged demonstrating the safety and efficacy of the technique in comparison to other conventional surgical approaches, with the same or better clinical and radiological results.[1,13,14,18,19]

Older patients with significant comorbidities who are unable to tolerate large, disruptive surgeries are among the biggest beneficiaries of lateral access surgery.[20] The most rewarding indications for these patients are adjacent segment degeneration and degenerative scoliosis. For adjacent level disease, the lateral approach avoids the previously operated approach pathway, either dorsally or ventrally, preventing access to scarred tissues. Moreover, the reconstruction of the anterior column is accomplished by the large interbody cage implanted laterally, which avoids injury to muscle groups accessed during the posterior approach,[21] and abdominal organs and vasculature that are more vulnerable in the anterior approach.[22,23]

Table 8.1 Clinical studies on MIS LLIF and open fusion for adjacent segment disease

Author (year)	Level	Study	Type	No. of patients	OR time	EBL	LOS	Fusion	Findings
Rodgers et al (2007)	III	Prospective	MIS	100	n/a	Average 1.34 g ↓	1.13 d	Average Lenke score 2.0 at 6 mo	No documented infections w/ improved VAS scores in 70% of patients at 6 mo
Karikari et al (2011)	III	Prospective	MIS	22	n/a	227	4.8 d	95%	5 of 22 patients treated for ASD w/ 95% of total patients showing radiologic evidence of fusion w/ improved clinical benefits
Le et al (2012)	IV	Retrospective	MIS	101	n/a	n/a	n/a	n/a	6 of 101 XLIF patients showing post-op complications (3 hardware failure, 3 VB fx)
Youssef et al (2010)	IV	Retrospective	MIS	84	199 min	155 mL	2.6 d	81%	Favorable fusion rate and improvement in pre-op VAS and functional scores w/ 6% post-op complication rate
Chen et al (2001)	IV	Retrospective	Open	39	n/a	n/a	n/a	94.9%	77% of patients experiencing clinical benefits and pain improvement at 2-year follow-up, 5 of 39 patients having further ASD, 2 requiring third fusion procedure

Abbreviations: EBL, estimated blood loss; LLIF, lateral lumbar interbody fusion; LOS, length of stay; MIS, minimally invasive surgery; OR, operation room; VAS, visual analog scale; XLIF, extreme lateral interbody fusion.

8.4 Advantages of Open Surgery

Open surgery for the treatment of ASDis should be considered the default technique for addressing virtually any type of pathology that can be encountered. This is particularly true for patients with adjacent level stenosis with or without some form of instability. The principles of revision decompression are well known to most spine surgeons.

While minimally invasive surgical techniques such as LLIF purport advantages of avoiding previous areas of surgical scar, thoughtful posterior surgical maneuvers can be performed to work within a previously operated field. Of most importance is appreciating that the anatomical plane between the dural sac and operative scar is tightly adherent. In our practice, this plane is left intact when possible in order to avoid dural injury and cerebrospinal fluid leak.

In cases of adjacent level stenosis, as is presented in this chapter's case, usually there has not been decompression previously performed at the new (adjacent) area of stenosis. Thus, any previously decompressed areas (provided that decompression remains adequate) do not require extensive epidural dissection. Instead, these areas are left "buried" within the scarified field, while the areas of new stenosis are carefully dissected free.

This consideration highlights a distinction in posterior revision decompression surgery that can be helpful. Cases of adjacent level stenosis are usually well addressed by a so-called fake revision laminectomy. In other words, despite the presence of operative scar, the interlaminar space with adjacent level stenosis has not been previously operated. Thus, once the laminae have been exposed (albeit through scar), the interlaminar window should be relatively virginal, with little reason to expect that the ligamentum flavum will be scared to the underlying dural sac. Illustratively, one can imagine the very typical case of adjacent level stenosis that occurs at L3–L4 years following an L4–L5 laminectomy and fusion. Provided that the previous decompression maintained the superior aspect of the L4 and did not enter the L3–L4 interspace, the surgeons should expect a "fake" revision at the L3–L4 level.

This can be distinguished from "true" revision laminectomy. Had the patient above undergone a full L4 laminectomy (from the bottom of L3 to the top of L5) with fusion only of L4–L5 and subsequently developed recurrent stenosis at L3–L4 secondary to ASDeg, the surgeon must dissect within the scarred dural sac from the bony borders of the previous decompression prior to revision laminectomy or facetectomy.

The primary advantages of posterior open surgery are versatility and direct decompression of the neural elements. As discussed above, regardless of the extent and location of the epidural scar, the bony borders can be defined and revision decompression can be performed. Moreover, decompression does *not* rely on any type of realignment. Whereas LLIF increases disc space height, which then is believed to indirectly decompress the spinal canal by tensioning redundant ligamentum flavum, posterior open revision laminectomy (whether "fake" or "true") does not require anatomical realignment. While proponents of LLIF extol its ability to reduce low-grade spondylolistheses via insertion of a tall interbody device, one should keep in mind that this can also be performed through a posterior approach (e.g., transforaminal lumbar interbody fusion [TLIF]). What is contestable, however, is the clinical benefit of reducing such mild deformities, particularly when the overall global balance of the spine is satisfactory. It is in fact our routine practice to not perform any substantial deformity correction unless indicated based on global sagittal alignment measurements. In further demonstration of open surgery's superiority, one can consider the common case of isolated foraminal stenosis in an area of previous decompression that is not associated with any significant deformity or misalignment. This can arise from hypertrophy of an unfused facet joint. In this case, it would be difficult to imagine how performing an LLIF procedure would affect any neural decompression. It is, however, easy to envision how an open revision foraminotomy and extension of the fusion can be an effective procedure.

The above arguments have only considered the advantages of open surgery for decompression. Similar arguments can be made for open surgery being the better approach to address issues involving the fusion. By nature of the diagnosis of ASDis, a previous fusion has been performed adjacent to a level of new pathology. In most cases encountered, fusion has been stabilized with pedicle screws. With the fear of sounding too obvious, what has been inserted through a posterior approach (i.e., pedicle screws) can be revised through an open posterior approach. While there might be a few, technically gifted and adventurous surgeons who would venture to extend a previous posterior pedicle screw construct through a minimally invasive approach, this is by no means something that is widely accepted. Justifiably, this is also not what has been proposed by Dr. Pimenta and his colleague in this chapter. It appears they would be satisfied with the stabilizing effects of the interbody cage alone, or perhaps with a lateral plate. It would only be in the rare cases in which no previous posterior instrumentation had been placed that one could expect the average spine surgeon to insert percutaneous pedicle screws at the adjacent level for stabilization.

8.5 Case Illustration

The images in ▶ Fig. 8.1 are that of a 61-year-old woman with a history of previous lumbar laminectomy and fusion from L3–L5 10 years prior to presentation. The patient's current complaints are of both back and bilateral leg pain, both of which she rates 8 of 10 on most days that are primarily claudicant in nature. She does have some pain in her back that is aggravated with sitting and standing for long periods of time, but her leg pain arises with ambulation. She has failed an exhaustive attempt at nonoperative treatment including physical therapy, epidural steroids injections, and acupuncture. On clinical examination, she presents with no neurological deficits, but has walking and standing intolerance.

Imaging studies show evidence of solid fusion from L3 to L5 without lucency around the pedicle screws. Importantly, on the T2 sagittal MRI images, central canal and bilateral foraminal stenosis (▶ Fig. 8.1d, left paramedian image; ▶ Fig. 8.1e, right paramedian image) is present at L2–L3 disc, which is suprajacent to the previous fusion. On axial T2 images, the central and bilateral stenosis is confirmed. CT sagittal reconstructions

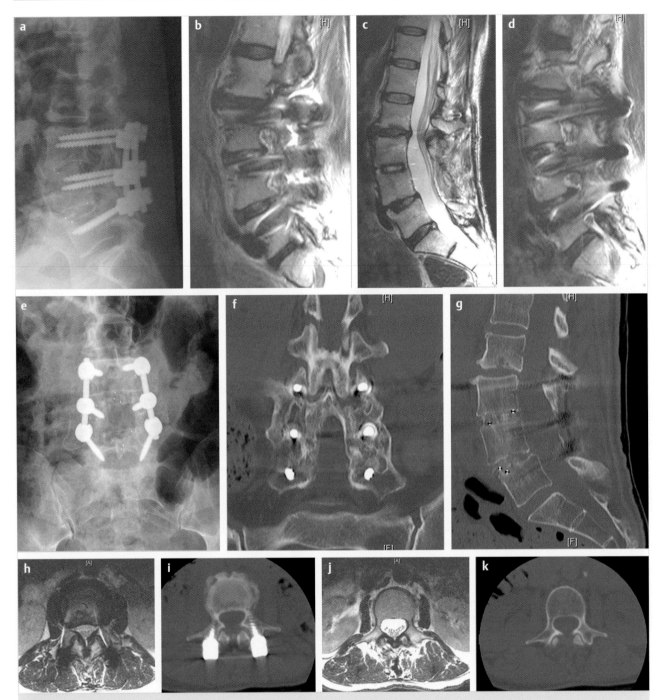

Fig. 8.1 **(a)** Standing lateral radiograph of the lumbar spine. **(b)** Left-sided paramedian MR image through the neural foramina. **(c)** Sagittal T2-weighted MR image of the lumbar spine. **(d)** Right-sided paramedian MR image through the neural foramina. **(e)** Standing anteroposterior radiograph of the lumbar spine. **(f)** Coronal CT reconstruction through lumbar spine. **(g)** Sagittal CT reconstruction through lumbar spine. **(h)** MR image at the level of the L2–L3 disc space. **(i)** Axial CT image through the level of the L2–L3 disc space. **(j)** MR image at the level of the L2 pedicle. **(k)** Axial CT image through the level of the L2 pedicle.

show a retrolisthesis of L2 on L3, while on standing lateral radiographs there is suggestion of local lumbar kyphosis at this segment. Flexion/extension views demonstrated no appreciable dynamic changes at L2–L3. Of note, it appears that the lamina of L3 is still present and that the previous decompression did not enter the L2–L3 interlaminar space (▶ Fig. 8.1**h**). This is noted on both the MRI and CT images.

8.6 Surgical Technique in Minimally Invasive Surgery

8.6.1 Patient Positioning

In the operating room, the first step is the placement of surface electrodes from an electromyography system that monitors the lumbar plexus during the psoas traverse, which is mandatory in this procedure. Four muscle groups per side are monitored as they represent spinal nerve distributions from L2–S2: vastus medialis, anterior tibialis, biceps femoris, and medial gastrocnemius. Also, a reference electrode is placed upper to the lateral thigh, and a return electrode is placed superior to the operative site, such as on the latissimus dorsi muscle. Proper skin preparation ensures good electrical conductivity. The patient is transferred onto a radiopaque bendable surgical table in a direct lateral decubitus position (90°), perpendicular to the table, with the greater trochanter directly positioned over the table break and with legs and knees slightly bent. The four adhesive strips to attach the patient are: (1) torso, (2) iliac crest, (3) leg and knee, and (4) knee and foot. This configuration increases the space between iliac crest and ribs, especially relevant when accessing thoracolumbar junction or L4–L5 level.

The ideal positioning is confirmed by fluoroscopy, ensuring that when at 0° the C-arm provides a true anteroposterior (AP) image and when at 90° a true lateral image. It is substantial that the lateral fluoroscopic images show both vertebral plateaus and superior pedicles aligned, presented as a single line, and that the AP image reveals the spinous processes in a middle position, and pedicles as circumferences.

8.6.2 Lateral Retroperitoneal Access

Over the skin, the iliac crest, the transition between the last rib and the posterior abdominal wall, and the quadratus lumborum muscles must be marked. After skin asepsis, the central position of the targeted disc can be identified using two Kirschner wires and lateral fluoroscopic images, making a marking that covers the center of the affected disc space. Afterward, a longitudinal skin incision is made, over the intersection between the posterolateral muscles of the abdominal wall (abdominal internal oblique, abdominal external oblique, and transverse abdominis). A first fascia incision is made to permit the surgeon to introduce the index finger into the retroperitoneal space and gently create a pathway and releases all attachments of the peritoneum, providing a safe lateral entry. Once the retroperitoneal space is identified, a second fascia incision is made below the first skin mark to introduce the initial dilator. The index finger will safely guide all dilators up to the psoas muscle, protecting abdominal structures.

8.6.3 Psoas Traverse

The first dilator is placed upon the posterior third of the L2–L3 disc, as confirmed by AP and lateral fluoroscopy. Then, the fibers are gently separated by the initial blunt dilator, with concomitant EMG monitoring for assessing the closeness to the lumbar plexus. The dilator must be rotated in position to determine proximity and spatial distribution of nerves. The dilators in sequence are placed over the previous, always checking the EMG, until the final placement of the closed retractor. The working portal is connected to a suspension arm in order to prevent unwanted movement. After confirming the ideal position by fluoroscopy, the blades can be selectively adjusted to the desired diameter. A bifurcated optical fiber cable is attached to the retractor for optimal direct visualization of the exposure. Moreover, the retractor opening must be minimal, with the duration of muscle spreading as short as possible, since the lumbar plexus must be compressed during psoas traverse.

8.6.4 Disc Space Preparation

The L2–L3 discectomy is performed using standard instruments under direct visualization. The anterior and posterior portions of the disc containing the longitudinal ligaments must be preserved in order to keep intact the anterior and posterior longitudinal ligaments, responsible for ligamentotaxis and indirect decompression of the neural structures.[12,17,24] Contralateral disc removal and release of the annular ring with a Cobb are essential to ensure symmetrical distraction and proper bilateral decompression and to avoid coronal iatrogenic changes. Furthermore, this maneuver allows for placement of an implant that covers both side edges of the cortical apophyseal ring, maximizing the spinal plateau support. The complete removal of cartilage and rasping the cortical bone layer provides blood precursor cells and bone growth factors that facilitate bone ingrowth.

8.6.5 Device Insertion

Implant trials determine the proper cage height, length, and angle that must be utilized to reach the stipulated objectives. The entire process must be guided by fluoroscopic imaging. The ideal placement of the device is centered across the disc space from an AP view, and between the anterior third and middle third of the disc space from a lateral view. The ideal implant positioning also restores focal lordosis, especially at L4–L5.[25] The use of synthetic bone grafts instead of autologous bone is recommended, avoiding major postoperative morbidity. The final position of the implant must be checked by AP and lateral fluoroscopy. A lateral plate can be placed after graft insertion to supplement fusion, with care being taken to avoid existing pedicle screws during screw insertion.

8.6.6 Closure

The surgical site is washed and the retractor is closed. The portal must be slowly removed in order to observe the psoas muscle closure and confirm hemostasis. The incisions are closed in a standard fashion. No drain is required. The construct may be supplemented with the internal fixation system of choice, if indicated.

8.7 Surgical Technique in Open Surgery

8.7.1 Patient Positioning

After general endotracheal intubation, the patient is carefully positioned prone on a radiolucent, four posterior table. The abdomen is allowed to freely hang and all other pressure points are well padded and protected. The previous incision is marked. Using fluoroscopy, the level of the L2 pedicle is then delineated with a cross mark. The previous midline incision is then marked to extend approximately 2 cm above this mark.

8.7.2 Surgical Exposure

After sterile preparation and draping, incision is made and the exposure performed. Exposing the previously operated segment involves the following steps. First, dissection is taken within the midline down until the tips of the spinous processes of L2 and L5 can be seen. Because there are no spinous processes present at L3 and L4, the depth of the dissection must be inferred based on the upper and lower intact levels. Dissection then proceeds on either side of the spinous processes and is maintained in the plane between the paraspinal muscles and deep (epidural) scar. This proceeds anterolaterally until the pedicle screws at L3, L4, and L5 are exposed. Proximally, dissection extends in a similar manner to exposure the L1–L2 facet joint. Importantly, this joint should not be violated given it will not be fused in the planned construct.

Next, dissection is taken lateral to the L1–L2 facet joint and pedicle screws to expose the transverse processes and previous fusion mass (if present), respectively. The continuity of the fusion mass can be assessed at this time. Following this step, the end caps for the screws can be removed, followed by the rod. All of the screws are then assessed to ensure that they still have adequate fixation. If any screws are loose, they should be replaced with a larger diameter screw to gain stable fixation. In this case, a nonunion of the previous fusion mass should be strongly suspected, which does not appear to be likely in the presented case.

8.7.3 Revision Decompression

With these steps being completed, attention is now paid to carefully exposing the lamina of L2 and L3 as well as the intervening facet joint. The lamina and pars of L2 are first uncovered given they lie farthest away from previous decompression. Next, dissection is taken along the inferior aspect of the L2–L3 facet joint until the L3 lamina is visualized. This step is planned based on the imaging studies, which clearly demonstrate that there is a large residual L3 posterior arch remaining. The caudal aspect of L3 is left buried in epidural scar because this is an area of bone that does not need to be removed and will have dense adhesions with the underlying dural sac.

With these bony landmarks exposed, a "fake" revision laminectomy can now be performed in a similar manner to a virgin procedure. A large rongeur is used to remove the inferior half of the L2 spinous process and thin the corresponding lamina. If there is any L3 spinous process remaining (which does not appear to be in this case), the superior aspect can be removed at this time to reveal the interlaminar window.

Next, the ligamentum flavum is released from the inferior aspect of the lamina of L2 and medial aspects of the inferior articular process of L2. A Kerrison rongeur is used to complete the laminectomy cranially until the edge (i.e., insertion) of the ligamentum flavum can be seen. Laterally, as fusion and instrumentation is planned, the entire inferior articular process is removed. All resected bone is saved for autogenous bone grafting.

At this time, a curette is used to release the ligamentum flavum from the superior aspect of the L3 lamina and the medial aspect of the superior articular processes of L3. If there are going to be adhesions related to the previous decompression, they will most likely be encountered along the L3 lamina, so ensuring that there is a free plane between the flavum/dura and the bone prior to bone resection is paramount. The majority of the superior articular processes are removed with a Kerrison rongeur. The superior aspect of the L3 lamina is removed until the distal edge of the flavum appears to be released. If substantial foraminal decompression is needed, the entire superior articular process can be resected at this time.

With bone removal complete, the flavum is then mobilized starting in the midline. Using a Woodson elevator deep to the flavum in the midline, a #15 blade scalpel is used to vertically incise this structure. A pituitary rongeur is then used to retract one side of the flavum posterolaterally, while a Penfield 4 elevator is used to release any adhesions and ensure that there is a free plane between the flavum and the dura. If adequate bone removal has been performed, the ligamentum flavum should easily be removed en bloc and should demonstrate a well-decompressed central canal, lateral recess, and foramina. If adhesions are encountered, they may be carefully dissected free. If a plane is not achievable between the flavum and the dura, removal of the surrounding bone should allow the flavum to float posteriorly.

8.7.4 Extension of Fusion

Once decompression is complete, a burr is then used to decorticate the transverse processes of L2 and the proximal fusion mass of L3. Next, under fluoroscopic guidance, pedicle screws are inserted into the L2 pedicles. After confirmation of the placement of these implants, a rod is selected and inserted to span from the L2 to L5 screws. The construct is final tightened. Following wound irrigation with 3 L of normal saline, the salvaged local bone, having been meticulously cleaned of all soft tissue, is then packed over the decorticated posterolateral elements. If additional graft is needed, synthetic bone extenders may be used.

8.7.5 Closure

A subfascial drain is inserted through a separate stab wound incision. The wound is then closed in multilayer fashion. In revision cases, it is our preference to use nylon suture for skin closure.

8.8 Discussion of Minimally Invasive Surgery

Spinal arthrodesis has been utilized for several segmental spinal conditions, but its use alters the biomechanics and kinematics of the lumbar spine, increasing mobility of the adjacent levels.[26] The degeneration of a segment adjacent to a previous fusion has inherent complications that make surgical treatment difficult. The success of a revision spine surgery ranges from 60 to 80%.[25] Approaching laterally, the surgeon avoids extension of the previous instrumentation, scar tissue, and adherences. This itself reduces surgical time and its related morbidity that, allied to the characteristics inherent to the lateral procedure, has been shown to be effective in the treatment of several pathologies of the spine, including ASDis.[13,18,27,28,29] However, no comparative studies have been done in order to prove that lateral access surgery is superior to open approaches in the treatment of adjacent segment degeneration.

8.8.1 Level I Evidence in Minimally Invasive Surgery

There are no level I studies available.

8.8.2 Level II Evidence in Minimally Invasive Surgery

There are no prospective comparative cohort studies using minimally invasive approach specifically for the treatment of ASDis.

8.8.3 Level III and IV Evidence in Minimally Invasive Surgery

Rodgers et al[30] conducted the only specific study regarding lateral access surgery for the treatment of ASDis. They prospectively treated a case series of 100 patients with adjacent segment degeneration after prior lumbar fusion using the lateral approach. Of this cohort, 79 had undergone prior instrumented posterior fusion procedures, 15 had undergone prior uninstrumented posterior fusion procedures, and 6 had undergone anterior lumbar interbody fusion procedures. The authors documented little intraoperative blood loss, and the mean length of hospital stay was only 1.13 days. There were gains in disc height and slippage reduction in cases of spondylolisthesis. Lenke score showed good progression of fusion, while clinical outcomes improved significantly at all follow-up points. While this experience is very limited without a large number of level I and II studies, current results are encouraging. Karikari et al[31] reported a prospective case series of 22 patients that included 5 cases of adjacent segment disease in the thoracic spine. There were no neural, vascular, or visceral injuries or death. Clinical benefit was seen in 95.5% of all enrolled patients at a mean follow-up of 16.4 months, with the same percentage of fusion. Acosta et al[32] reviewed images from 36 patients who underwent fusion procedure by lateral approach, 5 of them operated due adjacent level disease.

Le et al[33] conducted a retrospective analysis of 101 patients who underwent LLIF with supplemental lateral plates for degenerative conditions, including ASD after prior lumbar fusion. The authors have found a 5.9% of surgical complication that included three cases of dislodged lock nut and lateral plate, and three cases of vertebral body fracture, all occurring in multilevel constructions. Youssef et al,[34] in a chart cohort review of patients, enrolled 84 subjects for several spinal conditions, including ASD, but the number of patients enrolled for each condition was not noted. Patients reached a mean follow-up period of 15.7 months, with 68 patients showing solid fusion and 14 patients with developing arthrodesis. The authors found significant improvements in clinical outcomes scores, radiographic measures, and cost effectiveness, with low complication rate and short operating room times, minimal estimated blood loss, and few complications. They found favorable long-term outcomes, with maintained improvements in patient-reported pain and function scores as well as radiographic parameters, including high rates of fusion, which makes the lateral access surgery a favorable alternative treatment for adjacent segment disease. Pimenta[35] presented his study's results in a 2013 Brazilian Spine Society Meeting, indicating that adjacent level disease must be the choice for a surgeon's first lateral access surgery. The recommendation was based on the fact that degenerative changes in upper lumbar levels are usually related to previous adjacent fusion, and due to the difficulties inherent in this kind procedure, the possibility to address the pathology from a different pathway will allow the surgeon to avoid previous scar tissue, facilitating the procedure. Another favorable feature described by the author is the fact that the lumbar plexus in upper lumbar levels are more posterior, making transpsoas surgery safer and easier.[36]

8.9 Complications in Minimally Invasive Surgery

A literature review mostly demonstrates low rates of complications in the immediate postoperative period, including hip flexion weakness or numbness ipsilateral to the surgical access (psoas weakness), and less frequently sensory changes in the lower limb, all resolved within 6 months.[1,12,29] Transient plexopathies (motor or sensory) and hip flexor weakness are the most commonly reported complication associated with lateral access surgery.[37,38] Sensory deficits are more prevalent than motor abnormalities, and transient psoas weakness is more prevalent than both. About 40 to 90% of these cases can expect resolution of their symptoms within 90 days; very few patients have symptoms lasting more than 12 months.[37,38] Manipulation of the psoas muscle is an obvious cause of hip flexor weakness in the absence of neurological etiologies. Thus, inhibition of the muscular contraction is expected postoperatively even without any intraoperative neural damage. Otherwise, the reports did not find a higher prevalence of thigh symptoms based on the number of levels that underwent transpsoas approach, or with the utilization of multiple procedures and approaches to achieve positive outcomes.

Subsidence is another well-described complication related to anterior fusion surgery. It is usually related to standalone constructs, and has been correlated to instability at the index level, possibly due to resection of the anterior and posterior longitudinal ligaments. Subsidence decreases distraction of the disc space and the indirect decompression of the neural structures. Also, it can cause a spinal imbalance, not reaching the proper correction of sagittal alignment. The implantation of wider interbody spacers by lateral approach has been proved to maximize the end plate support and allow a standalone construction with a lower incidence of severe cage subsidence, preventing acute pain onset and preserving surgical gains such as disc space distraction, sagittal alignment, and their effects on neural decompression.[39]

8.10 Conclusion of Minimally Invasive Surgery

Government and private payers are increasing their scrutiny of spine surgeries due to perceived overutilization and lack of level I data in support of such surgeries. This is ironic for several reasons. (1) It is very difficult to create randomized clinical trials for spine surgeries. (Who would agree to participate in such a trial?) (2) There are a host of newer technologies that are demonstrating proven results, yet payers continue to try to classify them as investigational or experimental.

Minimally invasive approach surgeons are finding that newer, less invasive technologies are proving to reduce operating times and patient length of stay, minimize damage to adjacent tissue, and improve patient satisfaction. This is particularly relevant to spinal deformities, stenosis, herniated discs, and fusions. In addition, reduced operative time and hospital stay associated with faster return to daily living activities are directly related to a reduction in surgery expenses. The lateral approach has been shown to be a safe and effective procedure to the thoracolumbar spine. Although the technique is not free of complications, its rate has been lower than other traditional methods of surgical treatment, being in most cases transient and related to the psoas muscle. Midterm follow-up results demonstrate that the technique stimulates spinal arthrodesis through a minimal invasive lateral approach, decreasing pain, aligning the spine in coronal and in sagittal planes, indirectly decompressing the neural elements by disc and foraminal height restoration, and treating the most varied spinal conditions with minimum blood loss and tissue scarring, but no level I studies are found in the literature.

There are no level I or II studies demonstrating safety and efficacy of LLIF for ASDis. There are a number of prospective case series and cohort studies providing level III evidence of the benefit of minimally invasive surgery (MIS) lateral fusion in the setting ASDis. Level III studies indicate a decreased length of hospital stay and excellent radiographic fusion rate when utilizing an MIS approach. In addition, there is level III evidence supporting low-complication rates with MIS lateral fusion. Using the Guyatt et al grading scale, the data provide a Grade 2B recommendation that MIS lateral fusion provides equivalent fusion rates and surgical complication rates when compared to open fusion for adjacent segment disease.[40]

Going forward, it is imperative that surgeons and their professional associations continually assess the value of the care we deliver using methods that allow us to compare one surgical intervention versus another, and also with nonsurgical disciplines and interventions. This is the new environment that we live in, and we must adapt.

8.11 Discussion of Open Surgery

8.11.1 Level I Evidence in Open Surgery

There are no level I studies comparing open surgery to MIS for the treatment of ASDis.

8.11.2 Level II Evidence in Open Surgery

There are no level II studies (i.e., prospective comparative cohort or lesser quality randomized controlled trial) comparing open surgery to MIS for the treatment of ASDis.

8.11.3 Level III and IV Evidence in Open Surgery

There are a number of lower level studies that have documented the results of open revision decompression for recurrent stenosis. However, these data can be difficult to interpret because of the various different procedures that have been used. In one cohort study of elderly patients undergoing nonfusion procedures, 36% were "very" or "somewhat satisfied," although significant improvements in VAS (visual analog scale) pain scores were noted.[41] In another study of 124 patients with an average follow-up of 37 months, 83% had "success," although the investigators did not use validated outcome measurements.[42]

There are a number of factors that influence the outcomes of revision lumbar spine surgery (LSS) surgery in ASDis. Adogwa et al found that a higher preoperative Zung depression score was associated with less improvement in Oswestry Disability Index (ODI) at 2 years after revision surgery for adjacent segment disease, pseudoarthrosis, or recurrent stenosis.[43] This was independent of other potentially variables such as age, BMI (body mass index), symptom duration, smoking, comorbidities, and level of preoperative symptoms.

Unfortunately, outcomes of surgery for ASD tend to be lumped together, despite the fact that this "diagnosis" encompasses a wide range of symptomatology and clinical diagnoses. Therefore, interpretation of available data is difficult. Chen et al[25] showed good or excellent clinical results in nearly 80% of patients treated with autogenous bone graft and pedicle screw fixation for ASDis. Unfortunately, a number of these patients ultimately developed additional levels of ASDis, almost half of whom required another operation.

8.12 Complications of Open Surgery

As with all spinal procedures, there are numerous adverse events that can occur. Commensurate with both experience and the literature, revision lumbar surgery seems to be associated with a higher risk of complications. Among others, the most notable are dural tears, new-onset postoperative neurological deficits, and wound infections.

Dural tears can occur during any lumbar decompressive procedure. There is conflicting data regarding an increase of dural tear with revision decompression. Tafazal and Sell[44] found 13% of revision discectomies were complicated by dural tears in comparison to 3.5% in primary cases. Contrastingly, Wang et al[45] did not find a substantial difference between revision versus primary lumbar surgery. Furthermore, this group found that outcomes were not significantly affected by the occurrence of a dural tear that could be repaired primarily.[45] While MIS proponents report that dural tears do not require repair owing to the smaller incisions and dead space with their approach, tears with open surgery necessitate more careful attention.

Although rare, iatrogenic neurological injuries following revision open lumbar surgery can be disabling and permanent. Usually, it is limited to a single nerve root injury that results in varying degrees of weakness or anesthesia. It is not entirely clear that neurological injuries are significantly more common with revision decompression procedures that do not involve substantial deformity correction. What has been more commonly reported is nerve injury related to misplacement of pedicle screws. In one study, the rate of nerve injury with pedicle screw fixation in both primary and revision surgery was about 4%, half of which were permanent.[46] Pedicle screw misplacement may be more difficult with revision procedures if anatomical landmarks are obfuscated by scar or distortion of bony landmarks. The use of image guidance, whether by standard fluoroscopy or more complex navigational systems, can help reduce misplacement.

The risk of postoperative wound infection is increased with revision lumbar surgery.[47] This is thought to be the result of a number of factors. First, work is performed within a previously operated field that can have a compromised blood supply from dense scar and possible soft-tissue defects. Second, surgical duration is often longer with revision surgeries, which can predispose to infection. Early identification of postoperative infections is paramount, with deep infections requiring a thorough surgical debridement and an appropriate course of antibiotic therapy tailored to intraoperative cultures.

8.13 Conclusion of Open Surgery

From the arguments presented above, the reader should conclude that open surgery is the ideal treatment for symptomatic ASDis not only in this patient but also in nearly all patients with this condition. While minimally invasive techniques such as LLIF can be utilized in specific situations of ASDis that are uniquely amenable, open surgery can be used in all cases. In the case presented, it is reasonable to expect that LLIF can achieve fusion of the L2–L3 segment and, at least in the short term, produce some indirect decompression of the canal and foramina via height restoration. However, this relies on the absence of any subsidence and loss of fixation. Furthermore, it is not clear how the posterior pedicle screw construct can be extended to L2 using minimally invasive techniques.

What is more clear is that following an open "fake revision" laminectomy of the L2–L3 segment, the spine surgeon will be confident that the central canal, lateral recesses, and foramina are widely decompressed, which can be performed with near-complete avoidance of epidural scar. It should be clear to the reader that inserting two new pedicle screws into L2 is a familiar task that, again, will be performed in nearly virginal tissue. Although it would be our preference to perform a simple posterolateral (i.e., intertransverse) fusion in the presented case, a

TLIF could also be readily performed if desired. With the described techniques, this can be done safely and efficiently with minimal blood loss and reasonable expectations for symptom relief.

Based on the literature cited above, there are no level I or II studies investigating clinical outcomes of open fusion for ASD in comparison to MIS techniques. Level III studies do not lend significant focus on the efficacy of open fusion in the treatment of adjacent segment disease or its benefit over an MIS approach. Using the Guyett et al grading scale, the data provide a Grade 2B recommendation for improved pain relief and functionality following open fusion for ASD. However, the data provide a Grade 2C recommendation for the efficacy of open fusion over MIS techniques in superior clinical outcomes and radiologic evidence of fusion.

8.14 Editors' Commentary
8.14.1 Minimally Invasive Surgery

When considering whether to approach adjacent level degeneration through an MIS or an open approach, multiple factors must be taken into account. These include the patient's age, habitus, and comorbidities, what technique was used for the previous surgery (surgeries), if previous instrumentation will interfere with a particular approach, whether the patient has undergone previous intra-abdominal surgery, and the surgeon's experience with specific required skills for the procedure. It must also be kept in mind that regardless of whether a technique will be performed posteriorly or anteriorly, it can be done through either an open or an MIS technique.

The case presented here represents an interesting example of "supra-adjacent" degeneration resulting in lumbar stenosis without instability and consequent claudication. One option to consider is to do a simple MIS decompression of stenosis. This could be considered in that the pathology is not unstable and is not immediately adjacent to a nonmobile segment. Technically, the posterior rods would not obscure the approach and the procedure itself would not create instability at that level. This would transform a large operation into an outpatient or overnight procedure, and would not burn any bridges should another procedure be necessary in the future.

However, many would argue that in the presence of the previous two-level fusion, it is mandatory that the fusion be extended to this degenerative level. If one accepts this argument, then a host of questions must be addressed. One MIS option would be to perform stand-alone LLIF procedures at L2/L3 and L3/L4. If successful, this would enable a very minimally invasive procedure for the patient. However, even with ligamentotaxis, the ability to adequately decompress the central canal is limited. Moreover, the risk of subsidence of the grafts, particularly in elderly or osteoporotic patients, is not insignificant. In addition to the LLIF procedures, one might consider augmentation with posterior instrumentation. If the posterior instrumentation had been inserted using percutaneous MIS technique, then the instrumentation could similarly be extended using MIS technique. However, if the posterior instrumentation was placed using open technique and/or if the bone placed for posterior fusion has grown over the top of the rods/screws, then MIS technique would not be possible.

Finally, especially if the previous fusion and instrumentation was performed with MIS technique, then an entirely posterior procedure combining TLIF with extension of the posterior instrumentation could also be performed. With MIS technique, it is quite easy to remove the entire posterior instrumentation system, perform the decompression and fusion procedure without obstruction, and replace the instrumentation under direct vision.

8.14.2 Open Surgery

The treatment of adjacent level disease after spinal fusion is a relatively common procedure and one that is managed easily with any technique given the adjacent level has usually not undergone previous central decompression. The difficulty in avoiding a dural injury is often at the junction of the previous decompression and adjacent undecompressed bony and soft-tissue elements. The goals of an adjacent level procedure are typically stabilization and decompression. The case example used in this chapter is typical and describes single-level degeneration with stenosis. In a discussion of techniques which can be used to manage this single-level problem, the surgeon must first establish the need to improve or maintain sagittal balance. This raises the question of the need for an interbody procedure. The literature supporting the use of interbody fusion compared to posterolateral fusion alone is very scant, unless, of course, sagittal alignment needs to be improved; it is probably safe to say that the patient presented in this case has no strong indication for the use of interbody support. In addition, a stand-alone interbody device and indirect decompression is not a practical solution for patients with central stenosis and would be an even worse choice in patients with osteoporosis or osteopenia due to the increased risk of interbody cage subsidence. The track record of lateral plating (which is easily accomplished through the lateral approach used to place the cage) is mixed and numerous coronal plane vertebral fractures have been reported, many in osteoporotic patients who would benefit most from additional stabilization. Although the use of an interbody cage without posterior stabilization is appealing because of the potential for avoiding technically difficult revision posterior surgery, this treatment strategy will likely result in an unacceptably high failure rate if applied broadly.

References

[1] Marchi L, Oliveira L, Amaral R, et al. Lateral interbody fusion for treatment of discogenic low back pain: minimally invasive surgical techniques. Adv Orthop. 2012; 2012:282068

[2] Hoogendoorn RJW, Helder MN, Wuisman PIJM, Bank RA, Everts VE, Smit TH. Adjacent segment degeneration: observations in a goat spinal fusion study. Spine. 2008; 33(12):1337–1343

[3] Glassman SD, Carreon LY, Djurasovic M, et al. Lumbar fusion outcomes stratified by specific diagnostic indication. Spine J. 2009; 9(1):13–21

[4] Kim J-H, Kim S-S, Suk S-I. Incidence of proximal adjacent failure in adult lumbar deformity correction based on proximal fusion level. Asian Spine J. 2007; 1(1):19–26

[5] Lee DY, Lee S-H, Maeng DH. Two-level anterior lumbar interbody fusion with percutaneous pedicle screw fixation: a minimum 3-year follow-up study. Neurol Med Chir (Tokyo). 2010; 50(8):645–650

[6] Zencica P, Chaloupka R, Hladíková J, Krbec M. Adjacent segment degeneration after lumbosacral fusion in spondylolisthesis: a retrospective radiological and clinical analysis [in Czech]. Acta Chir Orthop Traumatol Cech. 2010; 77(2): 124–130

[7] Cheh G, Bridwell KH, Lenke LG, et al. Adjacent segment disease followinglumbar/thoracolumbar fusion with pedicle screw instrumentation: a minimum 5-year follow-up. Spine. 2007; 32(20):2253–2257

[8] Kaito T, Hosono N, Mukai Y, Makino T, Fuji T, Yonenobu K. Induction of early degeneration of the adjacent segment after posterior lumbar interbody fusion by excessive distraction of lumbar disc space. J Neurosurg Spine. 2010; 12(6):671–679

[9] Kim KH, Lee S-H, Shim CS, et al. Adjacent segment disease after interbody fusion and pedicle screw fixations for isolated L4-L5 spondylolisthesis: a minimum five-year follow-up. Spine. 2010; 35(6):625–634

[10] Park P, Garton HJ, Gala VC, Hoff JT, McGillicuddy JE. Adjacent segment disease after lumbar or lumbosacral fusion: review of the literature. Spine. 2004; 29 (17):1938–1944

[11] Ozgur BM, Aryan HE, Pimenta L, Taylor WR. Extreme lateral interbody fusion (XLIF): a novel surgical technique for anterior lumbar interbody fusion. Spine J. 2006; 6(4):435–443

[12] Oliveira L, Marchi L, Coutinho E, Pimenta L. A radiographic assessment of the ability of the extreme lateral interbody fusion procedure to indirectly decompress the neural elements. Spine. 2010; 35(26) Suppl:S331–S337

[13] Dakwar E, Cardona RF, Smith DA, Uribe JS. Early outcomes and safety of the minimally invasive, lateral retroperitoneal transpsoas approach for adult degenerative scoliosis. Neurosurg Focus. 2010; 28(3):E8

[14] Rodgers WB, Cox C, Gerber E. Experience and Early Results with a Minimally Invasive Technique for Anterior Column Support Through eXtreme Lateral Interbody Fusion (XLIF®). US Musculoskelet Rev. 2007; 2:28–32

[15] Pimenta L, Díaz RC, Guerrero LG. Charité lumbar artificial disc retrieval: use of a lateral minimally invasive technique. Technical note. J Neurosurg Spine. 2006; 5(6):556–561

[16] McAfee PC, Phillips FM, Andersson G, et al. Minimally invasive spine surgery. Spine. 2010; 35(26) Suppl:S271–S273

[17] Marchi L, Abdala N, Oliveira L, Amaral R, Coutinho E, Pimenta L. Stand-alone lateral interbody fusion for the treatment of low-grade degenerative spondylolisthesis. Sci World J. 2012; 2012:456346

[18] Pimenta L, Marchi L, Oliveira L, Coutinho E, Amaral R. A prospective, randomized, controlled trial comparing radiographic and clinical outcomes between stand-alone lateral interbody lumbar fusion with either silicate calcium phosphate or rh-BMP2. J Neurol Surg A Cent Eur Neurosurg. 2013; 74 (6):343–350

[19] Uribe JS, Smith WD, Pimenta L, et al. Minimally invasive lateral approach for symptomatic thoracic disc herniation: initial multicenter clinical experience. J Neurosurg Spine. 2012; 16(3):264–279

[20] Rodgers WB, Gerber EJ, Rodgers JA. Lumbar fusion in octogenarians: the promise of minimally invasive surgery. Spine. 2010; 35(26) Suppl:S355–S360

[21] Chrastil J, Patel AA. Complications associated with posterior and transforaminal lumbar interbody fusion. J Am Acad Orthop Surg. 2012; 20(5): 283–291

[22] Garg J, Woo K, Hirsch J, Bruffey JD, Dilley RB. Vascular complications of exposure for anterior lumbar interbody fusion. J Vasc Surg. 2010; 51(4):946–950, discussion 950

[23] Rajaraman V, Vingan R, Roth P, Heary RF, Conklin L, Jacobs GB. Visceral and vascular complications resulting from anterior lumbar interbody fusion. J Neurosurg. 1999; 91(1) Suppl:60–64

[24] Deukmedjian AR, Dakwar E, Ahmadian A, Smith DA, Uribe JS. Early outcomes of minimally invasive anterior longitudinal ligament release for correction of sagittal imbalance in patients with adult spinal deformity. Sci World J. 2012; 2012:789698

[25] Chen WJ, Lai PL, Niu CC, Chen LH, Fu TS, Wong CB. Surgical treatment of adjacent instability after lumbar spine fusion. Spine. 2001; 26(22):E519–E524

[26] Akamaru T, Kawahara N, Tim Yoon S, et al. Adjacent segment motion after a simulated lumbar fusion in different sagittal alignments: a biomechanical analysis. Spine. 2003; 28(14):1560–1566

[27] Amaral R, Marchi L, Oliveira L, et al. Minimally invasive lateral alternative for thoracolumbar interbody fusion. Coluna/Columna. 2011; 10(3):239–243

[28] Berjano P, Damilano M, Lamartina C. Sagittal alignment correction and reconstruction of lumbar post-traumatic kyphosis via MIS lateral approach. Eur Spine J. 2012; 21(12):2718–2720

[29] Marchi L, Oliveira L, Amaral R, et al. Anterior elongation as a minimally invasive alternative for sagittal imbalance-a case series. HSS J. 2012; 8(2): 122–127

[30] Rodgers W, Cox C, Gerber E. Minimally invasive treatment (XLIF) of adjacent segment disease after prior lumbar fusions. Internet J Minim Invasive Spinal Technol 2008;3(4). Available at: http://ispub.com/IJMIST/3/4/7005

[31] Karikari IO, Nimjee SM, Hardin CA, et al. Extreme lateral interbody fusion approach for isolated thoracic and thoracolumbar spine diseases: initial clinical experience and early outcomes. J Spinal Disord Tech. 2011; 24(6):368–375

[32] Acosta FL, Liu J, Slimack N, Moller D, Fessler R, Koski T. Changes in coronal and sagittal plane alignment following minimally invasive direct lateral interbody fusion for the treatment of degenerative lumbar disease in adults: a radiographic study. J Neurosurg Spine. 2011; 15(1):92–96

[33] Le TV, Smith DA, Greenberg MS, Dakwar E, Baaj AA, Uribe JS. Complications of lateral plating in the minimally invasive lateral transpsoas approach. J Neurosurg Spine. 2012; 16(3):302–307

[34] Youssef JA, McAfee PC, Patty CA, et al. Minimally invasive surgery: lateral approach interbody fusion: results and review. Spine. 2010; 35(26) Suppl: S302–S311

[35] Pimenta L. Adjacent Segment Disease. 2013

[36] Uribe JS, Arredondo N, Dakwar E, Vale FL. Defining the safe working zones using the minimally invasive lateral retroperitoneal transpsoas approach: an anatomical study. J Neurosurg Spine. 2010; 13(2):260–266

[37] Cummock MD, Vanni S, Levi AD, Yu Y, Wang MY. An analysis of postoperative thigh symptoms after minimally invasive transpsoas lumbar interbody fusion. J Neurosurg Spine. 2011; 15(1):11–18

[38] Le TV, Burkett CJ, Deukmedjian AR, Uribe JS. Postoperative lumbar plexus injury after lumbar retroperitoneal transpsoas minimally invasive lateral interbody fusion. Spine. 2013; 38(1):E13–E20

[39] Marchi L, Abdala N, Oliveira L, Amaral R, Coutinho E, Pimenta L. Radiographic and clinical evaluation of cage subsidence after stand-alone lateral interbody fusion. J Neurosurg Spine. 2013; 19(1):110–118

[40] Guyatt G, Schünemann H, Cook D, Jaeschke R, Pauker S, Bucher H; American College of Chest Physicians. Grades of recommendation for antithrombotic agents. Chest 2001;119(1, Suppl):3S7S

[41] Shabat S, Arinzon Z, Gepstein R, Folman Y. Long-term follow-up of revision decompressive lumbar spinal surgery in elderly patients. J Spinal Disord Tech. 2011; 24(3):142–145

[42] Wong C-B, Chen W-J, Chen L-H, Niu C-C, Lai P-L. Clinical outcomes of revision lumbar spinal surgery: 124 patients with a minimum of two years of follow-up. Chang Gung Med J. 2002; 25(3):175–182

[43] Adogwa O, Parker SL, Shau DN, et al. Preoperative Zung Depression Scale predicts outcome after revision lumbar surgery for adjacent segment disease, recurrent stenosis, and pseudarthrosis. Spine J. 2012; 12(3): 179–185

[44] Tafazal SI, Sell PJ. Incidental durotomy in lumbar spine surgery: incidence and management. Eur Spine J. 2005; 14(3):287–290

[45] Wang JC, Bohlman HH, Riew KD. Dural tears secondary to operations on the lumbar spine. Management and results after a two-year-minimum follow-up of eighty-eight patients. J Bone Joint Surg Am. 1998; 80(12): 1728–1732

[46] Hadjipavlou A, Enker P, Dupuis P, Katzman S, Silver J. The causes of failure of lumbar transpedicular spinal instrumentation and fusion: a prospective study. Int Orthop. 1996; 20(1):35–42

[47] Smith JS, Shaffrey CI, Sansur CA, et al. Scoliosis Research Society Morbidity and Mortality Committee. Rates of infection after spine surgery based on 108,419 procedures: a report from the Scoliosis Research Society Morbidity and Mortality Committee. Spine. 2011; 36(7):556–563

9 Degenerative Scoliosis: Is There an Advantage to Using Minimally Invasive Techniques to Treat Degenerative Scoliosis?

MIS: Chun-Po Yen and Juan S. Uribe
Open: Christopher I. Shaffrey

9.1 Introduction

Adult scoliosis is a spinal deformity in skeletally mature patients with a Cobb angle of greater than 10° in the coronal plane. Based on the pathogenesis, adult scoliosis can be classified into the following: type 1, primary (de novo) degenerative scoliosis (DS); type 2, progressive idiopathic scoliosis in adult life; and type 3, secondary DS consequent to idiopathic scoliosis, pelvic obliquity, or metabolic bone diseases (such as osteoporosis).[1] DS begins with asymmetric degeneration of the intervertebral discs. Subsequently, the lack of competency in the facets and asymmetric compression fracture of osteoporotic vertebrae cause progression of the curve. Spondylolisthesis and translational or rotational dislocations are often associated with DS and further complicate the deformity.

9.2 Indications of Surgery for Adult Degenerative Scoliosis

Conservative treatment might be adequate and should be tried in the majority of patients with DS. With a gradual shift to an aging society and a longer life expectancy, there is a rise in the prevalence of adult DS and increasing demand from the patients for a better quality of life (QOL). To this end, surgical intervention has been increasingly utilized to treat DS, although the risks of surgeries have traditionally been considered higher compared to those for adolescent idiopathic scoliosis (AIS) given the old age, medical comorbidities, and deficient bone stock in adults. Studies have shown that surgically treated patients with adult DS had a significantly greater improvement in back or leg pain and QOL when compared with nonoperatively managed patients.[2,3,4] In general, patients with the following conditions are candidates for surgery: claudication or radicular symptoms due to canal, lateral recess, or foraminal stenosis; back pain related to degenerated discs/facets or muscular fatigue that failed conservative management; neurological deficits; instability; and progression of curve. Surgeries usually consist of decompression, instrumentation, fusion, realignment, or a combination of all of these based on patient's symptoms, degree of instability, severity and flexibility of curve, and presence of sagittal imbalance.

Unlike AIS, adult DS are usually rigid and may require a combined anteroposterior approach, especially in those with advanced disease. Silva and Lenke provided a graded treatment recommendation for selection of surgical procedures based on the clinical and radiological findings of DS patients.[5] Level I treatment consists of limited decompression for those with only claudication or radiculopathy caused by stenosis. Radiographically, suitable patients are those with anterior osteophytes, scoliosis less than 30°, and subluxation less than 2 mm without sagittal imbalance. This is with a caveat that progression of scoliosis might occur. Level II treatment involves addition of limited posterior lumbar instrumented fusion and is indicated in patients with stenosis requiring a wide decompression but without anterior osteophytes. Level III treatment involves instrumented fusion of lumbar curve and is indicated in patients with primary symptom of back pain and radiographically with significant curve and subluxation without sagittal imbalance. Level IV treatment involves addition of anterior spinal fusion and is indicated in patients with loss of lumbar lordosis. Level V treatment involves extension of instrumented fusion to thoracic region and is indicated in patients with flexible sagittal imbalance. Level VI treatment involves osteotomy and is indicated in patients with stiff or fixed sagittal imbalance.

9.3 Advantages of Minimally Invasive Surgery

Minimally invasive surgery (MIS) is intended to achieve the same goals of open surgery while minimizing the collateral damage from the access. Decompression is usually accomplished in an indirect manner through placement of large footprint interbody cages and is usually selected for patients with mild to moderate stenosis. This technique has the benefits of avoiding prior surgical scar and obviating nerve root injury and unintentional durotomy.

MIS technique for DS relies heavily on anterior column manipulation and support. Direct manipulation of the anterior and middle columns permits a potentially greater degree of deformity correction compared with posterior approach alone. This is advantageous for osteoporotic patients given the large footprint cages placed across the hard apophyseal ring reduce the risk of subsidence and loss of indirect decompression. The anterior column support can be achieved through a mini-open anterior or lateral approach. MIS lateral approach has been gaining significant interests, as the approach does not require an access surgeon. In patients with significant sagittal imbalance, an anterior longitudinal ligament (ALL) release and placement of a hyperlordotic cage can achieve a 15° or more lordosis and can be performed at multiple levels without significant blood loss or nerve manipulation.[6]

Posterior instrumentation is usually required to augment the stability and maintain the correction. Placement of percutaneous screws for long segment has been proved feasible with the aims of minimizing paraspinal muscular injury and preserving posterior tension band.

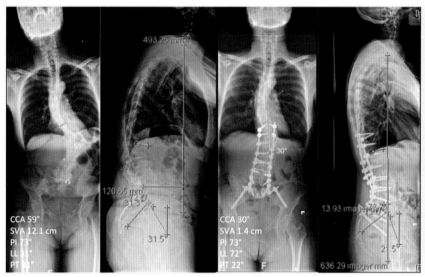

Fig. 9.1 Preoperative and postoperative 36-inch long-cassette radiographs of a 48-year-old woman with lumbar degenerative scoliosis. She underwent a hybrid minimally invasive correction of adult degenerative scoliosis and kyphosis. The coronal Cobb angle improved from 59° to 30°, the lumbar lordosis increased from 31° to 72°, and the pelvic tilt decreased from 31° to 22°.

9.4 Advantages of Open Surgery

The open posterior approach remains the workhorse for correcting adult DS. All surgical procedures can be performed in a single position, and the posterior anatomy is certainly more familiar to the spine surgeons.

DS patients with severe stenosis usually require a wide decompression, which can be adequately addressed under direct visualization in an open setting. Interbody fusion is usually performed through a transforaminal lumbar interbody fusion (TLIF). Compared to posterior lumbar interbody fusion, a unilateral approach with less dural/nerve retraction allows for an anterior placement of a large lordotic cage. In cases undergoing anterior-placed TLIF cages, posterior column osteotomy, and compression, an increase in segmental lordosis can range from 6° at L1/L2 level to 22° at L5/S1 level.[7] For patients with rigid or fixed DS and those with sagittal imbalance, posterior column osteotomy and three-column osteotomy such as pedicle subtraction osteotomy (PSO) or vertebral column resection (VCR) are powerful tools to realign the spine in both coronal and sagittal planes.

Placement of pedicle screws under direct visualization reduces the use of imaging guidance and lowers radiation exposure of the surgeons and patients. Manipulation of posterior rods to correct the three-dimensional deformity is more feasible in an open fashion. In addition, a wide exposure of posterior spinal structure allows robust posterolateral fusion.

9.5 Case Illustration

A 48-year-old woman presented with back pain and progression of kyphoscoliosis. She had a history of AIS, and underwent a placement of the Harrington rod at the age of 15 years. The rod "popped out" 2 years later and was subsequently removed. She stated that she has been "relatively straight" until 3 years ago when she started to lean to the right and forward. Clinically, she presented with mid- and low back pain and anterior thigh pain without other neurological deficits.

On 36-inch long-cassette X-rays, she had a coronal Cobb angle of 59°, lumbar lordosis of 31°, pelvic incidence of 73°, and pelvic tilt of 31° (▶ Fig. 9.1). Computed tomography (CT) demonstrated posterolateral fusion mass from T4 to L3 with pseudoarthrosis between T12 and L3 (▶ Fig. 9.2). Magnetic resonance imaging (MRI) demonstrated multilevel moderate foraminal stenosis on the concave side of the curve.

Based on the history and imaging findings, the patient is likely to have partially corrected AIS with secondary DS in the lumbar region. Given her symptoms and progression of kyphoscoliosis, she was considered a candidate for correction surgery.

9.6 Surgical Technique in Minimally Invasive Surgery

The patient underwent a two-stage surgery. The first stage was performed in a posterior open fashion. She was placed in a prone position on a Jackson table, with exposure of posterior elements from T11 to iliac crest. Bilateral T11 to S1 pedicle screws and iliac bolts were placed under the assistance of fluoroscope, followed by L1/L2, L2/L3, and L3/L4 posterior column osteotomy to remove the prior fusion mass, and L4/L5 and L5/S1 medial facetectomy. Two temporary rods were placed across L1 to L4 pedicle screws. Three days later, the patient was brought back to the operating room and underwent the second stage surgery, which included a mini-open L5/S1 anterior lumbar interbody fusion (ALIF) with placement of a 30° hyperlordotic cage in supine position; right L1/L2, L2/L3, L3/L4, and L4/L5 lateral lumbar interbody fusion (LLIF) with 10° lordotic cages in lateral position; and placement of posterior rods from T11 to ilium in posterior position. At 6-month follow-up, long-cassette X-rays demonstrated improved radiographic parameters. The Cobb angle reduced to 30°, lumbar lordosis increased to 72°, and pelvic tilt reduced to 22°. Her pain improved significantly (▶ Fig. 9.1; ▶ Fig. 9.3).

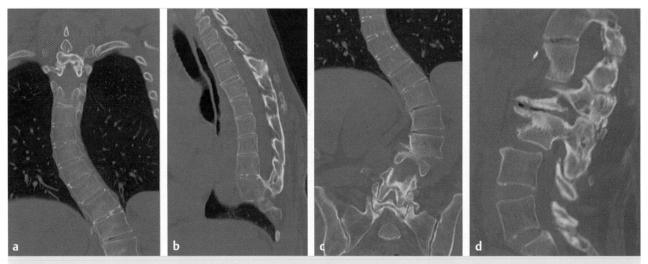

Fig. 9.2 (a,b) Preoperative thoracic and lumbar and (c,d) spine computed tomography images demonstrated fusion mass from T4 to L3 with pseudoarthrosis between T12 and L3.

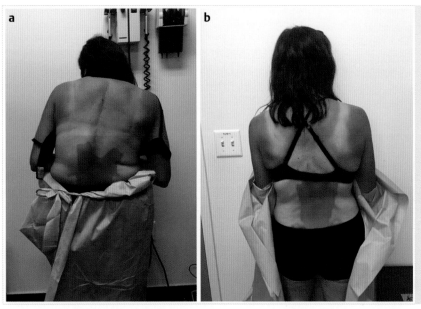

Fig. 9.3 (a) Pre- and (b) postoperative photographs of the patient.

9.7 Surgical Technique in Open Surgery

The patient was placed in a prone position on a Jackson table. The abdomen was left hanging free to increase the venous blood return and reduce intraoperative bleeding. A longitudinal skin incision was followed by a subperiosteal dissection of the paravertebral muscles to complete exposure of the bony structures. Pedicle screws are inserted from T10 to S1 and iliac screws were placed bilaterally using a combination of anatomic landmarks and fluoroscopic guidance. Multilevel posterior column osteotomy was performed from T12 to S1. A temporary rod was placed on the convex side from L4 to S1 under distraction. A distractor attached to the pedicle screws on the concave side where the TLIF was planned further opens the disc space between L4/L5 and L5/S1. The inferior facets of L4 and L5 and cranial part of superior facets of L5 and S1 were removed to expose the Kambin triangles. After adequate discectomy and preparation of the end plates, the hyperlordotic cages filled with recombinant human bone morphogenetic protein 2 (rhBMP-2) (Infuse; Medtronic Sofamor Danek, Inc., Memphis, TN) and autografts were placed to the ventral part of intervertebral space at L4/L5 and L5/S1. The use of rhBMP-2 was an off-label indication in the TLIF procedure. Autologous bone graft was packed in the residual disc space. Permanent rods contoured as desired were then placed and secured with compression across the levels of TLIF. Further rod rotation, intersegmental compression/distraction, and in-situ rod bending were performed to correct kyphoscoliosis. Decortication of posterior elements was performed followed by placement of rhBMP-2 along with autografts and allografts to reinforce fusion.

9.8 Discussion of Minimally Invasive Surgery

MIS techniques use specialized instruments to minimize approach-related soft-tissue damage. The techniques reduce blood loss, minimize postsurgical pain, and expedite patient's recovery. In addition, wound infections are reduced because of limited surgical exposure. Given the adults with DS are more likely to have medical comorbidities, less blood loss and fluid requirement reduces cardiopulmonary and renal burden; early mobilization decreases risk of venous thromboembolism; and less narcotics consumption reduces occurrence of ileus.

For patients with mild to moderate stenosis associated with DS, indirect decompression can be accomplished by restoration of disc height following the placement of a large footprint interbody cage through a mini-open anterior, lateral, or posterolateral approaches. For those with severe stenosis, a direct decompression might be needed and can be accomplished through a tubular retractor or a small incision.

Unlike adolescent spinal curves, adult scoliotic deformities are usually rigid and often require a combined anteroposterior approach. Anterior column surgeries provide access to the load-bearing elements of the spine and allows for greater corrective forces to be applied. Combining the use of interbody cages, the anterior approach provides structural stability, decreases stress on pedicle screws, improves fusion rates, offers better lumbar lordosis, and thereby potentially necessitates fewer surgical levels to treat the deformities.[8] The anterior column surgeries can be performed through mini-open ALIF and LLIF.

ALIF has long been considered the gold standard technique for interbody fusion. It affords a direct access for discectomy, release of ALL to restore lordosis, and placement of a large cage for arthrodesis. For patients with DS, augmentation of the lumbosacral segment in long constructs with interbody fusion at L5–S1 improves biomechanical stability and reduces the risk of lumbosacral pseudoarthrosis.[9,10] The procedure can be performed through a mini-open or laparoscopic approach with minimal access-related complications.

LLIF uses a retroperitoneal transpsoas corridor to perform a lumbar interbody fusion without violating ALL, posterior longitudinal ligament, and the posterior tension band.[11,12] Bilateral annulus release combined with lateral insertion of wide cages in coronally asymmetric discs provides a strong corrective force to segmentally restore coronal alignment. Further coronal correction in discs surrounded by asymmetrical vertebral bodies can be achieved by the use of coronally asymmetrical cages. The large footprint cages spanning the apophyseal ring reduce the risk of cage subsidence especially in patients with osteoporosis.

Pedicle screws allow spine surgeons to correct kyphoscoliosis and secure spine fixation. Placement of percutaneous pedicle screws through multiple small paramedian incisions reduces the severity of paraspinal muscle injury. Preservation of posterior tension has been reported to lower the risk of proximal junctional kyphosis.[13] In patients with DS, the fusion can be stopped at L5 if possible, as apex of scoliosis is usually located between L2 and L4. However, in patients with fractional curves, spondylolisthesis, prior laminectomy, or severe degenerative disc disease at L5/S1, additional fixation to sacrum and pelvis

can be performed percutaneously to further stabilize long fusion construct.

Historically, the circumferential MIS approach has been satisfactory in terms of correcting coronal curve but often falls short on correcting sagittal imbalance. Recently developed ALL release technique allows for larger degrees of anterior column realignment.[6] Alternatively, a hybrid MIS technique, which involves the incorporation of the aforementioned MIS decompression and interbody fusion with open posterior surgeries such as posterior column osteotomies and open instrumentation, enhances the effect of anterior column reconstruction and restoration of sagittal balance and spinopelvic parameters.[14]

9.8.1 Level I Evidence in Minimally Invasive Surgery

There are no level I studies available.

9.8.2 Level II Evidence in Minimally Invasive Surgery

Two recent prospective studies are available for review (▶ Table 9.1). Phillips et al, in a prospective, multicenter, single-arm study including 107 DS patients treated with extreme lateral lumbar interbody fusion (XLIF) with or without supplemental posterior fixation, reported significant improvement in all clinical outcome measures as well as lumbar lordosis and coronal Cobb's angle at 24-month follow-up.[15] The authors concluded that XLIF is associated with similar clinical and radiographical results as are reported in the literature after traditional open surgical procedures, while having a substantially lower complication rate.

Scheufler et al prospectively enrolled 30 DS patients with back pain, radiculopathy, or claudication. Patients were treated with MIS multilevel TLIF and placement of pedicle screws under fluoroscopic guidance or CT-based navigation.[16,17] The authors reported significant coronal and sagittal plane correction, and patients improved clinically based on Oswestry Disability Index (ODI), visual analog score (VAS), and Short Form-12 questionnaire (SF-12). The authors emphasized the accuracy of CT-based navigation and elimination of radiation exposure to the surgeon using the technique.

9.8.3 Level III and IV Evidence in Minimally Invasive Surgery

Summary of recently published retrospective studies investigating the outcomes and complications of MIS technique for adult DS are listed in ▶ Table 9.1.[18,19,20,21,22,23,24] The case numbers in MIS series tend to be small with a relatively short follow-up so far. Most of the series utilized a combination of lateral approach (LLIF, XLIF, DLIF) and posterior instrumentation to manage DS. All series reported improved ODI and significant correction of coronal Cobb's angle. The study from Tempel et al showed that the increase of lumbar lordosis is not significant.[23] In the study from Dakwar et al, one-third of patients failed to achieve sagittal balance.[21]

Table 9.1 Summary of minimally invasive approach series for adult degenerative scoliosis

Authors (year)	Level of evidence	Study design	Type	No.	Follow-up (mo)	Clinical outcome	Coronal Cobb's angle (°)	Lumbar lordosis (°)	Cx (%)	Fusion (%)
Castro et al (2014)[20]	IV	Retrospective	MIS (XLIF stand-alone)	35	24	Improved ODI, VAS ODI, 51 to 29	21 to 12	33 to 41	Subsidence in 29	84
Tempel et al (2014)[23]	IV	Retrospective	MIS hybrid (LLIF + PSIF)	26	12	Improved ODI, VAS ODI, 48 to 38	41 to 15	43 to 49	42	96
Khajavi and Shen (2014)[22]	IV	Retrospective	MIS (XLIF with or without perc screws)	21	24	Improved ODI, VAS, SF-36 ODI, 48 to 24	28 to 17	32 to 44	5	100
Anand et al (2014)[18]	IV	Retrospective	MIS (DLIF with or without perc screws)	54	39	Improved ODI, VAS, SF-36 ODI improvement, 21	20 to 11		23	94
Phillips et al (2013)[15]	II	Prospective	MIS XLIF with or without pedicle screws	107	24	Improved ODI, VAS, SF Mean ODI improved, 22	21 to 15	28 to 34	24	92
Caputo et al (2013)[19]	IV	Retrospective	MIS XLIF with pedicle screws	30	14	N/A	20 to 6	44 to 48	26	88
Dakwar et al (2010)[21]	IV	Retrospective	MIS (XLIF with or without pedicle screws)	25	11	Improved ODI, VAS ODI, 54 to 30	21 to 6	One-third not achieving sagittal balance	12	80
Scheufler et al (2010)[16,17]	II	Prospective	MIS (TLIF with perc screws)	30	20	Improved ODI, VAS, SF-12 ODI, 57 to 25	45 to 11	−9 to 36	Major, 23 Minor, 60	93
Wang and Mummaneni (2010)[24]	IV	Retrospective	MIS (DLIF with perc screws)	23	13	Improved VAS	31 to 12	37 to 46	17	Interbody, 100 Posterolateral, 71

Abbreviations: DLIF, direct lateral lumbar interbody fusion; LLIF, lateral lumbar interbody fusion; MIS, minimally invasive surgery; ODI, Oswestry Disability Index; perc, percutaneous; PSIF, posterior segmental instrumentation and fusion; SF-12, short form 12; SF-36, short form 36; TLIF, transforaminal lumbar interbody fusion; VAS, visual analogue scale; XLIF, extreme lateral lumbar interbody fusion.

Overall, the complication rate seems to be low, ranging from 12 to 26% in most series (except for the 60% minor complication rates in series from Scheufler et al[16,17] and 42% in the series of Tempel et al,[23] in which a hybrid approach was used). Depending on the definition and modalities used to evaluate fusion, the fusion rates range from 80 to 100%.[25]

9.9 Complications in Minimally Invasive Surgery

Although MIS technique aims to minimize approach-related morbidities, each technique has its own set of possible complications. ALIF has been associated with vascular and visceral injuries, and the risk of retrograde ejaculation is well known. Several comparative studies have shown that no marked difference exists between laparoscopic ALIF and the open or mini-open ALIF in terms of short-term efficacy, such as operative time, blood loss, and length of hospital stay. With regard to the complication rate, however, there was a higher incidence of retrograde ejaculation in laparoscopic ALIF.[25]

LLIF uses the transpsoas route and can cause psoas syndrome that consists of hip flexion weakness or thigh sensory symptoms such as pain, numbness, and dysesthesia. The most dreadful complication of lumbar plexus, bowel, and vascular injuries are low but the incidence may increase given the anatomical variation of DS patients with significant vertebral rotation.[26,27,28] The incidence of psoas symptoms varied between 4 and 34% and the majority of them are transient. The risk of true femoral/obturator nerve injury was reported in the range of 0 to 4%.

The MIS percutaneous screws' placement relies on image guidance through either fluoroscope or other forms of navigation. The radiation remains a concern for the surgeons and the patients. Posterolateral fusion is often compromised in MIS technique due to limited exposure. As mentioned earlier, correction of sagittal imbalance through a circumferential MIS approach may be deficient.

9.10 Conclusion of Minimally Invasive Surgery

MIS approach has been gaining popularity in treating adult DS in the hope of minimizing approach-related complications while achieving the surgical goals of its open counterpart. Recent publications especially those using LLIF have shown promising results, although follow-up is relative short. Secondary to the anatomical constraint of the iliac crest, the L5–S1 disc space is not easily or safely approachable with this technique. There is, in addition, a higher reported risk of lumbar plexus injury using LLIF at L4/L5 level. The risk can be alleviated with the use of real-time intraoperative EMG neuromonitoring. Given the anatomical variations in DS patients, a careful evaluation of anatomy on preoperative imaging is critical. If supplemental posterior instrumentation or direct decompression is required, a separate posterior incision and approach might be needed. Changing patient positioning could be cumbersome at times, although ALIF and percutaneous pedicle screws' placement can be performed in a lateral position. Nevertheless, the placement of ALIF cage and trajectories of percutaneous screws

might not be ideal. In addition, there is a steep learning curve associated with the MIS approach, and further training might be required.

The increasing popularity of minimally invasive techniques over the last two decades has led to its expanded use in pathologies previously dominated by open surgery. Over the last several years, a wealth of research has expanded our knowledge on the application of these minimally invasive techniques in the correction of scoliosis and sagittal imbalance. Numerous retrospective cohort studies, in addition to a limited number of prospective studies, have indicated that anterior and posterior MIS techniques can provide adequate deformity correction with similar clinical outcomes (VAS, ODI score) and fusion rates when compared with historical open studies. Based on these data, a Grade 1C recommendation using the Guyatt et al grading scale may be given to evidence supporting similar efficacy of MIS and open techniques in addressing spinal deformity with improvements in pain and QOL.[29]

9.11 Discussion of Open Surgery

Open surgeries can be implemented through an anterior-only, posterior-only, or combined approach. The anterior-only approach is occasionally used for young adults with a relatively flexible curve. Anterior interbody support in conjunction with anterior instrumentation up and down to the neutral vertebrae can be performed to correct scoliosis and obtain fusion. The benefit of anterior approach is its superior correction, fewer motion segments fused, and a low incidence of nonunion.[30]

Posterior approach remains the workhorse for scoliosis surgery. Single positioning of the patients allows for decompression, instrumentation, fusion, and realignment with an overall shorter surgery time. In DS patients with moderate to severe stenosis, a direct decompression is usually required. The decompression can be accomplished under direct visualization, and impinging material can be removed.

Dorsally based interbody fusion can be performed through a posterior or transforaminal approach to correct kyphoscoliosis and enhance fusion. Advantages of TLIF include a familiar posterior anatomy and direct decompression of neural structures. However, the constrained corridor usually limits the size of implants. These smaller footprint implants resting on the weaker central part of the vertebral end plate are more susceptible to subsidence. Recent advance of expandable interbody cage devices has overcome some of the limitations while facilitating alignment and stability. For DS patient, the cages may be biased to the concavity of the scoliosis to address the coronal plane deformity.

Occasionally, the lower instrumented fusion can end at L5. The fusion, however, might have to be extended to the sacrum if there is a fractional curves > 15°, advanced degeneration of the L5/S1 intervertebral disc, L5/S1 spondylolysis, or previous decompression at this segment. Additional augmentation of the lumbosacral reconstruction in long constructs with anterior column support in the form of interbody fusion at L5–S1 improves biomechanical stability and reduces the risk of lumbosacral pseudoarthrosis.[10] In contrast to ALIF, which require mobilization of viscera and great vessels, and LLIF in which L5/S1 is inaccessible due to the constraint of iliac crest, an anterior structural graft at L5–S1 can easily be achieved with TLIF to restore sagittal balance.

Patients with DS often have combined sagittal plane deformity. Those with positive sagittal imbalance often reported worse pain, function, and self-image as found on the health-related QOL questionnaires. Therefore, restoration of sagittal imbalance is critical in addition to the correction of scoliosis. Correction of sagittal imbalance can be performed through a graded osteotomy ranging from posterior column osteotomy (such as Ponte or Smith-Petersen osteotomy) to three-column osteotomy (such as PSO or VCR).[31] Asymmetrical PSO and VCR remain the most powerful tools in correcting rigid biplanar deformities.

9.11.1 Level I Evidence in Open Surgery

There are no level I studies available.

9.11.2 Level II Evidence in Open Surgery

Two recent published prospective studies were available for review. Bridwell et al, in a prospective comparative cohort analysis of 160 patients with adult symptomatic lumbar scoliosis who were treated either nonoperatively or operatively, reported that the operative cohort significantly improved in all QOL measures at minimum 2-year follow-up.[2] The nonoperative cohort did not improve and nonsignificant decline in QOL scores was common. Crandall and Revella compared the clinical and radiographic outcomes in 40 consecutive DS patients treated with posterior instrumented correction and fusion with additional ALIF versus TLIF and reported improving pain (VAS), function (ODI), and deformity (curve correction).[32] There was no difference in clinical outcomes or curve correction in patients treated with ALIF versus TLIF. There was no statistical difference between the ALIF and TLIF groups for nonunions, adjacent fractures, adjacent level disease, and infections.

9.11.3 Level III and IV Evidence in Open Surgery

Summary of recently published retrospective studies investigating the outcomes and complications of open technique for adult DS are listed in ▶ Table 9.2.[33,34,35,36,37,38,39] Cho et al, Faldini et al, and Wang et al compared DS patients undergoing short versus long segment fusion. In general, all patients had improvement of function based on ODI, and patients undergoing long fusion tend to have more correction of coronal and sagittal Cobb's angle. Transfeldt et al compared three groups of DS patients with radiculopathy undergoing decompression alone, decompression and limited fusion, and decompression and full-curve fusion.[36] The coronal and sagittal Cobb's angles improved significantly in the group with full-curve fusion but remained unchanged in the decompression only and limited fusion groups. Improved ODI scores were seen in decompression alone and decompression and limited fusion, but not in decompression and full-curve fusion. In contrast, the satisfaction questionnaire showed the highest success to be in the full-curve fusion group and the lowest in the decompression-only group. The complication rate was highest (56%) in the full fusion group,

40% in the limited fusion group, and 10% in the decompression alone group.

Based on the major series published after 2008, the overall complication rates range from 10 to 66% and rates of pseudoarthrosis range from 0 to 20% (▶ Table 9.2).

9.12 Complications in Open Surgery

Traditional open surgery has been associated with a complication rate as high as 20 to 80%, even at specialized centers.[24,40,41,42] In their series of patients undergoing posterior fusion and instrumentation for DS, Cho et al reported an overall complication rate of 68% including an early perioperative complication rate of 30% and late complication rate of 38%.[43] One of the main risk factors that increased the early perioperative complications in this study was a blood loss of more than 2 L.

In a retrospective review of a cohort of 5,470 adult scoliosis patients undergoing surgeries, Shaw et al reported an overall complication rate of 13.5% and mortality rate of 0.3%.[44] Patients who experienced complications were significantly older than those without complications.

Charosky et al, in a large multi centric retrospective study of 306 primary adult scoliosis patients treated surgically, reported an overall 39% complication rate.[45] The general or medical complication rate was 13.7%; infection occurred in 5.2%; neurological complications were present in 7%; and mechanical complications such as hardware failure, pseudoarthrosis, or aggravation of deformity were 24%. Twenty-six percent of the patients were reoperated for mechanical or neurological complications. Risk factors for mechanical or neurological complications were number of instrumented vertebra, fusion to the sacrum, PSO, and a high preoperative pelvic tilt of 26° or more.

9.13 Conclusion in Open Surgery

Adult DS is a complex three-dimensional deformity of the spine, and all three planes need to be addressed to maximize patient outcomes. For patients with severe and rigid deformity, an open approach remains the most powerful technique to achieve the surgical goals. The open procedures tend to be lengthy and invasive due to the need to expose and fuse a large portion of the spine. They are also more morbid to older patients who tend to have more underlying medical diseases. However, the elderly, despite having a greater risk of complications, tend to obtain a greater improvement in disability and pain with surgery compared to the young patients.[46] The open technique is a time-tested technique that will remain the most important tool in the spine surgeons' armamentarium for correction of DS. However, wisely chosen or combined MIS techniques, if feasible, are expected to reach the same outcome while reducing the risk of complications. The data obtained from an extensive number of retrospective and prospective studies provide a Grade 1C recommendation that open surgical techniques lead to improved long-term pain relief and QOL while adequately correcting spinal deformity in patients with DS when compared to conservative treatment.

Table 9.2 Summary of open approach for adult degenerative scoliosis

Authors (year)	Level of evidence	Study design	Type	No.	Follow-up	Clinical outcome	Coronal Cobb's angle	Lumbar lordosis	Cx	Pseudo (%)
Wang et al (2016)[38]	III	Retrospective	Open (short vs. long fusion)	108	34 mo	Short ODI, 62.5 to 21.8 SRS-22, 44.8 to 70.9 Long ODI, 73.4 to 30.4 SRS-22, 45.4 to 68.8	Short, 22° to 17° Long, 41° to 26°	Short 17° to 20° Long 5° to 16°	19%	5
Faldini et al (2015)[34]	III	Retrospective	Open (short vs. long fusion)	81	4 y	Improved RMDQ Short, 15 to 4 Long, 15 to 4	Short, 24° to 12° Long, 45° to 10°	Short 45° to 60° Long 24° to 55°	19%	5
Hsieh et al (2015)[35]	III	Retrospective	Open (combined vs. posterior approach)	110	53 mo	Improved ODI and VAS back/leg Combined, 28.8 to 6.4 Posterior, 29.1 to 6.2	Combined, 41 to 9° Posterior, 39° to 21°	Combined 3° to 36° Posterior 6° to 16°	11%	0
Zhu et al (2014)[39]	III	Retrospective	Open (PSIF with TLIF)	95	7.8 y	ODI, 32.2 to 11.1	31.1 to 8.3	9.3 to 30.1	37%	2
Tsai et al (2011)[37]	III	Retrospective	Open (PLIF)	58	39 mo	ODI, 28.1 to 12.2	19.3 to 7.7	30 to 29	N/A	N/A
Transfeldt et al (2010)[36]	III	Retrospective	Open (decompression vs. short vs. long fusion)	85	4.8 y	Improved ODI except long fusion group Decomp, 39.5 to 31.6 Short, 33.9 to 26.3 Long, 39.5 to 39.1	Decomp unchanged Short unchanged Long, 39° to 19°	Decomp unchanged Short unchanged Long 40° to 50°	Decomp, 10% Short, 40% Long, 56%	0 5 20
Crandall and Revella (2009)[32]	II	Prospective	Open (PSIF with ALIF vs. TLIF)	40	38 mo	Improved ODI and VAS ODI ALIF, 52 to 28.2 TLIF, 46.5 to 27.9	ALIF, 31° to 9° TLIF, 24° to 8°	ALIF 31° to 32° TLIF 45° to 48°	4 medical 2 neurological 3 infection 8 adjacent degeneration	15
Bridwell et al (2009)[2]	II	Prospective	Open (op vs. non-op)	85/75	2 y	Improved ODI, SRS QOL scores, NRS back and leg in op group ODI op, 34 to 20 ODI non-op, 30 to 32	Op, 56 to 27 Non-op, 50 to 51	N/A	36%	N/A
Cho et al (2008)[33]	III	Retrospective	Open (short vs. long fusion)	50	4.3 y	ODI Short, 65.3 to 48.6 Long, 71 to 47.8	Short, 16° to 10° Long, 22° to 6°	Short 3° to 32° Long 26° to 22°	66%	2

Abbreviations: ALIF, anterior lumbar interbody fusion; Decomp, decompression; LLIF, lateral lumbar interbody fusion; Non-op, nonoperative management; NRS, numeric rating scale; ODI, Oswestry Disability Index; Op, operative; PLIF, posterior lumbar interbody fusion; PSIF, posterior segmental instrumentation and fusion; QOL, quality of life; RMDQ, Roland–Morris Disability Questionnaire; SRS-22, Scoliosis Research Society 22 questionnaire; TLIF, transforaminal interbody fusion; VAS, visual analog scale.

9.14 Editors' Commentary

9.14.1 Minimally Invasive Surgery

MIS correction of deformity is the most recent application of MIS technique to spinal surgery. In line with the observations that "the bigger the operation, the more advantageous is MIS," the impact of MIS technique on correction of deformity is proving to be huge. Multiple reports have now demonstrated that the use of MIS technique decreases blood loss, the need for transfusion, infection rate, complications, hospitalization, intensive care, return to normal activities, and cost. It has, however, been reported that open technique corrects sagittal balance better than MIS technique. Despite this, clinical results (as measured by VAS and ODI) are equivalent using either technique. Moreover, hyperlordotic cages and novel rod contouring techniques are eliminating the discrepancy in sagittal correction between open and MIS surgery. As the experience with MIS deformity correction grows, it will progressively take over a larger and larger proportion of deformity correction surgery.

9.14.2 Open Surgery

Treatment of DS inherently lends itself to the use of an open procedure because of the importance of bone grafting, the requirement to place rods with coronal plane bend given curve stiffness and inability to achieve full correction, and the frequent need for concomitant multilevel decompression to treat associated spinal stenosis. The surgical technique described above for "MIS" includes two additional surgical approaches (anterior retroperitoneal for placement of L5–S1 interbody device, lateral approach for placement of lumbar interbody devices) as well as a similar open posterior approach. Compared to placement of cages using a transforaminal approach during an open posterior procedure, adopting an MIS procedure as described above seems more invasive rather than less. The additional time under anesthesia is disadvantageous both for the patient and from a cost-effectiveness standpoint, and the advantages of a multi-procedure approach are uncertain. There is little evidence that laterally placed cages introduce more sagittal plane segmental correction than TLIF; concern for sagittal plane correction should prompt surgeons to consider multilevel ALIF via a retroperitoneal approach or osteotomy.

Lateral approach surgery at the L4–L5 level is associated with a rate of lumbar plexus injury, which far exceeds that associated with all-posterior-based procedures in many reports. This risk of neurologic injury is unnecessary and can easily be avoided using a TLIF approach when interbody support is necessary. In those situations when bone density is a concern, placement of two TLIF cages achieves a similar footprint to laterally placed cages to guard against cage subsidence and involves little additional time or risk. A traditional open procedure is the best approach for the treatment of DS.

References

[1] Aebi M. The adult scoliosis. Eur Spine J. 2005; 14(10):925–948

[2] Bridwell KH, Glassman S, Horton W, et al. Does treatment (nonoperative and operative) improve the two-year quality of life in patients with adult symptomatic lumbar scoliosis: a prospective multicenter evidence-based medicine study. Spine. 2009; 34(20):2171–2178

[3] Smith JS, Shaffrey CI, Berven S, et al. Spinal Deformity Study Group. Improvement of back pain with operative and nonoperative treatment in adults with scoliosis. Neurosurgery. 2009; 65(1):86–93, discussion 93–94

[4] Smith JS, Shaffrey CI, Berven S, et al. Spinal Deformity Study Group. Operative versus nonoperative treatment of leg pain in adults with scoliosis: a retrospective review of a prospective multicenter database with two-year follow-up. Spine. 2009; 34(16):1693–1698

[5] Silva FE, Lenke LG. Adult degenerative scoliosis: evaluation and management. Neurosurg Focus. 2010; 28(3):E1

[6] Deukmedjian AR, Dakwar E, Ahmadian A, Smith DA, Uribe JS. Early outcomes of minimally invasive anterior longitudinal ligament release for correction of sagittal imbalance in patients with adult spinal deformity. Sci World J. 2012; 2012:789698

[7] Jagannathan J, Sansur CA, Oskouian RJ, Jr, Fu KM, Shaffrey CI. Radiographic restoration of lumbar alignment after transforaminal lumbar interbody fusion. Neurosurgery. 2009; 64(5):955–963, discussion 963–964

[8] Shamji MF, Isaacs RE. Anterior-only approaches to scoliosis. Neurosurgery. 2008; 63(3) Suppl:139–148

[9] Polly DW, Jr, Klemme WR, Cunningham BW, Burnette JB, Haggerty CJ, Oda I. The biomechanical significance of anterior column support in a simulated single-level spinal fusion. J Spinal Disord. 2000; 13(1):58–62

[10] Kuklo TR, Bridwell KH, Lewis SJ, et al. Minimum 2-year analysis of sacropelvic fixation and L5-S1 fusion using S1 and iliac screws. Spine. 2001; 26(18):1976–1983

[11] Ozgur BM, Aryan HE, Pimenta L, Taylor WR. Extreme lateral interbody fusion (XLIF): a novel surgical technique for anterior lumbar interbody fusion. Spine J. 2006; 6(4):435–443

[12] Uribe JS, Arredondo N, Dakwar E, Vale FL. Defining the safe working zones using the minimally invasive lateral retroperitoneal transpsoas approach: an anatomical study. J Neurosurg Spine. 2010; 13(2):260–266

[13] Mummaneni PV, Park P, Fu K-M, et al. International Spine Study Group. Does minimally invasive percutaneous posterior instrumentation reduce risk of proximal junctional kyphosis in adult spinal deformity surgery? A propensity- matched cohort analysis. Neurosurgery. 2016; 78 (1):101–108

[14] Kanter AS, Tempel ZJ, Ozpinar A, Okonkwo DO. A review of minimally invasive procedures for the treatment of adult spinal deformity. Spine. 2016; 41 Suppl 8:S59–S65

[15] Phillips FM, Isaacs RE, Rodgers WB, et al. Adult degenerative scoliosis treated with XLIF: clinical and radiographical results of a prospective multicenter study with 24-month follow-up. Spine. 2013; 38(21):1853–1861

[16] Scheufler KM, Cyron D, Dohmen H, Eckardt A. Less invasive surgical correction of adult degenerative scoliosis, part I: technique and radiographic results. Neurosurgery. 2010; 67(3):696–710

[17] Scheufler KM, Cyron D, Dohmen H, Eckardt A. Less invasive surgical correction of adult degenerative scoliosis. Part II: complications and clinical outcome. Neurosurgery. 2010; 67(6):1609–1621, discussion 1621

[18] Anand N, Baron EM, Khandehroo B. Is circumferential minimally invasive surgery effective in the treatment of moderate adult idiopathic scoliosis? Clin Orthop Relat Res. 2014; 472(6):1762–1768

[19] Caputo AM, Michael KW, Chapman TM, et al. Extreme lateral interbody fusion for the treatment of adult degenerative scoliosis. J Clin Neurosci. 2013; 20(11):1558–1563

[20] Castro C, Oliveira L, Amaral R, Marchi L, Pimenta L. Is the lateral transpsoas approach feasible for the treatment of adult degenerative scoliosis? Clin Orthop Relat Res. 2014; 472(6):1776–1783

[21] Dakwar E, Cardona RF, Smith DA, Uribe JS. Early outcomes and safety of the minimally invasive, lateral retroperitoneal transpsoas approach for adult degenerative scoliosis. Neurosurg Focus. 2010; 28(3):E8

[22] Khajavi K, Shen AY. Two-year radiographic and clinical outcomes of a minimally invasive, lateral, transpsoas approach for anterior lumbar interbody fusion in the treatment of adult degenerative scoliosis. Eur Spine J. 2014; 23(6):1215–1223

[23] Tempel ZJ, Gandhoke GS, Bonfield CM, Okonkwo DO, Kanter AS. Radiographic and clinical outcomes following combined lateral lumbar interbody fusion and posterior segmental stabilization in patients with adult degenerative scoliosis. Neurosurg Focus. 2014; 36(5):E11

[24] Wang MY, Mummaneni PV. Minimally invasive surgery for thoracolumbar spinal deformity: initial clinical experience with clinical and radiographic outcomes. Neurosurg Focus. 2010; 28(3):E9

[25] Inamasu J, Guiot BH. Laparoscopic anterior lumbar interbody fusion: a review of outcome studies. Minim Invasive Neurosurg. 2005; 48(6):340–347

[26] Assina R, Majmundar NJ, Herschman Y, Heary RF. First report of major vascular injury due to lateral transpsoas approach leading to fatality. J Neurosurg Spine. 2014; 21(5):794–798

[27] Tormenti MJ, Maserati MB, Bonfield CM, Okonkwo DO, Kanter AS. Complications and radiographic correction in adult scoliosis following combined transpsoas extreme lateral interbody fusion and posterior pedicle screw instrumentation. Neurosurg Focus. 2010; 28(3):E7

[28] Regev GJ, Kim CW. Safety and the anatomy of the retroperitoneal lateral corridor with respect to the minimally invasive lateral lumbar intervertebral fusion approach. Neurosurg Clin N Am. 2014; 25(2):211–218

[29] Guyatt G, Schunëmann H, Cook D, Jaeschke R, Pauker S, Bucher H; American College of Chest Physicians. Grades of recommendation for antithrombotic agents. Chest 2001;119(1, Suppl):3S7S

[30] Bradford DS, Tay BK, Hu SS. Adult scoliosis: surgical indications, operative management, complications, and outcomes. Spine. 1999; 24(24):2617–2629

[31] Schwab F, Blondel B, Chay E, et al. The comprehensive anatomical spinal osteotomy classification. Neurosurgery. 2014; 74 1:112–120

[32] Crandall DG, Revella J. Transforaminal lumbar interbody fusion versus anterior lumbar interbody fusion as an adjunct to posterior instrumented correction of degenerative lumbar scoliosis: three year clinical and radiographic outcomes. Spine. 2009; 34(20):2126–2133

[33] Cho KJ, Suk SI, Park SR, et al. Short fusion versus long fusion for degenerative lumbar scoliosis. Eur Spine J. 2008; 17(5):650–656

[34] Faldini C, Di Martino A, Borghi R, Perna F, Toscano A, Traina F. Long vs. short fusions for adult lumbar degenerative scoliosis: does balance matters? Eur Spine J. 2015; 24 Suppl 7:887–892

[35] Hsieh MK, Chen LH, Niu CC, Fu TS, Lai PL, Chen WJ. Combined anterior lumbar interbody fusion and instrumented posterolateral fusion for degenerative lumbar scoliosis: indication and surgical outcomes. BMC Surg. 2015; 15:26

[36] Transfeldt EE, Topp R, Mehbod AA, Winter RB. Surgical outcomes of decompression, decompression with limited fusion, and decompression with full curve fusion for degenerative scoliosis with radiculopathy. Spine. 2010; 35(20):1872–1875

[37] Tsai TH, Huang TY, Lieu AS, et al. Functional outcome analysis: instrumented posterior lumbar interbody fusion for degenerative lumbar scoliosis. Acta Neurochir (Wien). 2011; 153(3):547–555

[38] Wang G, Cui X, Jiang Z, Li T, Liu X, Sun J. Evaluation and surgical management of adult degenerative scoliosis associated with lumbar stenosis. Medicine (Baltimore). 2016; 95(15):e3394

[39] Zhu Y, Wang B, Wang H, Jin Z, Zhu Z, Liu H. Long-term clinical outcomes of selective segmental transforaminal lumbar interbody fusion combined with posterior spinal fusion for degenerative lumbar scoliosis. ANZ J Surg. 2014; 84(10):781–785

[40] Carreon LY, Puno RM, Dimar JR, II, Glassman SD, Johnson JR. Perioperative complications of posterior lumbar decompression and arthrodesis in older adults. J Bone Joint Surg Am. 2003; 85-A(11):2089–2092

[41] Zurbriggen C, Markwalder TM, Wyss S. Long-term results in patients treated with posterior instrumentation and fusion for degenerative scoliosis of the lumbar spine. Acta Neurochir (Wien). 1999; 141(1):21–26

[42] Marchesi DG, Aebi M. Pedicle fixation devices in the treatment of adult lumbar scoliosis. Spine. 1992; 17(8) Suppl:S304–S309

[43] Cho KJ, Suk SI, Park SR, et al. Complications in posterior fusion and instrumentation for degenerative lumbar scoliosis. Spine. 2007; 32(20): 2232–2237

[44] Shaw R, Skovrlj B, Cho SK. Association between age and complications in adult scoliosis surgery: an analysis of the scoliosis research society morbidity and mortality database. Spine. 2016; 41(6):508–514

[45] Charosky S, Guigui P, Blamoutier A, Roussouly P, Chopin D, Study Group on Scoliosis. Complications and risk factors of primary adult scoliosis surgery: a multicenter study of 306 patients. Spine. 2012; 37(8):693–700

[46] Smith JS, Shaffrey CI, Glassman SD, et al. Spinal Deformity Study Group. Risk-benefit assessment of surgery for adult scoliosis: an analysis based on patient age. Spine. 2011; 36(10):817–824

10 Flatback Syndrome: Can Lumbar Flatback Syndrome Be Treated Adequately with Minimally Invasive Techniques?

MIS: Navid R. Arandi and Gregory M. Mundis Jr.
Open: Randa El Mallah and Ahmad Nassr

10.1 Introduction

In 1973, Doherty[1] first outlined sagittal plane deformities in patients with adult spinal deformity (ASD) with thoracolumbar scoliosis. He noted postural complications and loss of lumbar lordosis (LL) in patients following posterior spinal fusion and Harrington's instrumentation. Subsequently in 1977, Moe and Denis[2] popularized the term "flatback syndrome" and reported satisfactory short-term results with closing wedge osteotomies in 16 patients. Flatback is characterized by a decline in LL, which leads to a fixed sagittal plane deformity, failure to stand upright without knee flexion and hip hyperextension, stooped forward posture of the torso, and pain. Patients often try to compensate by hyperextending their hips and flexing their knees in order to maintain their gaze at level with the horizon. The constant strain required to maintain sagittal equilibrium leads to pain and fatigue along the spine, thighs, and buttocks.

Flatback syndrome has been extensively studied over the last decade and has evolved to a clinical diagnosis known as sagittal imbalance. This has been defined as a distinct clinical entity that has strong correlations with spino-pelvic radiographic parameters. As such, they warrant careful consideration, as treatment recommendations are made and operative plans are created and executed. Glassman et al demonstrated that adult deformity patients with a positive sagittal vertical alignment (SVA > 5 cm) have worse health-related quality of life (HRQOL) scores and that a linear relationship exists between function scores and increasing magnitude of sagittal imbalance.[3,4] Pelvic tilt (PT), pelvic incidence (PI), and sacral slope are also essential preoperative parameters to consider. PI is a morphologic parameter that remains constant once skeletal maturity is achieved. Its value is fundamental in the understanding of an individual's ideal physiologic LL. HRQOL has been found to significantly worsen when PI–LL is greater than 10°. PT is the major compensatory mechanisms of the pelvis to maintain horizontal gaze with worsening sagittal balance. A PT greater than 20° has also been established as an independent predictor of HRQOL and may even be a primary indication for surgery.[5,6] Schwab et al[5] recently validated a comprehensive and clinically based classification system for ASD (▶ Fig. 10.1). The Scoliosis Research Society (SRS)-Schwab classification for ASD characterizes four different curve types along with three sagittal and pelvic modifiers and was developed using radiographic and HRQOL outcomes. Their classification system should be considered in all deformity cases for preoperative planning to achieve optimal deformity correction.

10.2 Indications

A thorough preoperative history is necessary to gauge the duration and progression of deformity, prior treatment, and the extent of leg and back pain. Physical exam should assess the flexibility of the deformity and the integrity of the extensor spinal musculature. Hip and knee flexion contractures should be identified as they can undermine surgical outcomes if left untreated. Patient's general health along with their clinical presentation and ability to withstand extensive reconstructive surgery must also be considered when deciding on a treatment plan. Although debatable, nonoperative treatment plays only a minor role in the management of a patient with sagittal imbalance including medications for symptomatic pain relief, physical therapy to strengthen core musculature, and bracing. Prolonged bracing, however, can contribute to atrophy of the paraspinal musculature and does not play a significant role in the definitive treatment of sagittal imbalance.

Surgery is the only definitive form of treatment for flatback. Surgical goals are not only to reduce pain, improve function, and achieve arthrodesis but also to restore sagittal balance with PI–LL ratio within 10°, PT less than 20°, and SVA < 5 cm.[5,6] Traditional methods for the treatment of flatback syndrome have been open surgical osteotomies including Smith-Petersen osteotomy (SPO), pedicle subtraction osteotomy (PSO), and vertebral column resection (VCR). Although these techniques have a proven track record, the associated morbidity is often a deterrent for patients to subject themselves to reconstruction.

Recent technological advancements in conjunction with efforts to decrease perioperative morbidity, hospital costs, and recovery times have led to heightened interest in minimally invasive techniques as viable modalities of treatment.

10.3 Advantages of Minimally Invasive Surgery

Despite the reliability of conventional open techniques at correcting sagittal deformity, they carry a high complication profile and can result in significant perioperative morbidity, and

Coronal Curve Types	Sagittal Modifiers		
	PI minus LL		
T: Thoracic ONLY With lumbar curve <30°	0	within 10°	
	+	Moderate 10-20°	
	++	Marked >20°	
L: TL/Lumbar ONLY With thoracic curve < 30°	**Global Alignment**		
	0	SVA < 4cm	
D: Double Curve With T and TL/L curves >30°	+	SVA 4 to 9.5cm	
	++	SVA > 9.5cm	
N: No major coronal Deformity All coronal curves <30°	**Pelvic Tilt**		
	0	PT < 20°	
	+	PT 20-30°	
	++	PT > 30°	

Fig. 10.1 Scoliosis Research Society (SRS)-Schwab classification for adult spinal deformity. LL, lumbar lordosis; PI, pelvic incidence; PT, pelvic tilt; SVA, sagittal vertical axis; TL, thoracolumbar. From Akbarnia B, Mundis G, Moazzaz P, et al. Anterior Column Realignment (ACR) for Focal Kyphotic Spinal Deformity Using a Lateral Transpsoas Approach and ALL Release. J Spinal Disord Tech. 2014 Feb;27(1):29-39, used with permission.

require supraphysiologic demands to recover.[7,8,9] Recovering from a three-column osteotomy can last as long as a year or more with significant convalescence and need for prolonged perioperative skilled nursing. The rehabilitation process is demanding not only of the medical community at large but also of the patient's family and caregivers. Minimally invasive techniques reduce the morbidity of the surgery itself without affecting the long-term outcome that can be achieved with open techniques. Minimally invasive surgery (MIS) accomplishes this by reducing intraoperative blood loss, decreasing transfusion rates, and inflicting less collateral damage to surrounding tissues, thereby subsequently incurring fewer complications and ultimately reducing cost. Cost is further driven down by decreasing the need for ICU care and shortening the postoperative convalescence and need for prolonged skilled nursing and rehab.[10,11,12,13,14,15,16,17,18,19,20]

A decade ago, the lateral retroperitoneal approach was reintroduced to the spine community using a mini-open approach and minimally invasive retractors to gain access to the anterior spinal column and perform a minimally invasive lateral interbody fusion (LLIF). While initially used for single-level degenerative disorders, it quickly found significance in spinal deformity surgery by decreasing the perioperative morbidity and enhancing recovery time compared to traditional anterior open techniques.[10,12,14,17,18,19] Akbarnia et al recently introduced anterior column realignment (ACR) as an evolution of LLIF to treat focal kyphotic deformity by adding a complete anterior release to the traditional LLIF procedure.[10] Early results are promising; however, larger cohorts with longer follow-up and direct comparisons to open techniques are needed to gauge its true potential.

10.4 Advantages of Open Surgery

Open techniques for the treatment of flatback syndrome and fixed sagittal deformities have been the mainstay of treatment for these disorders. While technically challenging, they have been shown to result in excellent outcomes for patients with significant sagittal plane deformity.[21,22,23,24,25] Open surgery offers direct visualization of the neural elements and allows for powerful reduction techniques to be employed to achieve correction of the deformity. The open techniques also expose the entirety of the posterior elements, allowing for a large surface area to achieve fusion. While complication rates are still significantly high in this patient population, many studies have demonstrated durable results with these techniques.[23,25,26,27,28]

Minimally invasive techniques being applied to the treatment of flatback deformities is a relatively new concept. Although these techniques may provide short-term benefits such as reduced intraoperative blood loss and faster postoperative recovery, there are many factors keeping them from being widely adopted. These techniques often rely on the use of interbody grafting techniques to achieve both reduction and fusion. The current surgical tools to achieve reduction are still not optimized for the treatment of deformity due to their limited ability to perform compression and distraction maneuvers.[12,14] The associated learning curve and high implant costs associated with these techniques are also other impediments to their widespread adoption.

10.5 Case Illustration

A 66-year-old man with a history of progressive back and leg pain radiating to the upper thighs. He has suffered a significant decline in overall function, with numerous attempts at conservative nonsurgical management proving unsuccessful at alleviating his symptoms or restoring function. On physical exam, he exhibits grossly positive sagittal and coronal imbalance with no hip flexion contractures (▶ Fig. 10.2**a,b**). Scoliosis radiographs show an LL of+2°, thoracolumbar kyphosis of 66° (T10–L3), T1 sagittal pelvic inclination (T1SPI) of 4°, SVA of+18 cm, and PT and PI of 48° and 60°, respectively (▶ Fig. 10.2**c,d**). There is a 62° PI–LL mismatch. Multilevel reconstructive surgery was mutually agreed upon.

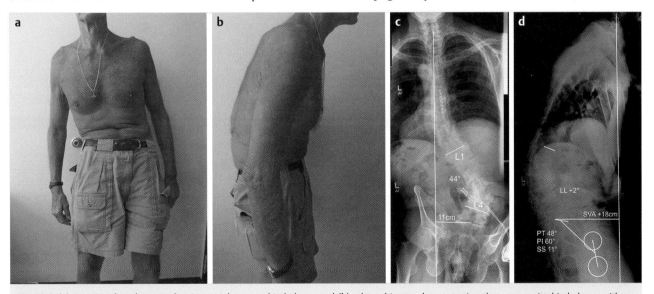

Fig. 10.2 (a) Anterior clinical image showing a right coronal imbalance and (b) a lateral image demonstrating the gross sagittal imbalance with a stooped forward posture. (c) Posteroanterior and (d) lateral X-rays further elucidating the severity of the sagittal and coronal imbalance. From Akbarnia B, Mundis G, Moazzaz P, et al. Anterior Column Realignment (ACR) for Focal Kyphotic Spinal Deformity Using a Lateral Transpsoas Approach and ALL Release. J Spinal Disord Tech. 2014 Feb;27(1):29-39, used with permission.

10.6 Surgical Technique in Minimally Invasive Surgery

Selecting the right patient is crucial and depends on the severity of deformity, region and number of involved levels, prior surgery, and flexibility. The lateral retroperitoneal transpsoas approach is best utilized for treating segmental and global kyphotic deformities from T12 to L5 with or without anterior longitudinal ligament (ALL) release. For more severe regional deformities, multilevel ACRs can be supplemented with posterior osteotomies (i.e., PSO) in order to achieve the desired correction.

ACR is a modification of the minimally invasive LLIF technique using the lateral retroperitoneal approach, hyperlordotic interbody cages, and complete anterior release, including release of the ALL, for the treatment of sagittal plane deformity. There have been considerable advancements in the technique since its introduction in 2006 by Ozgur et al[19] and the recently described ACR technique published by Akbarnia et al.[10]

Work-up of the patient for their sagittal plane deformity includes obtaining 36-inch radiographs that must include the femoral heads and the cervical spine. Supine hyperextension lateral radiographs are utilized to assess flexibility at the apical intervertebral disc, the site of the desired ACR. Magnetic resonance imaging (MRI) and/or a computed tomography (CT) myelograms are also used preoperatively to localize the psoas muscle and lumbar plexus, visualize the vascular anatomy, and to assess the posterior bony structures for facet arthropathy and fusion, and the anterior disc space for ankylosis and large osteophytes. The MRI will also help determine if patients may need a direct posterior decompression in addition to their realignment procedure. Dual-energy X-ray absorptiometry (DEXA) scans are obtained on all patients, and if the T-score is less than –2.5, the patient must be treated for their osteoporosis before the spine is reconstructed. Consideration should be given to vitamin D and calcium supplementation among all patients.

After the administration of anesthesia, the patient is placed in a lateral decubitus position on an operating table that has a break in it. The patient is padded appropriately to ensure that all pressure points are cushioned. Anteroposterior and lateral fluoroscopy is used to locate the intervertebral disc space. Excessive flexion of the operating table should be avoided in order to prevent undue tension on the psoas muscle and lumbar plexus. A lateral retroperitoneal approach is made to the disc space with concurrent directional eletromyographic (EMG) neuromonitoring to ensure safe passage through the psoas. The target of the first dilator and guidewire is the posterior one-third of the disc space to ensure a complete anterior release and to facilitate the cage placement. Many transpsoas exposure systems and monitoring systems exist. The surgeon must be familiar with the particular characteristics of each. The ACR technique was developed in conjunction with Nuvasive XLIF-ACR (eXtreme lateral interbody fusion [XLIF]; Nuvasive Inc., San Diego, CA) as the procedure requires specialized instruments designed specifically for this procedure.

Following sequential dilations, the retractor is secured to the operating table with a mounting bracket. A shim (retaining pin) is used to maintain the position of the retractor and prevent its anterior migration. The retractor is opened to the margins of the disc space, just enough to perform the initial discectomy. Once the discectomy is complete with release of the contralateral annulus, the disc space is prepared for an appropriate-size implant. Ideally, 24 mm of disc space exposure is obtained to accommodate a 22-mm wide interbody cage used in ACR. The anterior retractor is placed between the ALL and the anterior vasculature. The gentle development of the plane anterior to the ALL is critical for the proper retraction of the vascular structures. Fluoroscopy is used to confirm if the retractor reaches the contralateral pedicle. A sufficiently wide anterior retractor is used to ensure that the anterior retractor does not fall into the disc space after the ALL is released. Any additional disc material behind the anterior annulus and ALL is removed in order to sequester the ALL and ensure its safe release. The ALL is then released using a custom knife. A paddle distractor can also be used to confirm a satisfactory release of the ALL. Incomplete release of the ALL or a partially intact contralateral annulus can result in persistent tension during distraction. One must reassess and assure that these structures are fully released before continuing with trialing.

Sequential trialing is performed with standard 22-mm trials up to an anterior height of 12 mm. The ACR trial implants, which come in 20° and 30°, are then inserted. The amount of lordosis needed should be predetermined from preoperative planning. The appropriate sized cage is then prepared on the back table with the biologic of choice. The implant is then placed while attached to the posterior blade of the retractor to ensure that the implant is placed at the desired location within the disc space. The position of the interbody cage is confirmed with biplanar fluoroscopy. A screw is placed through the cephalad flange abutting the end plate of the cephalad vertebral body. This helps prevent expulsion of the implant and allows for unobstructed placement of pedicle screws.

The wound is closed in a layered technique. A small Hemovac drain is placed overlying the psoas to prevent hematoma formation. It is removed once the patient starts to ambulate the following day.

10.7 Surgical Technique in Open Surgery

Open approaches to flatback syndrome consist of anterior and posterior approaches and combinations of the two. The surgical approach is determined by the rigidity of the deformity and surgeon preference. The posterior approach often involves a posterior column–shortening procedure to allow for reestablishment of lordosis. An anterior approach involves increasing the anterior column height to reduce the deformity. These approaches may be combined or done in isolation. Indications for a combined approach include large-angle coronal deformities and imbalance, lumbar pseudoarthrosis, osteopenia, and planned fusion across the lumbosacral junction.[28] Posterior options for correction of fixed deformity include the SPO, PSO, and VCR.

10.7.1 Smith-Petersen Osteotomy

The SPO is a posterior closing wedge osteotomy that results in lengthening of the anterior column. The facets and ligamentum flavum are resected and then closed utilizing compression techniques to achieve deformity correction. It was previously common to use this technique in the treatment of the fused spine with a forced osteoclasis of the anterior column. This has been largely abandoned due to vascular and visceral complications due to the anterior distraction in those cases. With a mobile disc space and preserved disc height, it is possible to achieve 1° of deformity correction with each millimeter of posterior bone resection. Multiple osteotomies are often employed to achieve the degree of deformity correction that is needed. More distal osteotomies generate a larger degree of deformity correction. Anterior spinal fusion may be necessary if a large anterior gap is created to prevent pseudarthrosis and instability.[26,29] An SPO will achieve approximately 10° of lordosis at one segment.[26]

10.7.2 Pedicle Subtraction Osteotomy

From the posterior approach, a wedge-shaped portion of the vertebral body and both pedicles are resected. The posterior column is shortened without elongation of the anterior column. As a result, the apex of the wedge removed is the anterior margin of the vertebral body with the base at the spinous processes. This technique was originally described by Thomasen[30] and was felt to have less potential for vascular injury due to anterior stretch in comparison to the SPO. A single PSO in the lumbar spine will typically result in approximately 30° of lordotic correction.[26]

The first part of the procedure involves resection of the posterior elements above and below the planned pedicle resection. The transverse processes are then detached from the vertebral body. The posts of the pedicles are left in place to protect the nerve roots and dura. De-cancellation of the vertebral body in a wedge shape is then performed through the pedicles with the use of large curettes. The anterior cortex and ALL are preserved as the hinge for the osteotomy. The pedicles are then resected until they are flush with the posterior vertebrae. Dissection is then carried out lateral to the vertebral body. The lateral vertebral wall is then resected according to the planned osteotomy angle. The posterior vertebral wall is then impacted ventrally to complete the osteotomy. Frequent neurophysiologic monitoring and sometimes an interoperative wake-up test are utilized to ensure adequate space for the neural elements.[22,30]

10.7.3 Vertebral Column Resection

In cases of severe rigid deformity, VCR can be utilized to achieve even further correction than is possible with other types of osteotomies. One or more vertebral segments are removed (including the posterior elements, pedicles, entire vertebral body, and discs above and below). A cage is placed anteriorly to act as a fulcrum for deformity correction. This can be performed through a combined anterior and posterior approach; however, all posterior techniques have gained popularity due to the ability to directly control the spine after the osteotomy is created.[23,31] Up to 80° of correction can be achieved utilizing this technique.[24]

10.8 Discussion of Minimally Invasive Surgery

Sagittal imbalance is a major source of pain and dysfunction among patients with ASD.[3,4,17,32] Historically, open posterior and/or anterior procedures have been used to reconstruct the spine despite their inherently high complication profile.[7,9] When considering open procedure, due diligence must be paid to patient's age, comorbidities, potential for blood loss, and complication risk.

The literature on MIS in the treatment of ASD has traditionally been centered around coronal plane correction,[18,33] with incomplete data to truly assess the sagittal plane.[12,34] Direct comparisons with traditional open procedures is also lacking in the current literature. Despite its potential benefits in adult deformity correction, prospective studies with large cohorts and longer clinical and radiographic follow-up are needed in order to characterize the true potential of MIS in the treatment of sagittal plane deformities.

One of the confounding variables in performing ACR is its frequent supplementation with an open posterior release at the ACR level and/or open pedicle screw fixation in an effort to achieve optimal sagittal plane correction. Furthermore, randomization of patients into an MIS or open group is unethical and attempts to gain institutional approval will be futile. Thus, it is challenging to perform quality comparative studies on purely minimally invasive ACR versus open reconstruction for the treatment of sagittal plane deformities.[35]

10.8.1 Level I and II Evidence in Minimally Invasive Surgery

There are currently no level I or II studies available.

10.8.2 Level III and IV Evidence in Minimally Invasive Surgery

Akbarnia et al[10] were the first to report their midterm experience with ACR for the treatment of focal kyphotic deformity. Everyone in our cohort of 17 consecutive patients underwent ACR procedure followed by open posterior pedicle screw fixation. There were 12 women and 5 men, with average age of 63 years and average follow-up of 24 months. Of the 17 patients, 82% (14) had prior spine surgery, 71% (12) of which were spinal fusions. The procedure was staged with mean intraoperative blood loss of 111 mL for ACR and 1,484 mL during the posterior procedures. Indications for surgery included degenerative scoliosis, progressive focal sagittal plane deformity, instability at the level of the focal deformity, decreased QOL, and pain. Motion segment angle (measured from superior end plate of the upper end vertebrae to the lower end plate of the lower end vertebrae) improved from a mean of 9° preoperatively to –19° (28° change) after ACR and –26° (35° change) after posterior surgery, which are similar to the segmental correction achieved via open methods (▶ Fig. 10.3). Preoperative LL improved from –16° to –38° and –45° after ACR and posterior instrumentation, respectively, and was maintained at –51° at final follow-up ($p < 0.05$). PT improved from 34° preoperatively to 24° following ACR and remained stable at 25° at the latest follow-up. The T1SPI (as described by Legaye et al[36]) was used as a surrogate for sagittal vertical axis to avoid calibration errors. Results were divided into two groups based on baseline preoperative values of T1SPI. Patients with negative preoperative T1SPI averaged –6° and corrected to –0.6° after ACR with posterior

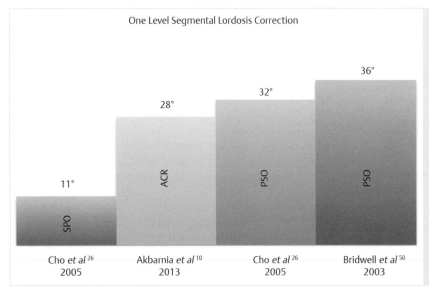

One Level Segmental Lordosis Correction

36°
32°
28°
11°

SPO — Cho et al[26] 2005
ACR — Akbarnia et al[10] 2013
PSO — Cho et al[26] 2005
PSO — Bridwell et al[50] 2003

Fig. 10.3 Comparison of single-level ACR vs. single-level PSOs and SPOs in literature. Mean degrees of segmental lordosis correction following single-level ACR was comparable to traditional open procedures such as SPO and PSO. ACR, anterior column realignment; PSO, pedicle subtraction osteotomy; SPO, Smith-Petersen osteotomy. (From Behrooz, A, Mundis, G, Moazzaz, P: Anterior Column Realignment (ACR) For Focal Kyphotic Spinal Deformity Using a Lateral Traspsoas Approach and ALL Release J Spinal Disord Tech. 2014 Feb;27(1):29-39 Wolters Kluwer Heatlh, with permission.)

instrumentation and –2° at final follow-up. Those with positive or zero T1SPI averaged + 5° and corrected to –0.5° after ACR with posterior instrumentation and –3° at final follow-up. Mean SRS-22 score improved from 2.42 preoperatively to 3.14 ($p < 0.05$) at final follow-up. Mean visual analog scale improved significantly from baseline to final follow-up (6.8 to 4.1, $p < 0.05$).

Deukmedjian et al[13] recently reported their early experience with ACR in their cohort of seven patients with sagittal imbalance. LLIF with ALL release was followed by posterior percutaneous pedicle screw fixation in seven patients and by open posterior pedicle screw fixation in one patient. Global LL improved an average of 24°, while the authors reported a mean of 17° improvement in segmental LL per level of ALL release. SVA improved from 9 cm preoperatively to 4.1 cm at final follow-up, and PT decreased by an average of 7° overall. Average improvement in SRS-22 and ODI was 26.2 and 18.3%, respectively, at 9 months postoperatively. The authors concluded that this technique was a practical option in sagittal deformity correction.

Marchi et al[14] used LLIF and hyperlordotic cages without ALL release to treat eight patients with sagittal deformity. Mean preoperative global and segmental lordosis improved from 17.7° and 2.3° to 39° and 27.1°, respectively. Mean preoperative SVA was 11.8 cm, which improved to 6.2 cm at final follow-up. PT showed an average of 11.4° improvement at final visit.

Global and segmental LL were further analyzed by Le et al[34] in a 35 patient cohort with stand-alone LLIF and 10° lordotic interbody cages without ALL release. Despite a mean 11° to 13° improvement in segmental lordosis, the authors did not find significant improvement in global LL. They concluded that greater global LL can be achieved using hyperlordotic cages with concurrent release of the ALL.

In a cadaveric study, Uribe et al[32] also examined changes in global and segmental LL. In their study, lumbar spines were subjected to one of several treatments, which involved placement of increasingly lordotic cages (10°, 20°, or 30°) with or without ALL release and no posterior fixation. The authors found the greatest segmental LL correction was achieved when using 30° cages with ALL release (11.6° mean increase) which is comparable to reported segmental correction achieved by

SPO.[37] Subsequent placement of lordotic cages at L1–L5 and ALL release lead to a mean global LL increase of 3.2° using 10° cages, 12° using 20° cages, and 20.3° using 30° cages.

In a prospective review of 107 patients with degenerative scoliosis, Phillips et al[15] demonstrated good clinical and radiological outcomes following surgical management. All patients were treated with LLIF (XLIF) and no ALL release, with or without posterior instrumentation. In a subset of patients ($n = 36$) with preoperative hypolordosis, global LL significantly improved from 27.7° to 33.6° at 2-year follow-up. They also reported statistically significant improvements in the HRQOL outcomes at 2-year follow-up.

10.9 Complications of Minimally Invasive Surgery

ASD surgery has been reported to carry a 2.4% mortality risk.[38] The complication rate for ASD with traditional open procedures is reportedly between 35 and 86%.[7,9,39,40] Regardless of etiology, a high complication profile can be expected in the treatment of sagittal plane deformity. Moreover, it is imperative to distinguish approach-related transient complications associated with MIS. If the surgical approach persistently derives transient neurological events (i.e., lower extremity paresthesias or weakness), then these events are more likely an anticipated by-product of the approach rather than a complication. Nevertheless, there continues to be a lack of consistency with which MIS complications are reported in the current literature.

Approach-related postoperative thigh paresthesias and weakness are common following the lateral transpsoas approach, with reports ranging from 0.6 to 75%.[15,17,18,33,41,42] This wide discrepancy can be associated with surgeon experience, operative time, the levels treated, and small sample sizes.[15,42] A report of neurological events in 235 LLIF patients by Pumberger et al[42] showed that the prevalence of sensory-, mechanical-, and lumbar plexus–related motor deficits were 28.7, 13.1, and 4.9%, respectively, at 6 weeks postoperatively. At 1-year follow-up, these numbers had decreased to 1.6, 1.6, and 2.9%, respectively. The largest study to analyze peri- and postoperative complications following LIF was performed by Rodgers and colleagues.[20] In their single-center review of 600 adult patients treated with XLIF, they reported an overall 6.2% complication rate (intraoperatively up to 6 weeks postoperation) with a 0.7% incidence of transient neurological complication. Interestingly, the authors did not find a significant correlation with age, comorbidities, and increased complication rate. Prior spinal fusion and treatment of L4–L5, however, were found to be significant cofactors in the occurrence of complications in those with a complication. Furthermore, the authors reported no wound infections or vascular injuries, and only 1.8% incidence events requiring a reoperation.

In our 17 patient cohort treated with ACR, 8 patients (47%) had a neurological complication, 4 patients (24%) after ACR and 6 patients (35%) after the posterior procedure.[10] Major and minor complications were defined based on the duration of symptoms. Transient dysesthesia or paresthesia in the ilioinguinal, iliohypogastric, genitofemoral, lateral femoral cutaneous, or anterior cutaneous nerve distributions persistent beyond 1 month but less than 3 months postoperatively was defined as minor. Major complications were defined as persistent dysesthesia, paresthesia, or radiculopathy continuing beyond 1 month after surgery, requiring a revision surgery, neurological weakness isolated to a specific nerve root, or persistent iliopsoas weakness continuing after the first postoperative visit. It is important to note that three of the four complications associated with ACR were transient and resolved postoperatively. Further breakdown of complications by the level of ACR showed a complication rate of 38% (3 of 8) at L4/L5 and 11% (1 out of 9) for the remainder of the levels (L1–L4).

Anand et al[11] reviewed 71 ASD patients who underwent MIS corrective surgery and reported a 19.7% (14/71) complications rate (medical and surgical) requiring a revision surgery. The most common transient postoperative complication among those who underwent a lateral retroperitoneal approach was thigh numbness. Phillips et al[15] performed a similar analysis in which they showed a 24.3% overall complication rate (95% confidence interval: 17.2–33.2%) in their 107 patient cohort who were treated with XLIF. Twelve percent of their patients required a revision surgery during the course of a 2-year follow-up. Transient lower extremity motor weakness was reported in 34% (36 of 107) of patients in the immediate postoperative period which was attributed to psoas trauma during the passage of the retractors. At 1-year follow-up, only 5% of those patients exhibited persistent lower extremity weakness. Interestingly, the authors found that mean operative time was significantly longer in those with motor weakness ($p = 0.03$).

10.10 Conclusion of Minimally Invasive Surgery

"An MIS procedure is one that by virtue of the extent and means of surgical technique results in less collateral tissue damage, resulting in measurable decrease in morbidity and more rapid functional recovery than traditional procedures, without differentiation in the intended surgical goal."[35] Open techniques for the treatment of flatback in ASD have a proven track record for improved patient outcomes. However, they also have proven track record of an unacceptably high complication rate,

postoperative morbidity, and need for revision surgery. In light of the growing elderly population and the increasing health care costs, MIS must not be neglected as a viable treatment option. Long-term clinical, biomechanical, and economical studies are needed in order to assess the true potential of MIS in the treatment of not only sagittal imbalance but also ASD as a whole.

There is currently no level I or II evidence to corroborate its use in adult deformity correction. The reported ACR literature to date has been level III or IV with small sample sizes and early to midterm follow-up. Much of the evidence has to be inferred from LLIF studies performed not only because of their power, but also because of the common approach shared by both ACR and LLIF. ACR is a new minimally invasive technique and still in the early stages of development. It has great promise to provide an alternative treatment to three-column osteotomies in the nonrigid spine and currently merits only a Grade 2C recommendation.

10.11 Discussion of Open Surgery

In 1945, Smith-Petersen were the first to use a posterior osteotomy for the correction of fixed sagittal deformity. This was performed on patients with rheumatoid arthritis.[29] These extension osteotomies were also used for the correction of ankylosing spondylitis, although these techniques are associated with anterior distraction which has been associated with visceral and vascular injury. Smith-Petersen osteotomies are most commonly utilized when the intervertebral disc spaces are mobile. This allows for partial correction of the deformity after posterior closure of the osteotomy through the flexible disc.

La Chapelle[43] modified this technique by adding an anterior release to the extension osteotomy. This would further enhance the hyperextension created by the extension osteotomy, and involved packing tibial bone into the disc space to maintain the opening.

Another approach to sagittal deformities is the use of polysegmental osteotomies. Wilson and Turkell[44] introduced this to correct sagittal balance. Polysegmental osteotomies obtained correction without rupture of the ALL. They involved correction at several levels by removing facet joints and compressing the posterior elements to create the hyperextension of the lumbar spine (lordosis). Unlike extension osteotomies, polysegmental osteotomies did not create an elongation of the anterior column, thus avoiding putting neurovascular structures at risk.

Closing wedge osteotomies were next described to correct the fixed sagittal deformity without lengthening the anterior spine. Scudese and Calabro[45] first described a monosegmental intravertebral closing wedge osteotomy of the lumbar spine. This technique has been used for fixed sagittal plane deformities ranging from ankylosing spondylitis to trauma to flatback deformity.

A version of the closing wedge osteotomy, the PSO, has gained popularity in correcting sagittal and coronal plane deformities. It is thought to provide a more extensive correction that can be obtained with a single posterior approach, irrespective of spine flexibility.[22]

VCR has been described for the management severe rigid spinal deformities. Osteotomies such as the SPO and PSO may not provide the desired amount of correction in very severe deformities. VCR provides an option, albeit a more challenging one, for the correction of these severe deformities with limited flexibility. It allows for translational and rotational correction of the spinal column as well as controlled manipulation of the anterior and posterior column via an anterior and posterior approach.[46] Suk et al were first to discuss a posterior-only approach for VCR to minimize operative time as well as complications.[31]

The amount of correction needed in the sagittal deformity governs the surgical procedure performed, as each provides a different degree of correction.

10.11.1 Level I Evidence in Open Surgery

There is no published level I evidence regarding the treatment of flatback syndrome.

10.11.2 Level II Evidence in Open Surgery

There is limited level II evidence regarding the treatment of flatback syndrome. There is no published evidence comparing the use of MIS and open surgery in flatback syndrome.

A study by Cho et al[26] prospectively collected clinical data comparing the use of different open techniques for the treatment of flatback syndrome. The SPO was compared to the PSO. When comparing the use of Smith-Petersen osteotomies at three or more levels to a PSO at one level, there was a near-identical correction in the lumbar kyphosis (33° vs. 31.7°). The SPO provided about 10° of correction per segment. Therefore, three SPOs are comparable to one PSO. The PSO group showed a significant improvement in sagittal plane correction (11.2 cm) over the SPO group (5.49 cm). There was an overall mean improvement in the Oswestry score in both groups, but this was not statistically significant ($p = 0.35$). Blood loss was noted to be substantially greater in the PSO group (approximately 1 L more). The substantial bleeding occurs from resection of pedicles and osteotomy through the vertebral body, as well as disruption of fragile epidural veins superior to each pedicle being resected. It can be concluded that at a single vertebral level, a PSO provides a greater degree of correction, at the expense of more blood loss.

Bridwell et al conducted a prospective observational study on patients with symptomatic lumbar scoliosis to determine the improvement nonoperative and operative treatment make on QOL. Eighty-five patients who were treated operatively demonstrated a statistically significant improvement in the SRS QOL score. In the 75 patients treated nonoperatively (with physical therapy, medication, or observation), there was no improvement in the QOL that was statistically significant.[47]

Schwab et al[48] conducted a multicenter prospective study on 947 patients with thoracic, thoracolumbar, and lumbar deformities. In the study, they determined the impact of lordosis and intervertebral subluxation on outcome measures (ODI/SRS). In the thoracolumbar and lumbar patient group, loss of lordosis was associated with higher ODI scores and lower SRS pain/function scores. This was also seen in patients with increased intervertebral subluxation. In those with predominantly thoracic deformities, degree of LL did not significantly affect outcome scores.

10.11.3 Level III and IV Evidence in Open Surgery

Several reports provide evidence for the use of PSO in the correction of flatback deformity. Hyun and Rhim[49] conducted a retrospective analysis of 13 patients treated with PSOs for fixed sagittal imbalances in thoracic and lumbar vertebrae. They presented with back pain and were resistant to nonoperative forms of treatment. PSOs were performed at T12, L1, L3, and L4. The mean increase in LL was 34.4° ($p < 0.0001$), and the average C7 plumb line value improved from 11.5 to 3.2 cm ($p < 0.0001$). Ten patients completed the ODI questionnaire, and there was a statistically significant overall improvement in score after surgery. This is level III evidence.

Bridwell et al[22] studied 27 patients with sagittal imbalance treated with lumbar PSO. Average increase in lordosis was 34.5° and average improvement in the sagittal plumb line was 13.5 cm. No substantial loss in correction was seen, except in one patient who developed increased kyphosis caudal to the fusion, resulting in loss of some of the sagittal correction. Twenty patients demonstrated improvements in the overall Oswestry score (mean 15 points). Sixteen patients exhibited an improvement on the pain scale of 2 or more points on a 9-point scale. Complications included development of lumbar and thoracic pseudoarthrosis in one patient and six patients, respectively.

Buchowski et al[27] assessed 108 patients who underwent lumbar PSOs over a period of 10 years. Neurologic deficits (both intraoperative and postoperative) were seen in 12 of the patients, of which 3 developed permanent deficit. They were all unilateral and the majority did not correspond to the level of the osteotomy. They were not detected by intraoperative neuromonitoring, which included SSEP (somatosensory evoked potential), NMEP, and occasionally EMG. These deficits, thought to be caused by a combination of dural buckling, subluxation, and residual dorsal impingement, included motor weakness of the tibialis anterior, quadriceps, and extensor hallucis longus. Four patients reported having weakness of multiple muscle groups. In 9 out of the 12 patients, additional surgical intervention consisting of central enlargement and further decompression was performed to correct the deficits. The neurologic deficits were most common in the degenerative sagittal imbalance group versus other spinal deformities, but the observed correlation was not statistically significant ($p < 0.503$). However, all patients who developed permanent neurologic deficits had degenerative sagittal imbalance, suggesting that the condition has a risk of developing neurologic deficit.

Bridwell et al[50] reviewed 33 patients who underwent PSO for fixed sagittal imbalance. The clinical and radiographic results were analyzed retrospectively. The mean correction for the PSO was 34.5°, with an average 1.6° loss of correction on 2- to 5-year follow-up. The mean C7 plumb line improvement was 14.9 cm immediately postoperatively and 12.7 cm at follow-up. Mean blood loss was 2,386 mL and average operative time was 12.2 hours. There were no permanent neurologic deficits associated with the PSOs. There was a statistically significant improvement in the average Oswestry Disability Index (OWI) and pain scores. Based on the SRS questionnaire, 24 patients felt their pain had improved following the PSO. Four patients felt that their pain had not changed, and a further four felt their pain had increased. Overall, there was an improvement in the health outcome measures at long-term follow-up in this group of patients.

VCR plays a role in deformities that are more severe, particularly sharper and more angulated kyphoses as well as very large scoliosis deformities. The use of VCR, particularly via a posterior-only approach, has had limited discussion in the literature. Suk et al[31] were one of the first to promote VCR via a posterior-only approach. They retrospectively reviewed 70 patients diagnosed with adult scoliosis (7 patients), congenital kyphoscoliosis (38 patients), or postinfectious kyphosis (25 patients). Sagittal spinal imbalance was determined by the C7 plumb line distance from the posterior superior corner of S1, with an imbalance considered as a trunk shift of more than 2 cm in the coronal or sagittal plane. VCR was carried out at the apex of the deformity. Indication for VCR was a coronal or sagittal imbalance with limited flexibility in which a translation of the column was necessary for deformity correction and restoration of trunk balance. In the patients with adult scoliosis, a range of one to three vertebral segments were removed with an average correction of 54° at final follow-up. In those with kyphoscoliosis, a range of one to two vertebral segments were removed with an average correction of 40° at final follow-up. In the postinfectious kyphosis group, a range of one to seven vertebral segments were removed with an average of 53° correction at final follow-up. On follow-up, five patients experienced fixation failures, of which two needed revision surgery and three needed a prolonged localized cast for 6 months.

Lenke et al[23] conducted a retrospective reviewed of 43 patients who underwent a VCR via a posterior-only approach for rigid spinal deformity. The categories of patients included severe scoliosis, global kyphosis, angular kyphosis, and combined kyphoscoliosis. Thirty-seven of the patients had a single-stage procedure, while the remaining were treated with a two-part procedure. A two-stage procedure was performed if the VCR was not started within 5 to 6 hours of commencing the operation. All the patients demonstrated a correction in their curvature. The average curve correction was a combined 109° for the patients with kyphoscoliosis, 57° for those with scoliosis, 45° for global kyphosis, and 49° for angular kyphosis. The average estimated blood loss for the patients was 1,103 mL. No patients showed a permanent deterioration in spinal cord function as monitored by intraoperative motor evoked potentials. No patients had required revision surgery for instrumentation or fusion complications.

Wang et al[51] reported the use of a multilevel modified VCR. This combined a VCR and a transpedicular eggshell osteotomy via a posterior-only approach. Thirteen cases of congenital kyphoscoliosis were treated by this technique and retrospectively studied. At 2-year follow-up, deformity correction was 33.7° in the coronal plane and 32° in the sagittal plane. There was a statistically significant improvement ($p < 0.05$) in pain, function, and level of activity.

Wang et al[24] used the same multilevel modified VCR technique via a posterior approach on nine patients with severe Pott's kyphosis. These patients had a kyphosis of the lower thoracic or upper lumbar spine with Konstam angle greater than 90°. The main complaints included fatigue, back pain, and cosmetic problems. Postoperatively, there was a mean correction of 80° of the kyphotic deformity ($p < 0.001$). Average operative blood loss was 2,933 mL. Neurological complications were observed in one patient; there was postoperative paraplegia below T9 that recovered following 8 months of rehabilitation.

Hamzaoglu et al conducted a retrospective analysis of 102 patients who have undergone posterior VCR for severe deformities, including hypolordotic deformities of the lumbar spine. This level IV evidence demonstrated an average improvement in the thoracic kyphosis of 47°. In patients with hypolordotic deformity, the average correction in lordosis was 17°. The preoperative sagittal imbalance improved by 71%. Complications included postoperative infection, hematoma, nerve root palsies, and changes in motor evoked potentials.[46]

Studies have also shown a decrease in pain following surgery for sagittal imbalance/flatback syndrome. A study by Booth et al showed that 79% of patients described a decrease in pain as a direct result of surgical treatment with osteotomies. Fifty percent reported increased function and 57% reported increased self-image; 86% were either extremely or somewhat satisfied with the results of the surgery.[25]

Glassman et al[4] studied the impact of positive sagittal balance in ASD on health status, pain, and function. In total, 352 patients with a C7 plumb line deviation ranging from 1 to 271 mm were identified. Health status was determined by scores such as ODI, SRS-29, and SF-12 physical health composite score. As the magnitude of positive sagittal balance increased, there was evidence of decreased function and increased pain as highlighted by poorer health status scores. There was no statistically significant correlation noted in the SF-12 mental health composite score. It was also noted that a more distal region of maximal kyphosis generated a higher disability score on ODI. With progressive sagittal imbalance, there is a correlated increase in severity of symptoms.

A similar study was performed by Glassman et al to assess the correlation between radiographic appearances and health outcome scores. A total of 298 patients were studied, of whom 172 had no prior surgery and 126 had undergone prior spine fusion. In those with no prior surgery, a coronal shift of greater than 4 cm corresponded with poorer outcomes on SRS-22, SF-12, and ODI health outcome measures. In patients with prior spinal fusion, those with a positive sagittal balance had poorer health outcome measures such as pain, function, and self-image.[3]

Rose et al[52] analyzed 40 patients to determine the ideal spinopelvic parameters to regain sagittal balance after PSO. It was determined that using both thoracic kyphosis and PI measurements was the most sensitive in determining optimal LL in each patient. This provided a 91% sensitivity for predicting PSO success. (LL predicted by the formula LL < 45° – TK – PI).

10.12 Complications in Open Surgery

Complications associated with the open correction of flatback syndrome vary according to the technique used. Global complications include deep wound infection, pseudoarthrosis, deep venous thrombosis, coronal imbalance, and insufficient sagittal correction.[25]

The use of the SPO technique carries with it a risk of significant morbidity and mortality. Because it involves lengthening of the anterior column, there is a risk of injury to the neurovascular structures anterior to the vertebrae. Forceful hyperextension during this approach may result in rupture of the aorta or inferior vena cava. This risk is increased in patients with ankylosing spondylitis who have frequently calcified vessels. This lengthening is also associated with an increased incidence of emesis and aspiration due to stretch or disruption of gastrointestinal structures. These complications are less prevalent in PSOs because there is no lengthening of the anterior column.[53]

Osteotomies are often associated with a significant amount of blood loss. Reports of average blood loss vary in the literature. According to the previously mentioned study by Cho et al, average postoperative blood loss for an SPO is 1,400 mL.[26] Yang et al studied their patients undergoing PSO. Their average postoperative blood loss for PSO was 5,300 mL and average duration in ICU was 9.5 days following the procedure. Fifteen percent of patients who underwent lumbar PSO showed radiographic evidence of instrumentation failure following the initial 90-day postoperative period.[21]

Hyun and Rhim assessed 13 patients who underwent PSOs for fixed sagittal imbalance. Intraoperative complications involved one dural tear and bleeding of greater than 5,000 mL. Perioperative complications included transient paraplegia and CSF leakage. Four patients (30%) developed late-onset kyphosis progression, and there were six instrumentation failures.[49]

Bridwell et al's review of 33 patients who underwent PSOs demonstrated 2 patients with breakdown and kyphosis at segments proximal to the instrumented fusion on follow-up. One patient presented 6 weeks postoperatively with a T10 compression fracture and was treated with a brace. The other presented 4 months postoperatively with a T11 burst fracture. This required reoperation to extend the fusion and instrumentation in the upper thoracic spine. Six patients developed pseudoarthrosis proximal to the osteotomy.[50]

VCRs carry a high risk of serious complications, such as neurological injuries. These can result from direct injury during bone resection or compression by residual bone and soft tissue following correction. Complications can also occur secondary to dural buckling and subluxation of the spinal column. A VCR via a posterior-only approach allows for reduced operating time and amount of blood loss.[46] According to Lenke et al's study of posterior-only VCR, two patients suffered transient nerve root palsies postoperatively, with both recovering completely within 6 months.[23] In Suk et al's study,[31] serious complications included fixation failure, complete cord injury, root injuries, and hematomas associated with cauda equina syndrome.

10.13 Conclusion of Open Surgery

Based on the level II evidence available, PSO provides roughly 30° and SPO provides approximately 10° correction per segment. The level III and IV evidence shows that VCR provides the greatest degree of correction per level for thoracic kyphotic deformities. Pedicle subtraction osteotomies were shown to be more corrective for hypolordotic deformities.

Open techniques have long been the mainstay of surgical treatment for flatback syndrome, while minimally invasive techniques are relatively new to the field of sagittal plane deformities. From the limited literature, it seems that minimally invasive improvements in lordosis and sagittal balance have not been widely demonstrated.[12,14] As a result, it is difficult to provide an adequate comparison, given there is a paucity of literature directly comparing MIS and open techniques; the majority is focused on the outcomes of individual open techniques. At this point of time, there is abundantly more information on the use of open techniques.

10.14 Editors' Commentary

10.14.1 Minimally Invasive Surgery

One must always be cautious when stating what "cannot" be done when speaking of new and evolving techniques and technologies. History is full of quotes uttered by famous people that, over time, became absurdities. Consider, for example, the emphatic statement of Marshall Ferdinand Foch, French military strategist and WWI commander, who proclaimed "Airplanes are interesting toys, but of no military value."

Over the last several years, three changes have occurred which invalidate the claim that sagittal plane deformity (of which "flatback" syndrome is one manifestation) cannot adequately be corrected using MIS techniques. First, hyperlordotic cages for use both anteriorly and laterally have enabled segmental correction of 20 to 25° per level. Second, section of the ALL further enables even greater segmental correction. Finally, alternative rod bending techniques, such as in vivo rod bending using the "push through" technique, combined with posterior osteotomies have enabled correction of sagittal plane deformity equivalent to that achieved with open technique. Furthermore, it has been done while maintaining the now well-known advantages of MIS surgery, such as less blood loss, less pain, faster recovery, lower infection rates, and overall complication rates. The lesson to be learned, then, is when considering newly evolving techniques and technologies, look to the future, not the past.

10.14.2 Open Surgery

The correction of flatback deformity is one of the most challenging surgical endeavors in the field of spine surgery. The advantage of pedicle subtraction osteotomy is a large degree of sagittal plane correction that can be obtained with a single approach at one level, which eliminates the need for multiple posterior column osteotomies over an extended surface area. The MIS section of this discussion suggests that posterior corrective techniques are often still required after MIS anterior approach surgery to achieve sufficient correction. A properly performed PSO obviates the need for segmental correction using an anterior approach. An anterior lumbar interbody fusion that utilizes hyperlordotic implants may improve sagittal alignment more so than traditional interbody cages but places the anterior great vessels and segments at risk due to the need for vessel manipulation with compromised visualization. This procedure has the similar risk of visceral and vascular injury as open procedures but with only a limited corridor to visualize and protect these structures. Injury of either the bowel or great vessels would likely require immediate, and possibly emergent, conversion to an open procedure. Spine surgeons without extensive general surgery training would benefit from having a general surgeon standing by during the more dangerous parts of these procedures.

If an MIS procedure requires an additional posterior approach to accomplish sagittal correction, then its benefit as a minimally invasive procedure is somewhat diluted compared to a procedure that can be performed through a single posterior approach (PSO) with similar corrective outcomes.

In summary, in the setting of spinal disease which requires a significant corrective maneuver to alter sagittal alignment, MIS interventions at this time appears to be more risky and less efficacious than a standard open posterior corrective osteotomy.

References

[1] Doherty J. Complications of fusion in lumbar scoliosis. Proceedings of the Scoliosis Research Society. J Bone Joint Surg Am. 1973; 55:438

[2] Moe JH, Denis F. The iatrogenic loss of lumbar lordosis. Orthop Trans. 1977; 1 (2):131

[3] Glassman SD, Berven S, Bridwell K, Horton W, Dimar JR. Correlation of radiographic parameters and clinical symptoms in adult scoliosis. Spine. 2005; 30(6):682–688

[4] Glassman SD, Bridwell K, Dimar JR, Horton W, Berven S, Schwab F. The impact of positive sagittal balance in adult spinal deformity. Spine. 2005; 30 (18):2024–2029

[5] Lafage V, Bharucha NJ, Schwab F, et al. Multicenter validation of a formula predicting postoperative spinopelvic alignment. J Neurosurg Spine. 2012; 16 (1):15–21

[6] Schwab F, Lafage V, Patel A, Farcy JP. Sagittal plane considerations and the pelvis in the adult patient. Spine. 2009; 34(17):1828–1833

[7] Auerbach JD, Lenke LG, Bridwell KH, et al. Major complications and comparison between 3-column osteotomy techniques in 105 consecutive spinal deformity procedures. Spine. 2012; 37(14):1198–1210

[8] Kim YB, Lenke LG, Kim YJ, et al. The morbidity of an anterior thoracolumbar approach: adult spinal deformity patients with greater than five-year follow-up. Spine. 2009; 34(8):822–826

[9] Cho SK, Bridwell KH, Lenke LG, et al. Comparative analysis of clinical outcome and complications in primary versus revision adult scoliosis surgery. Spine. 2012; 37(5):393–401

[10] Akbarnia BA, Mundis GM, Jr, Moazzaz P, et al. Anterior column realignment (ACR) for focal kyphotic spinal deformity using a lateral transpsoas approach and ALL release. J Spinal Disord Tech. 2014; 27(1):29–3

[11] Anand N, Baron EM, Khandehroo B, Kahwaty S. Long-term 2- to 5-year clinical and functional outcomes of minimally invasive surgery for adult scoliosis. Spine. 2013; 38(18):1566–1575

[12] Dakwar E, Cardona RF, Smith DA, Uribe JS. Early outcomes and safety of the minimally invasive, lateral retroperitoneal transpsoas approach for adult degenerative scoliosis. Neurosurg Focus. 2010; 28(3):E8

[13] Deukmedjian AR, Dakwar E, Ahmadian A, Smith DA, Uribe JS. Early outcomes of minimally invasive anterior longitudinal ligament release for correction of sagittal imbalance in patients with adult spinal deformity. Sci World J. 2012; 2012:789698

[14] Marchi L, Oliveira L, Amaral R, et al. Anterior elongation as a minimally invasive alternative for sagittal imbalance-a case series. HSS J. 2012; 8(2):122–127

[15] Phillips FM, Isaacs RE, Rodgers WB, et al. Adult degenerative scoliosis treated with XLIF: clinical and radiographical results of a prospective multicenter study with 24-month follow-up. Spine. 2013; 38(21):1853–1861

[16] Rodgers WB, Gerber EJ, Rodgers JA. Lumbar fusion in octogenarians: the promise of minimally invasive surgery. Spine. 2010; 35(26) Suppl:S355–S360

[17] Mundis GM, Akbarnia BA, Phillips FM. Adult deformity correction through minimally invasive lateral approach techniques. Spine. 2010; 35(26) Suppl: S312–S321

[18] Youssef JA, McAfee PC, Patty CA, et al. Minimally invasive surgery: lateral approach interbody fusion: results and review. Spine. 2010; 35(26) Suppl: S302–S311

[19] Ozgur BM, Aryan HE, Pimenta L, Taylor WR. Extreme Lateral Interbody Fusion (XLIF): a novel surgical technique for anterior lumbar interbody fusion. Spine J. 2006; 6(4):435–443

[20] Rodgers WB, Gerber EJ, Patterson J. Intraoperative and early postoperative complications in extreme lateral interbody fusion: an analysis of 600 cases. Spine. 2011; 36(1):26–32

[21] Yang BP, Ondra SL, Chen LA, Jung HS, Koski TR, Salehi SA. Clinical and radiographic outcomes of thoracic and lumbar pedicle subtraction osteotomy for fixed sagittal imbalance. J Neurosurg Spine. 2006; 5(1):9–17

[22] Bridwell KH, Lewis SJ, Rinella A, Lenke LG, Baldus C, Blanke K. Pedicle subtraction osteotomy for the treatment of fixed sagittal imbalance. Surgical technique. J Bone Joint Surg Am. 2004; 86-A Suppl 1:44–50

[23] Lenke LG, Sides BA, Koester LA, Hensley M, Blanke KM. Vertebral column resection for the treatment of severe spinal deformity. Clin Orthop Relat Res. 2010; 468(3):687–699

[24] Wang Y, Zhang Y, Zhang X, et al. Posterior-only multilevel modified vertebral column resection for extremely severe Pott's kyphotic deformity. Eur Spine J. 2009; 18(10):1436–1441

[25] Booth KC, Bridwell KH, Lenke LG, Baldus CR, Blanke KM. Complications and predictive factors for the successful treatment of flatback deformity (fixed sagittal imbalance). Spine. 1999; 24(16):1712–1720

[26] Cho KJ, Bridwell KH, Lenke LG, Berra A, Baldus C. Comparison of Smith-Petersen versus pedicle subtraction osteotomy for the correction of fixed sagittal imbalance. Spine. 2005; 30(18):2030–2037, discussion 2038

[27] Buchowski JM, Bridwell KH, Lenke LG, et al. Neurologic complications of lumbar pedicle subtraction osteotomy: a 10-year assessment. Spine. 2007; 32 (20):2245–2252

[28] Berven SH, Deviren V, Smith JA, Hu SH, Bradford DS. Management of fixed sagittal plane deformity: outcome of combined anterior and posterior surgery. Spine. 2003; 28(15):1710–1715, discussion 1716

[29] Smith-Petersen MN, Larson CB, Aufranc OE. Osteotomy of the spine for correction of flexion deformity in rheumatoid arthritis. Clin Orthop Relat Res. 1969; 66(66):6–9

[30] Thomasen E. Vertebral osteotomy for correction of kyphosis in ankylosing spondylitis. Clin Orthop Relat Res. 1985(194):142–152

[31] Suk SI, Kim JH, Kim WJ, Lee SM, Chung ER, Nah KH. Posterior vertebral column resection for severe spinal deformities. Spine. 2002; 27(21):2374–2382

[32] Uribe JS, Smith DA, Dakwar E, et al. Lordosis restoration after anterior longitudinal ligament release and placement of lateral hyperlordotic interbody cages during the minimally invasive lateral transpsoas approach: a radiographic study in cadavers. J Neurosurg Spine. 2012; 17(5):476–485

[33] Isaacs RE, Hyde J, Goodrich JA, Rodgers WB, Phillips FM. A prospective, nonrandomized, multicenter evaluation of extreme lateral interbody fusion for the treatment of adult degenerative scoliosis: perioperative outcomes and complications. Spine. 2010; 35(26) Suppl:S322–S330

[34] Le TV, Vivas AC, Dakwar E, Baaj AA, Uribe JS. The effect of the retroperitoneal transpsoas minimally invasive lateral interbody fusion on segmental and regional lumbar lordosis. Sci World J. 2012; 2012:516706

[35] McAfee PC, Phillips FM, Andersson G, et al. Minimally invasive spine surgery. Spine. 2010; 35(26) Suppl:S271–S273

[36] Legaye J, Hecquet J, Marty C, Duval-beaupere G. Equilibre Sagittal du Rachis: relations entre bassin et courbures rachidiennes sagittales en position debout. Rachis. 1993; 5:215–226

[37] Bridwell KH. Decision making regarding Smith-Petersen vs. pedicle subtraction osteotomy vs. vertebral column resection for spinal deformity. Spine. 2006; 31(19) Suppl:S171–S178

[38] Pateder DB, Gonzales RA, Kebaish KM, Cohen DB, Chang JY, Kostuik JP. Short-term mortality and its association with independent risk factors in adult spinal deformity surgery. Spine. 2008; 33(11):1224–1228

[39] Lapp MA, Bridwell KH, Lenke LG, et al. Long-term complications in adult spinal deformity patients having combined surgery a comparison of primary to revision patients. Spine. 2001; 26(8):973–983

[40] Cho SK, Bridwell KH, Lenke LG, et al. Major complications in revision adult deformity surgery: risk factors and clinical outcomes with 2- to 7-year follow-up. Spine. 2012; 37(6):489–500

[41] Anand N, Rosemann R, Khalsa B, Baron EM. Mid-term to long-term clinical and functional outcomes of minimally invasive correction and fusion for adults with scoliosis. Neurosurg Focus. 2010; 28(3):E6

[42] Pumberger M, Hughes AP, Huang RR, Sama AA, Cammisa FP, Girardi FP. Neurologic deficit following lateral lumbar interbody fusion. Eur Spine J. 2012; 21(6):1192–1199

[43] La Chapelle EH. Osteotomy of the lumbar spine for correction of kyphosis in a case of ankylosing spondylarthritis. J Bone Joint Surg Am. 1946; 28(4):851–858

[44] Wilson MJ, Turkell JH. Multiple spinal wedge osteotomy; its use in a case of Marie-Strumpell spondylitis. Am J Surg. 1949; 77(6):777–782

[45] Scudese VA, Calabro JJ. Vertebral wedge osteotomy. Correction of rheumatoid (ankylosing) spondylitis. JAMA. 1963; 186:627–631

[46] Hamzaoglu A, Alanay A, Ozturk C, Sarier M, Karadereler S, Ganiyusufoglu K. Posterior vertebral column resection in severe spinal deformities: a total of 102 cases. Spine. 2011; 36(5):E340–E344

[47] Bridwell KH, Glassman S, Horton W, et al. Does treatment (nonoperative and operative) improve the two-year quality of life in patients with adult symptomatic lumbar scoliosis: a prospective multicenter evidence-based medicine study. Spine. 2009; 34(20):2171–2178

[48] Schwab F, Farcy JP, Bridwell K, et al. A clinical impact classification of scoliosis in the adult. Spine. 2006; 31(18):2109–2114

[49] Hyun SJ, Rhim SC. Clinical outcomes and complications after pedicle subtraction osteotomy for fixed sagittal imbalance patients : a long-term follow-up data. J Korean Neurosurg Soc. 2010; 47(2):95–101

[50] Bridwell KH, Lewis SJ, Edwards C, et al. Complications and outcomes of pedicle subtraction osteotomies for fixed sagittal imbalance. Spine. 2003; 28 (18):2093–2101

[51] Wang Y, Zhang Y, Zhang X, et al. A single posterior approach for multilevel modified vertebral column resection in adults with severe rigid congenital kyphoscoliosis: a retrospective study of 13 cases. Eur Spine J. 2008; 17(3): 361–372

[52] Rose PS, Bridwell KH, Lenke LG, et al. Role of pelvic incidence, thoracic kyphosis, and patient factors on sagittal plane correction following pedicle subtraction osteotomy. Spine. 2009; 34(8):785–791

[53] McMaster MJ, Coventry MB. Spinal osteotomy in akylosing spondylitis. Technique, complications, and long-term results. Mayo Clin Proc. 1973; 48 (7):476–486

11 Can Thoracic Disc Herniation Be Effectively Treated Using Minimally Invasive Techniques?

MIS: Paul W. Millhouse, Troy I. Mounts, and Kristen E. Radcliff
Open: Alexander A. Theologis and Vedat Deviren

11.1 Introduction

The diagnosis and treatment of thoracic disc herniations (TDHs) has always been challenging.[1] Although asymptomatic TDHs are quite common,[1,2] the incidence of symptomatic TDHs is low, accounting for 0.1 to 4% of all surgically treated disc herniations.[2,3,4] Herniated thoracic discs present equally in both sexes and can occur medially, laterally, or centrolaterally. The symptoms vary widely and include axial pain, radicular pain, and/or myelopathy. This protean presentation contributes to delays in diagnosis.[4]

The thoracic spine lies in close proximity to the thoracic visceral organs and articulates with the rib cage through costovertebral joints. The thoracic spinal cord is unique due to the watershed blood supply, the limited space available in the spinal canal, and the kyphotic alignment.[5] Thus, TDHs pose unique technical challenges for surgeons. Therefore, operative intervention for thoracic spine pathology is typically reserved for patients with debilitating symptoms refractory to conservative treatment.[5] The role of surgery for localized or axial pain in the presence of a TDH remains controversial because the herniation may be an incidental finding.[6] However, for a symptomatic herniated disc, involving neurologic deficit or intractable pain not responsive to conservative measures, surgery is regarded as the treatment of choice to prevent the sequelae of compressive myelopathy.[7]

Given the anatomical considerations and variations in pathology and patient considerations, a plethora of surgical approaches and techniques have been developed to treat TDH.[1,5] A variety of anterior and posterolateral procedures remain in use today. Traditional anterior thoracotomy exposures provide direct visualization of the disc space but risk injury to the intrathoracic elements. Posterolateral approaches afford greater access to the posterior structures, the potential for circumferential decompression, the ability to place segmental instrumentation for stabilization, and the possibility of providing deformity correction. The disadvantage of posterolateral approaches includes diminished access to the ventral cord and disc space. A dorsolateral path can also entail excessive muscle dissection and removal of bony elements with a potential risk of iatrogenic instability. Minimally invasive procedures have been tailored for use in the thoracic spine and are reportedly associated with decreased soft-tissue injury, less operative blood loss, shorter hospitalization, and quicker recovery.[5] However, there is a substantial learning curve with the thoracoscopic techniques, as well as a limited field of vision and diminished ability to address potential complications. Muscle-sparing lumbar retractors have been adapted to the thorax recently, but are also associated with some technical difficulty. In this chapter, the authors discuss surgical alternatives, including the advantages and disadvantages of open versus minimally invasive surgery (MIS) for TDHs and propose recommendations for future improvements and considerations for treating this rare disorder.

11.2 Indications

Indications for surgical excision of TDHs include myelopathy, radiculopathy, and severe intractable axial pain.[8] Myelopathy is the clearest indication for surgery to prevent further compression and irreversible spinal cord damage.[9] Among the myelopathic patients, acute myelopathy is the strongest consideration for surgery and best predictor for neurologic improvement.[8] Another primary indication for surgical intervention is protracted, disabling radicular pain refractory to conservative treatment.[9] Radiculopathy, defined as axial pain or pain radiating to a dermatomal area of distribution, is a relative indication and often responds to nonsurgical therapy.[8] Most of the patients with purely axial pain can be managed nonoperatively.[8] Surgery for axial back pain in the presence of a TDH is controversial. Many TDHs discovered on magnetic resonance imaging (MRI) may be incidental, and additional studies, such as computed tomography (CT) myelography, must be done to correlate the finding with pain.

11.3 Advantages of Minimally Invasive Surgery

After one decides to intervene surgically on a TDH, the next critical question to address is how the decompression will be performed. A multitude of surgical techniques and approaches have been described to treat TDHs. They include anterior/anterolateral (i.e., transthoracic transpleural, transthoracic extrapleural), posterolateral (i.e., costotransversectomy [CTVS]/lateral extracavitary, transpedicular, transfacet/pedicle-sparing), and posterior (laminectomy) approaches. There is no perfect approach, as each technique is associated with unique advantages and disadvantages.

11.3.1 Minimally Invasive Anterior/Anterolateral Approaches

Although traditional open anterior approaches to the thoracic spine allow for access to all types of disc herniations below T4, direct visualization of the dura-disc interval, and decompression of the canal with the least manipulation of neurologic structures, they have been associated with significant perioperative discomfort, difficult ventilation, shoulder girdle dysfunction, wound healing problems, and pulmonary complications (i.e., pulmonary emboli, parenchymal tears, pneumonia).[10,11,12,13,14] With the goal to decrease pulmonary complications and improve patient outcomes, MIS techniques performed via an anterior/anterolateral approach were developed. The two most common MIS techniques to address TDHs are thoracoscopy and mini-open anterior approaches and their modifications, including the mini-open lateral approach. One of the most common indications for thoracoscopic spine surgery is thoracic discectomy.[12,15,16,17,18] Using thoracoscopy, a discectomy is performed through three or four small portals. As the portals are situated between the ribs, the need to retract and/or resect a rib is eliminated, which decreases the incidence of intercostal neuralgia (ICN) compared to open procedures.[18] Additional intraoperative advantages of thoracoscopy include enhanced visualization to the surgeons and operative team, direct visualization of the ventral spinal surface without the need to take down the diaphragm, and reduced intraoperative blood loss.[9,19,20,21,22] Many of the intraoperative benefits correlate to postoperative advantages, which include a better cosmetic result, improved shoulder girdle function, less postoperative pain and narcotic use with improved ventilatory excursion, shorter chest tube use, shorter hospital length of stay (LOS), and faster recovery times.[9,12,15,19,20,21,22] While previous thoracotomy and pleural adhesions have been stated as contraindications to the use of thoracoscopic intervention,[12] it has been used successfully and safely for reoperation of thoracic discs in the presence of pleural adhesions and distorted spinal anatomy after previous thoracotomy.[23] Despite these advantages, there are no prospective studies that compare thoracoscopy to open thoracotomy in myelopathic patients with thoracic disc disease.

Mayer first described the mini-thoracotomy approach (mini-TTA), which represents a middle ground between open and thoracoscopic approaches.[24] The approach combines the resection of a rib, single-lung ventilation, and the use of a surgical microscope. This setup provides the unique advantage of direct visualization and magnification of the surgical field. In contrast to thoracoscopy, which involves 2D visualization of 3D pathology, the microscope allows for 3D visualization. The mini-TTA also allows for the most direct and shortest route to the anterior thoracic spine and is associated with a reduction in postoperative thoracic pain and pulmonary complications relative to open approaches.[25,26,27] The mini-TTA has been used with great success and has had few major associated complications in the treatment of TDH that occupy greater than 40% of the spinal canal diameter, also known as "giant thoracic disc herniations" (GTDHs).[24,25]

The most recently developed MIS approach to the thoracic spine is the mini-open lateral approach, which represents a modification to the mini-TTA. The strength of this technique is that a standard anterior discectomy and fusion with instrumentation can be performed while avoiding collateral approach-related complications. The mini-open lateral approach can be a retropleural technique, which allows for canal exposure without sacrificing intercostal nerves, avoids the potential risk of intraforaminal radiculomedullary artery occlusion, and optimizes spinal exposure by limiting aorta or vena cava spinal coverage compared to standard open thoracotomy.[25] In addition, the use of a retropleural retractor system eliminates the need to deflate the ipsilateral lung, theoretically decreasing the risk of postoperative atelectasis and pulmonary complications and minimizing overall perioperative morbidity. The mini-open lateral approach also does not involve a microscope, avoids rib resection, and allows for performance of the procedure under

direct vision with concomitant control of the pathologic process and the essential anatomic structures. As this approach allows for direct visualization and conventional surgical techniques, there is no need for highly trained staff and the learning curve is theoretically also shorter than that for thoracoscopy, although this has not been demonstrated in a clinical series.

11.3.2 Minimally Invasive Posterolateral Approaches

Traditional posterolateral approaches to the thoracic spine are popular among spine surgeons, as they can be performed independently without the assistance from an "approach surgeon." However, in order to access a TDH via these approaches, extensive muscle dissection and ligamentous detachment are required. The working area required to adequately visualize pathology and manipulate surgical instruments is much larger than the actual area of pathology.[26,28,29] Another disadvantage of traditional posterolateral approaches is that their use is limited to the treatment of lateral, soft TDHs, as surgical decompression of the ventral spinal cord is often performed blindly. Thus, in an attempt to minimize soft-tissue disruption, avoid complications associated with anterior thoracic approaches, decrease incision length, and improve visualization, posterolateral MIS approaches to the thoracic spine were developed.

Creation of MIS posterolateral approaches can be credited to Jho and Fessler.[28] Since their first descriptions, MIS approaches have been used for the transpedicular,[28,30,31] transfacet/pedicle-sparing,[32,33] and CTVS[34,35] approaches with the aid of tubular retractors for exposure and the endoscope and/or microscope for visualization.[28,30,31,32,33,34,35] Access via tubular retractors (i.e., 18 and 20 mm) requires incisions that range in size from 2 to 4 cm,[28,30,31,32,35] which are significantly smaller than the traditionally sized incisions that range from 7 to 10 cm in length. The importance of a smaller incision cannot be overlooked, given it results in minimal muscular and ligamentous trauma, thereby decreasing postoperative pain, hospital LOS, and overall morbidity.[28,30,31,32,35] For example, an MIS CTVS approach avoids the need for rib resection, pleural retraction, and the violation of the costal neurovascular bundle and pleural cavity. Therefore, it is associated with less intraoperative estimated blood loss (EBL), shorter operative time (ORT), avoidance for the need of a chest tube, fewer blood transfusions, shorter hospital LOS, and lower overall complication rates compared to a traditional open CTVS approach.[35]

The use of the endoscope is also an important advantage of MIS posterolateral techniques, as it allows for safe access and decompression of areas around the spinal cord that were traditionally thought to be too dangerous to access with an open posterolateral approach. For example, Jho described the use of a 70°-angled endoscope and curved surgical instruments introduced through a transpedicular route to directly visualize and safely decompress the ventral spinal cord.[30,31] The use of a microscope provides the unique advantage of performing thoracic disc decompression using traditional discectomy instruments under 3D visualization.[28] In addition, the microscope's stereoscopic views allow surgeons to drill in a more controlled and safer manner than if the endoscope were used.[30] However, the views of an endoscope can be enhanced if a 3D endoscope is used with a high-definition video monitor.[30] The advantages described herein for MIS posterolateral approaches have allowed many surgeons to treat a variety of TDHs with excellent outcomes and a limited risk profile.

11.4 Advantages of Open Surgery

Anterior thoracotomy is the gold standard procedure to treat TDH. The greatest risks with intrathoracic procedures (open or MIS) are great vessel, cardiac, lung, and/or esophageal injury. Of these, the most common catastrophic complication involves hemorrhage and death from an aortic or segmental vessel injury. The open anterior exposure offers unparalleled ability to identify, dissect, and control the vessels safely and prevent lethal hemorrhage compared to an MIS approach. If a vascular injury occurs during an MIS procedure, the operative field often is obscured with blood, which makes control of the injury exceedingly difficult. Emergent conversion to an open thoracotomy due to vascular injury and/or extensive bleeding has been reported as an adverse event of MIS techniques.[36]

The second advantage of open thoracotomy for thoracic discectomy includes a greater appreciation of thoracic and spinal canal anatomy. Following open thoracotomy, the surgeon has excellent visualization of the vertebral bodies, end plates, and disc. If an MIS approach is performed, the surgeon may lose appropriate orientation due to loss of visualization of 3D surface landmarks. This latter complication may be particularly concerning if the patient is malrotated, which is common in the lateral decubitus position. Instrumentation can also be more carefully applied in open cases. Thoracic disc pathology differs from the lumbar spine, where disc herniations frequently are composed of "soft" nucleus pulposis and are easily amenable to treatment through a smaller approach. TDHs are usually not "soft" herniations, as they are extruded, sequestered, and/or calcified. TDHs frequently occur in the setting of ossification of the posterior longitudinal ligament (OPLL). Careful resection of the osteophytes and occasionally the vertebral body end plates is required to adequately decompress the spinal cord. An open approach affords the surgeon the best opportunity to perform a "partial corpectomy" to confidently resect all the osteophytes.

Posterolateral approaches are increasingly common in the treatment of complex thoracic pathology, including tumor metastases and epidural abscess. With each of these approaches, the surgeon can stabilize spinal elements, place segmental instrumentation, perform a partial or complete corpectomy with an expandable cage, and correct a deformity. In contrast to lumbar discectomies, retraction of the thecal sac to access anterior pathology is impractical in the thoracic spine. Instead, the anterior epidural space is accessed through a pedicular zone or extrapedicular corridor, thus avoiding cord manipulation. A transpedicular approach avoids damage to the radicular vessels[4]; however, it involves the resection of the pedicle and lateral vertebral wall.[4] A transfacet approach has the advantage of sparing resection of the pedicle. Maintaining the structural integrity of the pedicle may reduce postoperative back pain and improve spinal stability.[2] This technique is not suitable for midline disc herniations.[37] Open posterolateral approaches are safer than MIS cannulated discectomy through the lateral recess, given the latter requires thecal

sac retraction and the associated risk of spinal cord injury. Due to the complex costovertebral anatomy, endoscopic discectomy through the neural foramen and Kambin's triangle is not possible in the thoracic spine. Minimally invasive tubular transpedicular decompression is potentially very difficult due to poor visualization from the pedicle's bleeding cancellous bone. In addition, placement of instrumentation and stabilization through a percutaneous approach is technically demanding.

In summary, in comparison to MIS counterparts, open anterior and posterolateral approaches to the thoracic spine are safer and provide a greater ability to address thoracic spine pathology, visualize and control potential blood vessel injuries, as well as place spinal instrumentation.

11.5 Case Illustration

The patient was a 59-year-old woman with a long history of chronic back pain and prior cervical, thoracic, and lumbar surgeries who presented with persistent back pain and upper abdominal numbness and radicular pain. Pertinent physical examination findings included bilateral lower extremity numbness and weakness (4/5 in proximal muscle groups). After clinical examination and review of appropriate radiographic imaging, it was evident that her symptoms were due to chronic, severe thoracic myelopathy from a large midline, calcified T9–T10 disc herniation (▶ Fig. 11.1). Given that the patient had exhausted multiple conservative methods of management, surgical intervention was recommended. The goals of surgery were to arrest the progression of myelopathy and to improve her thoracolumbar radicular pain.

11.6 Surgical Technique in Minimally Invasive Surgery

The patient is brought to the operating room. The procedure is performed under general anesthesia. The patient is intubated with a regular endotracheal tube rather than a double-lumen tube. Neuromonitoring modalities, including SSEP (somatosensory evoked potential), MEP (motor evoked potential), and EMG (electromyogram), are placed. The patient is then positioned in the lateral decubitus position with the left-side up. The patient is secured to the table with 4-inch tape and the table is flexed to help open the space between the ribs at the affected level.

The surgical field is widely prepped so that the incision could be extended to a regular thoracotomy if necessary. The junction of the posterior and middle thirds of the desired disc space is marked over the skin using fluoroscopy. A 4-cm incision is centered over the mark. The subcutaneous tissue and the intercostal muscles are divided with electrocautery. The ribs are identified with gentle subperiosteal dissection. The thoracic cavity is entered through the superior edge of the rib overlying the desired disc space in order to avoid the neurovascular bundle at the superior aspect of the intercostal space. Approximately 2 inches of the rib are resected, and with blunt dissection, the pleura is mobilized over the rib cage. The parietal pleura is carefully deflected from the inner thoracic wall. The desired level is verified with fluoroscopy, and the dilators are placed over the affected disc space. The retropleural retractor system

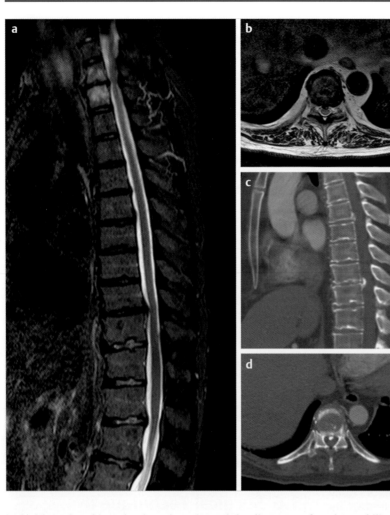

Fig. 11.1 (a) Preoperative sagittal and (b) axial MRI images, and (c) sagittal and (d) axial CT radiographs at affected level.

is then introduced into the thoracic cavity and the disc space of interest is exposed. After confirmation of the level, the segmental vessels are ligated over the vertebral body. The vessels are mobilized and the anterior border of the spine is exposed along with the posterior border of the disc space and the rib heads. The rib head covering the affected disc spaces is resected. The disc is then removed with a pituitary rongeur, curettes, Kerrison rongeurs, and disc cutters. The anterior and posterior annuli are left intact. After the discectomy is completed, attention is turned to cord decompression. A partial corpectomy may be performed with wedge resections. The disc space is prepared and a cage filled with local bone graft is placed into the disc space. The spine is instrumented with an anterior single-rod construct spanning the index disc space. The wound is irrigated, a small chest tube drain is placed over the extrapleural space, and the wound is closed in layers.

11.7 Surgical Technique in Open Surgery

The anterior transthoracic approach is usually performed with the assistance of an "approach surgeon." After adequate general anesthesia, a patient is intubated with a double-lumen endotracheal tube and placed in the lateral decubitus position. A left lateral thoracotomy incision is made over the planned level of exposure in the midaxillary line, extended anteriorly toward

the umbilicus and then carried posterior and proximally. The dissection is carried through the skin and subcutaneous tissues to the latissimus dorsi and serratus anterior, which are divided sequentially to expose the thoracic cage and intercostal muscles. The rib is dissected from the surrounding structures using electrocautery and a periosteal elevator. The thoracic cavity can be entered through an intercostal space or by costal resection. The ribs are retracted using a Finochietto retractor. The ipsilateral lung is deflated and retracted anteriorly, although this is not necessary for TDHs in the lower thoracic spine. The pleura overlying the thoracic spine is incised and dissected toward the aorta, which is retracted medially and anteriorly. Fluoroscopy is then obtained to verify the proper level, and the intercostal vessels overlying the disc are then clipped and divided.

A partial corpectomy may be necessary for large TDHs that protrude posterior to the vertebral body and impinge on the ventral spinal cord. These procedures are typically performed through an anterior transthoracic approach to the spine with the patient placed in the lateral decubitus position. The dissection is performed in the same manner as described above. The majority of the disc and the cartilaginous end plate are removed. A partial vertebrectomy is performed by careful dissection of the posterior vertebral cortices, herniated disc material, and posterior longitudinal ligament off the dura.[37] The extent of bone resection is dependent on the size and location of the herniation.[37] A strut graft or a cage packed with autologous bone graft is then inserted. The spine is instrumented with an anterior single-rod construct spanning the index disc space.

11.8 Discussion of Minimally Invasive Surgery

TDHs are a challenging clinical entity that can be treated via a multitude of surgical approaches. As a result of an unacceptably high risk profile associated with traditional open anterior and posterolateral approaches, MIS surgical approaches were designed and refined over the last 20 years. Currently, MIS anterior and posterolateral approaches to the thoracic spine provide a spine surgeon with unique, safe, and effective options for the treatment of TDHs. However, comparative data of open approaches to MIS approaches for the treatment of TDHs are limited. The literature presented below represents the current evidence of MIS anterior and posterolateral thoracic approaches for the treatment of TDHs. Studies that report on the use of MIS anterior thoracic approaches for thoracic pathology of another nature (i.e., tumor, infection) are omitted from this discussion.

11.8.1 Level I Evidence in Minimally Invasive Surgery

There are no level I studies available.

11.8.2 Level II Evidence in Minimally Invasive Surgery

There are no level II studies available.

11.8.3 Level III Evidence in Minimally Invasive Surgery

Thoracoscopic surgery was originally used by cardiothoracic surgeons to treat tumors, autonomic disturbances, and infectious diseases of the chest.[12] In 1993, Mack et al presented the first clinical series of the use of thoracoscopy for patients with thoracic spine disease, which ranged from TDH to spinal deformity.[12,38] Since that initial report, several more homogeneous clinical cohort studies have been published regarding the efficacy of thoracoscopy in the treatment of TDH. Regan et al in 1998 presented a landmark retrospective cohort analysis of 29 patients with 32 TDHs between T5 and L1, and compared the results to 10 patients who had previously undergone treatment for TDH with a traditional anterior approach.[12] The minimum follow-up was 1 year (range, 12–24 months).[12] In comparison to open procedures, the authors found a significantly shorter ORT, EBL, ICU, and hospital LOS with thoracoscopy.[12] In patients treated with thoracoscopy, there was also a significant improvement in disability related to radiculopathy and myelopathy, as assessed by the Oswestry Disability Index.[12] In the thoracoscopy group, narcotic usage was significantly reduced and/or eliminated postoperatively, and 75.8% of patients were satisfied with their outcomes.[12] This study was one of the first series to demonstrate the advantages of thoracoscopy for the treatment of symptomatic TDHs in comparison to open approaches.

A second important study was published in 1998 by Rosenthal and Dickman, who compared thoracoscopy to thoracotomy and CTVS.[9] The authors studied 55 patients who underwent thoracoscopy for TDHs between T3 and T12, of which 36 patients had myelopathy and 19 patients had radiculopathy.[9] Thirteen of the thoracoscopic procedures were performed after a previously unsuccessful attempt at decompression via a transpedicular, transfacet/pedicle-sparing, CTVS, or thoracotomy approach.[9] The thoracoscopy patients were compared to 18 patients who underwent thoracotomy and 15 patients who underwent CTVS, all of whom had similar characteristics.[9] The authors found that the patients treated with thoracoscopy in comparison to thoracotomy patients had at least an hour-shorter ORT, 350 mL less EBL, 18 mg/day less narcotic use, 2-day shorter chest tube use, and a shorter hospital LOS by 10 days.[9] In comparison to the CTVS group, thoracoscopy had 75 minutes shorter ORT and an equivalent EBL, chest tube use duration, narcotic usage, and hospital LOS.[9] Importantly, 61% of the patients with myelopathy and 79% of patients with radiculopathy treated with thoracoscopy had a full neurologic recovery.[9] These results suggested that patients with recurrent TDHs treated with thoracoscopy had good outcomes and significantly less intraoperative and in-hospital morbidity compared to open approaches.

Another, more recent retrospective cohort analysis was performed by Oppenlander et al, who compared outcomes of patients with TDHs treated with thoracoscopy, thoracotomy, and posterolateral approaches.[39] The authors' cohort consisted of 56 patients who underwent 62 procedures for 130 TDHs.[39] A thoracotomy was performed in 23 patients, thoracoscopy in 26 patients, and a posterolateral approach in 13 patients.[39] The approach utilized was based on the disc's characteristics, that is, patients who underwent thoracotomy were more likely to have multilevel, calcified, central, giant, and/or intradural herniations.[39] Presenting symptoms persisted for an average of 28 months (range: 0.1–180 months) and included myelopathy (82%), radiculopathy (64%), and mixed symptomatology (43%).[39] Patients treated with thoracoscopy in comparison to thoracotomy were found to have a lower EBL, shorter hospital LOS, fewer instrumented fusions, and an equivalent requirement for blood transfusions.[39] While the analysis by Oppenlander et al demonstrated several advantages of treating TDHs with thoracoscopy, the advantages should be critically considered in the setting of the open approaches being used to treat more difficult pathology.

The first study to compare thoracoscopy to another MIS approach was presented by Bartels and Peul in 2007, as a retrospective cohort analysis.[40] The authors in this study compared the intraoperative data and morbidity between thoracoscopy ($n = 7$) and mini-TTA ($n = 21$) for the treatment of 30 TDHs between T5 and T12.[40] All the patients presented with myelopathic symptoms and had either partially or completely calcified discs.[40] The authors reported no difference in patient characteristics, duration of surgery, chest tube duration, EBL, ICU or hospital LOS, and neurologic changes between the two groups.[40]

Of the posterolateral approaches to the thoracic spine, the transpedicular approach is the least invasive. It was first described for the treatment of a TDH in 1978 by Patterson and Arbit.[41] The first modification of the technique was reported in

1995 by Stillerman et al, which involved a transfacet approach via a skin incision 4 cm in length.[42] More recently in 1997, Jho presented a modification of the two techniques that involved the use of an endoscope with a 70°-angled lens inserted through a 2-cm transverse incision.[31] The first two cases presented using this technique were of a 31-year-old woman with a T9–T10 disc herniation and myelopathy and a 52-year-old woman with a T10–T11 disc herniation and radiculopathy.[31] Both patients had no postoperative complications and had a full neurologic recovery.[31] Since that initial report, Jho published a larger case series consisting of 25 patients with TDH between T1 and T12 treated with the same endoscopic transpedicular technique.[30] A total of 7 patients presented with myelopathy, 6 patients had radiculomyelopathy, 10 patients had radiculopathy, and 2 patients had axial pain.[30] The author reported that 12 out of the 13 patients with myelopathy had "excellent" results, and none of the patients experienced a complication postoperatively.[30]

Chi et al in 2008 published a retrospective cohort analysis of seven patients with TDHs treated with a mini-open transpedicular approach (3- to 4-cm incision) using a microscope compared to four patients with TDHs treated with a traditional open transpedicular approach.[28] Of the seven patients treated with the mini-open technique, six patients presented with myelopathy and two patients had calcified discs.[28] Of the four patients treated with the traditional open technique, three patients presented with myelopathy and two patients had calcified discs.[28] There was no statistically significant difference between the two groups in regard to hospital LOS (mini-open: 3.5 days vs. open: 4.1 days).[28] The authors found that the mini-open approach was associated with less EBL and lower postoperatively morbidity, as assessed by modified Prolo scores (a 20-point scoring system based on pain, functional status, ability to work, and quantity of pain medication usage) compared to the open approach.[28]

CTVS was first described in 1960 for the treatment of TDH by Hulme.[35,43] Given the open CTVS was initially developed to improve exposure relative to transpedicular and transfacet approaches, it involves a large posterolateral incision, removal of a large segment of rib, mobilization and retraction of the pleura, division of the intercostal neurovascular bundle, and placement of a chest tube. Therefore, it is relatively moribund. A minimally invasive extracavitary approach minimizes soft-tissue disruption, as it is performed with a 15° endoscope through a 1-cm incision. Thus, it avoids the aforementioned soft-tissue and osseous retraction while preserving the exposure's visualization of pathology. Khoo et al published a comparison of a minimally invasive lateral extracavitary approach (MI-LECA) and open thoracotomy for the treatment of noncalcified TDH (level III).[35] The MI-LECA approach was via uni- or bilateral hemilaminotomy. Interbody cage placement is achieved through a 20-mm working tubular access portal and a 2-cm paramedian incision using a microscope. The 13 patients treated with MI-LECA had a total of 15 paracentral TDH located between T5 and T12.[35] In comparison to open thoracotomy, the MI-LECA was found to have significantly shorter ORT times (93.8 vs. 175 minutes), less EBL (33 vs. 295 mL), fewer chest tubes placed (0/13 vs. 11/11 patients), shorter duration of ICU stay, fewer transfusions (0/13 vs. 6/11 patients), and fewer postoperative complications (4.2 times higher for open

thoracotomy patients).[35] No difference between the two groups in regard to neurologic outcomes was reported.[35]

There are no level III studies available regarding the use of the mini-open lateral and transfacet/pedicle-sparing approaches for the treatment of TDHs.

11.9 Complications of Minimally Invasive Surgery

Disadvantages of a surgical technique are determinants of approach-related intraoperative and postoperative surgical complications. In contrast to open approaches that maximize visualization of pathology by exposing a wide field of anatomy, MIS approaches inherently rely on smaller working fields. In addition, MIS approaches are relatively new techniques that require time and practice to develop efficiency with the relationship of the surgical equipment and relative anatomy. Therefore, major criticism and reported disadvantages of MIS techniques are centered around a limited assessment of anatomy and a more difficult and potentially inadequate ability to address pathology and intraoperative complications. This is a particular concern in surgeons with limited experience with MIS techniques and equipment. However, in the hands of experienced surgeons adept at MIS techniques, the limited exposure provided by MIS approaches consistently results in shorter ORTs, less intraoperative blood loss, and fewer intraoperative and postoperative complications.

11.9.1 Anterior Approaches

Because anterior approaches to the thoracic spine inherently involve penetration through the chest wall and manipulation of the thoracic cavity's contents, they are coupled with unique and important complications. Intraoperative complications associated with thoracoscopy include excessive bleeding, trocar placement through the hemidiaphragm requiring intraoperative repair, pericardial penetration, screw malposition, and dural tear.[12,19,36,44] Postoperative complications experienced after thoracoscopy for TDH include residual disc herniation, neurologic deterioration, pseudarthrosis, spinal instability, atelectasis, loculated pleural effusion requiring thoracentesis, pleuritic pain, pneumothorax, hemothorax, pneumonia, pleural effusion, chylothorax, and ICN requiring intercostal nerve blocks.[9,12,15,19,40,45] Several of the complications observed with thoracoscopy are likely related to how the procedure is technically performed. Portal placement is critical for a successful procedure. If placed in inappropriate positions, the trocars and instruments are more difficult to maneuver and there is a higher risk of penetrating vital anatomic structures, i.e., the great vessels. The control of vascular injuries is problematic through a limited exposure, and often necessitates conversion to an open approach.[46] A greater incidence of temporary neurologic dysfunction with MIS techniques is postulated to be due to increased difficulty with "gentle treatment of nerve roots and certain homeostasis techniques" relative to open techniques.[1]

Many of the reported complications associated with thoracoscopy, particularly pulmonary and ICN, are also observed with the open thoracotomy, although the frequency of complications is lower with thoracoscopy. For example, Rosenthal and Dickman reported the complications of patients treated with thoracoscopy, thoracotomy, and CTVS.[9] Compared to patients treated with an open thoracotomy, fewer patients after thoracoscopy had atelectasis (7 vs. 33%), pleural effusions (4 vs. 6%), chylothorax (0 vs. 6%), hemothorax (4 vs. 6%), infections (0 vs. 6%), and ICN (16 vs. 50%).[9] In addition, Johnson et al reported greater than a 100% complication rate with open thoracotomy and a 31% complication rate with thoracoscopy in patients treated for TDH, OPLL, and thoracic discitis.[22] More specifically, patients treated with thoracoscopy in comparison to thoracotomy had a lower rate of pneumonia (6 vs. 25%), ICN (14 vs. 75%), chylothorax (3 vs. 13%), and additional neurologic deficit (3 vs. 13%).[22]

The complications associated with the mini-open anterior transthoracic approaches, including the mini-TTA and the mini-open lateral approach, are similar to those reported for thoracoscopy and traditional anterior approaches. The mini-TTA has resulted in dural tears and subsequent cerebrospinal fluid (CSF) leaks and ICN.[24,40] In addition to the potential complications associated with traditional thoracotomy, injury to the azygos and hemiazygous vein, segmental vessels, aorta, and intercostal vessels is possible with the mini-TTA.[46] The mini-open lateral approach has resulted in ICN, pleural tears, pneumonia, atelectasis, pleural effusions, wound infections, dural tears, and thromboembolic events.[6,10,47] The true complication profile for each of the mini-open anterior/anterolateral techniques is yet to be fully understood and appreciated, as few studies have been published regarding their use for TDH and no studies have directly compared the mini-open lateral approach to other MIS anterior thoracic approaches.

11.9.2 Posterolateral Approaches

Although thoracoscopy is associated with fewer complications than traditional open anterior thoracic approaches, thoracoscopy is not a benign approach. In fact, complication rates of thoracoscopic surgery have been reported to be as high as 45%.[1,36,48] Alternatively, MIS posterolateral approaches have a significantly lower rate of complications.

MIS transpedicular and transfacet/pedicle-sparing approaches have been utilized without reported complication when used to treat TDH.[30,31,32,33] While no intraoperative neurologic complications were observed in studies using a 70°-angled endoscope, as described by Jho, the author warns his readers of the potential of spinal cord damage using the endoscope through a transpedicular approach.[30] During this approach, neuromonitoring is recommended, although the use of neuromonitoring does not preclude the development of a catastrophic neurologic event. The risk of spinal cord injury using a 70°-angled endoscope via a transpedicular approach is higher when used by an inexperienced surgeon. Therefore, Jho recommends that a surgeon inexperienced with the 70° endoscope first approach a TDH via a lateral extracavitary approach so as to develop familiarity with this unique endoscope.[30] It is important to use a 70°-angled endoscope during the MIS transpedicular approach, as nerve root damage is more likely when a conventional 0°-angled endoscope is used for exposure.[30] To optimize visualization and minimize the risk of injury to neurologic structures, a microscope may be utilized.

Transpedicular exposure with the use of a microscope was first presented by Chi et al.[28] Of the seven patients treated with the modified mini-open transpedicular approach, the authors observed no intraoperative or postoperative complications.[28] Khoo et al reported their experience treating TDH with the microscope via an MIS lateral extracavitary approach.[35] The authors documented five complications, which consisted of two patients with unilateral radicular numbness and a stitch abscess, two patients with abdominal wall hyperesthesia and a unilateral abdominal wall flaccid paralysis, and an intraoperative incidental durotomy, which was repaired using 4–0 Nurolon stitches and Tisseel-Duragen patch.[35] CSF leaks may be particularly difficult to repair with MIS approaches given the size of the approach,[28] particularly with calcified TDHs, which have a tendency to adhere to the dura.[2] To avoid this complication, the disc may be incompletely resected.[49] Alternatively, if a dural tear develops during an MIS approach, the less invasive tissue dissection may protect the patient from the development of a pseudomeningocele.[28]

11.10 Conclusion of Minimally Invasive Surgery

Thoracic spine surgery is an evolving field with an interesting history and an exciting future. Building on negative experiences with the laminectomy for TDHs, spine surgeons have searched for the ideal surgical approach to the thoracic spine. The anterior thoracotomy is the gold-standard approach. However, it is associated with significant perioperative morbidity. Numerous iterations of thoracic surgical approaches are a testament to the spine surgeon's desire to maximize the quality of life of patients with pathology of the thoracic spine. Thoracic MIS approaches are the youngest additions to the field and represent an important new practice. Since their introduction less than 20 years ago, relatively few reports have documented their effectiveness in the treatment of TDHs. Nonetheless, investigations that have been published comparing open and MIS approaches illustrate some distinct advantages to the use of MIS approaches for the treatment of TDHs.

MIS anterior options for the surgeon include thoracoscopy and modifications of the mini-open transthoracic approach, including the mini-open lateral approach. Despite having a steep learning curve and relatively costly equipment, thoracoscopy is an effective and relatively safe alternative to open thoracotomy. Importantly, it provides outstanding cosmetic results, minimal shoulder girdle dysfunction, low postoperative morbidity, and short hospital stays and recovery times. The mini-open lateral approach is the most recently developed MIS anterior exposure and is our preferred technique for the treatment of TDH. As it utilizes familiar XLIF retractors and allows for retropleural exposure and dual-lung ventilation, it offers a surgeon an unprecedented opportunity to address diverse thoracic spinal pathologies.

Posterolateral approaches using MIS techniques represent promising alternatives to traditionally moribund approaches. Transpedicular, transfacet/pedicle-sparing, and lateral extracavitary MIS approaches using the endoscope and microscope can be performed through incisions less than 4 cm in length. A 70°-angled endoscope allows for decompression of the ventral spinal canal, while the microscope provides the unique advantage of performing decompressions under 3D visualization. Few complications have been associated with each of these techniques; however, a more accurate profile of the techniques' risks will surface as the literature grows with individual surgeon's experiences and large multicenter studies. A grade IIC recommendation can be made for MIS techniques to help avoid approach-related morbidities associated with open thoracotomy and traditional posterior approaches.

Just as the last decade has witnessed an extraordinary revolution in the treatment of patients with TDHs using minimally invasive methods, the next decade is anticipated to produce even shorter LOS in the hospital and better outcomes for these patients. In order to minimize risks and fully appreciate the benefits of MIS, surgeons treating patients with TDHs using MIS approaches should have adequate training and consistent surgical experience with endoscopic and microscopic tools. These are particularly important considerations in our current and evolving health care system.

11.11 Discussion of Open Surgery

11.11.1 Level I Evidence in Open Surgery

There are no level I studies available.

11.11.2 Level II Evidence in Open Surgery

There are no level II studies available.

11.11.3 Level III Evidence in Open Surgery

Open exposures for the treatment of symptomatic disc herniation have a long track record of successful clinical results. Anterior transthoracic approaches were first used in the 1960s. They provide outstanding visualization of the thoracic spine with minimal risk of nerve root or spinal cord injury.[4,10,50] A wide variety of anterior, lateral, and posterolateral approaches have been adapted and used to treat diverse thoracic spine pathology. This extensive history illustrates the importance of the operative approach in achieving desirable outcomes.[50] While these exposures have been amenable to modification with advanced surgical techniques, open surgery continues to be the most widely used method to treat TDHs.

Surgical approaches to address TDHs are presented in ▶ Table 11.1. The table highlights the progression of techniques. A laminectomy intended for access to a TDH is rarely performed now due to incomplete decompression and the risk of spinal cord injury. Significant spinal cord manipulation is necessary to access the disc space with a laminectomy.[27] Since its first description in 1964, the open anterior thoracotomy continues to be the workhorse approach for TDH, as it provides the most reliable and effective approach to address broad central or centrolateral, calcified, and/or multilevel TDHs. For lateral TDHs, a variety of posterolateral techniques, such as CTVS, transfacet, transpedicular, and their muscle-sparing variants exist. They are each utilized based on the type of pathology and a surgeon's preference. Therefore, two primary open surgical approaches—

transthoracic and posterolateral—are used commonly today.[39] The traditional open thoracotomy exposure has withstood the test of time and continues to be used for the widest range of pathology and patient considerations.

What is the optimal method to treat symptomatic TDHs? Unfortunately, there are no prospective, randomized investigations (level I or level II) comparing open and minimally invasive approaches for the treatment of TDHs. The evidence is therefore derived from literature reviews and level III and level IV investigations. The majority of the literature suggests that MIS approaches are associated with comparable complication rates and achieve similar intermediate and long-term results compared to open procedures. Many of the studies focus on the approaches used for a variety of heterogeneous diagnoses including tumor metastases, osteomyelitis, traumatic lesions, and degenerative disc disease.[51] Although this heterogeneity likely confounds the interpretation of each approach's reoperation, morbidity, and mortality rates for TDHs, the literature provides important insight into each approach's limitations and complications. Furthermore, all the studies are not randomized and do not compare approaches to one another. Nonetheless, these studies provide the best available data on complication rates and outcome measures for surgical approaches commonly used to treat TDH.

Lubelski et al published a systematic review comparing the CTVS, lateral extracavitary, and transthoracic thoracotomy approaches.[51] Their review identified 4,677 articles and analyzed 31 studies.[51] The vast majority of the studies included in the aforementioned systematic review are considered level III evidence. This study is the only systematic review conducted regarding surgical approaches to the thoracic spine.[51] This review was not limited to the use of these three approaches for TDH, given that it included reports on various other pathologies, including spinal metastases. The authors acknowledge that the heterogeneity of the data and surgeon experiences may be confounding variables. Nevertheless, they reported a mean complication rate of 15% for CTVS, 17% for lateral extracavitary, and 39% for transthoracic thoracotomy.[51] Thoracotomy was associated with the highest average reoperation rate (3.5%) and mortality rate (1.5%).[51] The high total complication rate for thoracotomy was influenced by two investigations—one by Johnson et al[22] and one by Khoo et al[35]—each of which reported complication rates for thoracotomy that exceeded 100% (i.e., more than one complication per patient). If these manuscripts are considered outliers, the total complication rate for open thoracotomy would range from 16 to 33%, and the neurological complication rates would range from 4 to 14%.[51] Aside from the inconsistencies between investigators, the authors recommend that the high overall complication rate associated with open transthoracic thoracotomy be interpreted with caution, as greater than 25% of the patients underwent the procedures for spinal metastases.[51] Patients with cancer differ vastly from those with trauma or degenerative disc disease due to the inhibitory effect of oncologic burden on postoperative recovery.[51] Overall, the neurological outcomes were similar between the CTVS, LECA, and transthoracic approaches.[51] The transthoracic thoracotomy approach was associated with an average ORT of 244 minutes, 630 mL of EBL, and an average LOS of 7.8 days.[51] For CTVS, the following was reported: an average mortality rate of 1.2%, a reoperation rate of 4.3%, an average

Table 11.1 Procedures by publication date (more patient, outcome information)

Author	Year	Level	Approach	Exposure
Love and Kiefer[59]	1950	IV	Lami	Open
Epstein[60]	1954	IV	Lami	Open
Perot and Munro[61]	1969	IV	TTA	Open
Albrand and Corkill[62]	1979	IV	TTA, CTVS	Open
Maiman et al[63]	1984	IV	LECA	Open
Otani et al[29]	1988	IV	TT-IBF	Open
el-Kalliny et al[64]	1991	III	TFacet, TPed, TTA	Open
Singounas et al[65]	1992	IV	CTVS	Mini-open
Simpson et al[66]	1993	IV	Mod-CTVS	Open
Le Roux et al[67]	1993	IV	TForam	Open
Dietze and Fessler[68]	1993	IV	LECA	Open
Currier et al[7]	1994	IV	TTA-IBF	Open
Stillerman et al[42]	1995	IV	TFacet	Mini-open
Regan et al[12]	1998	IV	VATS, TTA	Both
Stillerman et al[69]	1998	IV	TTA, LECA, CTVS	Open
Rosenthal and Dickman[9]	1998	III	TScope, CTVS, TTA	Both
Jho[70]	1999	IV	TForam	Endo
Dickman et al[23]	1999	III	VATS, TTA	Endo
Bilsky[2]	2000	IV	TForam	Open
Kim et al[71]	2000	IV	IG-CTVS	Open
Johnson et al[22]	2000	III	TTA, TScope	Both
McCormick et al[27]	2000	III	Review	Open
Dinh et al[72]	2001	IV	TCostVert	Open
Han et al[73]	2002	III	TScope	Endo
Anand and Regan[15]	2002	III	VATS	Endo
Perez-Cruet et al[32]	2004	IV	TFacet	Mini-open
Oskouian and Johnson[74]	2005	III	TScope	Endo
Hott et al[52]	2005	IV	TTA, CTVS	Open
Bartels and Peul[40]	2007	III	TScope, mini-TTA	Endo and mini
Chi et al[28]	2008	III	TForam, CTVS	Mini-open
D'Aliberti et al[75]	2008	IV	TTA	Open
Bransford et al[3]	2010	III	TFacet, TTA	Open
Machino et al[76]	2010	IV	TForam, TTA	Open
Ayhan et al[1]	2010	III	TTA	Open
Bransford et al[77]	2010	IV	TFacet	Open
Khoo et al[35]	2011	III	MI-LECA, TTA	Both
Uribe et al[10]	2012	III	MI lat (micro)	Mini-open
Moran et al[25]	2012	IV	mini-TTA	Mini-open
Quint et al[45]	2012	III	TScope	Endo
Russo et al[24]	2012	IV	TForam (micro)	Mini-open
Oppenlander et al[39]	2013	III	TTA, TScope, TFacet, CTVS	Both
Lubelski et al[51]	2013	III	LECA, CTVS, TTA	Open
Zhao et al[58]	2013	IV	TTA	Open
Smith et al.[33]	2013	IV	TFacet (micro)	Mini-open

Abbreviations: CTVS, costotransversectomy; IG, image guided; Lami, laminectomy; LECA, lateral extracavitary approach; TCostVert, transcostovertebral; MI, minimally invasive; TFacet, transfacet; TForm, transforaminal; TPed, transpedicular; TScope, thoracoscopic; TTA, transthoracic approach; TT-IBF, transthoracic with interbody fusion; VATS, video-assisted thoracoscopic surgery.

ORT of 405 minutes, mean EBL of 2.0 L, and LOS of 6.7 days.[51] Therefore, the conclusion of the systemic review by Lubelski et al was that CTVS, LECA, and transthoracic thoracotomy approaches "are safe and rarely associated with neurological deterioration" in historical contrast to laminectomy.[51] It provides level III evidence about the safety and efficacy of these exposures to the thoracic spine.[51]

Another recent meta-analysis was published by Uribe et al describing the results of open versus MIS approaches to the thoracic spine.[10] The overall clinical results for the open approaches included the following: average ORT of 229.3 minutes, average EBL of 562.9 mL, a mean LOS of 8.6 days, a reoperation rate of 4.3%, and a total complication rate of 36.7%.[10] For MIS approaches, clinical data included an average ORT of 199.8 minutes, an average EBL of 307.1 mL, a mean LOS of 3.8 days, a reoperation rate of 5.9%, and an average total complication rate of 28.4%.[10] These numbers were based on a wide range of approaches, including laminectomy, CTVS, LECA, transfacet, transforaminal, and transthoracic.[10] The data from Johnson et al[22] and Khoo et al[35] were also included in the analysis of the open approaches' data,[10] which as previously described likely significantly increased the complication rates of open approaches. Of note, the number of thoracic levels of pathology addressed with open procedures ranged from 1 to 5, while the MIS exposures treated 1 to 2 levels.[10] This report provides level III evidence about outcome measures and follow-up data associated with various minimally invasive and open procedures used to treat TDHs.[10]

The anterior and posterolateral approaches to the thoracic spine are different procedures, each with specific surgical indications based on the location, size, and quality of a TDH. For example, an open anterior exposure is more likely to be utilized for a large, midline, calcified, and/or multilevel TDH. For small, central, one- or two-level TDH, an MIS anterior exposure is often employed. For small, soft, lateral TDHs, a posterolateral approach may be most effective. Because of this heterogeneity, complication rates and outcomes of each approach should ideally be compared separately based on the approach and in the context of each patient's pathology. However, much of the data regarding approaches to the thoracic spine are retrospective series that do not control for the multiple variables involved in the treatment of TDHs. For example, the size and nature of the disc pathology as well as the patient's symptoms often differ between patient groups. For example, Rosenthal and Dickman's study comparing thoracotomy to thoracoscopy and CTVS reported that those selected for CTVS tended to have smaller, more focal, eccentrically located TDH.[9] In contrast, the open thoracotomy was utilized for larger, broad-based central, and calcified discs, and the patients treated with an open thoracotomy had a higher incidence of severe myelopathy.[9] In addition, several patients who were initially scheduled to undergo thoracoscopy were switched to undergo thoracotomy due to medical and surgical factors. In a report by Johnson et al, there were large disparities in patient symptoms and sizes of lesions despite the general characteristics (i.e., age and sex) of the two groups being similar.[22] Of those treated with an open thoracotomy, all patients presented with myelopathy and a calcified disc herniation, half had OPLL, and an average of 4.5 levels were treated.[22] This is in contrast to the patients who underwent thoracoscopy who did not have myelopathy, who had soft disc

herniations, and an average of 1.2 levels of pathology were addressed. The authors acknowledge that patient selection criteria were based on the number of involved levels, complexity of pathology, the presence of OPLL, and prior transthoracic disc surgery.[22] Other studies similarly used less invasive exposures selectively. Oppenlander et al reported 220 cases of surgically treated TDHs in which the "surgical approach was dictated by disc size, consistency, and location."[39] Based on historical data and on their experience with 82 symptomatic TDHs, Stillerman et al found that no single approach was best suited for all herniations, and that no criteria existed to help surgeons choose an approach.[42] Therefore, they designed a "surgical selection guideline" that considered multiple factors, including presenting clinical symptoms, medical history, herniation size and location, degree of calcification, extent of spinal cord deformation, and dural involvement.[42]

Surgical selection is particularly important for the treatment of giant herniated thoracic discs because they are often calcified and have intradural extension.[25,52] Hott et al analyzed 20 cases of GTDH that were treated surgically and had an average postoperative follow-up of 2.6 years.[52] Ninety-five percent of these patients initially presented with myelopathy.[52] The patients were treated with thoracoscopy ($n = 8$), an open thoracotomy ($n = 8$), or a posterolateral approach ($n = 4$).[52] Compared to open thoracotomy, the patients treated with thoracoscopy exhibited worse short- and long-term outcomes and had a greater average EBL (850 vs. 700 mL).[52] There were no differences in outcomes between the thoracoscopy and open thoracotomy approach for patients with smaller midline discs.[52] The authors discussed the difficulty and impracticality of separating calcified material from the dura piecemeal, as is necessary when using the endoscope, and therefore, they concluded that an open anterior approach with corpectomy and fusion was preferred for GTDHs.[52] Barbanera et al subsequently reported a series of seven patients with calcified GTDHs, 95% of whom had myelopathy likely as a result of a delayed presentation.[53] The authors agreed with the conclusions proposed by Hott et al,[52] and added that an anterior approach with direct stereoscopic visualization was "mandatory" for calcified discs.[53] The reports by Hott et al and Barbanera et al provide level IV evidence that GTDHs are managed more safely with an open procedure than an MIS approach.[52,53]

A commonly reported disadvantage of MIS approaches (i.e., thoracoscopy) is the time, effort, and cost required to acquire the skills to perform the procedure. Thoracoscopy equipment may be borrowed in some hospital settings; however, this arrangement is not an ideal, reliable, or sustainable practice pattern. As the specialized instruments used for thoracoscopy are long and difficult to use and the operative ports may impede manipulation,[22] a substantial amount of time and dedication are required to become accustomed to performing transthoracic surgery without the customary tactile feedback and/or familiar direct visualization of pertinent anatomy.[54] Thus, procedures performed when "learning the technique" may have longer ORTs, higher complication rates, and greater morbidity than traditional open approaches.[54] As the incidence of symptomatic TDHs is low, surgeons may find it difficult to gain sufficient experience with MIS techniques to incorporate them into their daily surgical repertoire.[40] If a surgeon has familiarity with an MIS technique, it is imperative that said surgeon continue to use the technique at a sufficient frequency so as to maintain an appropriate proficiency.[22]

The "learning curve," technical difficulty, and overall costs associated with thoracoscopy raise concerns about the cost-effectiveness of its use for the treatment of TDHs. Newton et al investigated the question of the cost-effectiveness of thoracoscopy in TDH by comparing its use to open thoracotomy in 14 pediatric patients with pediatric deformity.[55] The authors found that the overall hospital cost for patients treated with thoracoscopy was on average $4,585 more expensive than that for patients treated with an open thoracotomy.[55] Of note, the charges related to operating room facilities, including the endoscopic equipment, accounted for the majority of the increased cost.[55] They also reported a substantial decrease in the average ORT for thoracoscopy as surgeon experience increased, that is, 220 minutes for the first seven cases and 162 minutes for the last seven cases performed.[55] The overall average ORT for thoracoscopy was significantly longer that for open thoracotomy despite other similar intraoperative parameters, including number of discs excised and EBL, between the two groups.[55] The complication rates and hospital LOS were similar between the two groups.[55] The study by Newton et al provides level III evidence that endoscopic approaches to the thoracic spine are associated with a steep "learning curve" and a significant financial burden to a hospital.[55]

11.12 Complications in Open Surgery

A wide range of complications have been reported in association with the treatment of TDH, which include spinal cord injury, neuralgia, dural tears, paresis or paralysis, pulmonary complications, infection, wrong-level surgery or misdiagnosis, and postoperative instability or kyphosis.[56] Among the most often cited complications of the anterior and lateral procedures are ICN, also known as anesthesia dolorosa, and the postthoracotomy pain syndrome. The development of ICN can be minimized by the use of a preoperative local nerve block consisting of 1% Marcaine with epinephrine. Postoperative ICN can be treated with an intercostal nerve block and/or radiofrequency rhizotomy.[54] Because anterior exposures necessitate invasion of the thoracic cavity and the use of single-lung ventilation, pleural effusions and chylothorax are also common complications of the anterior approaches. Postoperatively, atelectasis and pneumonia also often develop as a result of splinting from thoracic pain. The incidence of complications is similar between the different open approaches.

The aforementioned systematic review by Lubelski et al discussed complications unique to each thoracic exposure.[51] The two most common complications for an open thoracotomy were pneumonia (4.2%) and ICN (5.1%).[51] The two most common complications associated with CTVS were wound infection (3.7%) and thromboembolic events (3.7%).[51] As the approaches evaluated were for the treatment of various thoracic pathology, the morbidity from procedures exclusively used to address TDHs may be lower. Fessler and Sturgill reviewed the complications associated with surgery for thoracic disc disease in patients older than 60 years; the review included 18 qualifying articles.[57] The authors reported that after laminectomy was

abandoned as a treatment for TDH, none of the other approaches were associated with a mortality or catastrophic paresis and paralysis.[57] Surgical wound infections accounted for the total morbidity associated with the transpedicular (9%) and CTVS approaches (12%).[57] The overall postoperative complication rate associated with LECA was 12%, and consisted of pneumonia or atelectasis (4%), wound infections (3%), intraoperative pleural tears (4%), and postoperative ICN (3%).[57] LECA was found to be the only approach associated with pleural tears[57]; however, iatrogenic pleural violation is also an anticipated complication of a traditional open thoracotomy. Of the 88 patients who had a transthoracic approach, 11% suffered a complication.[57] Two percent of the patients developed pneumonia or atelectasis, 3% suffered wound infections, 1% had a pulmonary embolus, 1% had an occult compression fracture, and 1% had a postoperative seizure.[57] The authors concluded that the morbidity and mortality associated with a traditional open thoracotomy and the posterolateral approaches were "virtually identical" and that a selected surgical approach should therefore depend on the location of the herniation, the patients' health, and surgeon experience.[57]

In 2000, McCormick et al also published an article regarding complications associated with only open surgical approaches for TDHs and discussed methods for complication avoidance.[27] While data on laminectomy for TDH were included in the authors' analysis, a discussion of the laminectomy results has been omitted in this discussion. The overall rates of postoperative instability were 4.6% for a transfacet/pedicle-sparing approach and 2.1% for transthoracic approaches.[27] The authors added that instability typically resulted when there was an underlying disease or prior procedure, and that interbody fusion was not necessary with the anterior approach unless the decompression was particularly aggressive.[27] Pulmonary embolism occurred in 2.1% of the patients treated with transthoracic approaches; pleural effusion occurred in 1.8% of patients treated with CTVS and in 0.7% of patients treated via a transthoracic approach.[27] ICN was the highest reported complication for LECA (2.8%) and transthoracic approaches (7.1%).[27] They also found no difference in surgical site infection rates between the different approaches analyzed.[27] Overall, the authors found that there were no differences in morbidity and mortality between anterior and thoracic exposures.[27] The analyses concluded that no complication was conclusively associated with a single approach.[27] The authors suggested that the relatively low complication rates associated with some approaches were likely due to surgeon selection based on herniated disc location and consistency.[27] The article by McCormick et al[27] provides level III evidence for the complication rates among the variety of open procedures for thoracic disc disease.

While the aforementioned studies are literature reviews comparing the various surgical approaches to the thoracic spine, case series that present the results of the use of individual approaches also exist.[58] Most recently, Zhao et al presented a series of 15 consecutive patients who underwent an open transthoracic decompression and instrumented interbody fusion for large calcified herniated discs.[58] The authors found a mean ORT of 179 minutes, an average EBL of 840 mL, no dural tears or CSF leaks, and no postoperative neurologic deterioration.[58] There were a total of four complications (26.7%).[58] Two of the complications were due to postoperative pain at the incision site, which improved with conservative measures and an intercostal nerve block.[58] One patient suffered a "cardiac event" and one developed pneumonia.[58] This study provides level IV evidence on operative data and complications associated with the open anterior approach for large calcified TDHs.[58]

Oppenlander et al recently presented a series of 220 consecutive patients with TDHs who were surgically treated via a thoracotomy, thoracoscopy, or posterolateral exposures.[39] The complication rate for all the procedures was 23%.[39] Thoracoscopy was associated with a 15% total complication rate, of which half were due to pleural effusions.[39] In contrast, thoracotomy was associated with a 39% total complication rate, which included pleural effusions (13%), chylothorax (9%), residual disc material requiring reoperation (9%), incidental durotomies (4%), and other minor/miscellaneous complications (4%).[39] The higher complication rate for the open transthoracic approaches may have been a result of these approaches being disproportionately utilized for large and calcified herniations, with 39% of the procedures involving three or more levels of pathology.[39] For the posterolateral approach, an 8% total complication rate was reported, which was attributable to one incidental durotomy.[39] The authors concluded that multilevel decompression more often required thoracotomy and instrumented fusion, involved greater blood loss, and resulted in a higher complication rate than single-level operations.[39] Postoperative follow-up data were analyzed and reported according to the binary variable of the number of levels treated (single-level vs. multilevel) and rates of symptom improvement and/or resolution.[39] The group with large and complex TDH had excellent long-term neurological outcomes regardless of exposure.[39] This report provides level III evidence on complication rates and long-term follow-up for a large and complex group of patients treated with three procedures commonly utilized for symptomatic TDH.[39]

In summary, the average total complication rates associated with open approaches to the thoracic spine range from 9 to 39%. These data must be considered in context and are influenced by patient considerations and large or complex pathology. For an open thoracotomy, the most common complications are postoperative incision-site pain or ICN, with an average occurrence ranging between 5.1 and 13.3%. Other notable complications associated with the open transthoracic approaches consist of pneumonia or atelectasis (2.3–13.3%), pleural effusions (0.7–13%), chylothorax (13%), thromboembolic events (1.1–2.1%), and instability (1.1–2.1%). Complications associated with open posterolateral approaches include ICN (2.6–2.8%), pneumonia or atelectasis (3.9%), pleural effusion (1.8%), wound infection (3.7–9.1%), thromboembolic events (3.7%), and postoperative instability (4.6%). These data are comparable to complication rates associated with comparable minimally invasive approaches. There are presently limited data to compare the complications associated with cannulated or retractor-based anterior approaches to traditional open thoracotomy.

11.13 Conclusion of Open Surgery

Today, the vast majority of procedures for thoracic spine pathology are performed through anterior and posterolateral exposures. Small central TDH are adequately treated via an MIS anterior approach. A posterolateral approach is well suited to address a lateral TDH. For broad, medial, calcified, and multilevel herniations, an anterior open transthoracic approach is the best option, given that it is easily expansile.

The relevant literature on the topic of approaches for the treatment of TDH is considered level III or IV evidence and involves various procedures used to treat heterogeneous pathology. The methods are subject to bias and the compiled results are difficult to interpret. Therefore, there is no high-level comparative evidence that establishes a benefit to MIS approaches for TDHs compared to open approaches. Although these data may become available in the future, there is currently no compelling evidence to justify the technical difficulty, cost, and potential for catastrophic vascular complications associated with a minimally invasive approach. If patient-based outcomes are comparable, practice considerations and surgeon preferences determine whether assimilating the techniques would be advantageous for this low-incidence pathology. Because these approaches are all very different operations with characteristic indications and complication profiles, each approach should be compared separately. A grade IIB recommendation is made for open thoracic discectomy to effectively treat symptomatic TDHs. More prospective, randomized, matched cohort and other higher quality studies are recommended to explore these surgical options.

11.14 Editors' Commentary

11.14.1 Minimally Invasive Surgery

Having spent my career learning and developing many of the techniques for thoracic discectomy, I have a "worldly view" of this interesting and difficult problem. I have evolved through laminectomy, thoracotomy, CTVS, and transpedicular thoracic discectomy techniques. And I have developed or participated in the development of the open lateral extrapleural approach and transthoracic endoscopic approach prior to developing the MIS tubular lateral extrapleural approach and finally the tubular transpedicular technique. Having personally used each of these techniques, there is absolutely no question in my mind that the optimal technique for lateral disc herniations is the tubular transpedicular approach, and the optimal technique for more centralized herniations is the tubular lateral extrapleural approach. In each case, these techniques have transformed major surgical procedures requiring multiple days of hospitalization and prolonged recovery to outpatient procedures. The beneficial impact on the patient is almost beyond comprehension and is among the most dramatic in any comparison of open versus MIS technique.

11.14.2 Open Surgery

Treatment of symptomatic soft TDHs or small posterior lateral/foraminal disc osteophytes can likely be done safely and successfully after an appropriate learning curve through MIS techniques. These procedures have relatively high risk profiles and already are technically difficult before unfamiliar instrumentation and devices are used. The unpopular video-assisted thoracoscopic surgery (VATS) followed a similar appeal by a minority of surgeons who had spent considerable time developing the skill set necessary to perform the surgery. VATS never became popular, largely because the skill set using unfamiliar techniques and expensive equipment created a substantial learning barrier for surgeons. The MIS procedures described are rarely required in a spine surgeon's practice and therefore few surgeons may be willing to invest the necessary time learning such a technically challenging and risky procedure. If these surgeries were commonly performed, there would be an obvious incentive to develop the safe skills required to address this pathology minimally invasively. However, this is not the case.

Minimizing the size of an incision to perform the same surgery such as is described above for the "mini-open" thoracotomy is more an intellectual extension of the traditional "open" technique than something fundamentally different enough to label a unique MIS procedure, particularly when a rib resection is required. Utilizing a retractor system that is branded for MIS surgery does not change the underlying invasiveness of the procedure.

References

[1] Ayhan S, Nelson C, Gok B, et al. Transthoracic surgical treatment for centrally located thoracic disc herniations presenting with myelopathy: a 5-year institutional experience. J Spinal Disord Tech. 2010; 23(2):79–88

[2] Bilsky MH. Transpedicular approach for thoracic disc herniations. Neurosurg Focus. 2000; 9(4):e3

[3] Bransford RJ, Zhang F, Bellabarba C, Lee MJ. Treating thoracic-disc herniations: Do we always have to go anteriorly? Evid Based Spine Care J. 2010; 1(1):21–28

[4] Burke TG, Caputy AJ. Treatment of thoracic disc herniation: evolution toward the minimally invasive thoracoscopic technique. Neurosurg Focus. 2000; 9(4):e9

[5] Sheikh H, Samartzis D, Perez-Cruet MJ. Techniques for the operative management of thoracic disc herniation: minimally invasive thoracic microdiscectomy. Orthop Clin North Am. 2007; 38(3):351–361, abstract vi

[6] Deviren V, Kuelling FA, Poulter G, Pekmezci M. Minimal invasive anterolateral transthoracic transpleural approach: a novel technique for thoracic disc herniation. A review of the literature, description of a new surgical technique and experience with first 12 consecutive patients. J Spinal Disord Tech. 2011; 24(5):E40–E48

[7] Currier BL, Eismont FJ, Green BA. Transthoracic disc excision and fusion for herniated thoracic discs. Spine. 1994; 19(3):323–328

[8] Shah R, Grauer J. Thoracoscopic excision of thoracic herniated disc. In: Vaccaro A, Bono C, eds. Minimally Invasive Spine Surgery. New York, NY: Informa Healthcare; 2007:73–80

[9] Rosenthal D, Dickman CA. Thoracoscopic microsurgical excision of herniated thoracic discs. J Neurosurg. 1998; 89(2):224–235

[10] Uribe JS, Smith WD, Pimenta L, et al. Minimally invasive lateral approach for symptomatic thoracic disc herniation: initial multicenter clinical experience. J Neurosurg Spine. 2012; 16(3):264–279

[11] Faciszewski T, Winter RB, Lonstein JE, Denis F, Johnson L. The surgical and medical perioperative complications of anterior spinal fusion surgery in the thoracic and lumbar spine in adults. A review of 1223 procedures. Spine. 1995; 20(14):1592–1599

[12] Regan JJ, Ben-Yishay A, Mack MJ. Video-assisted thoracoscopic excision of herniated thoracic disc: description of technique and preliminary experience in the first 29 cases. J Spinal Disord. 1998; 11(3):183–191

[13] Naunheim KS, Barnett MG, Crandall DG, Vaca KJ, Burkus JK. Anterior exposure of the thoracic spine. Ann Thorac Surg. 1994; 57(6):1436–1439

[14] Sundaresan N, Shah J, Foley KM, Rosen G. An anterior surgical approach to the upper thoracic vertebrae. J Neurosurg. 1984; 61(4):686–690

[15] Anand N, Regan JJ. Video-assisted thoracoscopic surgery for thoracic disc disease: classification and outcome study of 100 consecutive cases with a 2-year minimum follow-up period. Spine. 2002; 27(8):871–879

[16] Horowitz MB, Moossy JJ, Julian T, Ferson PF, Huneke K. Thoracic discectomy using video assisted thoracoscopy. Spine. 1994; 19(9):1082–1086

[17] Mack MJ, Regan JJ, McAfee PC, Picetti G, Ben-Yishay A, Acuff TE. Video-assisted thoracic surgery for the anterior approach to the thoracic spine. Ann Thorac Surg. 1995; 59(5):1100–1106

[18] McAfee PC, Regan JR, Zdeblick T, et al. The incidence of complications in endoscopic anterior thoracolumbar spinal reconstructive surgery. A prospective multicenter study comprising the first 100 consecutive cases. Spine. 1995; 20(14):1624–1632

[19] Dickman CA, Karahalios DG. Thoracoscopic spinal surgery. Clin Neurosurg. 1996; 43:392–422

[20] Dickman CA, Rosenthal D, Karahalios DG, et al. Thoracic vertebrectomy and reconstruction using a microsurgical thoracoscopic approach. Neurosurgery. 1996; 38(2):279–293

[21] Landreneau RJ, Hazelrigg SR, Mack MJ, et al. Postoperative pain-related morbidity: video-assisted thoracic surgery versus thoracotomy. Ann Thorac Surg. 1993; 56(6):1285–1289

[22] Johnson JP, Filler AG, Mc Bride DQ. Endoscopic thoracic discectomy. Neurosurg Focus. 2000; 9(4):e11

[23] Dickman CA, Rosenthal D, Regan JJ. Reoperation for herniated thoracic discs. J Neurosurg. 1999; 91(2) Suppl:157–162

[24] Russo A, Balamurali G, Nowicki R, Boszczyk BM. Anterior thoracic foraminotomy through mini-thoracotomy for the treatment of giant thoracic disc herniations. Eur Spine J. 2012; 21 Suppl 2:S212–S220

[25] Moran C, Ali Z, McEvoy L, Bolger C. Mini-open retropleural transthoracic approach for the treatment of giant thoracic disc herniation. Spine. 2012; 37 (17):E1079–E1084

[26] McCormick PC. Retropleural approach to the thoracic and thoracolumbar spine. Neurosurgery. 1995; 37(5):908–914

[27] McCormick WE, Will SF, Benzel EC. Surgery for thoracic disc disease. Complication avoidance: overview and management. Neurosurg Focus. 2000; 9(4):e13

[28] Chi JH, Dhall SS, Kanter AS, Mummaneni PV. The mini-open transpedicular thoracic discectomy: surgical technique and assessment. Neurosurg Focus. 2008; 25(2):E5

[29] Otani K, Yoshida M, Fujii E, Nakai S, Shibasaki K. Thoracic disc herniation. Surgical treatment in 23 patients. Spine. 1988; 13(11):1262–1267

[30] Jho HD. Endoscopic transpedicular thoracic discectomy. Neurosurg Focus. 2000; 9(4):e4

[31] Jho HD. Endoscopic microscopic transpedicular thoracic discectomy. Technical note. J Neurosurg. 1997; 87(1):125–129

[32] Perez-Cruet MJ, Kim BS, Sandhu F, Samartzis D, Fessler RG. Thoracic microendoscopic discectomy. J Neurosurg Spine. 2004; 1(1):58–63

[33] Smith JS, Eichholz KM, Shafizadeh S, Ogden AT, O'Toole JE, Fessler RG. Minimally invasive thoracic microendoscopic diskectomy: surgical technique and case series. World Neurosurg. 2013; 80(3–4):421–427

[34] Lidar Z, Lifshutz J, Bhattacharjee S, Kurpad SN, Maiman DJ. Minimally invasive, extracavitary approach for thoracic disc herniation: technical report and preliminary results. Spine J. 2006; 6(2):157–163

[35] Khoo LT, Smith ZA, Asgarzadie F, et al. Minimally invasive extracavitary approach for thoracic discectomy and interbody fusion: 1-year clinical and radiographic outcomes in 13 patients compared with a cohort of traditional anterior transthoracic approaches. J Neurosurg Spine. 2011; 14(2):250–260

[36] Barbagallo GM, Piccini M, Gasbarrini A, Milone P, Albanese V. Subphrenic hematoma after thoracoscopic discectomy: description of a very rare adverse event and review of the literature on complications: case report. J Neurosurg Spine. 2013; 19(4):436–444

[37] Debnath UK, McConnell JR, Sengupta DK, Mehdian SM, Webb JK. Results of hemivertebrectomy and fusion for symptomatic thoracic disc herniation. Eur Spine J. 2003; 12(3):292–299

[38] Mack MJ, Regan JJ, Bobechko WP, Acuff TE. Application of thoracoscopy for diseases of the spine. Ann Thorac Surg. 1993; 56(3):736–738

[39] Oppenlander ME, Clark JC, Kalyvas J, Dickman CA. Surgical management and clinical outcomes of multiple-level symptomatic herniated thoracic discs. J Neurosurg Spine. 2013; 19(6):774–783

[40] Bartels RH, Peul WC. Mini-thoracotomy or thoracoscopic treatment for medially located thoracic herniated disc? Spine. 2007; 32(20):E581–E584

[41] Patterson RH, Jr, Arbit E. A surgical approach through the pedicle to protruded thoracic discs. J Neurosurg. 1978; 48(5):768–772

[42] Stillerman CB, Chen TC, Day JD, Couldwell WT, Weiss MH. The transfacet pedicle-sparing approach for thoracic disc removal: cadaveric morphometric analysis and preliminary clinical experience. J Neurosurg. 1995; 83(6):971–976

[43] Hulme A. The surgical approach to thoracic intervertebral disc protrusions. J Neurol Neurosurg Psychiatry. 1960; 23:133–137

[44] Huang TJ, Hsu RW, Sum CW, Liu HP. Complications in thoracoscopic spinal surgery: a study of 90 consecutive patients. Surg Endosc. 1999; 13(4):346–350

[45] Quint U, Bordon G, Preissl I, Sanner C, Rosenthal D. Thoracoscopic treatment for single level symptomatic thoracic disc herniation: a prospective followed cohort study in a group of 167 consecutive cases. Eur Spine J. 2012; 21(4): 637–645

[46] Mayer H. The microsurgical anterior approach to T5–T10 (mini-TTA). In: Minimally Invasive Spine Surgery. Berlin: Springer; 2000:59–66

[47] Nacar OA, Ulu MO, Pekmezci M, Deviren V. Surgical treatment of thoracic disc disease via minimally invasive lateral transthoracic trans/retropleural approach: analysis of 33 patients. Neurosurg Rev. 2013; 36(3):455–465

[48] Watanabe K, Yabuki S, Konno S, Kikuchi S. Complications of endoscopic spinal surgery: a retrospective study of thoracoscopy and retroperitoneoscopy. J Orthop Sci. 2007; 12(1):42–48

[49] Gille O, Soderlund C, Razafimahandri HJ, Mangione P, Vital JM. Analysis of hard thoracic herniated discs: review of 18 cases operated by thoracoscopy. Eur Spine J. 2006; 15(5):537–542

[50] Angevine PD, McCormick PC. Thoracic disc. J Neurosurg Spine. 2012; 16(3): 261–262, discussion 262–263

[51] Lubelski D, Abdullah KG, Steinmetz MP, et al. Lateral extracavitary, costotransversectomy, and transthoracic thoracotomy approaches to the thoracic spine: review of techniques and complications. J Spinal Disord Tech. 2013; 26(4):222–232

[52] Hott JS, Feiz-Erfan I, Kenny K, Dickman CA. Surgical management of giant herniated thoracic discs: analysis of 20 cases. J Neurosurg Spine. 2005; 3(3): 191–197

[53] Barbanera A, Serchi E, Fiorenza V, Nina P, Andreoli A. Giant calcified thoracic herniated disc: considerations aiming a proper surgical strategy. J Neurosurg Sci. 2009; 53(1):19–25, discussion 25–26

[54] Mitsunaga L, Kim C. Thoracoscopic corpectomy. In: Vaccaro A, Bono C, eds. Minimally Invasive Spine Surgery. New York, NY: Informa Healthcare; 2007:81–90

[55] Newton PO, Wenger DR, Mubarak SJ, Meyer RS. Anterior release and fusion in pediatric spinal deformity. A comparison of early outcome and cost of thoracoscopic and open thoracotomy approaches. Spine. 1997; 22(12):1398–1406

[56] Shirzadi A, Drazin D, Jeswani S, Lovely L, Liu J. Atypical presentation of thoracic disc herniation: case series and review of the literature. Case Rep Orthop. 2013; 2013:621476

[57] Fessler RG, Sturgill M. Review: complications of surgery for thoracic disc disease. Surg Neurol. 1998; 49(6):609–618

[58] Zhao Y, Wang Y, Xiao S, Zhang Y, Liu Z, Liu B. Transthoracic approach for the treatment of calcified giant herniated thoracic discs. Eur Spine J. 2013; 22 (11):2466–2473

[59] Love JG, Kiefer EJ. Root pain and paraplegia due to protrusions of thoracic intervertebral disks. J Neurosurg. 1950; 7(1):62–69, illust

[60] Epstein JA. The syndrome of herniation of the lower thoracic intervertebral discs with nerve root and spinal cord compression. A presentation of four cases with a review of literature, methods of diagnosis and treatment. J Neurosurg. 1954; 11(6):525–538

[61] Perot PL, Jr, Munro DD. Transthoracic removal of midline thoracic disc protrusions causing spinal cord compression. J Neurosurg. 1969; 31(4):452–458

[62] Albrand OW, Corkill G. Thoracic disc herniation. Treatment and prognosis. Spine. 1979; 4(1):41–46

[63] Maiman DJ, Larson SJ, Luck E, El-Ghatit A. Lateral extracavitary approach to the spine for thoracic disc herniation: report of 23 cases. Neurosurgery. 1984; 14(2):178–182

[64] el-Kalliny M, Tew JM, Jr, van Loveren H, Dunsker S. Surgical approaches to thoracic disc herniations. Acta Neurochir (Wien). 1991; 111(1–2):22–32

[65] Singounas EG, Kypriades EM, Kellerman AJ, Garvan N. Thoracic disc herniation. Analysis of 14 cases and review of the literature. Acta Neurochir (Wien). 1992; 116(1):49–52

[66] Simpson JM, Silveri CP, Simeone FA, Balderston RA, An HS. Thoracic disc herniation. Re-evaluation of the posterior approach using a modified costotransversectomy. Spine. 1993; 18(13):1872–1877

[67] Le Roux PD, Haglund MM, Harris AB. Thoracic disc disease: experience with the transpedicular approach in twenty consecutive patients. Neurosurgery. 1993; 33(1):58–66

[68] Dietze DD, Jr, Fessler RG. Thoracic disc herniations. Neurosurg Clin N Am. 1993; 4(1):75–90

[69] Stillerman CB, Chen TC, Couldwell WT, Zhang W, Weiss MH. Experience in the surgical management of 82 symptomatic herniated thoracic discs and review of the literature. J Neurosurg. 1998; 88(4):623–633

[70] Jho HD. Endoscopic transpedicular thoracic discectomy. J Neurosurg. 1999; 91(2) Suppl:151–156

[71] Kim KD, Babbitz JD, Mimbs J. Imaging-guided costotransversectomy for thoracic disc herniation. Neurosurg Focus. 2000; 9(4):e7

[72] Dinh DH, Tompkins J, Clark SB. Transcostovertebral approach for thoracic disc herniations. J Neurosurg. 2001; 94(1) Suppl:38–44

[73] Han PP, Kenny K, Dickman CA. Thoracoscopic approaches to the thoracic spine: experience with 241 surgical procedures. Neurosurgery. 2002; 51(5) Suppl:S88–S95

[74] Oskouian RJ, Johnson JP. Endoscopic thoracic microdiscectomy. J Neurosurg Spine. 2005; 3(6):459–464

[75] D'Aliberti G, Talamonti G, Villa F, et al. Anterior approach to thoracic and lumbar spine lesions: results in 145 consecutive cases. J Neurosurg Spine. 2008; 9(5):466–482

[76] Machino M, Yukawa Y, Ito K, Nakashima H, Kato F. A new thoracic reconstruction technique "transforaminal thoracic interbody fusion": a preliminary report of clinical outcomes. Spine. 2010; 35(19):E1000–E1005

[77] Bransford R, Zhang F, Bellabarba C, Konodi M, Chapman JR. Early experience treating thoracic disc herniations using a modified transfacet pedicle-sparing decompression and fusion. J Neurosurg Spine. 2010; 12(2):221–231

12 Posterior Cervical Foraminotomy

MIS: Tim Eugene Adamson
Open: Andrew C. Hecht and Steven Joseph McAnany

12.1 Introduction

Various surgical techniques have been described for the treatment of cervical radiculopathy. The surgeon must choose between an anterior or posterior approach based on the nature of the pathology and comfort level with a particular approach. The anterior approach to the cervical spine was first pioneered by Smith and Robinson[1] and was later modified by Cloward.[2] Multiple modifications over the years, including allografts, cages, and fixed and dynamic plating, have led many to consider it the gold standard for the treatment of cervical disc disease.

The use of a posterior approach for the treatment of cervical radiculopathy originated more than 65 years ago. Mixter was the first to report on the use of a posterior approach for the treatment of a cervical disc herniation.[3] The posterior cervical foraminotomy (PCF) was pioneered by Scoville et al and Frykholm.[4,5] In the 1980s, case series by Fager, Casotto, and Epstein et al popularized the so-called "key-hole" laminoforaminotomy with a success rate approaching 90%.[6,7,8] More recently, Jagannathan et al[9] found a 95% success rate in the resolution of radiculopathy. In spite of a proven track record of success with a favorable complication profile, anterior cervical discectomy and fusion (ACDF) remains a more popular procedure. Ruetten et al[10] showed that when treating radiculopathy alone, PCF and ACDF produce clinically equivalent results, as measured by visual analog scale, Hilibrand's criteria, and the North American Spine Society Instrument. Similarly, Wirth et al[11] demonstrated similar results, finding no significant differences in surgical complication rates or postoperative symptom relief between the two approaches.

Advantages of the posterior approach include better access to posterolateral-directed herniations, no risk for pseudarthrosis or graft subsidence, and decreased risk of iatrogenic kyphosis.[9,12] The complications reported with this approach include nerve root injury, dural tear, spinal cord injury with and without K-wire misplacement, same-segment and adjacent-segment syndrome, and spinal instability.[13,14,15]

The posterior laminoforaminotomy was initially developed as a midline approach, utilizing a subperiosteal lamina dissection to minimize bleeding. The open approach allows for excellent visualization and access to lateral disc herniations and bony foraminal compromise secondary to cervical spondylosis. Opponents of the open PCF cite postoperative neck pain and spasm as a disadvantage of the procedure. The development of the operative microscope resulted in a further refinement in technique but the traditional midline subperiosteal approach remained the same. In 1997, Foley and Smith introduced the lumbar microendoscopic discectomy technique and the muscle-splitting tubular retractor system.[16] As an alternative to these standard open approaches, endoscopic and minimally invasive techniques have been developed. Minimally invasive surgery (MIS) techniques allow for shorter hospital stays, same-day surgery, faster recovery times, and reduced blood loss.[13,17,18] Minimally invasive foraminotomy is an increasingly relied upon means of foraminal decompression, but whether it is superior to the open technique remains a matter of debate.

12.2 Indications for Posterior Cervical Foraminotomy

The management of cervical radiculopathy remains a controversial area within spine surgery. PCFs are typically indicated for patients with cervical radiculopathy due to foraminal stenosis that is refractory to at least 6 weeks of conservative management.

The posterior laminoforaminotomy is best utilized in the treatment of foraminal lesions or cases of posterolateral soft disc herniation that compresses the nerve root while lying lateral to the cord. The primary contraindications to PCF include segmental kyphosis or instability at the operative level. A relative contraindication to PCF is the presence of clinical or radiographic myelopathy or myelomalacia. A summary of the literature for open and MIS PCF can be found in ▶ Table 12.1.

Table 12.1 Literature summary of minimally invasive and open cervical foraminotomy

Study	Level of evidence	Number of patients	Summary of findings
Kim and Kim[19]	I	19 open 22 MIS	• Significantly lower length of stay, analgesic use, and length of skin incision in MIS group • Significantly lower VAS of neck pain in MIS group at 1 d, 5 d, and 4 wk • No differences in VAS of neck pain at 3 mo and beyond
Winder et al[20]	III	65 open 42 MIS	• Significantly less blood loss, analgesic use, and length of hospital stay in the MIS group • 7.1% complication rate in MIS group vs. 10.8% in open group
Fessler and Khoo[18]	III	25 MIS	• Noted increased blood loss, operative time, and complications during the initial learning curve
Wang et al[25]	III	178 open	• Index level reoperation with ACDF of 5% after average follow-up of 31.7 mo
Adamson[13]	III	100 MIS	• Excellent/good results in 97/100 • Two cases of dural tear
Hilton[22]	IV	222 MIS	• No incidence of dural tear in any patients

Abbreviations: ACDF, anterior cervical discectomy and fusion; MIS, minimally invasive surgery; VAS, visual analog scale.

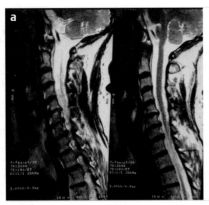 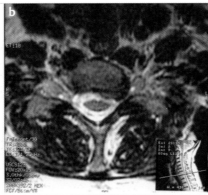

Fig. 12.1 (a) Sagittal and (b) axial T2-weighted magnetic resonance images demonstrating a left-sided disc osteophyte complex at C7–T1 causing severe foraminal stenosis with compression of the exiting C8 nerve root.

12.3 Advantages of the Minimally Invasive Surgery

All minimally invasive spinal surgery techniques, and especially those involving the cervical spine, result in less muscle damage and disruption than the traditional open techniques. By eliminating the subperiosteal dissection that detaches the muscular insertions on the posterior spinal elements and secondary denervation, the MIS approach, utilizing a muscle-splitting dilatation technique, results in less acute muscle injury and its consequences as well as less chronic muscular denervation, atrophy, and alteration to long-term cervical biomechanics.

Multiple studies have demonstrated a significant difference in the early indicators of muscle damage between open and MIS lumbar techniques focusing on the serum CPK (creatine phosphokinase) levels, which directly reflect the degree of muscle damage. In the cervical spine, this has also been shown to correlate with lower rates of postoperative pain, narcotic use, length of hospitalization, and wound infections. As would be expected, the same laminoforaminotomies done through different muscle approaches (MIS vs. open) have similar results for relief of radiculopathy.

Postoperative imaging more than 1 year after surgery reveals that the amount of long-term muscle change is markedly different between the two approaches. Unilateral atrophy of the multifidus muscle is not uncommon following an MIS approach given the direct disruption necessary to expose the lateral lamina and medial facet, but the more superficial musculature does not appear to be damaged. Following the subperiosteal dissection associated with an open approach, not only is the multifidus muscle directly affected, but also there is long-term atrophy of the semispinalis and more superficial musculature. The impact of this long-term asymmetry and potential change in function has not been studied in any detail.

12.4 Advantages of Open Surgery

The benefits of the open PCF have been detailed above. The posterior approach to the cervical spine is well known to most spinal surgeons. This familiarity provides the main benefit over the MIS technique, as it allows surgeons to avoid the steep learning curve that is associated with mastering an MIS approach. In addition, complications that are unique to the MIS approach include misplacement of the percutaneous Kirschner wire or Steinman pin, medial migration of the tubular retractor with injury to the spinal cord or nerve roots, and lateral migration of the tubular retractor with damage/injury to the exiting nerve root or vertebral artery.

12.5 Case Illustration

A 55-year-old man presented with a 1-year history of left arm pain, weakness, and paresthesias that have failed to respond to conservative treatment including physical therapy, NSAIDs (nonsteroidal anti-inflammatory drugs), and injections. Magnetic resonance imaging (MRI) revealed a C7–T1 posterolateral disc herniation with significant foraminal stenosis and compression of the left C8 nerve root (▶ Fig. 12.1). Surgical intervention was recommended to decompress the affected nerve root.

12.6 Surgical Technique in Minimally Invasive Surgery

Following the induction of anesthesia, the bed is positioned so that the operative side is away from the anesthesia equipment. The patient is then placed in a sitting or semirecumbent position utilizing a Mayfield-Kees head holder. The patient's blood pressure is carefully monitored as the back is elevated and the lower legs flexed to accomplish a "lounge chair" position. This allows the head to be positioned neutrally with respect to rotation and flexion. The posterior cervical region is positioned vertically and the head holder securely locked in place. The fluoroscopy arm is then brought in from the foot of the bed and positioned to allow a true lateral image. The posterior neck is then prepped and draped with a disposable cranial incise drape to take advantage of the drainage pouch. The fluoroscopy arm is draped into the field so that imaging can be obtained at any point during the procedure.

The target level is initially localized by placing a spinal needle lateral to the neck and checked fluoroscopically. The needle is then repositioned one fingerbreadth off of midline to the affected side and introduced through the skin. Fluoroscopy is then used to monitor the trajectory as the needle is introduced to the middle of the lamina cephalad to the targeted disc space.

The ideal trajectory is to angle slightly cephalad from the skin to the lamina. Once the bone is contacted and localization confirmed with fluoroscopy, the needle is removed and a 16- to 18-mm incision sharply incised. It is optimum to obliquely angle this to take advantage of the Langer line anatomy. A K-wire is then introduced through the skin incision and positioned back along the needle trajectory with fluoroscopic guidance. Positioning this in the middle of the cephalad lamina is the safest and avoids the potentially dangerous interlaminar space. Once confirmed to be on the lamina, the first dilator is passed over the wire to the bone, and the wire is then removed. The first dilator is then used to create a pocket of subperiosteal dissection, which makes the initial soft tissue steps much easier once the cylinder is in place. Before progressing to the next dilators, the superficial and deep fascia layers are relaxed by spreading a pair of scissors or a hemostat along the outside of the first dilator. The remaining dilators are then used to introduce the operative cylinder to the back of the lamina and then positioned caudally with fluoroscopic confirmation until they are centered over the target disc space before anchoring to the table-mounted arm.

The remaining muscle overlying the bone is removed with a pituitary rongeur. At this point, the microendoscope is brought in to use from the cephalad side for visualization. The medial facet and lateral lamina can usually be visualized at this point. Any remaining soft tissue obstructing the view is either removed or cauterized. The laminoforaminotomy is then initiated using a high-speed drill removing the outer cortical layer and cancellous bone of the lamina as well as the medial aspect of the facet. Once a small opening is made through the deep cortical bone over the lateral canal, a 2-mm Kerrison rongeur is used to complete the foraminotomy. Identifying the medial and cephalad margins of the pedicle is useful for medial/lateral orientation. The foraminotomy is extended laterally until the lateral margin of the pedicle begins to fall away. At this point, only a third to one-half of the medial facet has been removed and should not impact stability. A small laminotomy in the caudal lamina is useful to visualize the lateral margin of the thecal sac. This is the safest area to introduce a nerve hook under the sac and then rotate it medially and cephalad under the origin of the nerve root. This motion allows the safe mobilization of a divided root, even in the lower cervical levels where it is more common. The rotating motion also will mobilize disc fragments into the axilla where they can be removed with a micropituitary rongeur. Contained fragments may require the use of a down-angled curette to fully mobilize into the axilla. If a spondylotic spur is encountered, no additional work is done under the root but the foraminotomy is enlarged to ensure that the root is fully decompressed.

Once hemostasis is obtained with electrocautery or hemostatic foam, the wound is carefully irrigated and a pledget of Depo-Medrol-soaked Gelfoam is placed over the foraminotomy site. The operative cylinder is removed and the wound closed in a single layer with 2–0 Vicryl suture in an inverted interrupted fashion in the subcutaneous fascia. Twenty milliliters of 0.25% Marcaine is infiltrated around the incision and the skin is sealed with Dermabond. Following a short stay in the PACU (postanesthesia care unit), the patient is discharged to home 2 to 3 hours after the surgery is completed.

12.7 Surgical Technique in Open Surgery

The patient is brought to operating room where general endotracheal tube intubation is administered. The patient is then placed into the prone position with the head secured with a Mayfield positioner. The patient's neck is flexed to decrease cervical lordosis and to better expose the superior facet of the caudal vertebrae. The bed is then positioned in a slight reverse Trendelenburg position to help decrease bleeding. For the lower cervical levels, the shoulders may be taped in order to facilitate imaging. A lateral cervical radiograph is obtained to verify the appropriate spinal levels.

A midline skin incision is made centered over the spinous process of the tip of the most cephalad level. The skin incision should measure approximately 2 cm in length for a single-level foraminotomy. The ligamentum nuchae is divided longitudinally to expose the spinous processes. An intraoperative lateral radiograph is obtained to verify the correct operative level. The paravertebral muscles are subperiosteally elevated from the lamina on either side of the spinous process. A self-retaining retractor can be placed to allow for adequate exposure. The dissection is carried laterally over the lamina to the facet with attention paid to preserve the facet joint capsule.

Using a high-speed burr, the caudal edge of the lateral potion of the lamina cephalad to the interspace is drilled away. The medial edge of the facet may also be removed to facilitate exposure. A small Kerrison rongeur (1–2 mm) can be used to enlarge the space.

The ligamentum flavum is sharply incised with a Kerrison rongeur. The nerve root is identified within the space. Additional bone may be removed from the dorsal aspect of the foramen as well as cephalad and caudad to the nerve root.

An operative microscope can be used to improve visualization around the neural elements. The nerve root is gently retracted superiorly to expose the extruded disc fragments or distended posterior longitudinal ligament. Additional bone should be resected to improve visualization instead of placing excessive traction on the nerve root. Venous oozing can be controlled with bipolar cautery or thrombin soaked Gelfoam.

A discectomy can now be performed by incising the posterior longitudinal ligament over the herniated fragments. Once all visible disc fragments are removed, it is important to properly assess the disc space for additional fragments. Irrigation of the disc space, reverse angle curettes, and up-going pituitaries can be used to adequately remove any remaining fragments.

After fragment removal, the nerve root is assessed to confirm adequate decompression. If the foramen remains tight, additional bone can be removed from the articular facets.

A standard layer closure is then performed after achieving meticulous hemostasis.

12.8 Discussion of Minimally Invasive Surgery

Cervical radiculopathy is a very common medical condition that requires surgical intervention when conservative therapy measures such as physical therapy, chiropractic care, and epidural steroid injections fail to obtain relief. Many of these patients can be easily treated with motion-preserving posterior cervical laminoforaminotomy that does not require any expensive implants and routinely obtains good outcomes with low morbidity. The transition from an open midline subperiosteal approach to a muscle-sparing/splitting MIS approach is associated in the short term with less pain, shorter hospital stays, and lower risk of infection. In the long term, there is less muscle damage and atrophy, which may result in better long-term neck functioning and potentially lower risk of long-term problems (▶ Table 12.1).

12.8.1 Level I Evidence in Minimally Invasive Surgery

A randomized, single-surgeon study of 41 patients comparing open and MIS cervical laminoforaminotomy was reported by Kim and Kim in 2009.[19] After a mean follow-up of 34.2 months, they were able to demonstrate similar radiculopathy relief and complication rates between the 19 open and 22 MIS cases but found statistically significant differences in length of hospital stay, analgesic use, length of skin incision, and VAS (visual analog scale) neck pain scores at 1 day, 5 days, and 4 weeks in favor of the MIS group. At 3 months, there was no longer a significant difference in neck pain. Interestingly, the authors obtained postoperative computed tomography (CT) scans and measured the size of the foraminotomy created, and found no difference between the techniques.

12.8.2 Level II Evidence in Minimally Invasive Surgery

There are no level II studies available.

12.8.3 Level III Evidence in Minimally Invasive Surgery

A single-center retrospective review of 107 (65 open vs. 42 MIS) patients treated with posterior cervical laminoforaminotomy by Winder and Thomas[20] also found a statistically significant difference favoring the MIS approach when looking at operative blood loss, analgesic use, and length of hospital stay. Again, operative time was similar. The complication rate was lower for the MIS group compared with the open group but did not reach statistical significance.

Multiple case series reports have been published recently with MIS cervical laminoforaminotomy techniques utilizing both endoscope and microscope visualization. These series report similar outcomes and complication rates when compared to the large open series published over the past few decades. Over 90% of both techniques report good relief of radiculopathy symptoms and low complication rates. However, the series of Lawton et al,[21] Hilton,[22] and Adamson[13] report that the majority of patients are done on an outpatient basis. The difference in the postoperative analgesic use seems to explain this difference as manifested in the length of hospital stay as noted previously by Kim and Kim[19] and Winder et al.[20]

A recent large report by Gerard et al looking at postoperative surgical infections at a single center with 2,299 cases of lumbar discectomy, laminotomy, or transforaminal lumbar interbody fusion found the risk of infection in the open approaches was 5.77 times greater than the MIS approaches.[23] Although this is a lumbar study, it is of such a size that the implications are appropriate for all spinal procedures, including cervical.

12.9 Complications in Minimally Invasive Surgery

The potential complications with open and MIS cervical laminoforaminotomy are most worrisome when affecting the spinal cord or nerves. In our own experience, the rate of spinal cord injury or RSD (reflex sympathetic dystrophy) has been less than 1 in 1,200. The risk of infection or hematoma formation has been less than 1% in our experience and is comparable to the series discussed previously. Incidental durotomy that does not require postoperative treatment is reported by many authors but is self-limited.

In none of the series discussed has the complication rate for the MIS techniques been greater than the rate for open techniques.

12.10 Conclusion of Minimally Invasive Surgery

The role of the posterior cervical laminoforaminotomy for the surgical treatment of cervical radiculopathy has been well established for many decades. Recently, the open subperiosteal approach has evolved to an MIS muscle-splitting and muscle-sparing approach. After reviewing the level I and III data available, it appears that the surgical outcomes with respect to relief of the preoperative radiculopathy have been similar and the perioperative complications have been similar. There are level I and III data to suggest that postoperative pain, as manifested by analgesic use and length of hospital stay, is significantly less with the MIS approach. Level I data also exist to suggest that the postoperative VAS neck pain scores are significantly lower for 4 weeks after surgery with the MIS approach. The long-term differences between the two techniques may best be demonstrated by looking at postoperative CT imaging and comparing the muscular changes in the cervical musculature that is present. Further studies looking at the functional long-term consequences of these changes will need to be done.

Using the grading scale developed by Guyatt et al, there is sufficient level I evidence to support a Grade 1C recommendation that better short-term clinical outcomes, including shorter hospital stays, less blood loss, lower narcotic analgesia usage, and immediate postoperative pain improvement, are seen in patients undergoing minimally invasive over open cervical foraminotomies. A Grade 2A recommendation may be assigned to the conclusion that open and minimally invasive posterior cervical foraminotomies achieve similar long-term patient outcomes with low complication rates.

12.11 Discussion of Open Surgery

Cervical radiculopathy is one of the most common complaints seen by the spine surgeon. Failure of conservative treatment leaves several good surgical options. The decision on approach and the type of surgery to be performed is based on patient and surgeon specific considerations. Open PCF remains a viable surgical option, with outcomes equal to or better than those seen with an MIS foraminotomy approach. The purported advantages of MIS include shorter hospital stays, decreased blood loss, and quicker return to function. However, there is a significant learning curve with an increased complication rate and operative time during this period.[18]

12.11.1 Level I Evidence in Open Surgery

There is one level I study that directly compares the open and MIS foraminotomy technique. Kim and Kim[19] recently published the results of a randomized controlled trial wherein 19 patients underwent open foraminotomies and 22 underwent MIS foraminotomies. The length of incision, duration of hospital stay, and amount of postoperative narcotic use all favored the MIS group. However, there were no significant differences found in radicular pain at any time point, and the final outcomes were not different between to the two groups.

12.11.2 Level II Evidence in Open Surgery

There are no level II studies available.

12.11.3 Level III Evidence in Open Surgery

There are a limited number of level III studies comparing the results of open and MIS PCF. In one study comparing open and MIS PCF, Winder et al[20] found significant differences favoring the MIS cohort, including decreased intraoperative blood loss, postoperative analgesic use, and length of hospital stay ($p < 0.001$). However, there were no differences in operative time or operative complications. The authors, however, note that the results of the study do not take into consideration the associated learning curve of the individual surgeons, which could impact the observed complications rate.

The learning curve associated with mastering a minimally invasive approach cannot be understated. Fessler and Khoo[18] noted increased blood loss, operative time, and complications rate during the initial learning curve. In addition, the authors noted an initial durotomy rate of 9%, which decreased to 1% with subsequent experience.

The other parameters also improved as the surgeons gained experience with the technique. The findings are consistent with those seen with the minimally invasive transforaminal lumbar interbody fusion technique (MIS-TLIF). Lee et al[24] found that surgeons reached the end of their learning curve after performing 30 or more procedures.

In a recent study examining the reoperation rate following open posterior foraminotomy, Wang et al[25] reported an index level reoperation rate of 5% at an average follow-up of 31.7 months. The authors concluded that PCF is associated with a low reoperation rate, similar to the historical reoperation for ACDF.

12.12 Complications in Open Surgery

One of the most commonly cited reasons for performing MIS are the limited muscle dissection that the procedure allows. The midline incision in the open foraminotomy procedure involves extensive subperiosteal elevation of the muscle mass and has been associated with postoperative neck pain and spasm. Hosono et al,[26] in a retrospective review of 98 patients undergoing laminoplasty, found a postoperative rate of axial neck pain greater than 60%. Similarly, Ratliff and Cooper,[27] in a meta-analysis of 41 retrospective laminoplasty studies, found an incidence of postoperative neck pain ranging from 6 to 60%. However, Fessler and Khoo[18] noted no significant differences in postoperative neck pain between the open and MIS group.

The most common complications following open cervical foraminotomy include durotomy and cerebrospinal fluid (CSF) leak.[9,28,29,30,31] Reported rates range from 0 to 9%. When compared with the rates seen in MIS approaches, there does not appear to be a significant difference in the rate of durotomy or CSF leak between the two procedures. In fact, Kim and Kim,[19] in their prospective study, had no complications in either group.

12.13 Conclusion of Open Surgery

Based on the review of the literature presented above, there are a limited number of studies with comparative data between open and MIS cervical foraminotomy. There exists one level I study which found no significant difference in outcome between the two procedures. There are no level II studies available in the literature. There is one level III study available in the literature. There is level I and level III evidence that the MIS technique allows for decreased length of stay, operative time, and blood loss. In addition, there is level III evidence that there is a higher complication rate during the learning curve with MIS techniques. There is level I and level III evidence that the rate of neurological injury, CSF leak, and durotomy are not significantly different between open and MIS techniques. Using the grading scale of Guyatt et al, we suggest a Grade 2B recommendation that open and MIS cervical foraminotomy are equivalent in terms of clinical outcomes and reoperation rates.

12.14 Editors' Commentary

12.14.1 Minimally Invasive Surgery

Among the earliest operations to be converted from open to MIS technique, cervical foraminotomy has now been performed for nearly 20 years. Numerous peer-reviewed publications have demonstrated its safety and efficacy; thousands of patient operations are now reported in the literature. It has transformed a very painful cervical operation into an outpatient procedure. When performed in the sitting position, blood loss is negligible. Using an endoscope makes this position very comfortable for the surgeon. Because the tube tamponades the vasculature, fear of air embolism is eliminated. In the prone position, by using a microscope with the head elevated slightly, blood loss can still be minimized.

12.14.2 Open Surgery

Open laminoforaminotomy has no clinically significant disadvantages compared to MIS laminoforaminotomy and has a shorter associated learning curve. The technique descriptions above for the MIS and open procedures describe a difference in incision length of between 2 and 4 mm, distances which are likely clinically insignificant with respect to important metrics of patient recovery including postoperative pain, narcotic use, and return to work. Procedures such as open laminoforaminotomy which are less invasive are unattractive targets for the introduction of MIS technique as there is substantially less potential room for improvement. Posterior cervical laminoforaminotomy has no evidence to suggest MIS surgery provides an advantage to the patient other than imaging studies, which suggest persistent alterations in muscular anatomy without adverse clinical correlation. When comparing such closely matched surgeries, the success rate, complication rate, and length of recovery are much more likely to be determined by surgeon experience and technical skill than particulars of which approach is selected. Length of stay for laminoforaminotomy is often measured in hours regardless of approach; arguments about cost-savings due to avoiding inpatient stays carry little weight. Use of MIS techniques for posterior cervical laminoforaminotomy has not distinguished itself clinically as an improvement upon an already less invasive, successful surgical technique.

References

[1] Smith GW, Robinson RA. The treatment of certain cervical-spine disorders by anterior removal of the intervertebral disc and interbody fusion. J Bone Joint Surg Am. 1958; 40-A(3):607–624

[2] Cloward RB. The anterior approach for removal of ruptured cervical disks. J Neurosurg. 1958; 15(6):602–617

[3] Mixter WJ. Rupture of the intervertebral disk; a short history of this evolution as a syndrome of importance to the surgeon. J Am Med Assoc. 1949; 140(3):278–282

[4] Frykholm R. Lower cervical vertebrae and intervertebral discs; surgical anatomy and pathology. Acta Chir Scand. 1951; 101(5):345–359

[5] Scoville WB, Whitcomb BB, McLaurin R. The cervical ruptured disc; report of 115 operative cases. Trans Am Neurol Assoc. 1951; 56:222–224

[6] Casotto A, Buoncristiani P. Posterior approach in cervical spondylotic myeloradiculopathy. Acta Neurochir (Wien). 1981; 57(3–4):275–285

[7] Epstein JA, Janin Y, Carras R, Lavine LS. A comparative study of the treatment of cervical spondylotic myeloradiculopathy. Experience with 50 cases treated by means of extensive laminectomy, foraminotomy, and excision of osteophytes during the past 10 years. Acta Neurochir (Wien). 1982; 61(1–3): 89–104

[8] Fager CA. Posterolateral approach to ruptured median and paramedian cervical disk. Surg Neurol. 1983; 20(6):443–452

[9] Jagannathan J, Shaffrey CI, Oskouian RJ, et al. Radiographic and clinical outcomes following single-level anterior cervical discectomy and allograft fusion without plate placement or cervical collar. J Neurosurg Spine. 2008; 8 (5):420–428

[10] Ruetten S, Komp M, Merk H, Godolias G. Full-endoscopic interlaminar and transforaminal lumbar discectomy versus conventional microsurgical technique: a prospective, randomized, controlled study. Spine. 2008; 33(9): 931–939

[11] Wirth FP, Dowd GC, Sanders HF, Wirth C. Cervical discectomy. A prospective analysis of three operative techniques. Surg Neurol. 2000; 53(4):340–346, discussion 346–348

[12] Samartzis D, Shen FH, Lyon C, Phillips M, Goldberg EJ, An HS. Does rigid instrumentation increase the fusion rate in one-level anterior cervical discectomy and fusion? Spine J. 2004; 4(6):636–643

[13] Adamson TE. Microendoscopic posterior cervical laminoforaminotomy for unilateral radiculopathy: results of a new technique in 100 cases. J Neurosurg. 2001; 95(1) Suppl:51–57

[14] Kumar GR, Maurice-Williams RS, Bradford R. Cervical foraminotomy: an effective treatment for cervical spondylotic radiculopathy. Br J Neurosurg. 1998; 12(6):563–568

[15] Zdeblick TA, Zou D, Warden KE, McCabe R, Kunz D, Vanderby R. Cervical stability after foraminotomy. A biomechanical in vitro analysis. J Bone Joint Surg Am. 1992; 74(1):22–27

[16] Foley KT, Smith MM. Microendoscopic discectomy. Tech Neurosurg. 1997; 3: 301–307

[17] Coric D, Adamson T. Minimally invasive cervical microendoscopic laminoforaminotomy. Neurosurg Focus. 2008; 25(2):E2

[18] Fessler RG, Khoo LT. Minimally invasive cervical microendoscopic foraminotomy: an initial clinical experience. Neurosurgery. 2002; 51(5) Suppl:S37–S45

[19] Kim KT, Kim YB. Comparison between open procedure and tubular retractor assisted procedure for cervical radiculopathy: results of a randomized controlled study. J Korean Med Sci. 2009; 24(4):649–653

[20] Winder MJ, Thomas KC. Minimally invasive versus open approach for cervical laminoforaminotomy. Can J Neurol Sci. 2011; 38(2):262–267

[21] Lawton CD, Smith ZA, Lam SK, Habib A, Wong RH, Fessler RG. Clinical outcomes of microendoscopic foraminaotomy and decompression in the cervical spine. World Neurosurg 2014 Feb;81(2):422-7. doi: 10.1016/j.wneu.2012.12.008. Epub 2012 Dec 12.

[22] Hilton DL, Jr. Minimally invasive tubular access for posterior cervical foraminotomy with three-dimensional microscopic visualization and localization with anterior/posterior imaging. Spine J. 2007; 7(2):154–158

[23] Ee WWG, Lau WLJ, Yeo W, Bing YV, Yue WM. Does minimally invasive surgery have a lower risk of surgical site infections compared with open spinal surgery? Clin Orthop Relat Res 2014 Jun;472(6):17181724. Published online 2013 Jul 12. doi: 10.1007/s11999-013-3158-5

[24] Lee KH, Yue WM, Yeo W, Soeharno H, Tan SB. Clinical and radiological outcomes of open versus minimally invasive transforaminal lumbar interbody fusion. Eur Spine J. 2012; 21(11):2265–2270

[25] Wang TY, Lubelski D, Abdullah KG, Steinmetz MP, Benzel EC, Mroz TE. Rates of anterior cervical discectomy and fusion after initial posterior cervical foraminotomy. Spine J. 2015; 15(5):971–976

[26] Hosono N, Yonenobu K, Ono K. Neck and shoulder pain after laminoplasty. A noticeable complication. Spine. 1996; 21(17):1969–1973

[27] Ratliff JK, Cooper PR. Cervical laminoplasty: a critical review. J Neurosurg. 2003; 98(3) Suppl:230–238

[28] Aldrich F. Posterolateral microdisectomy for cervical monoradiculopathy caused by posterolateral soft cervical disc sequestration. J Neurosurg. 1990; 72(3):370–377

[29] Jödicke A, Daentzer D, Kästner S, Asamoto S, Böker DK. Risk factors for outcome and complications of dorsal foraminotomy in cervical disc herniation. Surg Neurol. 2003; 60(2):124–129, discussion 129–130

[30] Murphey F, Simmons JC, Brunson B. Surgical treatment of laterally ruptured cervical disc. Review of 648 cases, 1939 to 1972. J Neurosurg. 1973; 38(6): 679–683

[31] Parker WD. Cervical laminoforaminotomy. J Neurosurg. 2002; 96(2) Suppl: 254–, author reply 254–255

13 Complications of Instrumentation: Is There a Higher Complication Rate in Placing Instrumentation via a Minimally Invasive Technique Compared with an Open Technique?

MIS: Russell G. Strom and Anthony K. Frempong-Boadu
Open: Saad B. Chaudhary and Michael J. Vives

13.1 Introduction

Open exposure of the dorsal spinal elements is the gold standard for placement of posterior instrumentation, given that it facilitates identification of anatomic landmarks and trajectories for safe screw placement. However, open techniques require significant paraspinal muscle dissection, resulting in frequent postoperative pain, delayed mobilization, and muscle atrophy. Minimally invasive approaches utilizing serial dilators, tubular retractors, and image guidance have been developed to place posterior instrumentation throughout the spine. Minimally invasive surgery (MIS) techniques cause less immediate postoperative pain and allow faster recovery, but it is controversial whether they come at the cost of screw accuracy, construct strength, fusion rate, and long-term outcome.

13.2 Indications of Posterior Instrumentation

Posterior spinal instrumentation is placed to immobilize the spine and facilitate fusion during surgery for degenerative, traumatic, oncologic, rheumatologic, or structural disease. Atlantoaxial stabilization is indicated for C1–C2 instability and can be achieved through a variety of techniques including C1–C2 transarticular screws (TASs) and screw–rod constructs (C1 lateral mass screw with C2 pedicle, pars, or laminar screw). Subaxial posterior cervical fixation is most commonly achieved using lateral mass screws. Subaxial cervical pedicle screws can also be placed and have greater pullout strength, but placement is technically demanding with a higher risk of vertebral artery or nerve root injury. Subaxial cervical fixation using percutaneous transfacet screws has also been described. In the present era, stabilization of the thoracic and lumbar spine is typically achieved with pedicle screw–rod constructs, although pedicle or laminar hooks and wiring techniques may be used in cases with poor pedicle anatomy or as salvage strategies. Pedicle screws may be placed using a traditional open approach or percutaneously with anteroposterior (AP)–lateral fluoroscopy or computer-aided navigation. Lumbar translaminar facet screws and transfacet-transpedicular screws may also be placed percutaneously, often to supplement an anterior interbody fusion.

13.3 Advantages of Minimally Invasive Surgery

Open placement of posterior instrumentation requires significant paraspinal muscle dissection, leading to frequent postoperative pain, delayed mobilization, blood loss, and muscle atrophy. Less soft-tissue trauma occurs when instrumentation is placed with serial dilators and tubular retractors. As a result, MIS techniques are associated with less postoperative pain, shorter hospital stays, and faster return to activities of daily living. Percutaneous screw placement also spares the midline fascia and ligaments, and the preservation of this posterior tension band may potentially lower the risk of adjacent segment disease. Percutaneous pedicle screws, when properly placed, minimize dissection and exposure of the facet joint and could reduce the risk of adjacent segment disease.

13.4 Advantages of Open Surgery

The advantages of open surgery are primarily its familiarity and versatility. Virtually all contemporary spine surgeons are intimately familiar with the anatomy of open posterior spinal exposures and the techniques of posteriorly placed spinal instrumentation. Utilization of anatomic landmarks can help guide implant placement, particularly in cases with limited fluoroscopic visualization. Combining anatomic cues with limited fluoroscopy also fosters a balanced approach to patient safety and radiation exposure to the surgical team. Given that most of these techniques have been commonplace for up to two decades, the nuances and pitfalls have become well understood and reasonably documented. As such, the risks and expectations associated with these procedures can be communicated to patients with a fair amount of confidence.

In addition to their familiarity, open techniques are versatile. Standard midline approaches permit bilateral exposure to the lateral masses and pedicle entry sites. Levels can be easily added if planned fixation sites are compromised due to screw cutout or poor purchase. Alternative midline fixation techniques, such as C1–C2 sublaminar cables or C2/C7 translaminar screws, can also be utilized for bailout or augmentation. If midline laminectomy is not necessary, then the available bony surfaces for fusion are substantially greater. Conversely, because many patients undergoing posterior instrumented fusion also require decompression, the open midline approach is often selected anyway, and as a consequence will be utilized more frequently throughout most surgeons' careers. Volume fosters familiarity and familiarity has the advantages noted above.

13.5 Case Illustration

A 35-year-old woman presents with chronic progressive neck pain and 6 months of left hand weakness and paresthesias. The patient has mild left hand intrinsic weakness with a positive left Hoffman's sign. Computed tomography (CT) demonstrates a

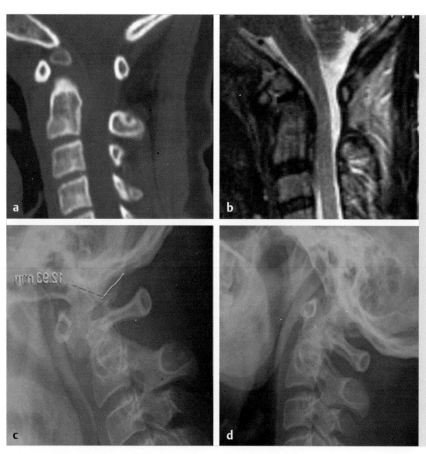

Fig. 13.1 **(a)** Sagittal CT and **(b)** T2-weighted MRI demonstrate os odontoideum associated with T2 signal abnormality. Lateral cervical spine X-rays demonstrate increased atlantodental interval on **(c)** flexion but not on **(d)** extension.

smooth dens separated from the body of the axis, consistent with os odontoideum (▶ Fig. 13.1a). No cord compression is seen on magnetic resonance imaging (MRI) with the neck in neutral position, but subtle T2 signal abnormality is present at C2 (▶ Fig. 13.1b). On lateral X-ray, an increased atlantodental interval is present on flexion but not on extension (▶ Fig. 13.1c,d).

13.6 Surgical Technique in Minimally Invasive Surgery

The patient is positioned prone in a Mayfield head holder with the neck extended to bring the atlas and axis in normal alignment.[1] A 2.5-cm paramedian incision is made overlying the C2 spinous process 2 cm lateral to midline. The fascia is incised, and under fluoroscopic guidance serial dilators are docked onto the lamina of C2. An expandable tubular retractor is placed over the largest dilator and fixed to the bed (▶ Fig. 13.2a). The retractor is then expanded, with the cephalad blade exposing the C1 lateral mass and the caudal blade exposing the C3 lateral mass. The C2 and C3 lateral masses are dissected with monopolar cautery (▶ Fig. 13.2b). The C2 nerve root is coagulated with bipolar cautery and cut to expose the C1–C2 facet joint and C1 lateral mass. C1 lateral mass and C2 pedicle screws are placed using standard entry points and trajectories with fluoroscopic guidance (▶ Fig. 13.2c,d). The C1–C2 joint is decorticated and filled with allograft chips and demineralized bone matrix. The

screws are secured to a rod, and the procedure is repeated contralaterally (▶ Fig. 13.2e).

13.7 Surgical Technique in Open Surgery

The patient is positioned similarly as described above. The shoulders can be taped to the table to eliminate redundant skin folds in the area of the exposure, if necessary. A midline skin incision is made from just above the foramen magnum to just below the tip of the C2 spinous process. Verification of the midline can be done by finger palpation before incising the nuchal fascia, as this minimizes bleeding. Initial exposure proceeds along the top of the C2 spinous process and lamina bilaterally, extending distally toward the C2–C3 facet joint and cephalad to expose the medial boarder of the C2 pedicle. Exposure of the bottom of the occiput in the midline can help establish the ventral depth of the exposure, as the tubercle of the atlas is not as easily palpated initially. Once the tubercle of the atlas can be palpated, subperiosteal dissection can proceed laterally to each side, up to 1.5 cm without risk to the vertebral artery. Gelfoam and bipolar electrocautery can be used to help control bleeding from the epidural venous plexus while exposing the C1 lateral mass and C1–C2 facet joint. The C2 nerve root can be retracted caudally with a Penfield or cut to aid with this exposure. C1 lateral mass and C2 pedicle screws are then placed with standard entry points and trajectories with the aid of fluoroscopy and

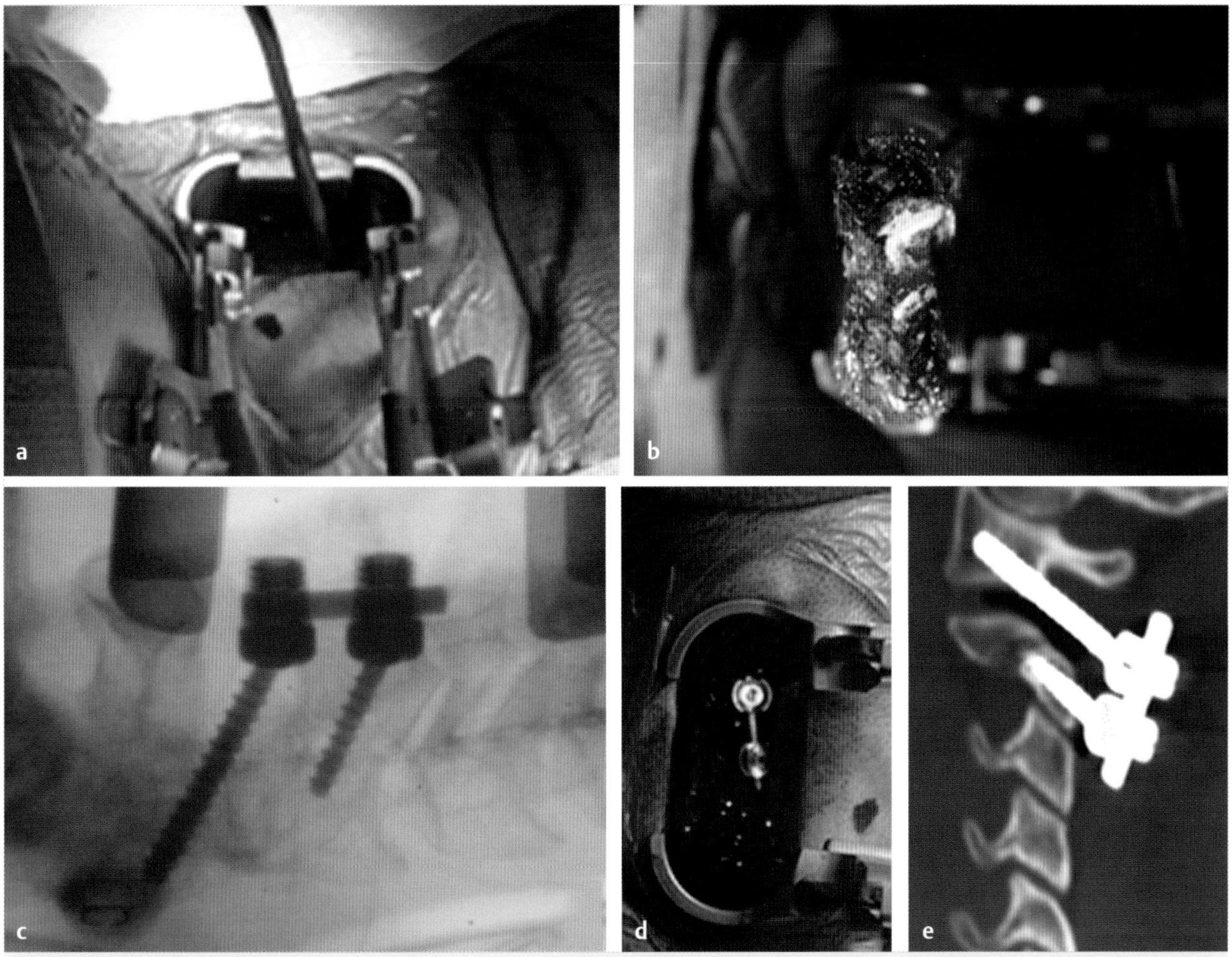

Fig. 13.2 Intraoperative photographs show placement of (a) expandable tubular retractor allowing exposure of (b) C1–C3 posterior spinal elements. (c) C1 lateral mass and C2 pedicle screws are placed through the retractor using standard starting points, trajectories, and fluoroscopic guidance. (d) The screws are secured to a rod, and (e) appropriate hardware placement is confirmed on postoperative imaging.

direct visualization (i.e., a Penfield or blunt nerve hook on the superomedial boarder of the C2 pedicle). If necessary, sublaminar wiring under the atlas can aid in the reduction of an anteriorly displaced dens fragment. A variety of C1–C2 wiring constructs or C2 translaminar screws can also be utilized if one of the originally selected fixation points becomes compromised intraoperatively. Decortication of the C1–C2 facets and, in selected cases, the posterior arch of C1 and C2 lamina provides adequate surface area for bony fusion. Copious irrigation of the wound, interval removal of the retractors, use of vancomycin powder in the wound bed, and meticulous closure all contribute to minimizing risk of surgical site infection.

13.8 Discussion of Minimally Invasive Surgery

Posterior segmental instrumentation may be placed throughout the spine using percutaneous or tubular retractor–based techniques. Atlantoaxial fixation may be achieved using C1 lateral mass and C2 pedicle/pars screws placed through tubular retractors. Subaxial cervical stabilization may performed using lateral mass screws through tubular retractors or using percutaneous

transfacet screws. Cervical pedicle screws may also be placed percutaneously. For thoracic and lumbar posterior stabilization, percutaneous pedicle screws may be placed using standard AP–lateral fluoroscopy or computer-guided stereotactic navigation. Lumbar translaminar facet and transfacet-transpedicular screws can be placed percutaneously or with a small mini-open exposure. There are many single-cohort studies reporting the feasibility and safety of these techniques. Several retrospective studies assess the complications and outcomes of MIS approaches compared to open stabilization. There are few prospective studies comparing MIS and open techniques (▶ Table 13.1; ▶ Table 13.2; ▶ Table 13.3).

13.8.1 Level I Evidence in Minimally Invasive Atlantoaxial Stabilization

There are no level I studies available.

13.8.2 Level II Evidence in Minimally Invasive Atlantoaxial Stabilization

There are no level II studies available.

Table 13.1 Summary of data on MIS posterior cervical instrumentation

Study	Level	Treatment groups	Outcomes
Joseffer et al[1]	IV	1 patient undergoing C1–C2 fixation with tubular retractor	• No perioperative complications • Early fusion of C1–C2 joint by 3 mo
Taghva et al[2]	IV	2 patients undergoing C1–C2 fixation with tubular retractor	• No perioperative complications, no breaches on CT • Improvement in pain and fusion at 2 y
Holly et al[3]	IV	6 patients undergoing C1–C2 fixation with tubular retractor	• No hardware malposition in the 4 patients undergoing CT • Solid fusion occurred in all patients, no complications
Wei et al[4]	III	22 patients undergoing open C1–C2 fusion, 22 undergoing MIS C1–C2 fusion	• No difference in screw accuracy • All cases achieved bony fusion, no hardware loosening • Similar JOA scores at last follow-up
Ahmad et al[5]	IV	3 patients undergoing percutaneous transfacet fixation following anterior fusion	• Demonstrated technical feasibility • No comparison group or long-term follow-up
Miyanji et al[6]	IV	Biomechanical study comparing transfacet vs. lateral mass fixation, 8 in each group	• Both groups had similar stability in flexion/extension, lateral bending, and axial torsion
Lee et al[7]	IV	Biomechanical study comparing transfacet vs. lateral mass fixation after multilevel corpectomy, 16 specimens	• Transfacet screw constructs had increased mobility and were associated with increased graft loading
Mikhael et al[8]	IV	Technical report describing lateral mass fixation using tubular retractors	• No report of complications, fusion rate, or outcomes
Fong and Duplessis[9]	IV	2 trauma patients undergoing lateral mass fixation with tubular retractors	• No reported complications but limited follow-up
Wang and Levi[10]	IV	18 patients undergoing lateral mass fixation with tubular retractor	• No bony violations on postop CT • Successful fusion in all cases
Schaefer et al[11]	IV	72 percutaneous cervical pedicle screws in 15 patients	• 76% placed without pedicle violations, no revision required • No long-term outcome or comparison group

Abbreviations: CT, computed tomography; JOA, Japanese Orthopaedic Association; MIS, minimally invasive surgery.

Table 13.2 Summary of data on percutaneous thoracolumbar pedicle screws

Study	Level	Treatment groups	Outcomes
Jiang et al[12]	I	31 percutaneous vs. 30 open pedicle screw patients with burst fractures	• Less blood loss, hospital stay in percutaneous group • No difference in screw accuracy or complications • Percutaneous group had better pain control and function at 3 mo, but no difference in long-term outcome
Li et al[13]	II	33 patients divided into percutaneous and open pedicle screw groups	• Less paraspinal muscle injury on EMG/CT in percutaneous group, mostly in the short term
King[14]	II	11 open vs. 8 percutaneous pedicle screw patients	• Lower blood loss and postoperative pain in percutaneous patients • Multifidus muscle cross-sectional area decreased post-op in open but not percutaneous group
Grossbach et al[15]	II	27 open vs. 11 percutaneous pedicle screw patients with flexion-distraction injury	• Shorter OR time and lower blood loss in percutaneous patients • No difference in complication rates • Limited follow-up period
Huang et al[16]	II	30 open vs. 30 percutaneous pedicle screw patients with burst fractures	• Percutaneous group had lower blood loss, length of stay • Percutaneous group had less pain at 3 mo • No difference in pain, disability, alignment at last follow-up (mean 2 y)
Yang et al[17]	II	Percutaneous pedicle screw fixation with computer-assisted navigation (42 patients) vs. conventional fluoroscopy (34 patients)	• Surgery faster and fewer pedicle breaches (3.0 vs. 7.2%) in guidance group
Lee et al[18]	III	27 open vs. 32 percutaneous pedicle screw patients with burst fractures	• Blood loss and operative time lower in percutaneous group • Percutaneous group had lower pain at 3 and 6 mo • No difference in alignment or clinical outcome at last follow-up
Kotani et al[19]	III	37 open vs. 43 percutaneous pedicle screw patients undergoing single-level fusion for degenerative disease	• Percutaneous group had lower blood loss and post-op pain • Disability scores were superior in percutaneous group as late as 24 mo post-op • No complications of screw placement, fusion rates equivalent

Table 13.2 (*continued*)

Study	Level	Treatment groups	Outcomes
Mobbs and Raley[20]	IV	Assessment for anterior breach with K-wire during placement of 525 percutaneous screws	• 7 cases of anterior breach with K-wire • 2 cases of retroperitoneal hematoma with ileus • No need for transfusion or surgical intervention
Jones-Quaidoo et al[21]	III	66 open vs. 66 percutaneous pedicle screw patients	• Higher percentage of percutaneous screws violated superior facet (6 vs. 13.6%)
Babu et al[22]	III	126 open vs. 153 percutaneous lumbar degenerative cases	• Superior facet violation more common in percutaneous patients
Yson et al[23]	III	245 open vs. 125 percutaneous screws placed with O-arm	• Superior facet violation more common in open group (26.5 vs. 4%)
Oh et al[24]	III	126 open vs. 111 percutaneous patients	• Incidence and severity of pedicle perforation similar between the two groups
Lau et al[25]	III	140 open vs. 142 percutaneous TLIFs	• No difference in rate of superior facet violation •
Houten et al[26]	III	141 percutaneous screws with standard fluoroscopy vs. 205 with O-arm	• Lower rate of pedicle perforation in navigated group (12.8 vs. 3%)
Fraser et al[27]	III	13 patients receiving percutaneous screws with standard fluoroscopy vs. 29 with navigation	• Lower rate of pedicle perforation in navigated group
Nakashima et al[28]	III	150 percutaneous screws with standard fluoroscopy vs. 150 with Iso-C	• Lower rate of pedicle perforation in navigated group (15.3 vs. 7.3%)

Abbreviations: CT, computed tomography; EMG, electromyogram; OR, operative; TLIF, tranforaminal lumbar interbody fusion.

Table 13.3 Summary of data on lumbar translaminar facet and transfacet screws

Study	Level	Treatment groups	Outcomes
Tuli et al[29]	II	40 translaminar facet vs. 37 open pedicle screw patients with degenerative disease	• Translaminar facet group had shorter length of stay and fewer perioperative complications • Translaminar facet group had greater need for reoperation for nonunion (7 of 40 vs. 1 of 37)
Hou et al[30]	IV	12 cadaveric specimens with two-level ALIF plus pedicle or translaminar facet screws	• Biomechanical strength similar in all types of motion tested
Burton et al[31]	IV	10 cadaveric specimens with interbody device plus pedicle or translaminar facet screws	• Biomechanical strength similar in all types of motion tested
Wang et al[32]	IV	Cadaveric specimens with two-level ALIF and either pedicle screws, translaminar facet screws, or transfacet screws	• Pedicle screw constructs more rigid than translaminar facet constructs, which were more rigid than transfacet constructs
Agarwala et al[33]	IV	2 groups of 7 cadaveric specimens instrumented with pedicle or transfacet screws	• Transfacet screws similar to pedicle screws in flexion–extension but weaker in lateral bending and rotation • Differences minimized when anterior instrumentation included
Amoretti et al[34]	IV	182 transfacet and 56 translaminar facet screws in patients undergoing ALIF	• No complications of screw placement • One translaminar facet screw failure, but radiographic fusion occurred in all patients at 1 y
Shim et al[35]	IV	20 patients undergoing translaminar facet fixation with ALIF	• One superior facet fracture from K-wire drilling • Fusion occurred in all patients
Aepli et al[36]	IV	476 patients undergoing translaminar facet fixation	• < 1% rate of screw breakage or loosening at average 10-y follow-up
Best and Sasso[37]	III	43 translaminar facet vs. 24 pedicle screw patients undergoing circumferential fusion	• Translaminar facet group had less blood loss and OR time • The two groups had similar outcomes at 2 y post-op • Reoperation more common in pedicle screw group
Jang and Lee[38]	III	44 facet screw vs. 40 pedicle screw patients undergoing ALIF	• No significant difference in disability index or fusion rates (average 2-y follow-up)

Abbreviations: ALIF, anterior lumbar interbody fusion; OR, operative.

13.8.3 Level III and IV Evidence in Minimally Invasive Atlantoaxial Stabilization

Joseffer et al[1] demonstrated that atlantoaxial fixation was technically feasible using a tubular retractor–based approach. C1 lateral mass and C2 pedicle screws were placed in one patient without complication, and early fusion was evident by 3 months. Taghva et al[2] reported two patients undergoing C1 lateral mass and C2 pedicle screw placement with expandable tubular retractors. Neither patient had any complication from surgery, and no breaches were noted on postoperative CT. Both patients had significant improvement in pain scores and had good fusion at 2-year follow-up. The advantages of this approach over open atlantoaxial fixation include preservation of the posterior tension band, less blood loss, and less postoperative pain.

Holly et al[3] reported six patients undergoing C1–C2 fusion using tubular retractors (five for type II dens fractures, one for os odontoideum). No patients suffered any complication, and solid fusion occurred in all patients (average follow-up time: 32 months). There was no hardware malposition found in the four of six patients undergoing postoperative CT. The authors noted that the techniques for placing instrumentation (entry points, trajectories) and the method of obtaining fusion do not substantially differ between open and tubular retractor techniques. As such, the long-term results would be expected to be similar, although the study did not have a comparison group of open patients.

Wei at el[4] performed a comparison study of MIS versus open C1–C2 fusion, with 22 atlantoaxial instability patients undergoing an MIS endoscopic approach and 22 undergoing open treatment. The two groups were similar in baseline characteristics, but the MIS group had lower blood loss, operation time, and incision length. There was no difference in foramen transversarium violation between the two groups. The patients were followed for a mean 25 months, and bony fusion without screw loosening or breakage was achieved in all cases. There was no significant difference in JOA (Japanese Orthopaedic Association) scores between the two groups at last follow-up. The authors concluded that MIS atlantoaxial fusion is equally effective as an open approach, with no increased risk of complications and less soft-tissue injury.

13.8.4 Level I Evidence in Minimally Invasive Subaxial Cervical Stabilization

There are no level I studies available.

13.8.5 Level II Evidence in Minimally Invasive Subaxial Cervical Stabilization

There are no level II studies available.

13.8.6 Level III and IV Evidence in Minimally Invasive Subaxial Cervical Stabilization

Percutaneous screws can be placed through the facet joints of the cervical spine to achieve stabilization without rod placement. Ahmad et al[5] reported three patients undergoing percutaneous cervical transfacet fixation without complication following multilevel anterior fusion. This study had no comparison group or long-term follow-up, and the authors noted that this technique is limited to supporting an anterior fusion until percutaneous bony fusion methods are developed. Miyanji et al[6] did a biomechanical study of human cervical spines, comparing transfacet versus lateral mass fixation ($n = 8$ in each group) in flexion/extension, lateral bending, and axial torsion. The transfacet group (with or without connecting rods) had similar biomechanical stability compared to the lateral mass group. On the other hand, some biomechanical data suggest that facet screws provide inferior stabilization once the spine has been destabilized by corpectomy. Lee et al[7] assessed the strength of transfacet versus lateral mass fixation following multilevel corpectomy. Corpectomy was performed in 16 cadaver cervical spines randomized to lateral mass or transfacet screw constructs. Transfacet screws were found to provide inferior spinal immobilization and were associated with increased graft loading.

Subaxial lateral mass screws may also be placed with MIS technique. Mikhael et al[8] wrote a technique article describing lateral mass screw placement through tubular retractors. There is no report of complications, fusion rate, or patient outcomes. Fong and Duplessis[9] described the feasibility of a tubular retractor system to achieve lateral mass fixation in two trauma patients. There were no reported complications. However, the screws were placed to supplement an anterior fusion, and no long-term follow-up was reported. Wang and Levi[10] reviewed 18 patients treated with lateral mass fixation using a tubular retractor. Postoperative CT showed no bony violations except for screws with bicortical purchase. All cases achieved fusion.

Pedicle screws may be inserted into the subaxial cervical spine using open or percutaneous approaches. Schaefer et al[11] demonstrated the feasibility of percutaneous cervical pedicle screw placement but revealed its limited accuracy. In total, 72 percutaneous cervical pedicle screws were placed, but only 76% had no bony violation on postoperative imaging. Still, there were no complications of posterior instrumentation, and no screw revision was required. There was no comparison to open pedicle screw placement.

13.8.7 Level I Evidence in Minimally Invasive Thoracolumbar Pedicle Screw Fixation

Jiang et al[12] performed a randomized controlled trial comparing percutaneous pedicle screw fixation ($n = 31$) with an open paraspinal muscle-splitting approach ($n = 30$) in the management of neurologically intact patients with thoracolumbar burst fractures. The percutaneous group had significantly less blood loss, operative time, and length of hospital stay, as well as superior pain control and function at 3 months. No screws required revision, and there was no difference in complications between the two groups. On the other hand, open surgery was associated with superior correction of kyphosis and restoration of vertebral body height. There were no significant differences in long-term clinical outcome.

13.8.8 Level II Evidence in Minimally Invasive Thoracolumbar Pedicle Screw Fixation

Studies of paraspinal muscle anatomy and function have demonstrated less muscle injury with percutaneous compared to open techniques. Li et al[13] assessed paraspinal muscle injury via electromyogram (EMG) and CT among 33 patients divided into percutaneous and open pedicle screw groups. Both procedures caused damage to paraspinal muscle, but less muscle injury was noted in the percutaneous group, mostly in the short term. King[14] prospectively followed 19 pedicle screw patients (11 open, 8 percutaneous) for a mean 21 months, assessing trunk extension strength and multifidus muscle cross-sectional area on axial imaging. The percutaneous patients had lower blood loss, less postoperative pain, and superior trunk extension strength (although the latter was not statistically significant). Postoperative versus preoperative multifidus muscle cross-sectional area significantly decreased in the open group ($p = 0.003$) but not in the percutaneous group ($p > 0.05$).

Grossbach et al[15] prospectively followed 38 patients undergoing surgery for flexion-distraction injury (27 with open pedicle screws, 11 with percutaneous screws). There was no significant difference in presenting ASIA (American Spinal Injury Association) scores or alignment. The MIS group had a shorter operative time and lower blood loss. There was no difference in perioperative complications between the groups. There were no cases of construct failure, although the follow-up period was short. In a similar report, Huang et al[16] compared percutaneous with traditional open pedicle screw fixation in neurologically intact patients with thoracolumbar burst fractures ($n = 30$ patients in each group). The percutaneous group had a significantly lower blood loss, length of hospital stay, and immediate postoperative pain (within 3 months of surgery). At last follow-up (average 2 years), there was no significant difference in kyphosis angle, vertebral height, pain as measured by VAS (visual analog scale), or disability as measured by ODI (Oswestry Disability Index).

Percutaneous pedicle screws are traditionally placed with AP–lateral fluoroscopy, but computer-assisted navigation techniques have also been developed. Yang et al[17] did a multicenter prospective study comparing 42 patients undergoing navigated percutaneous pedicle screw placement with 34 patients undergoing percutaneous screw placement with conventional fluoroscopic technique. Fluoroscopy time, time to place guidewire, and pedicle breach rate (3.0 vs. 7.2%) were superior in the guidance group. There was no comparison with open screw placement.

13.8.9 Level III and IV Evidence in Minimally Invasive Thoracolumbar Pedicle Screw Fixation

Several retrospective studies suggest that percutaneous pedicle screw fixation achieves similar long-term outcomes when compared to open screw placement, with less blood loss and postoperative pain and no increase in complications. Lee et al[18] compared 32 patients undergoing percutaneous fixation with

27 patients undergoing open fixation for thoracolumbar burst fractures. The percutaneous group had significantly less blood loss and operative time, as well as a significantly lower VAS score and superior LBOS (low back outcome score) at 3 and 6 months. At last follow-up, there was no significant difference in correction of kyphosis or clinical outcome. Kotani et al[19] did a retrospective review of 80 patients undergoing single-level posterolateral fusion for degenerative spondylolisthesis. Compared to open patients, the percutaneous group had significantly less blood loss and postoperative pain. The ODI and Roland–Morris Questionnaire (RMQ) scores were lower in the percutaneous group at 3, 6, 12, and 24 months postoperatively. The fusion rate was similar between the two groups (98 vs. 100%). There were no major complications of screw placement.

A few reports have associated percutaneous pedicle screw placement with certain complications. Mobbs and Raley[20] retrospectively assessed for anterior breaches with the K-wire during placement of 525 percutaneous screws. There were seven anterior breaches of the K-wire; two of these patients developed a retroperitoneal hematoma with ileus but neither required blood transfusion or surgical intervention. The authors concluded that the anterior breach with the K-wire is rare and generally of no long-term consequence, but surgeons must take care to avoid this event because catastrophic vascular or bowel injury are potential complications.

Another complication that some reports have associated with percutaneous pedicle screw fixation is violation of the adjacent unfused facet joint by the superior screw of the construct. Jones-Quaidoo et al[21] compared the incidence of superior facet disruption in 66 patients undergoing percutaneous fixation versus 66 undergoing open fixation. The percutaneous cohort was younger than the open group but otherwise well-matched. A significantly higher percentage of screws placed in the percutaneous group were in the facet joint compared to the open group (13.6 vs. 6%). Babu et al[22] also compared rates of superior facet violation during 126 open versus 153 percutaneous lumbar pedicle screw cases for degenerative disease. On postoperative CT, the percutaneous screws had a significantly higher rate of superior facet violation.

Other reports refute the claim that percutaneous pedicle screws are less accurate than open screws. Yson et al[23] compared the rate of superior facet violation among 245 open lumbar pedicle screws versus 125 percutaneous screws placed with three-dimensional CT-based guidance (O-arm). Facet violation by the cranial-most screws occurred significantly more frequently in the open group compared to the percutaneous group (26.5 vs. 4%). Oh et al[24] also did a retrospective cohort study assessing the accuracy of percutaneous versus open pedicle screw fixation in lumbosacral fusion (126 open patients, 111 percutaneous patients). Postoperative CTs were reviewed to assess the incidence and severity of breach. The incidence and severity of pedicle perforation were not significantly different between the two groups. Lau et al[25] compared the incidence of superior facet violation in percutaneous (142 patients) versus open (140 patients) pedicle screw placement during transforaminal lumbar interbody fusion. The rate of superior facet violation was similar in both groups.

There is some evidence that accuracy of percutaneous pedicle screws can be improved when intraoperative computer-based navigation is used instead of conventional fluoroscopic technique. Houten et al[26] retrospectively compared 141 percutaneous screws placed using standard fluoroscopic technique with 205 screws placed using O-arm computer-based navigation. The rate of pedicle perforation was 12.8% in the fluoroscopy group versus 3% in the O-arm group ($p < 0.001$). Screw placement was also faster in the O-arm group. Fraser et al[27] compared 29 patients undergoing percutaneous screw placement using three-dimensional navigation, with 13 undergoing screw placement using standard fluoroscopy. There was a significantly lower rate of pedicle perforation ($p = 0.04$) in the navigated group. Nakashima et al[28] retrospectively assessed percutaneous screw accuracy with conventional fluoroscopic technique ($n = 150$) versus three-dimensional fluoroscopy-based image guidance (Iso-C) ($n = 150$). On postoperative CT, 7.3% of the screws placed with Iso-C were outside the pedicle in comparison to 15.3% placed with fluoroscopy alone ($p < 0.05$).

13.8.10 Level I Evidence in Minimally Invasive Lumbar Translaminar Facet/Transfacet Fixation

There are no level I studies available.

13.8.11 Level II Evidence in Minimally Invasive Lumbar Translaminar Facet/Transfacet Fixation

Tuli et al[29] did a prospective cohort study comparing long-term outcomes in patients treated with translaminar facet screw fixation ($n = 40$) versus open pedicle screw fixation ($n = 37$) for degenerative lumbar disease. The translaminar facet screw group had a shorter length of stay, blood loss, and fewer perioperative complications. Nevertheless, facet screw patients had a greater need for reoperation for nonunion (7 of 40 vs. 1 of 37).

13.8.12 Level III and IV Evidence in Minimally Invasive Lumbar Translaminar Facet/Transfacet Fixation

Biomechanical studies suggest that translaminar facet fixation provides comparable strength to pedicle screw fixation following interbody fusion. Hou et al[30] compared the stiffness of translaminar facet versus pedicle screw constructs following two-level anterior lumbar interbody fusion (ALIF). A two-level ALIF was performed in 12 fresh human lumbar spines followed by placement of either pedicle screws or translaminar facet screws. There was no significant difference in stiffness during flexion, extension, lateral bending, or rotation. Burton et al[31] also compared translaminar facet versus pedicle screw fixation in 10 cadaveric specimens with an interbody graft. Translaminar facet screw fixation was equivalent to bilateral pedicle screw placement in compressive loading, flexion–extension, lateral bending, and axial torque.

Transfacet screw constructs have been shown to provide some degree of stabilization but are not as rigid as pedicle screw constructs. Wang et al[32] performed flexibility testing in fresh-frozen calf spines following two-level ALIF with either pedicle screws, translaminar facet screws, or transfacet screws. In lateral bending, pedicle and translaminar facet screw constructs had similar strength and were superior to transfacet screw constructs. In extension, pedicle screw constructs were more rigid than the other two. These results suggest that pedicle screws provide stronger fixation than translaminar facet screws, which in turn provide stronger fixation than transfacet screws. Similarly, Agarwala et al[33] studied two groups of seven human cadaver spines instrumented with either pedicle screws or transfacet screws, and examined strength in primary and circumferential fixation. Transfacet screws provided similar fixation in flexion–extension but inferior stiffness in lateral bending and rotation. These differences were minimized when anterior instrumentation was included.

While not providing the three-column fixation of pedicle screws, several studies have shown that translaminar facet screws and transfacet screws provide sufficient immobilization to facilitate successful ALIF. Amoretti et al[34] retrospectively assessed 182 percutaneous transfacet and 56 translaminar facet screws. All were placed with fluoroscopic guidance with one attempt following ALIF. Radiographic fusion occurred within 1 year in all patients despite one translaminar facet screw failure. Shim et al[35] reviewed 20 patients undergoing placement of 65 percutaneous translaminar facet screws with a mean follow-up time of 19.5 months. Eleven percent of the screws violated the laminar walls on postoperative imaging but none were neurologically symptomatic. There was one case of superior facet fracture from K-wire drilling. However, facet fixation was achieved in all levels, and fusion occurred in all treated levels. Aepli et al[36] demonstrated that translaminar facet screws are durable implants, with < 1% rate of screw breakage or loosening among 476 patients with average 10-year follow-up.

Retrospective comparative studies have demonstrated that both translaminar facet and transfacet fixation compare favorably to pedicle screw fixation in supporting ALIF. Best and Sasso[37] retrospectively compared 24 patients undergoing pedicle screw fixation with 43 undergoing translaminar facet fixation to support interbody fusion for discogenic back pain. The translaminar facet screw group had significantly less blood loss and operative time. At 2 years after surgery, the two groups had similar outcomes as measured by VAS. Reoperation was in fact more common in the pedicle screw group (37.5 vs. 4.7%, $p = 0.001$), although the study was likely subject to confounding variables. Similarly, Jang and Lee[38] retrospectively reviewed 44 patients undergoing percutaneous facet screw fixation and 40 undergoing pedicle screw fixation following ALIF. After 2 years of follow-up, there was no significant difference in ODI, and the fusion rates were similar (95.8 vs. 97.5%).

13.9 Complications in Minimally Invasive Surgery

Postoperative pain and delayed mobilization are frequent complications of spine surgery, but these issues appear to be less problematic with MIS compared to open thoracolumbar pedicle screw placement (level I evidence). Level II and III studies suggest the same for other types of MIS posterior instrumentation. Anatomic and functional studies have demonstrated less paraspinal muscle injury with MIS versus open screw placement (level II evidence). MIS posterior instrumentation may be placed with a high rate of screw accuracy comparable to open screw placement, with few procedural complications and a high rate of eventful fusion (level III evidence for atlantoaxial fixation, level IV for subaxial cervical lateral mass fixation, level I and II for thoracolumbar transpedicular fixation, level III for translaminar facet and transfacet fixation). Still, more prospective comparative studies are needed to assess the accuracy and efficacy of all types of MIS posterior instrumentation in comparison to the open gold standard.

There are limited data to support the efficacy of percutaneous cervical transfacet screws or the safety of percutaneous cervical pedicle screws. Biomechanical data suggest that cervical transfacet screws provide inferior immobilization compared to lateral mass screws following multilevel corpectomy. Still, they have been used successfully in a few patients. More clinical studies with long-term follow-up and control groups are required to assess the efficacy of cervical transfacet fixation with regard to maintenance of alignment and fusion rate. Similarly, there are limited data to support routine placement of percutaneous subaxial cervical pedicle screws. The accuracy of this technique has been reported to be only 76% in skilled hands.[11] While no cases of screw revision were required in that study, the risk of vertebral artery or nerve root injury is not insignificant. The benefits of MIS subaxial cervical pedicle screws are unclear given the existence of safer open and MIS fixation options, and the ability to combine these posterior techniques with anterior stabilization and fusion. Percutaneous cervical pedicle screw fixation should be performed only in select patient populations by surgeons with significant experience in this technique.

There are conflicting reports regarding percutaneous thoracolumbar pedicle screw accuracy, with some studies showing an increased rate of superior facet violation with the associated risk of adjacent segment disease. Other reports refute this finding and show equivalent or even superior screw accuracy with percutaneous screws, particularly when stereotactic navigation is utilized. The frequency of superior facet violation may be technique/surgeon dependent. Inserting the pedicle screw at the transverse process–facet junction (lateral starting point) rather than on the facet (medial starting point) may lower the risk of facet violation. More prospective multicenter studies assessing percutaneous versus open pedicle screws are needed to compare the rates of superior facet violation and the effect on adjacent level disease.

One complication of percutaneous pedicle screw placement is K-wire perforation beyond the anterior vertebral body, with the associated risk of vascular or bowel injury. A few cases of retroperitoneal hematoma and ileus have been reported. This risk can be minimized by surgeon attentiveness to the position of the K-wire at all times during pedicle cannulation.

Another potential complication of percutaneous screw placement is pseudarthrosis given that the posterior spinal elements are not exposed for decortication and graft placement. However, these screws are typically placed either to support an anterior fusion or promote healing of a vertebral body fracture. Several level II and III studies show similar rates of anterior fusion, maintenance of alignment, integrity of hardware, and long-term functional and pain outcomes with percutaneous versus open pedicle screw placement. Although lumbar

transfacet and translaminar facet screws provide less rigid fixation than pedicle screws, several level III studies show that this fixation is adequate to support anterior interbody fusion, with similar fusion rates and outcome indices when compared to pedicle screw fixation. Still, one level II study shows an increased rate of revision surgery when translaminar facet screws are used instead of pedicle screws for circumferential fusion. More long-term prospective studies are needed to compare the fusion rates and clinical outcomes from MIS versus open posterior instrumentation.

13.10 Conclusion of Minimally Invasive Surgery

Several reports suggest that MIS posterior instrumentation can be placed accurately and safely, with a similar rate of eventful fusion compared to open approaches. However, the number of studies addressing these issues is limited, and the quality of data is mixed (level I and II for thoracolumbar pedicle screws, level III for translaminar facet and transfacet screws, level III for atlantoaxial fixation, level IV for subaxial cervical lateral mass screws). Some level III studies suggest an increased incidence of superior facet violation with percutaneous lumbar pedicle screws. However, other studies show similar rates of facet violation, or even less violation with percutaneous screws. Use of computer-aided navigation may improve MIS screw accuracy compared to conventional fluoroscopic technique. Knowledge of proper technique and vigilance to patient anatomy may help prevent complications that have been associated with MIS screw placement (e.g., K-wire perforation into the retroperitoneum, superior facet violation). Lumbar translaminar facet and transfacet screws provide less rigid stabilization compared to pedicle screws, but level III studies suggest that this rigidity is adequate to promote anterior fusion. There is less evidence to support the safety of percutaneous cervical pedicle screws or the efficacy of cervical transfacet screws.

In conclusion, posterior instrumentation inserted using MIS techniques is associated with lower blood loss, less paraspinal muscle trauma, less immediate postoperative pain, and a shorter length of hospital stay compared to open approaches (level I evidence for thoracolumbar pedicle screws, level II for translaminar facet screws, level III for cervical screws). A Grade 1A can be made for thoracolumbar pedicle screw placement using MIS techniques, whereas a Grade 2C recommendation can be made for both MIS translaminar facet screws and cervical screws. More prospective studies are needed to assess the safety of all types of MIS posterior instrumentation in comparison to the open gold standard, both in the short term (screw accuracy, perioperative complications) and long term (ability to maintain alignment, support fusion, and avoid adjacent segment disease).

13.11 Discussion of Open Surgery

The minimally invasive techniques discussed above are virtually all recent modifications of the traditional open techniques for placement of rigid segmental instrumentation constructs that have widespread use. Despite long-standing and widespread use, most of these open techniques were not compared in prospective randomized controlled trials to the previous generation of less rigid spinal instrumentation constructs. The timeframes that saw their introduction and acceptance by the surgical community are now noted to be widely bereft of high-quality studies in the surgical sciences. Rigid cervical constructs such as C1 lateral mass–C2 pedicle/pars and subaxial lateral mass or pedicle screw constructs have obvious advantages over the previous generation of wiring constructs. These techniques have obviated the need for postoperative halo immobilization in the majority of cases. Therefore, despite the fact that most of the literature involving open cervical instrumentation techniques is level III and IV evidence, it would be difficult to justify conducting randomized controlled trials to compare this approach to earlier methods of cervical stabilization. Conversely, as minimally invasive techniques have only more recently been refined, the literature directly comparing these to the open counterparts is also sparse. The large body of lower level studies detailing the outcomes and complications of open posterior spinal instrumentation techniques, however, provides valuable information for the clinician. A representative overview is presented below.

13.11.1 Level I Evidence in Open Atlantoaxial Stabilization

There are no level I studies available.

13.11.2 Level II Evidence in Open Atlantoaxial Stabilization

There are no level II studies available.

13.11.3 Level III and IV Evidence in Open Atlantoaxial Stabilization

There are a fair number of level III and IV studies which report the results of patients undergoing open atlantoaxial stabilization, and a representative sample is presented in ▶ Table 13.4.[4,39,40,41,42,43,44,45,46,47,48,49,50,51,52,53,54] The only direct comparison between open and MIS C1–C2 stabilization is by Wei et al.[4] As presented above, the MIS group had lower blood loss, operation time, and incision length. From the information available to review, it is unclear whether these differences were clinically meaningful. There were no differences in rates of suboptimal screw placement, JOA scores, fusion rates, or late implant problems. This information is reassuring that C1–C2 stabilization appears to have similar rates of success and complications as the open approach, but the sample size of 22 patients in each group leaves open the possibility of a type II error in such an assumption.

Prior to advancements in understanding the anatomy of the C1 lateral mass to permit direct posterior access for screw placement, C1–C2 TAS fixation was the technique most widely utilized to obtain rigid fixation across this motion segment. Lee and colleagues performed a retrospective comparison of patients treated with posterior C1–C2 TAS fixation versus those treated with C1 lateral mass–C2 pedicle screw fixation by open techniques.[39] Twenty-eight patients were in the C1–C2 transar-

ticular group (group 1) and 27 patients in the C1 lateral mass–C2 pedicle screw group (group 2), with follow-up out to 24 months. The patients in group 2 had a fusion rate of 96% compared with 82% in group 1. One patient treated with open C1 lateral mass–C2 pedicle screw construct developed hardware failure with pseudarthrosis. One patient in this group also sustained a vertebral artery injury (VAI) during the dissection. Ninety-six percent of patients in this group reported no neck pain at final follow-up. All of these parameters compared favorably to the open C1–C2 transarticular comparison group.

The main body of literature on open C1–C2 stabilization consists essentially of uncontrolled case reports of various sizes. Several of these also include cases involving longer constructs than just C1–C2, and the relevant events are not necessarily stratified according to construct length. As such, comparing these series to the published case series on MIS atlantoaxial fusion has important limitations, which are not discussed here. The first report on the technique of C1 lateral mass screws was published by Goel and Laheri in 1994.[55] Their technique involved sectioning the C2 nerve root to facilitate placement of the screw in the midportion of the C1 lateral mass (near the C1–C2 joint) through a rigid plate combined with a C2 pedicle screw. In 2002, Goel et al published a larger series utilizing this technique in 160 patients.[40] They reported no vascular or infectious complications. They offered a 100% fusion rate based on flexion–extension radiographs, although one patient was found to have a broken screw at 18 months. They did not routinely perform CT scanning postoperatively, citing anticipated metal artifact. Eighteen patients reported sensory loss in the distribution of the C2 nerve root.

Harms and Melcher reported their modifications to this technique in 2001.[41] Rather than sectioning the C2 nerve root, they retracted it caudally and utilized polyaxial screws at C1 and C2 connected by a top-loading rod. They reported on 37 patients undergoing this procedure, with 3 patients not reaching 6-month follow-up and the remainder followed from 6 months to over 2 years. They reported no instances of dural laceration or VAI. One patient experienced a deep wound infection. They felt screw placement was satisfactory in all patients, although they did not comment on the use of postoperative CT imaging. All patients were deemed fused at final follow-up using radiographic criteria. They reported that no instances of occipital neuralgia were observed, and felt that the use of a screw with an unthreaded upper portion at C1 helped avoid irritation of the nearby C2 nerve root. Toward this goal, others reported variation of the C1 starting point partially or completely through the C1 posterior arch.[56,57] Since this time, the literature has featured debate regarding the merits and shortcomings of these variations.

Since minimally invasive stabilization at C1–C2 is typically done through expandable tubular retractors, routine sectioning of the C2 nerve root and a starting point below the posterior arch may have technical advantages. Examining such variations in the larger body of open C1–C2 surgical literature may therefore help anticipate how similar techniques used in MIS approach will fare in expanded use. One of the co-authors of the present chapter (A. K. F.-B.) recently conducted extensive meta-analyses to evaluate the biomechanical impact of the starting point of the C1 lateral mass screws and the impact of the C2 nerve status on the safety and accuracy of their

Table 13.4 Summary of representative data on open C1–C2 fusion (screw–rod constructs)

Study	Level	Treatment groups	Outcomes
Wei et al[4]	III	22 patients undergoing open C1–C2 fusion, 22 undergoing MIS C1–C2 fusion	• No difference in screw accuracy • All cases achieved bony fusion, no hardware loosening • Similar JOA scores at last follow-up
Lee et al[39]	III	27 patients undergoing C1–C2 fusion w/ SRC compared to 28 patients undergoing C1–C2 TAS	• SRC had 96% fusion • 1 pseudarthrosis/implant failure • 1 VAI
Goel et al[40]	IV	160 patients open C1–C2 by screw-plate construct	• 100% fusion by X-ray • No VAI, infections, or misplaced screws
Harms and Melcher[41]	IV	37 patients open C1–C2	• 100% fusion • Infection rate 2.7% • No VAI or misplaced screws
Chen et al[42]	IV	11 patients open C1–C2	• 100% fusion • No VAI, misplaced screws, or infections
El Masry et al[43]	IV	13 patients open C1–C2	• 100% fusion • No VAI, misplaced screws, or infections
Stulik et al[44]	IV	28 patients open C1–C2	• 100% fusion • Infections rate 3.6% • No VAI or misplaced screws
Li et al[45]	IV	23 patients open C1–C2	• 100% fusion • No VAI, misplaced screws, or infections
De Iure et al[46]	IV	13 patients open C1–C2	• 92.3% fusion • No VAI, misplaced screws, or infections
Payer et al[47]	IV	12 patients open C1–C2	• 91.7% fusion • No VAI, misplaced screws, or infections
Simsek et al[48]	IV	17 patients open C1–C2	• 100% fusion • Infection rate 5.9% • No VAI or misplaced screws
Pan et al[49]	IV	48 patients open C1–C2	• 100% fusion • No VAI, misplaced screws, or infections
Squires and Molinari[50]	IV	23 patients open C1–C2	• 100% fusion • No VAI, misplaced screws, or infections
Thomas et al[51]	IV	26 patients open C1–C2	• 100% fusion • No VAI, misplaced screws, or infections
Wang et al[52]	IV	319 patients open C1–C2	• 100% fusion • Infection rate 0.6% • No VAI or misplaced screws
Hamilton et al[53]	IV	44 patients open C1–C2	• 96.7% fusion • No VAI, misplaced screws, or infections
Kang et al[54]	IV	20 patients open C1–C2	• 100% fusion • Infection rate 10% • No VAI or misplaced screws

Abbreviations: JOA, Japanese Orthopaedic Association; MIS, minimally invasive surgery; SRC, screw–rod construct; VAI, vertebral artery injury.

placement.[58,59] Analyzing 34 studies that met their inclusion criteria, the authors were able to pool the results of 1,247 patients that underwent open C1–C2 fusion with a Goel–Harms technique. Variations in the starting point, including entry through the posterior arch of C1, did not demonstrate significant effect on the rate of successful arthrodesis. Regarding analysis of starting point and the C2 nerve status on the rates of screw malposition, VAI, and neurologic injury, 41 Class III studies involving 1,471 patients were analyzed. Three vertebral artery injuries were reported (0.1%). Five instances of clinically important screw malpositions were reported (0.2%). There were an additional 45 screws (1.6%) that were deemed malpositioned on postoperative imaging but were without clinical consequence. Upon meta-analysis, sacrifice of the C2 nerve root

was found to cause greater postoperative numbness but less neuralgia and fewer screw malpositions. When comparing posterior arch screws and those starting below the arch with C2 nerve preservation, the rates of screw malpositions and VAI were similar, but the latter had greater numbness and pain.

Another recent meta-analysis compared outcomes of patients treated with TASs and Goel–Harms type constructs for posterior atlantoaxial fusion.[60] This study searched online databases for English language articles on the subject from 1986 through 2011. Patients treated with either plates or polyaxial screws were considered together as the "screw–rod construct" (SRC) group. Twenty-four studies encompassing 1,073 patients fulfilled the inclusion criteria for the SRC group. All of the included studies were deemed level III evidence. The incidence of VAI in the SRC group was 2.0%, which was significantly less than the rate for TAS (4.1%). The incidence of malpositioned screws in the SRC group was 2.4%, which was also significantly lower than the TAS group (7.1%). The rate of fusion for the SRC was 97.5%, also significantly better than the TAS group (94.6%). The presence or absence of postoperative infection was documented for 92% of the patient cohort and amounted to an aggregate risk of 1% (range, 0–10%). Data concerning estimated blood loss (EBL) was only reported in 22% of SRC patients, with mean EBL calculated as 364 mL. Operative duration was only reported for 23% of the patients, with average duration calculated as 128 minutes. The authors acknowledged limitations such as lack of uniform imaging metrics to assess screw position or arthrodesis. In addition, differences in the grafting technique (autograft, allograft, structural/morselized, and the use of bone morphogenetic protein) may have impacted fusion outcomes. Despite these shortcomings, such meta-analyses generate large enough cohorts to give reasonable estimates as to the safety and efficacy of open C1–C2 fusion.

13.11.4 Level I Evidence in Open Subaxial Cervical Stabilization

There are no level I studies available.

13.11.5 Level II Evidence in Open Subaxial Cervical Stabilization

There are no level II studies available.

13.11.6 Level III and IV Evidence in Open Subaxial Cervical Stabilization

Several studies have reported implant-related complications in posterior open subaxial stabilization procedures and these are summarized in ▶ Table 13.5.[10,61,62,63,64,65,66,67,68,69,70,71,72,73] Roy-Camille et al first described the technique of posterior cervical fixation with lateral mass screws in 1979.[74] Since that time,

Table 13.5 Summary of representative studies detailing complications of open subaxial lateral mass fixation

Study	Level	Treatment groups	Outcomes/complications
Heller et al[61]	IV	78 patients, 654 screws with lateral mass plates	• 4 screws in 4 patients required revision due to nerve root injury • 4 late revisions due to pseudarthroses or screw/plate failure
Fehlings et al[62]	IV	44 patients, 210 screws	• No nerve root injury or early revisions • 3 patients required late revision due to pseudarthroses
Graham et al[63]	IV	21 patients, 164 screws	• 4 screws in 3 patients required revision due to nerve root injury • No pseudarthroses or late revisions required
Wellman et al[64]	IV	43 patients, 259 screws	• No nerve root injuries or early revisions • 1 late revision for pseudarthrosis
Sekhon[65]	IV	143 patients, 1,026 screws	• 8 facet joint violations, no nerve root injuries or early revisions • 6 late screw pullouts, 4 screw breakages, 1 plate breakage • 1 late reoperation for adjacent segment disease
Pateder and Carbone[66]	IV	29 patients, 198 screws	• 1 patient with late screw breakage and loss of reduction
Wang and Levi[10]	IV	18 patients, 77 screws	• No nerve root injuries or early revisions • No late implant complications or pseudarthroses
Roche et al[67]	IV	29 patients, 203 screws	• No nerve root injuries • 3 screw loosened, 3 dislodged, no late reoperations
Wu et al[68]	IV	115 patients, 673 screws	• No nerve root injuries or early revisions • 1 late screw pullout but no reoperations required
Stevens et al[69]	IV	34 patients, 267 screws	• 3 early reoperations due to wound infection • 3 late reoperations, 1 dislodged rod, 2 persistent pain
Katonis et al[70]	IV	225 patients, 1,662 screws, all evaluated by CT	• 3 screws in 3 patients required revision due to nerve root injury • 27 screws caused fracture of the involved lateral mass • 9 patients required late reoperation due to pseudarthrosis and late screw pullout
Audat et al[71]	IV	50 patients, 405 screws	• No nerve root injuries • 4 screw violated facet joint, 1 required revision • No late reoperations for implant complications or pseudarthroses
Inoue et al[72]	IV	94 patients, 457 screws, all evaluated by CT	• 9.6% screws contacted or breached transverse foramen • 2.8% screws violated facet joint • No VAI or nerve root injuries due to screw malpositioning
Kim et al[73]	IV	39 patients, 178 screws	• No nerve root injuries • 9% facet violations • No late reoperations for pseudarthroses

Abbreviations: CT, computed tomography; VAI, vertebral artery injury.

minor variations in the starting point and screw trajectories have been described by many authors. Earlier use of plates has been largely supplanted by the use of polyaxial screw–rod systems. Polyaxial screw–rod systems can better accommodate variable morphology of the lateral masses, permitting optimized screw position for each segment. Katonis and colleagues published a retrospective consecutive case series of 225 patients undergoing posterior cervical fixation with either screw-plate or polyaxial screw–rod constructs from 1999 to 2007, amounting to a total of 1,662 screws.[70] Screw position was evaluated by postoperative CT in all patients. Fracture of the lateral mass occurred during placement of 27 screws (1.6%). Using bicortical screws, three patients (1.3%) reported postoperative radiculopathy necessitating screw removal. Screw pullout occurred in three elderly patients (1.3%). The overall fusion rate was 97.4%. Two patients developed clinically significant wound hematoma requiring evacuation. No cases of VAI or wound infection were identified.

Wound-related issues aside, screw positioning is a leading factor contributing to complications. As lateral fluoroscopic imaging may be challenging in many patients in the mid and lower subaxial region, many surgeons utilize anatomic landmarks to guide screw trajectory. Inoue et al[72] recently published a large retrospective study examining the rate of screw-related complications with their technique of free-hand lateral mass screw placement. A total of 457 lateral mass screws in 94 patients were analyzed with postoperative CT. The authors utilized a modified Magerl technique with a starting point 1 mm medial to the midpoint of the lateral mass with a screw trajectory 30° laterally and superiorly (parallel to the facet joint). The superolateral quadrant was used as an "imaginary" target during drilling. Drilling was slowly advanced and bicortical screws were placed when feasible. The transverse foramen was contacted or breached by 9.6% of screws due to inadequate axial plane trajectory. The facet joint was violated by 2.8% of screws due to inappropriately low sagittal plane trajectories, most commonly at C6. None of these malpositioned screws resulted in vertebral artery or nerve root injury. Several other authors have published studies reporting use of anatomic landmarks for open screw placement, with malposition rates ranging from 0.3 to 9%.[67,69,73] The reported rates of clinically significant nerve root injury or radiculopathy attributable to screw malposition range from 0.6 to 1.4% of screws placed.

A recent meta-analysis examined screw-related complications with the use of lateral mass versus pedicle screws in the subaxial cervical spine.[75] Their literature search identified 28 eligible studies on lateral mass fixation, of which 18 studies were ultimately omitted due inclusion or exclusion criteria. One prospective and nine retrospective studies provided 766 patients in whom 5,328 screws were inserted from C3 to C7. The rate of each complication was calculated relative to the number of patients and screws involved. Perioperative complication rates were as follows: nerve root injury, 0.19% per screw and 1.36% per patient; SCI, 0% per screw and 0% per patient; VAI, 0% per screw and 0% per patient; fractures of the lateral mass, 1.62% per screw; facet violation, 0.62% per screw; and malposition requiring revision or removal, 0.38% per screw and 2.64% per patient. Late complication rates were calculated as screw loosening, 1.17% per screw; screw pullout 1.1% per patient; plate/rod breakage, 0.28% per patient; loss of reduction,

2.21% per patient; pseudarthrosis, 2.67% per patient; revision required, 2.81% per patient; and adjacent segment degeneration requiring surgery, 0.74% per patient. Upon comparison of these complication rates to those associated with subaxial cervical pedicle screws, the rates were similar uniformly. The distinct exception was the significantly higher rate of vertebral artery injuries (0.15% per screw and 0.61% per patient) associated with cervical pedicle screw placement.

While postoperative wound infection is a complication of open posterior subaxial instrumentation, many variables contribute to the risk of this occurrence. Infection rates are intuitively dependent on factors such as the magnitude of the surgery, including construct length and whether a laminectomy has been performed. These factors are typically associated with greater blood loss, larger postoperative dead space, and greater potential for residual postoperative bleeding and hematoma formation. Patient-related factors such as obesity, and index diagnoses such as infection or neoplasm presumably influence infection rates as well. A few studies have compared laminoplasty to laminectomy and fusion for the treatment of cervical spondylotic myelopathy.[76,77] Theoretically, the increased exposure and the presence of long implant constructs would suggest increased rates of infection for laminectomy and fusion compared with laminoplasty. Both studies reported slightly higher rates of infection in the fusion group (7.6 and 8.5% respectively). These differences were not significant; however, both studies were presumably at risk for a type II error on this comparison. Two other recent studies have examined the effect of intrawound vancomycin powder on surgical site infections after open posterior cervical fusion.[78,79] Both studies included comparator groups of open posterior cervical fusion predating the use of intrawound vancomycin powder which can serve as reasonable estimates of the risk for surgical site infection. The infection rates were reported as 15 and 10.9%.[78,79] Both studies reported significant reductions in surgical site infection with the application of vancomycin powder to the wound, with rates of 0 and 2.5%,[78,79] respectively. In addition to multilevel subaxial decompression and fusions for cervical spondylotic myelopathy, the latter study included occipitocervical/cervicothoracic fusions as well as procedures for tumors and infections.

While postoperative pain is not typically considered a complication, there is no doubt that techniques with less predicted postoperative pain are desirable. Unfortunately, this issue has not been studied routinely in the existing open posterior cervical literature in a way that fosters meaningful comparison to the limited data on MIS posterior cervical procedures. Once again, the open literature most commonly details multilevel constructs with associated laminectomy. Designing studies evaluating this issue in comparable procedures is necessary to truly understand the role for the MIS approach in this arena.

13.11.7 Level I Evidence in Open Thoracolumbar Pedicle Screw Fixation

Currently, no level I evidence is available comparing percutaneous pedicle screw fixation with a traditional open midline surgical approach and screw placement using either a free-hand technique or a fluoroscopic guided strategy. Jiang et al[12] devised a randomized control trial in Beijing, China, to compare navigation-guided percutaneous pedicle screw placement versus paraspinal screw fixation through a midline incision[80] for thoracolumbar burst fractures in neurologically intact patients. Although, the open technique employed in this paper is atypical, this study confirms some very important concepts. Open placement of pedicle screws did not result in any increased complication when compared with the percutaneous group. Four of 120 open screws and 6 of 124 percutaneous screws had screw misplacement and none required revisions or resulted in neurological complications. Furthermore, the open surgical technique resulted in improved overall sagittal alignment and fracture reduction when compared to the percutaneous approach. Surgical time was less in the percutaneous group, as was the intraoperative blood loss and hospital stay. However, there were no reported data suggesting a transfusion requirement in the open group. There were no significant differences in clinical outcomes at final follow-up (minimum of 3 years).

13.11.8 Level II Evidence in Open Thoracolumbar Pedicle Screw Fixation

A limited number of level II studies exist in the English language that address the outcomes of open versus minimally invasive strategies of managing spinal conditions, and a vast majority of them deal with fusion and trauma management. Evaluation of fusion quality between minimally invasive and open thoracolumbar surgeries is beyond the scope of this chapter and is better discussed elsewhere in the text. However, valuable information regarding instrumentation can be gleaned from these level II studies comparing open versus MIS thoracolumbar fusion surgeries. Kotani et al[19] prospectively performed conventional open versus minimally invasive posterolateral fusions (MIS-PLFs) with percutaneous screws for 80 consecutive patients with degenerative spondylolisthesis and stenosis. Their MIS-PLF group was performed with a small midline incision, but it did include a direct decompression/medial facetectomy and medial transverse process and facet decortication with iliac crest autograft harvest for fusion. In addition, they utilized bilateral parasagittal incisions for sextant screw placement. With this extensive technique, the authors reported a similar fusion rate between the open and the MIS PLF groups. They also reported an improved ODI and RMQ up to 2 years later in the "MIS-PLF" group versus the open group. The VAS group was only statistically superior on post-op day 3 in the MIS group and the only other statistical significant difference was a higher post-op hemoglobin of 10.8 ± 1.2 in the MIS group versus 10.2 ± 1.4 in the open group. The other parameters including CPK (creatine phosphokinase) levels and CRP (C-reactive protein) levels were equivalent. The differences in ODI and RMQ may simply be attributable to patient bias and perception as the patients themselves selected the technique of surgery based on their discussion with the surgeons. In addition to the nonrandomization limitation, the methodology of this study was imprecisely defined and it may be downgraded to a level III.

Grossbach et al[15] reported a short-term follow-up on 38 patients with flexion-distraction injuries that were treated either with open pedicle screw instrumentation and fusion (27 patients) or percutaneous/MIS fixation (11 patients). Mean duration of follow-up was 1.5 years for the open group and

9 months for the MIS group. There was no difference in the ASIA score or kyphotic angulation between the two treatment arms. Similarly, there was no statistical difference in the operative times or length of stay. There was significantly less blood loss in the percutaneous group when compared to the open cohort. The short-term follow-up provided by this study does not allow for appropriate assessment of long-term implant-related failures/complications, need for instrumentation removal, and maintenance of spinal alignment, especially in patients with ligamentous injury and no fusion. Other level II studies mentioned in support of the MIS group are not found in the English language and most have similar limitations.

Accuracy of pedicle screw insertion is most often determined by access to and use of imaging assistance. Recent advances in intraoperative imaging capacity and image guidance has allowed for an improved ability to accurately and safely place pedicle screw instrumentation. However, this technology is accompanied with higher irradiation, higher cost, extensive equipment, prolonged operative time, and lack of common accessibility and availability. Laine et al[81] reported their results on 100 consecutive patients randomized to pedicle screw fixation with conventional free-hand technique (50 patients) or to a computer-assisted group (41 patients). Due to methodological issues with nine dropout patients, this downgraded level II study did establish a statistically lower pedicle perforation rate of 13.6% in the free-hand conventional technique versus 4.6% in the computer-guided group. Moreover, the rate of pedicle perforation > 4 mm was 1.4% in the conventional group and none in the computer-assisted group. This improved accuracy is merely a reflection of improved/enhanced imaging capacity and has the same effect on accuracy regardless of open or percutaneous approach and does not favor the use of percutaneous over open strategy in spinal surgery.

13.11.9 Level III and IV Evidence in Open Thoracolumbar Pedicle Screw Fixation

The majority of the available literature assessing the safety profile of pedicle screw fixation comes from level III and level IV data. Lonstein et al[82] published their retrospective review of 4,790 pedicle screws in 875 patients revealing the safety profile and complications associated with open pedicle screw placement. Landmarks along with lateral radiographs were typically used for placement of screws. Laminectomy or laminotomies were utilized as needed for decompression and/or confirmation of screw placement. Patients routinely had PA and lateral radiographs intraoperatively or prior to discharge. In their single institution series, 95% of the pedicle screws were judged to be wholly positioned into the pedicles. Perforation was noted anteriorly in 2.8% (74% of these were in the sacrum and felt to be intentional for bicortical purchase); 1% lateral breach, 0.6% inferior breach, 0.4% medial breach, and 0.2% superior breach were reported. There was a 1% rate of nerve root irritation mostly associated with a medial breach and 8 out of 11 screws causing irritation were removed with a resolution of symptoms in most patients. There were no visceral or vascular injuries and other complications included pedicle fracture in 0.1% and screw fracture 0.5%. This classic paper was published during the early adoption of pedicle screws and the concept of percutaneous screw fixation was not yet available; however, to date, there are no comparative studies which show fluoroscopic-assisted percutaneous screw insertion to have a better hardware-related complication profile than Lonstein's open screw placement data.[83,84]

Kim et al[85] provide a more recent retrospective analysis of thoracic pedicle screw placement using an open free-hand technique. They reported on 3,204 thoracic pedicle screws, a vast majority of which were inserted for scoliosis/deformity patients. A random sample of 577 screws was evaluated postoperatively with a CT scan for analysis of screw-related complications. Thoracic screws were accurately placed in 93.8% by five surgeons. Moderate cortical perforation was evident in 6.2%; 1.7% violated the medial wall. Misplaced screws were accepted and left into position due to an absence of associated symptoms. There were no neurologic or vascular complications at up to 10 years of follow-up.

A comparative retrospective analysis of percutaneous and open pedicle screw fixation in lumbosacral fusion has been published by Oh et al.[24] The study group includes 237 patients and 1,056 screws. A total of 558 screws were placed using a fluoroscopic-assisted open technique and 498 screws were placed using a percutaneous strategy. Posterior instrumentation was performed in addition to either an anterior or transforaminal interbody fusion. Pedicle wall penetration was not statistically different in either group, with a 13.4% incidence in the open and a 14.3% incidence in the percutaneous group. There was a higher risk for medial and inferior penetration in the percutaneous group and a higher incidence of lateral perforation in the open group. In general, medial perforation has a higher risk for neurologic complications.[86,87]

In addition to the higher medial pedicle perforation, there are several authors who have reported on the increased rate and higher grade of facet violation with the percutaneous techniques. Jones-Quaidoo et al[21] and Babu et al[22] have both reported a significantly higher rate of superior facet violation using the percutaneous approach. This would result in increased stress and degeneration on the adjacent level above the fusion and may result in symptomatic adjacent level disease.

13.12 Conclusion of Open Surgery

Open placement of contemporary spinal instrumentation is currently the gold-standard approach for obtaining rigid posterior based fixation. The lack of level I studies notwithstanding, the large body of literature on these techniques gives reasonable estimates of complication rates in the practical setting. Still, a Grade 1C recommendation can be made for placement of screws using open techniques. By comparison, there is a much smaller body of literature to establish the risk of complications for minimally invasive approaches for cervical fixation. In high-volume centers, experienced surgeons may utilize these techniques with complication rates on par with open approaches. The ability to predict complication rates with more widespread use, however, is more nuanced. For example, one of the busiest spine trauma centers in North America recently published a study detailing their accuracy and complications associated with C1 fixation.[88] The authors' experience amounted to two to three cases requiring C1 instrumentation per month over the

6-year study period. This operation, however, is not nearly so commonly performed in general practice. It is unclear whether a less frequent operator would perform such procedures frequently enough to justify exposing patients to the learning curve inherent to the transition to the less invasive version of this technique, particularly when its benefits are more theoretical than proven.

Subaxial posterior cervical fixation, conversely, is much more commonly performed. The majority of these fusions, however, are multilevel constructs or done in concert with laminectomy, limiting the applicability of the minimally invasive technique. The main advantage of the minimally invasive approach for cervical stabilization would be expected to be lower rates of surgical site infection, which historically is the complication most likely to occur with open procedures. The rates of infection for open fusion, however, are impacted by factors such as construct length and associated laminectomy, so comparison to MIS one-level fusion without associated decompression has little validity. Hopefully, recently described adjuncts such as intrawound application of vancomycin powder will decrease this risk across the board.

The rationale for percutaneous thoracolumbar pedicle screws as an adjunct to anterior interbody fusion or as stabilization for fracture seems well founded given the amount of dissection required for open placement. The risk of superior facet joint violation, however, should not be understated and may necessitate more widespread use of surgical navigation to mitigate this occurrence (▶ Table 13.6).

13.13 Editors' Commentary
13.13.1 Minimally Invasive Surgery

More than being "technique"-dependent, complication rates are directly the result of four factors: (1) the complexity of the pathology, (2) the comorbidities associated with the patient, (3) the level of the spine being approached, and (4) the experience level of the surgeon. Certainly, the precision demanded in placement of instrumentation in the cervical spine is extreme, whether performed open or MIS. Except in very experienced hands, one might want to avoid the MIS technique in this anatomic area. On the other extreme, percutaneous placement of lumbar instrumentation is relatively easy and quite safe. Literature published early in the development of this technique suggested higher complications using the MIS technique than the open technique. However, this seems to have reflected both the relative infancy of the available instrumentation at that time and the inexperience of the surgeons performing the procedures. More recent publications have demonstrated lower complications rates using the MIS technique.

As with any surgical procedure, results improve and complications rates decrease with experience. Surgeons who are inexperienced or uncomfortable performing any procedure, open or MIS, should not be performing that procedure on patients. However, to relegate all new techniques to the "it is not as good as the old, tried and true, technique" would kill progress and innovation. With appropriate education and training, most surgeons can acquire the necessary skills to perform the more current MIS instrumentation techniques.

Table 13.6 Summary of representative data on open thoracolumbar pedicle screws

Study	Level	Treatment groups	Outcomes
Jiang et al[12]	I	31 percutaneous vs. 30 open pedicle screw patients with burst fractures	• Less blood loss, OR time, hospital stay in percutaneous group • No difference in screw accuracy or complications • Open group had improved alignment and fracture reduction • No difference in long-term outcome
Grossbach et al[15]	II	27 open vs. 11 percutaneous pedicle screw patients with flexion-distraction injury	• Shorter OR time and lower blood loss in percutaneous patients • No difference in complication rates • Limited follow-up period
Kotani et al[19]	II/III	37 open laminectomy and PLF vs. 43 MIS-PLF for patients undergoing single-level fusion for degenerative spondylolisthesis	• MIS group with midline incision + iliac crest autograft in the posterolateral gutters showed equivalent fusion as open group • Improved ODI and RMQ scores up to 24 mo post-op in MIS group • No complications of screw placement, CPK and CRP levels equivalent in both groups
Jones-Quaidoo et al[21]	III	66 open vs. 66 percutaneous pedicle screw patients	• Higher percentage of percutaneous screws violated superior facet (6 vs. 13.6%)
Babu et al[22]	III	126 open vs. 153 percutaneous lumbar degenerative cases	• Superior facet violation more common in percutaneous patients
Oh et al[24]	III	126 open vs. 111 percutaneous patients	• Incidence and severity of pedicle perforation similar between the two groups
Laine et al[81]	II	50 patients underwent open free-hand pedicle screw placement vs. 41 patients with computer-assisted open screw placement	• 13.6% perforation in free-hand technique vs. 4.6% rate in computer-assisted group • Pedicle perforation > 4 mm: 4.6% free-hand vs. 1.4% in navigation group
Lonstein et al[82]	IV	Retrospective review of 4,790 pedicle screws in 875 patients	• 95% accuracy of pedicle screw placement using open free-hand technique with lateral radiographic supplementation. • 1% lateral breach, 0.6% lateral breach, 0.4% medial breach. • No visceral injury. 1% nerve root irritation
Halm et al[83]	IV	Prospective clinical trial with 12 patients surgically treated for idiopathic scoliosis with open pedicle screw fixation	• 85/104 screws "within the pedicle" • Perforations: 10 screws lateral, 4 medial and 5 bilateral • No neurologic complications
Schizas et al[84]	III	CT analysis of 60 percutaneously placed pedicle screws in 15 consecutive patients s/p LS fusion	• 13% severe frank penetration, 80% some form of perforation • 1/15, 6.6%, suffered S1 root palsy due to breach
Kim et al[85]	IV	Retrospective review of 3,204 thoracic pedicle screws	• CT analysis revealed a 93.8% accuracy • 6.2% moderate perforation, 1.7% medial perforation

Abbreviations: CPK, creatine phosphokinase; CRP, C-reactive protein; CT, computed tomography; MIS-PLF, minimally invasive posterolateral fusion; ODI, Oswestry Disability Index; OR, operative; RMQ, Roland–Morris Questionnaire; s/p LS, LS-lumbosacral.

13.13.2 Open Surgery

In the most experienced hands, the rate of complications directly related to the placement of instrumentation is similar between open and MIS techniques. Navigating this steep learning curve in order to eventually achieve equivalence with a well-established open technique that has a more forgiving learning curve is often a tough sell for spine surgeons especially as patients like to feel that they are not being used as a learning example in an operating suite. It is unclear whether patients would be as eager to undergo MIS procedures if they understood the MIS learning curve and potential for associated complications. Because traditional open techniques form the basis for the majority of training during most spine fellowships, even experienced open surgeons will likely not be able to immediately replicate the published equivalence between these techniques. Similar studies documenting complication rates of surgeons at different stages of adopting MIS techniques would be more informative but potentially unsavory for participating surgeons to publish.

Many common procedures (such as most posterior cervical fusion procedures, aside from the less common scenario described in this chapter) require stabilization at multiple levels—less precise instrumentation placement is often the consequence of addressing multiple levels without repeatedly moving the retractor system. These same procedures, often with a mix of pedicle and lateral mass screw techniques, also provide a challenge for placement of rods without subjecting screws to high stresses which may result in cutout. In contrast, open surgery has a continuous surgical corridor without constraints on trajectory or entry point. Although not the focus of this chapter, the limitations in moving a retractor to allow ideal placement of instrumentation is also the same constraint which limits complementary procedures such as decortication and bone grafting during MIS fusion procedures.

References

[1] Joseffer SS, Post N, Cooper PR, Frempong-Boadu AK. Minimally invasive atlantoaxial fixation with a polyaxial screw-rod construct: technical case report. Neurosurgery. 2006; 58(4) Suppl 2:E375–, discussion E375

[2] Taghva A, Attenello FJ, Zada G, Khalessi AA, Hsieh PC. Minimally invasive posterior atlantoaxial fusion: a cadaveric and clinical feasibility study. World Neurosurg. 2013; 80(3)(–)(4):414–421

[3] Holly LT, Isaacs RE, Frempong-Boadu AK. Minimally invasive atlantoaxial fusion. Neurosurgery. 2010; 66(3) Suppl:193–197

[4] Wei W, Xiao Z, Lu W, Mai Y, Huang C, Hua S. Spinal pedicle screw internal fixation through endoscope-assisted posterior approach for treatment of traumatic atlantoaxial instability [in Chinese]. Zhongguo Xiu Fu Chong Jian Wai Ke Za Zhi. 2012; 26(11):1324–1329

[5] Ahmad F, Sherman JD, Wang MY. Percutaneous trans-facet screws for supplemental posterior cervical fixation. World Neurosurg. 2012; 78(6):716. e1–716.e4

[6] Miyanji F, Mahar A, Oka R, Newton P. Biomechanical differences between transfacet and lateral mass screw-rod constructs for multilevel posterior cervical spine stabilization. Spine. 2008; 33(23):E865–E869

[7] Lee YP, Robertson C, Mahar A, et al. Biomechanical evaluation of transfacet screw fixation for stabilization of multilevel cervical corpectomies. J Spinal Disord Tech. 2011; 24(4):258–263

[8] Mikhael MM, Celestre PC, Wolf CF, Mroz TE, Wang JC. Minimally invasive cervical spine foraminotomy and lateral mass screw placement. Spine. 2012; 37(5):E318–E322

[9] Fong S, Duplessis S. Minimally invasive lateral mass plating in the treatment of posterior cervical trauma: surgical technique. J Spinal Disord Tech. 2005; 18(3):224–228

[10] Wang MY, Levi AD. Minimally invasive lateral mass screw fixation in the cervical spine: initial clinical experience with long-term follow-up. Neurosurgery. 2006; 58(5):907–912, discussion 907–912

[11] Schaefer C, Begemann P, Fuhrhop I, et al. Percutaneous instrumentation of the cervical and cervico-thoracic spine using pedicle screws: preliminary clinical results and analysis of accuracy. Eur Spine J. 2011; 20(6):977–985

[12] Jiang XZ, Tian W, Liu B, et al. Comparison of a paraspinal approach with a percutaneous approach in the treatment of thoracolumbar burst fractures with posterior ligamentous complex injury: a prospective randomized controlled trial. J Int Med Res. 2012; 40(4):1343–1356

[13] Li C, Xu HZ, Wang XY, et al. Comparison of the paraspinal muscle change of percutaneous and open pedicle screw fixation in the treatment for thoracolumbar fractures [in Chinese]. Zhonghua Wai Ke Za Zhi. 2007; 45(14): 972–975

[14] King D. Internal fixation for lumbosacral fusion. J Bone Joint Surg Am. 1948; 30A(3):560–565

[15] Grossbach AJ, Dahdaleh NS, Abel TJ, Woods GD, Dlouhy BJ, Hitchon PW. Flexion-distraction injuries of the thoracolumbar spine: open fusion versus percutaneous pedicle screw fixation. Neurosurg Focus. 2013; 35(2):E2

[16] Huang QS, Chi YL, Wang XY, et al. [Comparative percutaneous with open pedicle screw fixation in the treatment of thoracolumbar burst fractures without neurological deficit]. Zhonghua Wai Ke Za Zhi. 2008; 46(2):112–114

[17] Yang BP, Wahl MM, Idler CS. Percutaneous lumbar pedicle screw placement aided by computer-assisted fluoroscopy-based navigation: perioperative results of a prospective, comparative, multicenter study. Spine. 2012; 37(24): 2055–2060

[18] Lee JK, Jang JW, Kim TW, Kim TS, Kim SH, Moon SJ. Percutaneous short-segment pedicle screw placement without fusion in the treatment of thoracolumbar burst fractures: is it effective?: comparative study with open short-segment pedicle screw fixation with posterolateral fusion. Acta Neurochir (Wien). 2013; 155(12):2305–2312, discussion 2312

[19] Kotani Y, Abumi K, Ito M, Sudo H, Abe Y, Minami A. Mid-term clinical results of minimally invasive decompression and posterolateral fusion with percutaneous pedicle screws versus conventional approach for degenerative spondylolisthesis with spinal stenosis. Eur Spine J. 2012; 21(6):1171–1177

[20] Mobbs RJ, Raley DA. Complications with k-wire insertion for percutaneous pedicle screws. J Spinal Disord Tech. 2014; 27(7):390–394

[21] Jones-Quaidoo SM, Djurasovic M, Owens RK, II, Carreon LY. Superior articulating facet violation: percutaneous versus open techniques. J Neurosurg Spine. 2013; 18(6):593–597

[22] Babu R, Park JG, Mehta AI, et al. Comparison of superior-level facet joint violations during open and percutaneous pedicle screw placement. Neurosurgery. 2012; 71(5):962–970

[23] Yson SC, Sembrano JN, Sanders PC, Santos ER, Ledonio CG, Polly DW, Jr. Comparison of cranial facet joint violation rates between open and percutaneous pedicle screw placement using intraoperative 3-D CT (O-arm) computer navigation. Spine. 2013; 38(4):E251–E258

[24] Oh HS, Kim JS, Lee SH, Liu WC, Hong SW. Comparison between the accuracy of percutaneous and open pedicle screw fixations in lumbosacral fusion. Spine J. 2013; 13(12):1751–1757

[25] Lau D, Terman SW, Patel R, La Marca F, Park P. Incidence of and risk factors for superior facet violation in minimally invasive versus open pedicle screw placement during transforaminal lumbar interbody fusion: a comparative analysis. J Neurosurg Spine. 2013; 18(4):356–361

[26] Houten JK, Nasser R, Baxi N. Clinical assessment of percutaneous lumbar pedicle screw placement using theO-arm multidimensional surgical imaging system. Neurosurgery. 2012; 70(4):990–995

[27] Fraser J, Gebhard H, Irie D, Parikh K, Härtl R. Iso-C/3-dimensional neuronavigation versus conventional fluoroscopy for minimally invasive pedicle screw placement in lumbar fusion. Minim Invasive Neurosurg. 2010; 53(4):184–190

[28] Nakashima H, Sato K, Ando T, Inoh H, Nakamura H. Comparison of the percutaneous screw placement precision of isocentric C-arm 3-dimensional fluoroscopy-navigated pedicle screw implantation and conventional fluoroscopy method with minimally invasive surgery. J Spinal Disord Tech. 2009; 22(7):468–472

[29] Tuli J, Tuli S, Eichler ME, Woodard EJ. A comparison of long-term outcomes of translaminar facet screw fixation and pedicle screw fixation: a prospective study. J Neurosurg Spine. 2007; 7(3):287–292

[30] Hou Y, Shen Y, Liu Z, Nie Z. Which posterior instrumentation is better for two-level anterior lumbar interbody fusion: translaminar facet screw or pedicle screw? Arch Orthop Trauma Surg. 2013; 133(1):37–42

[31] Burton D, McIff T, Fox T, Lark R, Asher MA, Glattes RC. Biomechanical analysis of posterior fixation techniques in a 360 degrees arthrodesis model. Spine. 2005; 30(24):2765–2771

[32] Wang M, Tang SJ, McGrady LM, Rao RD. Biomechanical comparison of supplemental posterior fixations for two-level anterior lumbar interbody fusion. Proc Inst Mech Eng H. 2013; 227(3):245–250

[33] Agarwala A, Bucklen B, Muzumdar A, Moldavsky M, Khalil S. Do facet screws provide the required stability in lumbar fixation? A biomechanical comparison of the Boucher technique and pedicular fixation in primary and circumferential fusions. Clin Biomech (Bristol, Avon). 2012; 27(1):64–70

[34] Amoretti N, Amoretti ME, Hovorka I, Hauger O, Boileau P, Huwart L. Percutaneous facet screw fixation of lumbar spine with CT and fluoroscopic guidance: a feasibility study. Radiology. 2013; 268(2):548–555

[35] Shim CS, Lee SH, Jung B, Sivasabaapathi P, Park SH, Shin SW. Fluoroscopically assisted percutaneous translaminar facet screw fixation following anterior lumbar interbody fusion: technical report. Spine. 2005; 30(7):838–843

[36] Aepli M, Mannion AF, Grob D. Translaminar screw fixation of the lumbar spine: long-term outcome. Spine. 2009; 34(14):1492–1498

[37] Best NM, Sasso RC. Efficacy of translaminar facet screw fixation in circumferential interbody fusions as compared to pedicle screw fixation. J Spinal Disord Tech. 2006; 19(2):98–103

[38] Jang JS, Lee SH. Clinical analysis of percutaneous facet screw fixation after anterior lumbar interbody fusion. J Neurosurg Spine. 2005; 3(1):40–46

[39] Lee SH, Kim ES, Sung JK, Park YM, Eoh W. Clinical and radiological comparison of treatment of atlantoaxial instability by posterior C1-C2 transarticular screw fixation or C1 lateral mass-C2 pedicle screw fixation. J Clin Neurosci. 2010; 17(7):886–892

[40] Goel A, Desai KI, Muzumdar DP. Atlantoaxial fixation using plate and screw method: a report of 160 treated patients. Neurosurgery. 2002; 51(6):1351–1356, discussion 1356–1357

[41] Harms J, Melcher RP. Posterior C1-C2 fusion with polyaxial screw and rod fixation. Spine. 2001; 26(22):2467–2471

[42] Chen JF, Wu CT, Lee SC, Lee ST. Posterior atlantoaxial transpedicular screw and plate fixation. Technical note. J Neurosurg Spine. 2005; 2(3):386–392

[43] El Masry MA, El Assuity WI, Sadek FZ, Salah H. Two methods of atlantoaxial stabilisation for atlantoaxial instability. Acta Orthop Belg. 2007; 73(6):741–746

[44] Stulik J, Vyskocil T, Sebesta P, Kryl J. Atlantoaxial fixation using the polyaxial screw-rod system. Eur Spine J. 2007; 16(4):479–484

[45] Li L, Zhou FH, Wang H, Cui SQ. Posterior fixation and fusion with atlas pedicle screw system for upper cervical diseases. Chin J Traumatol. 2008; 11(6):323–328

[46] De Iure F, Donthineni R, Boriani S. Outcomes of C1 and C2 posterior screw fixation for upper cervical spine fusion. Eur Spine J. 2009; 18 Suppl 1:2–6

[47] Payer M, Luzi M, Tessitore E. Posterior atlanto-axial fixation with polyaxial C1 lateral mass screws and C2 pars screws. Acta Neurochir (Wien). 2009; 151 (3):223–229, discussion 229

[48] Simsek S, Yigitkanli K, Seckin H, Akyol C, Belen D, Bavbek M. Freehand C1 lateral mass screw fixation technique: our experience. Surg Neurol. 2009; 72 (6):676–681

[49] Pan J, Li L, Qian L, Tan J, Sun G, Li X. C1 lateral mass screw insertion with protection of C1-C2 venous sinus: technical note and review of the literature. Spine. 2010; 35(21):E1133–E1136

[50] Squires J, Molinari RW. C1 lateral mass screw placement with intentional sacrifice of the C2 ganglion: functional outcomes and morbidity in elderly patients. Eur Spine J. 2010; 19(8):1318–1324

[51] Thomas JA, Tredway T, Fessler RG, Sandhu FA. An alternate method for placement of C-1 screws. J Neurosurg Spine. 2010; 12(4):337–341

[52] Wang S, Wang C, Wood KB, Yan M, Zhou H. Radiographic evaluation of the technique for C1 lateral mass and C2 pedicle screw fixation in three hundred nineteen cases. Spine. 2011; 36(1):3–8

[53] Hamilton DK, Smith JS, Sansur CA, Dumont AS, Shaffrey CI. C-2 neurectomy during atlantoaxial instrumented fusion in the elderly: patient satisfaction and surgical outcome. J Neurosurg Spine. 2011; 15(1):3–8

[54] Kang MM, Anderer EG, Elliott RE, Kalhorn SP, Frempong-Boadu A. C2 nerve root sectioning in posterior C1–2 instrumented fusions. World Neurosurg. 2012; 78(1)(–)(2):170–177

[55] Goel A, Laheri V. Plate and screw fixation for atlanto-axial subluxation. Acta Neurochir (Wien). 1994; 129(1)(–)(2):47–53

[56] Fiore AJ, Haid RW, Rodts GE, et al. Atlantal lateral mass screws for posterior spinal reconstruction: technical note and case series. Neurosurg Focus. 2002; 12(1):E5

[57] Resnick DK, Benzel EC. C1-C2 pedicle screw fixation with rigid cantilever beam construct: case report and technical note. Neurosurgery. 2002; 50(2):426–428

[58] Elliott RE, Tanweer O, Smith ML, Frempong-Boadu A. Impact of starting point and bicortical purchase of C1 lateral mass screws on atlantoaxial fusion: meta-analysis and review of the literature. J Spinal Disord Tech. 2015; 28(7):242–253

[59] Elliott RE, Tanweer O, Frempong-Boadu A, Smith ML. Impact of starting point and C2 nerve status on the safety and accuracy of C1 lateral mass screws: meta-analysis and review of the literature. J Spinal Disord Tech. 2015; 28(5):171–185

[60] Elliott RE, Tanweer O, Boah A, et al. Outcome comparison of atlantoaxial fusion with transarticular screws and screw-rod constructs: meta-analysis and review of literature. J Spinal Disord Tech. 2014; 27(1):11–28

[61] Heller JG, Silcox DH, III, Sutterlin CE, III. Complications of posterior cervical plating. Spine. 1995; 20(22):2442–2448

[62] Fehlings MG, Cooper PR, Errico TJ. Posterior plates in the management of cervical instability: long-term results in 44 patients. J Neurosurg. 1994; 81(3):341–349

[63] Graham AW, Swank ML, Kinard RE, Lowery GL, Dials BE. Posterior cervical arthrodesis and stabilization with a lateral mass plate. Clinical and computed tomographic evaluation of lateral mass screw placement and associated complications. Spine. 1996; 21(3):323–328, discussion 329

[64] Wellman BJ, Follett KA, Traynelis VC. Complications of posterior articular mass plate fixation of the subaxial cervical spine in 43 consecutive patients. Spine. 1998; 23(2):193–200

[65] Sekhon LH. Posterior cervical lateral mass screw fixation: analysis of 1026 consecutive screws in 143 patients. J Spinal Disord Tech. 2005; 18(4):297–303

[66] Pateder DB, Carbone JJ. Lateral mass screw fixation for cervical spine trauma: associated complications and efficacy in maintaining alignment. Spine J. 2006; 6(1):40–43

[67] Roche S, de Freitas DJ, Lenehan B, Street JT, McCabe JP. Posterior cervical screw placement without image guidance: a safe and reliable practice. J Spinal Disord Tech. 2006; 19(6):383–388

[68] Wu JC, Huang WC, Chen YC, Shih YH, Cheng H. Stabilization of subaxial cervical spines by lateral mass screw fixation with modified Magerl's technique. Surg Neurol. 2008; 70 Suppl 1:S1–, 25–33, discussion S1, 33

[69] Stevens QE, Majd ME, Kattner KA, Jones CL, Holt RT. Use of spinous processes to determine the optimal trajectory for placement of lateral mass screws: technical note. J Spinal Disord Tech. 2009; 22(5):347–352

[70] Katonis P, Papadakis SA, Galanakos S, et al. Lateral mass screw complications: analysis of 1662 screws. J Spinal Disord Tech. 2011; 24(7):415–420

[71] Audat ZA, Barbarawi MM, Obeidat MM. Posterior cervical decompressive laminectomy and lateral mass screw fixation. Neurosciences (Riyadh). 2011; 16(3):248–252

[72] Inoue S, Moriyama T, Tachibana T, et al. Cervical lateral mass screw fixation without fluoroscopic control: analysis of risk factors for complications associated with screw insertion. Arch Orthop Trauma Surg. 2012; 132(7):947–953

[73] Kim SH, Seo WD, Kim KH, Yeo HT, Choi GH, Kim DH. Clinical outcome of modified cervical lateral mass screw fixation technique. J Korean Neurosurg Soc. 2012; 52(2):114–119

[74] Roy-Camille R, Gaillant G, Bertreaux D. Early management of spinal injuries. In: McKibben B, ed. Recent Advances in Orthopedics. Edinburgh: Churchill-Livingstone; 1979:57–87

[75] Yoshihara H, Passias PG, Errico TJ. Screw-related complications in the subaxial cervical spine with the use of lateral mass versus cervical pedicle screws: a systematic review. J Neurosurg Spine. 2013; 19:614–623

[76] Fehlings MG, Smith JS, Kopjar B, et al. Perioperative and delayed complications associated with the surgical treatment of cervical spondylotic myelopathy based on 302 patients from the AOSpine North America Cervical Spondylotic Myelopathy Study. J Neurosurg Spine. 2012; 16(5):425–432

[77] Heller JG, Edwards CC, II, Murakami H, Rodts GE. Laminoplasty versus laminectomy and fusion for multilevel cervical myelopathy: an independent matched cohort analysis. Spine. 2001; 26(12):1330–1336

[78] Caroom C, Tullar JM, Benton EG, Jr, Jones JR, Chaput CD. Intrawound vancomycin powder reduces surgical site infections in posterior cervical fusion. Spine. 2013; 38(14):1183–1187

[79] Strom RG, Pacione D, Kalhorn SP, Frempong-Boadu AK. Decreased risk of wound infection after posterior cervical fusion with routine local application of vancomycin powder. Spine. 2013; 38(12):991–994

[80] Pang W, Zhang GL, Tian W, et al. Surgical treatment of thoracolumbar fracture through an approach via the paravertebral muscle. Orthop Surg. 2009; 1(3):184–188

[81] Laine T, Lund T, Ylikoski M, Lohikoski J, Schlenzka D. Accuracy of pedicle screw insertion with and without computer assistance: a randomised controlled clinical study in 100 consecutive patients. Eur Spine J. 2000; 9(3):235–240

[82] Lonstein JE, Denis F, Perra JH, Pinto MR, Smith MD, Winter RB. Complications associated with pedicle screws. J Bone Joint Surg Am. 1999; 81(11):1519–1528

[83] Halm H, Niemeyer T, Link T, Liljenqvist U. Segmental pedicle screw instrumentation in idiopathic thoracolumbar and lumbar scoliosis. Eur Spine J. 2000; 9(3):191–197

[84] Schizas C, Michel J, Kosmopoulos V, Theumann N. Computer tomography assessment of pedicle screw insertion in percutaneous posterior transpedicular stabilization. Eur Spine J. 2007; 16(5):613–617

[85] Kim YJ, Lenke LG, Bridwell KH, Cho YS, Riew KD. Free hand pedicle screw placement in the thoracic spine: is it safe? Spine. 2004; 29(3):333–342, discussion 342

[86] Söyüncü Y, Yildirim FB, Sekban H, Ozdemir H, Akyildiz F, Sindel M. Anatomic evaluation and relationship between the lumbar pedicle and adjacent neural structures: an anatomic study. J Spinal Disord Tech. 2005; 18(3):243–246

[87] Ebraheim NA, Xu R, Darwich M, Yeasting RA. Anatomic relations between the lumbar pedicle and the adjacent neural structures. Spine. 1997; 22(20):2338–2341

[88] Bransford RJ, Freeborn MA, Russo AJ, et al. Accuracy and complications associated with posterior C1 screw fixation techniques: a radiographic and clinical assessment. Spine J. 2012; 12(3):231–238

14 Dural Tears: Should a Minimally Invasive Complication Such as a Dural Tear Routinely Be Opened for Adequate Repair or Are There Safe and Reliable Minimally Invasive Techniques for Dural Closure?

MIS: John E. O'Toole
Open: Michelle J. Clarke

14.1 Introduction

The reported incidence of unintended durotomy during spine surgery in general ranges from 1.6 to 17.4%.[1,2,3,4,5,6,7,8,9] Minimally invasive surgery (MIS) techniques do not appear to increase this incidence, particularly when reported beyond surgeons' early learning curve with MIS.[6,10,11,12,13,14,15] The intraoperative management of unintended durotomy in traditional open spine surgery has been well explored, including the use of various methods of primary repair, fibrin glue, cerebrospinal fluid (CSF) diversion, epidural blood patch, and prolonged bedrest.[1,2,3,5,6,7,8,16,17,18,19,20] During MIS, however, primary dural closure using standard surgical instruments can be challenging due to the limited surgical corridor and working angles encountered using tubular retractors.

Concurrently, the evolution of and growing familiarity with MIS techniques have led to an increasing number of intradural pathologies addressed via MIS approaches, including intradural neoplasms, vascular malformations, syringomyelia, and tethered spinal cord.[21,22,23,24,25,26,27,28,29,30,31,32] In contrast to unintended durotomies, intended durotomies are often larger and thus may be more prone to cause postoperative complications if not properly closed. This chapter reviews the evidence concerning the management of both unintended and intended durotomies during MIS spinal surgery.

14.2 Indications for Repair of Durotomy during Minimally Invasive Surgery

A failure to achieve adequate dural closure after durotomy can lead to persistent CSF leak, pseudomeningocele, or CSF-cutaneous fistula with attendant headache, nausea, vomiting, and back pain. More severe complications including wound infection, meningitis, and even intracranial hemorrhage can be seen after insufficiently repaired durotomy.[1,3,6,33,34] A range of intraoperative dural injuries may occur including partial thickness (e.g., arachnoid intact), linear, stellate, root-sleeve, or avulsion. Each of these may be amenable to different strategies or techniques to manage them, but in each case, appropriate efforts should be made to control the egress of CSF to avoid postoperative complications.

14.3 Advantages of Minimally Invasive Surgery

By utilizing tissue dilation rather than subperiosteal dissection with a circumferentially solid retractor of a typically small diameter, multiple potential benefits are gained. The smaller working corridor and preservation of the normal paraspinal soft tissues allow the tissues to reapproximate at the end of the procedure, thereby obliterating potential dead space in which CSF might accumulate. Moreover, normal amounts of postoperative blood products layer over the dura and are contained just within the confines of the bony opening without significant extension into the paraspinal muscles, effectively functioning as a native "blood patch." Similarly, any muscle/fat graft or fibrin sealant placed over the dural defect is tightly contained. Finally, the solid tubular retractor and limited skin opening prevent introduction of skin flora that might impair wound healing or even produce a wound infection, either of which might perpetuate a CSF leak.

14.4 Advantages of Open Surgery

The advantage to open dural repair is access. By extending the incision, the surgeon is able to function without the constraints of the MIS retractor. This allows better visualization as the surgeon is able to simultaneously view a larger area. Thoroughly exposing the dural defect ensures the surgeon is able to safely tuck any herniated nerve roots back into the thecal sac to prevent further injury. Dural repair is made easier with unfettered access to the dural tear and without the need of special equipment for oversewing the rent within a narrow tube. Muscle and fat pledgets are easily harvested should the surgeon desire these to reinforce a primary repair of an unapposable tear. A tight, multilayered closure can then eliminate dead space and promote wound healing, and is the main line of defense against pseudomeningocele formation, transcutaneous CSF leak, and wound infection.

14.5 Case Illustration

A 63-year-old woman is undergoing an L4–L5 minimally invasive transforaminal interbody fusion via a 26-mm diameter tubular retractor. While removing the ligamentum flavum to expose the thecal sac and disc space, an unintended durotomy is created with a Kerrison rongeur. The durotomy is approximately 5 mm in length with CSF briskly emanating. Options for repair of the durotomy are considered.

14.6 Surgical Technique in Minimally Invasive Surgery

For the purposes of this discussion, standard access to the posterior spinal canal via a tubular retractor system is assumed.[35] Once a durotomy is created, either incidentally or intentionally for intradural access, efforts should be made to avoid excessive influx of blood products intradurally to limit the extent of inflammation and possible postoperative arachnoiditis.

Partial-thickness durotomies with intact arachnoid are typically treated with fibrin glue alone or with an additional tiny piece of Gelfoam (Pfizer, Kalamazoo, MI) soaked in local blood placed over the defect. For full-thickness unintended durotomies, the possibility of primary repair is assessed on a case-by-case basis. If the durotomy is not amenable to primary suture repair (e.g., located at the edge or undersurface of the bony opening or the ventral surface of the dura), a small blood-soaked piece of Gelfoam or dural substitute is laid over the dural defect (often gently tucked under the bony edge to secure it in place), followed by fibrin glue. For those durotomies that are amenable to primary repair (i.e., those more dorsally located), a variety of suture is available on appropriately sized needles, including 4–0 Nurolon, 5–0 Prolene, or 6–0 Gore-Tex sutures (Ethicon, Somerville, NJ). The latter suture has the advantage of the needle diameter being smaller than the suture diameter, resulting in fewer "stitch-hole leaks." The dura can be routinely closed using a commercially available, specialized set of dural repair instruments that includes two modified needle drivers, a bayoneted Chitwood Knot Pusher, and suture-cutting scissors (Scanlan International, St. Paul, MN).[7] These instruments have a bayoneted offset that allows proper microscopic visualization during needle driving and also allow the knots to be thrown outside the tubular retractor and seated down to the dura using the knot pusher. If the repair is not watertight to Valsalva's maneuver, a small piece of locally harvested paraspinal muscle can be sutured in as a buttress graft over the leak site. Fibrin glue is then routinely applied over the defect as well. After allowing the fibrin glue to congeal, the tubular retractor is slowly removed while obtaining hemostasis in the paraspinal musculature. The wound is then closed in layers using interrupted sutures for fascia and subcutaneous tissues followed by an adhesive sealant for the skin. No subarachnoid or subfascial drains are used. The patients are kept on bedrest overnight only and are allowed to fully mobilize on the morning of postoperative day 1.

14.7 Surgical Technique in Open Surgery

Upon noting the CSF leak, an initial attempt should be made to repair the dural defect and complete the surgery through the MIS approach as described above. However, in the rare case in which the surgical access limits the ability to repair the defect or

there are other complicating factors, one can consider transitioning to open surgery. Examples of situations in which open repair should be considered include nerve roots herniated from the defect that are difficult to reinsert into the thecal sac or a defect that extends beyond the area visualized by the retractors.

Once the decision has been made to convert to an open approach to aid in the dural repair, the wound is extended and retractors swapped to ensure excellent visualization. Of note, based on the original surgical trajectory (often a Wiltse or transmuscular approach), exposure will likely be more lateral than a standard open midline approach. While a standard open procedure involves stripping the muscular attachments to the posterior elements, opening laterally entails a less familiar transmuscular approach. The surgeons should take pains to separate the muscles longitudinally and take advantage of the natural plane between the multifidus and longissimus components of the sacrospinalis muscle as in the Wiltse approach.[36] The surgeon may also choose to close the original MIS incision and perform a true midline open approach and resection of appropriate bony elements for a broader exposure as the remaining spinous process and muscle mass medial to the MIS incision may continue to hinder visualization.

To complete an adequate repair the surgeon must completely define the durotomy edges. Often, durotomies occur under the laminectomy defect or near the insertion of the yellow ligament.[37] This is an awkward location to visualize, and further bone removal may be necessary. Care is taken to avoid injuring any herniated nerve roots. Nerve roots should be reduced and held in place with a surgical patty to prevent reherniation and minimize further CSF egress while the area around the defect is prepared. If the nerve roots are not reducible and are being strangulated in the defect, the durotomy may be enlarged and CSF drained to allow the roots to be safely tucked into the thecal sac.

Once the durotomy margins are defined, suture is used to close the defect in a watertight fashion as above. In most cases, a simple figure-of-eight or running suture will completely occlude the leak site. However, in cases where a portion of dura is missing, a dural patch graft can be used, or a muscle pledget can be oversewn without pulling the dural leaves together completely. At this point, a Valsalva maneuver is used to confirm the watertight repair. A dural sealant may be added as well.

The most important component of the open repair is watertight wound closure. Once the surgery is completed, a tight, multilayer closure is required to reduce dead space and the potential for pseudomeningocele formation. If a subfascial drain is required, instructions should be relayed to floor and house staff to be mindful of the possibility of ongoing CSF leak, and to remove the drain from suction should that be suspected. A tight fascial closure is performed with interrupted suture. This is followed by a running suture over the interrupted suture line to ensure this layer is watertight. The remainder of the incision is closed in standard fashion. The patient is kept on bedrest overnight and mobilized the morning following surgery.

14.8 Discussion of Minimally Invasive Surgery

A search of the National Library of Medicine via PubMed was performed using the following search strategy: spinal surgery

OR spine surgery AND durotomy OR dural tear OR cerebrospinal fluid leak OR cerebrospinal fluid cutaneous fistula OR CSF cutaneous fistula OR CSF leak AND minimally invasive as well as spinal surgery OR spine surgery AND open versus minimally invasive. These generated 147 references, of which the titles and abstracts were reviewed for relevance. Full text papers were then reviewed for relevance and their bibliographies searched for additional relevant publications. Studies that discussed the management of intraoperative durotomies during MIS surgery (with or without comparison to open surgery) with methods consistent with evidence levels I to IV were included. Solitary case reports were excluded. A total of 14 publications meeting the above criteria were identified. Key information from each selected manuscript is abstracted in the evidence table (▶ Table 14.1).

In general, the literature pertaining to the optimal management and clinical outcome of durotomies in MIS spinal surgery is scarce. The majority of publications directly examining MIS versus open techniques in spinal surgery do not focus on the issue of intraoperative durotomy. Many of these studies report rates of durotomy for each group but rarely describe details of repair technique or postoperative sequelae. Those that provide such data generally show no statistical differences in rates of unintended durotomy or postoperative CSF-related complications.[10,12,13,14,15]

14.8.1 Level I Evidence in Minimally Invasive Surgery

There is no level I evidence available regarding the management of durotomy during MIS surgery.

14.8.2 Level II Evidence in Minimally Invasive Surgery

There is no level II evidence available regarding the management of durotomy during MIS surgery.

14.8.3 Level III and IV Evidence in Minimally Invasive Surgery

Wong et al reported a retrospective comparative cohort study examining symptomatic CSF leaks between patients undergoing one-level or two-level lumbar foraminotomy, discectomy, or laminectomy using MIS versus open techniques at a single institution over 5 years.[11] A total of 863 patients were reviewed (319 MIS, 544 open). MIS patients were slightly older, and there were a nonsignificant slightly higher number of revision cases in the open group. Sixty-four patients had an unintended durotomy resulting in an incidence of 9.0% in the open group and 4.7% in the MIS group ($p = 0.02$). For revision cases in particular, the incidence was 14.4% for open and 7.8% for MIS. The surgeons suture-repaired the majority of open durotomies (27 out of 49) but only 2 out of 15 MIS durotomies, instead relying on Gelfoam, artificial dural onlay, and/or sealants to treat the durotomies. There was no difference in operative times for durotomy cases between open and MIS. Total hospital length of stay was 33% shorter in the MIS group than the open group. Within

each cohort, durotomy significantly extended length of stay. MIS durotomy cases required 46% fewer days of bedrest than the open durotomy patients. Eight open durotomy patients (1.5% of total, 16% of all open durotomy) required lumbar drain placement, whereas none of the MIS durotomy patients required lumbar drainage. Reoperation for persistent CSF leak was required in 25% of open durotomy cases versus none of the MIS durotomy cases ($p < 0.01$). Multivariate logistic regression analysis including numerous potentially related variables revealed that open surgery patients had an odds ratio of 2.3 (confidence interval [CI] = 1.2–3.7) for unintended durotomy compared to MIS. This publication provides level III evidence that during lumbar decompressive procedures, there is an increased incidence of unintended durotomy and durotomy-related postoperative complications (reoperation) during open surgery compared to MIS surgery.

In addition to this level III study, there are five unintended durotomy and eight intended durotomy level IV studies describing the management of durotomy during MIS surgery. Details of these can be found in the evidence table with citations on MIS unintended durotomies listed first followed by publications on MIS intended durotomies (▶ Table 14.1). Summing all of the literature in the evidence table, a total of 169 patients with MIS durotomies are studied, 99 unintended and 70 intended. Of all these MIS durotomy patients, only one of the unintended (transient meningismus) and two of the intended (one reoperation for cutaneous leak; one reoperation for pseudomeningocele) had postoperative sequelae of the durotomy resulting in a total 1.9% rate of postoperative CSF-related complications from durotomy (1.0% for unintended and 2.9% for intended). This rate is below the typically reported rates of postdurotomy complications from open spine surgery,[1,2,3] as highlighted in the large prospective cohort study by McMahon et al.[6]

14.9 Complications in Minimally Invasive Surgery

In theory, inadequate dural closure could lead to persistent CSF leak, but as described above, this has not been reported with any increased frequency in the MIS literature. Unique rates of nerve injury or other untoward complications from difficulties with dural closure during MIS are also not apparent in the available literature.

14.10 Conclusion of Minimally Invasive Surgery

There is adequate level III and IV evidence to support a Grade 1C recommendation that durotomies during MIS surgery can be managed safely and successfully using MIS techniques. Experience with postoperative complications from durotomies during open spinal surgery (and the very low incidence of these complications after MIS durotomies) further suggests that conversion to an open procedure after MIS durotomy not only provides no apparent benefit, but might, in fact, *increase* the risk for postoperative CSF-related problems.

Table 14.1 Literature on management of durotomy during MIS surgery

Authors (year)	Study design	Level	No. of patients	Findings	Comments
Wong et al (2014)[11]	Retrospective comparative cohort	III	863 (319 MIS, 544 open); 11 surgeons	Durotomy rates: open 9%, MIS 4.7% (OR, 2.3). Reoperation for persistent CSF leak in 25% open and 0% MIS durotomies	Increased incidence of durotomy and subsequent complications from durotomy in open vs. MIS
Senker et al (2013)[45]	Retrospective case series	IV	10 patients with MIS unintended durotomies (out of 72 total MIS TLIFs)	5/10 suture repaired. One patient with transient meningismus. No reoperations	Wide range of days of bedrest used
McMahon et al (2012)[6]	Prospective cohort	IV	104 unintended durotomies in 3,000 spinal procedures. 9/271 MIS (3.3%) and 95/2,729 open (3.5%)	No difference in incidence of durotomy between open and MIS. Post-op CSF-related complications seen in 7% of open vs. 0% of MIS durotomies	No statistics performed comparing open to MIS. All MIS durotomies managed with dural replacement onlay only
Ruban and O'Toole (2011)[7]	Retrospective case series	IV	53 patients with MIS unintended durotomies (out of 563 total MIS cases)	No conversion to open. Less than 24 h bedrest used. No cases of post-op symptomatic CSF leak or need for reoperation	Authors present algorithm for intraoperative management of MIS durotomy
Song and Park (2011)[18]	Retrospective case series	IV	7 patients with MIS unintended durotomies	U-clips used to repair durotomy. No post-op CSF-related symptoms or complications	6 out of 7 patients discharged on day of surgery
Than et al (2008)[19]	Retrospective case series	IV	5 patients with MIS unintended durotomies	4/5 treated with dural substitute and sealant. No post-op CSF-related symptoms or complications	Less than 48 h bedrest used
Gandhi and German (2013)[23]	Retrospective case series	IV	26 patients with MIS intended durotomy for a variety of intradural pathology	No post-op CSF-related symptoms or complications. Repair with either suture or dural substitute	Less than 24 h bedrest
Nzokou et al (2013)[27]	Retrospective case series	IV	4 patients with MIS intended durotomy for intradural neoplasms	No post-op CSF-related symptoms or complications. Dural repair with suture	
Haque et al (2013)[25]	Retrospective case series	IV	2 patients with MIS intended durotomy for intradural neoplasms	No post-op CSF-related symptoms or complications. Dural repair with suture	Authors emphasize type of suture used
Haji et al (2011)[24]	Retrospective case series	IV	15 patients with MIS intended durotomy for intradural neoplasms	1 out of 15 patients required open reoperation for persistent CSF leak. No other post-op CSF-related issues in other 14 patients	All patients with primary suture repair
Mannion et al (2011)[26]	Retrospective case series	IV	11 patients with MIS intended durotomy for intradural neoplasms	Only post-op CSF-related complication was cutaneous leak in 1 patient that was converted to open during index surgery for adequate tumor removal. No CSF-related issues in MIS cases	Three different dural repair strategies used
Potts et al (2010)[30]	Retrospective comparative cohort	IV	3 patients with MIS intended durotomy for tethered spinal cord release compared to 3 open releases	No statistically significant differences in EBL or LOS. Shorter incision in MIS cases. One MIS patient had reoperation for pseudomeningocele	Extremely small number of patients and paucity of detail downgrades study to level IV and disallows useful comparisons
Tredway et al (2006)[32]	Retrospective case series	IV	6 patients with MIS intended durotomy for intradural neoplasms	No post-op CSF-related symptoms or complications. Dural repair with suture	
Tredway et al (2007)[31]	Retrospective case series	IV	3 patients with MIS intended durotomy for tethered spinal cord release	No post-op CSF-related symptoms or complications. Dural repair with suture	

Abbreviations: CSF, cerebrospinal fluid; EBL, estimated blood loss; LOS, length of stay; MIS, minimally invasive surgery; TLIFs, transforaminal lumbar interbody fusions.

Note: Unintended durotomy literature is listed first, followed by intended durotomy literature.

14.11 Discussion of Open Surgery

Similarly, a search of the National Library of Medicine via PubMed was performed using the following search strategy: spinal surgery OR spine surgery AND durotomy OR dural tear OR cerebrospinal fluid leak OR cerebrospinal fluid cutaneous fistula OR CSF cutaneous fistula OR CSF leak AND spinal surgery OR spine surgery AND open versus minimally invasive. These generated 882 references, of which the titles and abstracts were reviewed for relevance as described above. A total of three publications comparing MIS and open repair for CSF leak were noted,[6,11,30] although there was no direct study of converting an MIS case to open following durotomy (▶ Table 14.1).

14.11.1 Level I Evidence in Open Surgery

There is no level I evidence available regarding the conversion to an open approach following durotomy during MIS surgery.

14.11.2 Level II Evidence in Open Surgery

There is no level II evidence available regarding the conversion to an open approach following durotomy during MIS surgery.

14.11.3 Level III and IV Evidence in Open Surgery

There is no evidence supporting the need to convert from MIS to open surgery in the event of a dural tear. The three cohort studies noted in the MIS section were the only direct comparison of complications in MIS and open surgery following CSF leak, although there is a large amount of literature regarding the detrimental effect of CSF leak in open surgery. Thus, the discussion regarding conversion of an MIS to open surgery following unintended durotomy is hypothetical.

Of the three cohort studies, few conclusions can be made. In all cases the rate of CSF-related complications is higher in the open cohorts; however, each study had serious flaws. Potts et al studied the rate of complications following tethered cord repair, but details and patient numbers were too few to draw meaningful conclusions.[30] McMahon et al studied the incidence of unintended durotomies and did note that no MIS durotomy lead to a CSF-related complication[6]; however, there is no direct comparison between MIS and open surgery or attempts to control for case type, making conclusions more difficult. Finally, Wong et al studied a cohort of open and MIS surgeries,[11] noting a far higher incidence of complications in the open group. However, questions raised over the open surgeons' general experience level and high rate of reoperation make true comparison questionable. As noted above, the CSF-related complication rate following durotomy in MIS surgery appears to be lower than that in open surgery. Most importantly, there is no evidence that converting an MIS case to open would increase or decrease the rate or severity of complications.

The historical experience with open cases is larger than MIS, with far more than 169 open durotomies recorded in the literature. This has provided the opportunity to report rarer complications such as late nerve root entrapment in incompletely repaired dural tears.[38,39,40,41,42,43] It is theorized that the nerve root herniates due to the intradural–extradural pressure gradient. Therefore, the risk of these complications may be reduced with the dead space elimination of MIS surgery; however, symptomatic postprocedure root herniations have been reported following lumbar puncture,[44] in which there is virtually no dead space. Unfortunately, strangled roots can result in lasting radicular symptoms. Thus, it is important that herniated roots are reduced and contained within the thecal sac. If the nerve roots are irreducible and strangled in the defect, the durotomy may be lengthened and spinal fluid released to allow the rootlets to be tucked inside. In cases where this is impossible due to the access afforded by MIS equipment, open conversion may be worthwhile.

14.12 Complications in Open Surgery

The complications of dural tear in open surgery are well documented. These include postural headaches, wound problems including pseudomeningocele, dural-cutaneous CSF fistulas, and infections, nerve root entrapment injuries, and intracranial hemorrhages.

14.13 Conclusion of Open Surgery

In general, it is unlikely that an MIS durotomy would require conversion to an open procedure. Indeed, such a conversion would eliminate the reduced dead space, which is likely the primary defense against CSF-related complications. However, there are instances in which conversion may be required to increase the working area and facilitate a mandatory repair.

The main issues are CSF leaks with irreducible nerve roots, which are difficult to access outside the surgical field or under a bony edge. If attempts fail to reduce the roots, or the roots continually reherniate and the durotomy is inaccessible, the surgeon should consider converting the field to a more accessible surgical corridor. In this case, the surgeon is sacrificing a lower infection, pseudomeningocele, and CSF fistula rate of the MIS corridor to ensure that a nerve root is not harmed.

14.14 Editors' Commentary

14.14.1 Minimally Invasive Surgery

Contrary to our initial fears of the difficulty of correcting dural tears in MIS surgery, MIS technique has made durotomy a relatively insignificant event. There are two routine scenarios in which durotomy is encountered. The first is in common procedures such as discectomy, decompression of stenosis, or MIS fusions such as in the TLIF procedure. In most cases, these durotomies are accidental and relatively limited in size. In my experience over the past 20 years, direct closure of these durotomies is not necessary. The working channel tube size in these cases is usually small (between 14 and 25 mm), minimal soft tissue is dissected, and all of the remaining soft tissue is vascularized and innervated. The dura can simply be sealed with a patch of Gelfoam and dural sealant. When the tube is removed, there is no or minimal dead space remaining. The viable muscle closes down on the dural sealant and prevents pseudomeningocele formation. To help with the dural seal, I keep the patient on bedrest overnight. In the past 20 years, I have had only one case in which further treatment was required to seal a pseudomeningocele in this situation (a blood patch).

The second scenario is when greater soft-tissue retraction is required to perform more extensive surgeries, such as intradural tumor resection or vertebrectomy. In these cases, the amount of exposure created provides ample room to use standard dural closure techniques. Once again, however, the viable dilated muscle tissue helps seal the durotomy with minimal creation of dead space. Thus, contrary to our initial fears, dural tears are now of little concern in MIS surgery.

14.14.2 Open Surgery

An adequate dural seal following a CSF leak is important to prevent potential complications such as a symptomatic pseudomeningocele, spinal fluid headache and meningitis. Variables such as tear location, size, and ability to appose dural margins to facilitate primary repair provide wide variation in the difficulty of this task for the surgeon. The limited surgical corridor available during MIS procedures adds an extra layer of difficulty to this procedure not only in terms of manipulating needles and needle drivers to pass suture through the dura but also in terms of having an adequate safe zone where spinal fluid can be suctioned without undue risk to exposed nerve roots. Those surgeons who have an able assistant such as an upper level resident, fellow, or another surgeon also lose the advantage this arrangement provides because there is limited room when working within a tubular retractor. Many technique descriptions for MIS procedures mention dural repair as an afterthought and more commonly describe nonprimary repair strategies with a heavy reliance on Gelfoam and sealants, techniques only considered to be adjuvants in open dural repair. Any advantage that MIS provides in terms of reduction of dead space is likely lost by a compromised ability to repair dural injuries primarily. Future technologies may provide more successful methods to repair dural injuries within the confines of a limited surgical corridor but current strategies are lacking; the inability to adequately address associated complications is a red flag for adoption of a new procedure.

References

[1] Bosacco SJ, Gardner MJ, Guille JT. Evaluation and treatment of dural tears in lumbar spine surgery: a review. Clin Orthop Relat Res. 2001(389):238–247

[2] Cammisa FP, Jr, Girardi FP, Sangani PK, Parvataneni HK, Cadag S, Sandhu HS. Incidental durotomy in spine surgery. Spine. 2000; 25(20):2663–2667

[3] Eismont FJ, Wiesel SW, Rothman RH. Treatment of dural tears associated with spinal surgery. J Bone Joint Surg Am. 1981; 63(7):1132–1136

[4] Epstein NE. The frequency and etiology of intraoperative dural tears in 110 predominantly geriatric patients undergoing multilevel laminectomy with noninstrumented fusions. J Spinal Disord Tech. 2007; 20(5):380–386

[5] Khan MH, Rihn J, Steele G, et al. Postoperative management protocol for incidental dural tears during degenerative lumbar spine surgery: a review of 3,183 consecutive degenerative lumbar cases. Spine. 2006; 31(22):2609–2613

[6] McMahon P, Dididze M, Levi AD. Incidental durotomy after spinal surgery: a prospective study in an academic institution. J Neurosurg Spine. 2012; 17(1):30–36

[7] Ruban D, O'Toole JE. Management of incidental durotomy in minimally invasive spine surgery. Neurosurg Focus. 2011; 31(4):E15

[8] Tafazal SI, Sell PJ. Incidental durotomy in lumbar spine surgery: incidence and management. Eur Spine J. 2005; 14(3):287–290

[9] Williams BJ, Sansur CA, Smith JS, et al. Incidence of unintended durotomy in spine surgery based on 108,478 cases. Neurosurgery. 2011; 68(1):117–123, discussion 123–124

[10] Ang CL, Phak-Boon Tow B, Fook S, et al. Minimally invasive compared with open lumbar laminotomy: no functional benefits at 6 or 24 months after surgery. Spine J. 2015; 15(8):1705–1712

[11] Wong AP, Shih P, Smith TR, et al. Comparison of symptomatic cerebral spinal fluid leak between patients undergoing minimally invasive versus open lumbar foraminotomy, discectomy, or laminectomy. World Neurosurg. 2014; 81(3(–)(4):634–640

[12] Fourney DR, Dettori JR, Norvell DC, Dekutoski MB. Does minimal access tubular assisted spine surgery increase or decrease complications in spinal decompression or fusion? Spine. 2010; 35(9) Suppl:S57–S65

[13] Lee KH, Yue WM, Yeo W, Soeharno H, Tan SB. Clinical and radiological outcomes of open versus minimally invasive transforaminal lumbar interbody fusion. Eur Spine J. 2012; 21(11):2265–2270

[14] Lee P, Liu JC, Fessler RG. Perioperative results following open and minimally invasive single-level lumbar discectomy. J Clin Neurosci. 2011; 18(12):1667–1670

[15] Tian NF, Wu YS, Zhang XL, Xu HZ, Chi YL, Mao FM. Minimally invasive versus open transforaminal lumbar interbody fusion: a meta-analysis based on the current evidence. Eur Spine J. 2013; 22(8):1741–1749

[16] Chou D, Wang VY, Khan AS. Primary dural repair during minimally invasive microdiscectomy using standard operating room instruments. Neurosurgery. 2009; 64(5) Suppl 2:356–358, discussion 358–359

[17] Shaffrey CI, Spotnitz WD, Shaffrey ME, Jane JA. Neurosurgical applications of fibrin glue: augmentation of dural closure in 134 patients. Neurosurgery. 1990; 26(2):207–210

[18] Song D, Park P. Primary closure of inadvertent durotomies utilizing the U-Clip in minimally invasive spinal surgery. Spine. 2011; 36(26):E1753–E1757

[19] Than KD, Wang AC, Etame AB, La Marca F, Park P. Postoperative management of incidental durotomy in minimally invasive lumbar spinal surgery. Minim Invasive Neurosurg. 2008; 51(5):263–266

[20] Wang JC, Bohlman HH, Riew KD. Dural tears secondary to operations on the lumbar spine. Management and results after a two-year-minimum follow-up of eighty-eight patients. J Bone Joint Surg Am. 1998; 80(12):1728–1732

[21] Diaz Day J. Minimally invasive surgical closure of a spinal dural arteriovenous fistula. Minim Invasive Neurosurg. 2008; 51(3):183–186

[22] Fontes RB, Tan LA, O'Toole JE. Minimally invasive treatment of spinal dural arteriovenous fistula with the use of intraoperative indocyanine green angiography. Neurosurg Focus. 2013; 35(2) Suppl:5

[23] Gandhi RH, German JW. Minimally invasive approach for the treatment of intradural spinal pathology. Neurosurg Focus. 2013; 35(2):E5

[24] Haji FA, Cenic A, Crevier L, Murty N, Reddy K. Minimally invasive approach for the resection of spinal neoplasm. Spine. 2011; 36(15):E1018–E1026

[25] Haque RM, Hashmi SZ, Ahmed Y, Uddin O, Ogden AT, Fessler R. Primary dural repair in minimally invasive spine surgery. Case Rep Med. 2013; 2013:876351

[26] Mannion RJ, Nowitzke AM, Efendy J, Wood MJ. Safety and efficacy of intradural extramedullary spinal tumor removal using a minimally invasive approach. Neurosurgery. 2011; 68(1) Suppl Operative:208–216, discussion 216

[27] Nzokou A, Weil AG, Shedid D. Minimally invasive removal of thoracic and lumbar spinal tumors using a nonexpandable tubular retractor. J Neurosurg Spine. 2013; 19(6):708–715

[28] O'Toole JE, Eichholz KM, Fessler RG. Minimally invasive approaches to vertebral column and spinal cord tumors. Neurosurg Clin N Am. 2006; 17(4):491–506

[29] O'Toole JE, Eichholz KM, Fessler RG. Minimally invasive insertion of syringosubarachnoid shunt for posttraumatic syringomyelia: technical case report. Neurosurgery. 2007; 61(5) Suppl 2:E331–E332, discussion –E332

[30] Potts MB, Wu JC, Gupta N, Mummaneni PV. Minimally invasive tethered cord release in adults: a comparison of open and mini-open approaches. Neurosurg Focus. 2010; 29(1):E7

[31] Tredway TL, Musleh W, Christie SD, Khavkin Y, Fessler RG, Curry DJ. A novel minimally invasive technique for spinal cord untethering. Neurosurgery. 2007; 60(2) Suppl 1:ONS70–ONS74, discussion ONS74

[32] Tredway TL, Santiago P, Hrubes MR, Song JK, Christie SD, Fessler RG. Minimally invasive resection of intradural-extramedullary spinal neoplasms. Neurosurgery. 2006; 58(1) Suppl:ONS52–ONS58, discussion ONS52–ONS58

[33] Beier AD, Soo TM, Claybrooks R. Subdural hematoma after microdiscectomy: a case report and review of the literature. Spine J. 2009; 9(10):e9–e12

[34] Lu CH, Ho ST, Kong SS, Cherng CH, Wong CS. Intracranial subdural hematoma after unintended durotomy during spine surgery. Can J Anaesth. 2002; 49(1):100–102

[35] Holly LT, Schwender JD, Rouben DP, Foley KT. Minimally invasive transforaminal lumbar interbody fusion: indications, technique, and complications. Neurosurg Focus. 2006; 20(3):E6

[36] Vialle R, Wicart P, Drain O, Dubousset J, Court C. The Wiltse paraspinal approach to the lumbar spine revisited: an anatomic study. Clin Orthop Relat Res. 2006; 445(445):175–180

[37] Takahashi Y, Sato T, Hyodo H, et al. Incidental durotomy during lumbar spine surgery: risk factors and anatomic locations: clinical article. J Neurosurg Spine. 2013; 18(2):165–169

[38] Asha MJ, George KJ, Choksey M. Pseudomeningocele presenting with cauda equina syndrome: is a 'ball-valve' theory the answer? Br J Neurosurg. 2011; 25(6):766–768

[39] Choi JH, Kim JS, Jang JS, Lee DY. Transdural nerve rootlet entrapment in the intervertebral disc space through minimal dural tear : report of 4 cases. J Korean Neurosurg Soc. 2013; 53(1):52–56

[40] Hosono N, Yonenobu K, Ono K. Postoperative cervical pseudomeningocele with herniation of the spinal cord. Spine. 1995; 20(19):2147–2150

[41] Nishi S, Hashimoto N, Takagi Y, Tsukahara T. Herniation and entrapment of a nerve root secondary to an unrepaired small dural laceration at lumbar hemilaminectomies. Spine. 1995; 20(23):2576–2579

[42] Pavlou G, Bucur SD, van Hille PT. Entrapped spinal nerve roots in a pseudomeningocoele as a complication of previous spinal surgery. Acta Neurochir (Wien). 2006; 148(2):215–219, discussion 219–220

[43] Töppich HG, Feldmann H, Sandvoss G, Meyer F. Intervertebral space nerve root entrapment after lumbar disc surgery. Two cases. Spine. 1994; 19(2):249–250

[44] Hasegawa K, Yamamoto N. Nerve root herniation secondary to lumbar puncture in the patient with lumbar canal stenosis. A case report. Spine. 1999; 24(9):915–917

[45] Senker W, Meznik C, Avian A, Berghold A. The frequency of accidental dural tears in minimally invasive spinal fusion techniques. J Neurol Surg A Cent Eur Neurosurg. 2013; 74(6):373–377

15 Do Minimally Invasive Techniques Broaden the Scope for Geriatric Spine Surgery?

Michael Y. Wang

15.1 The Evolution of Modern Minimally Invasive Techniques

The development of minimally invasive surgery (MIS) techniques for spinal surgery was innovated in large part due to the hope of achieving similar surgical results with fewer attendant sequelae due to reduced soft-tissue trauma. If realized, the end result would be (1) reduced pain, (2) shorter hospitalization periods, (3) fewer complications, (4) reduced narcotic use, and (5) improved clinical outcomes.[1] However, to date there exists no level I evidence to indicate that these goals have been fully realized. Nevertheless, a large proportion of surgeons employ various MIS methods due to the significant morbidity associated with spinal surgeries.

These purported benefits of MIS would have a disproportionate positive impact when applied to compromised patient populations, such as those who are frail, immunosuppressed, or elderly. The limited functional reserve of these patients renders them more susceptible to complications and other untoward effects of surgery, and these patients typically have longer hospital stays and surgical recovery times.[2,3,4] Thus, the application of MIS spine surgery to the elderly may have beneficial effects not seen when analyzing data from a standard patient population.

15.2 Challenges with Applying the Principles of Evidence-Based Medicine

The principles of contemporary evidence-based medicine (EBM) are designed to achieve the laudable goals of providing input to clinical decision-making through the analysis of high-quality clinical research. However, the practical application of EBM criteria becomes problematic in the arena of MIS and in specialized populations for several reasons.

First, the quality standards for clinical studies rate randomized prospective studies as the highest and most authoritative level of clinical evidence. However, in actual practice it is extremely difficult to perform a randomized trial in an ethical manner. Patients will typically have strong opinions, right or wrong, about their desire to undergo a surgery in the traditional open manner or using an MIS method. This makes equivalent patient allocation in a randomized trial extremely difficult and results in a high rate of crossover or refusal to participate. Also, it is rare for a surgeon to truly have equal expertise in both open and MIS, particularly for complex operations. Most surgeons will have an inherent bias toward one approach or the other, rendering them more expert at one approach.

Second, there is a great diversity of MIS procedures available. The box below shows a sampling of common MIS procedures that I perform. There are countless more performed by surgeons throughout the world. In many instances, several MIS options exist for treating a distinct pathological entity (in addition to an open method). For example, for neurogenic claudication due to degenerative lumbar stenosis confined to the L4/L5 level without back pain, the open surgery may be a standard laminectomy. However, MIS options would include a hemilaminotomy with medial facetectomy for bilateral decompression or an interspinous spacer (among other methods). How, then, are we to compare these methods without a complex trial with high sample numbers?

Common MIS Spine Procedures

- Endoscopic transforaminal discectomy
- Interlaminar endoscopic discectomy
- Tubular interlaminar microdiscectomy
- Endoscopic-assisted tubular interlaminar microdiscectomy
- Tubular far lateral microdiscectomy
- Tubular stenosis decompression with hemilaminotomy + medial facetectomy
- Endoscopic awake lumbar interbody fusion
- Tubular minimally invasive transforaminal interbody fusion
- Lateral interbody fusion (XLIF/DLIF)
- Spinal deformities correction with multilevel MIS TLIF
- Spinal deformities correction with multilevel lateral interbody fusion
- Spinal deformities correction with mini-open pedicle subtraction osteotomy
- Vertebroplasty/kyphoplasty
- Percutaneous fixation for spinal trauma
- Tubular retropleural transthoracic vertebrectomy for metastatic cancer
- Nonfusion disc preserving anterior cervical decompression

Third, there is significant heterogeneity in how any given procedure is performed. This is due to intersurgeon differences in philosophy, training, skill level, and custom. For example, in the landmark trial by Arts et al, the participating European surgeons, experts in MIS, found no benefit from using a tubular dilator for lumbar discectomy.[5] However, the innovators of the tubular retractor have publicly stated that these devices were intended to be inserted through the muscle tissue, dilating it. This is in contradistinction to the investigators who placed the tube through a subperiosteal pocket. Could this difference have accounted for the negative findings of the study?

Finally, the field of spinal medicine is notorious for the heterogeneity of the patient population. Typical clinical studies will account for demographics, disease subtype, and severity to ensure randomization or allocation into equivalent groups. However, many spinal diseases are heterogeneous in presentation. Because so many of the key outcome indicators measure subjective data (pain and disability), the preoperative state must also be accounted for. Thus, a properly conducted study would ideally account for psychological, social, economic, and environmental factors that are not typically measured in surgical studies.

15.3 Existing Evidence

15.3.1 Vertebral Body Cement Augmentation

The advent of vertebral body augmentation (VBA) represents a significant advance in the treatment of the elderly spine. The initial report of the technique was for the treatment of vertebral body angioma.[6] However, in current application, VBA is used primarily for the treatment of painful osteoporotic vertebral body fractures without neurological deficits. The injectate is typically polymethyl methacrylate (PMMA), which is a viscous liquid that rapidly polymerizes to a solid after placement into the cancellous bone through a needle. The two most common techniques for VBA are vertebroplasty and kyphoplasty, the difference being that in kyphoplasty a cavity within the vertebral body is first created using a balloon to expand the vertebral body prior to cement injection.

VBA was a significant advance because it was a completely new surgical procedure. It was not intended to replace an "open" surgical option because painful osteoporotic fractures are seldom treated with surgery. This is because prior to VBA no viable therapeutic option existed besides bracing and medical management. The patients susceptible to these fragility fractures were typically medically compromised, and an open fusion operation would be suboptimal given high rates of metallic hardware pullout, pseudarthrosis, and adjacent level problems.

Thus, comparisons of VBA with open surgery have not been performed. However, numerous randomized trials have compared VBA to nonsurgical treatments (▶ Table 15.1). The VERTOS European trials were the first randomized controlled trials of vertebroplasty. The first VERTOS trial had 34 patients, with an emphasis on short-term results. VERTOS II followed shortly thereafter and randomized 202 patients (101 vertebroplasty, 101 conservative treatment). The vertebroplasty group experienced better pain relief than the conservative group, with a mean VAS (visual analog scale) drop of 5.2 with vertebroplasty as compared with 2.7 in the conservative group at 1-month follow-up. At 1 year, the change from baseline was 5.7 with vertebroplasty and 3.7 with conservative treatment.[7,8] This was followed by ongoing trials (VERTOS IV) designed to expand the sample size and utilize a sham control group as opposed to a conservatively treated comparator cohort.[9]

The positive effects were corroborated in a randomized controlled study by Blasco et al.[10] Patients were randomized to either vertebroplasty ($n = 64$) or conservative treatment ($n = 61$). While both groups showed improvement in VAS scores at 2 months, the effect was greater with vertebroplasty (mean 3.07 point drop vs. 1.59). This reflected a mean 42% reduction in pain with VBA versus 25% with conservative care. The Blasco study did, however, identify a higher rate of new fractures during the 12-month follow-up period: 29 new fractures in 17 patients treated with vertebroplasty versus 8 new fractures in 8 of the conservatively treated patients were seen.

However, two papers published simultaneously in the *New England Journal of Medicine* concluded that there was no significant benefit from VBA compared to a sham surgery. In the Kallmes et al's study, patients were randomized to either vertebroplasty ($n = 68$) or sham surgery ($n = 63$).[11] One month after surgery, there was no significant difference between the groups on SF-36, EQ-5D, Roland Morris Disability Questionnaire, Study of Osteoporotic Fractures–Activities of Daily Living (SOF–ADL), and VAS. However, there was a trend toward improvements in VAS with vertebroplasty (64 vs. 48%, $p = 0.06$). In the accompanying Buchbinder et al's trial, 78 patients were enrolled (38 in the vertebroplasty group and 40 in the placebo group). There was no significant improvement in the vertebroplasty group compared to placebo at any time point, but both groups experienced significant improvement. Improvements in pain for vertebroplasty versus placebo at 3 months were 2.6 and 1.9, respectively, which was not a statistically significant difference.[12]

15.3.2 Interspinous Spacers for Lumbar Stenosis

Interspinous spacers function by creating increased space and slight kyphosis between the adjacent spinous processes. Through this action, some stretching of the ligamentum flavum and opening of the neuroforamina occur. In this manner, neurogenic claudication can thus potentially be relieved through indirect decompression. This can result in 20 to 62% increase in central canal area.[13] This obviates the need for a direct decompression, which is achieved by actually removing the offending anatomy by performing a laminectomy or some variant of a laminectomy. Interspinous spacer surgery can also potentially be performed under local or regional anesthesia, thus making the surgery potentially much safer in elderly patients.

In order to obtain U.S. Food and Drug Administration (FDA) approval, the first commercially available interspinous spacer, the X-Stop (Medtronic; Memphis, TN), had to undergo an investigational device exemption (IDE) trial.[14] Thus, level I evidence exists for the application of this device for the treatment of neurogenic claudication. In that trial, 100 patients were randomized to surgical treatment, while 91 underwent conservative treatment including epidural injections. The primary outcome was the Zurich Claudication Questionnaire, an accepted patient-driven measure of neurogenic claudication. Patients were assessed at 6 weeks, 6 months, 1 year, and 2 years after treatment initiation. At every time point, the surgically treated patients did better than the conservatively treated patients, and at 2 years 45.4% of the surgically treated versus 7.4% of the conservatively treated patients had improved. During the follow-up, six of the X-Stop patients elected to undergo a laminectomy and 22 of the conservatively treated patients had a laminectomy. While this study and others have not compared interspinous spacers to open surgery, this MIS method has been validated as being superior to nonoperative treatment.

Strömqvist et al recently conducted a randomized prospective study using either interspinous spacers or a laminectomy to treat one- and two-level lumbar stenosis.[15] The mean age was 69 years (range, 49–89), so the group as a whole was elderly as expected. Fifty patients were randomized to each group. The results were similar on the Zurich Claudication Questionnaire at all time points up to 2 years. The authors found that in

Table 15.1 Summary of MIS approaches for the geriatric population

Authors	Level	Design	Patients	Outcome and Findings
Vertebral body augmentations				
Klazen et al[7]	I	Randomized and prospective	101 vertebroplasty 101 conservative care	VAS drop of 5.2 with vertebroplasty as compared with 2.7 in the conservative group
Blasco et al[10]	I	Randomized and prospective	64 vertebroplasty 61 conservative care	42% reduction in pain with vertebroplasty vs. 25% in conservatively treated patients
Kallmes et al[11]	I	Randomized and prospective	38 vertebroplasty 40 sham surgery	No significant difference identified on pain functional and QOL measures
Buchbinder et al[12]	I	Randomized and prospective	68 vertebroplasty 63 placebo	No difference in pain improvement on VAS at 3 months; 2.6 and 1.9 for vertebroplasty and placebo
Interspinous spacer				
Zucherman et al[14]	I	Randomized and prospective	100 X-Stop 91 nonoperative	45.4 vs. 7.4% improvement on Zurich score at 2 y, favoring X-Stop
Strömqvist et al[15]	I/II	Randomized and prospective	50 X-Stop 50 laminectomy	Both groups with similar Zurich scores at all time points Less blood loss and operative time with X-Stop 3 revisions with laminectomy, 13 with X-Stop
Hemilaminotomy				
Rosen et al[17]	IV	Case series	50 Hemilaminotomy	Mean drop in Oswestry scores from 48 to 27 Median hospital stay of 29 h
Mobbs et al[18]	I/II	Randomized and prospective	27 hemilaminotomy 27 laminectomy	Mean VAS drop of 5.6 vs. 3.9 favoring MIS Hospital stay of 55.1 vs. 100.8 h favoring MIS
Instrumented fusion (TLIF)				
Wu et al[19]	III	Comparative Case series	61: age 65 y and older 90: under age 65 y	All MIS: identical improvements in clinical outcome and fusion rates Higher complications (16.4 vs. 6.7%) in elderly patients
Archavlis et al[20]	III	Comparative Case series	24 MIS TLIF 25 open TLIF	Similar ODI and VAS outcome rates; no difference in complications Reduced blood loss and transfusion rates in MIS group
Uribe et al[21]	II	Propensity-matched cohort of deformity patients	20 MIS 20 hybrid 20 open	Intraoperative complications were 0, 5.3, and 25% in MIS, hybrid, and open cases, respectively. Postoperative complication rates were 30, 47, and 50%, respectively

Abbreviations: MIS, minimally invasive surgery; ODI, Oswestry Disability Index; QOL, quality of life; TLIF, transforaminal lumbar interbody fusion; VAS, visual analog scale.

the X-Stop group blood loss (54 vs. 262 mL) as well as the operative time (62 vs. 98 minutes) was less. However, 3 patients (6%) in the decompression group underwent further surgery, compared with 13 patients (26%) in the X-Stop group. All three durotomies were in the laminectomy group.

Due to the fact that interspinous spacers are intended to treat neurogenic claudication, all clinical reports of the technique involve elderly patients. However, high-quality studies on the extreme elderly have been limited. A report by Lee and colleagues involved treatment of 10 patients with a mean age of 71 years (range, 61–79).[16] The report identified 22.3% expansion of the dural sac and 36.5% enlargement of the foramina. Seventy percent of the patients were satisfied with the procedure.

15.3.3 Minimally Invasive Lumbar Stenosis Decompression

For direct central canal and neuroforaminal decompression, one of the more popular options is to perform a hemilaminotomy

and medial facetectomy. In this procedure, the approach is similar to a microdiscectomy. After a laminotomy is performed, the base of the spinous processes is removed with a high-speed drill. Leaving the ipsilateral yellow ligament intact to push the thecal sac ventrally minimizes the risk of a dural tear. The midline raphe of the yellow ligament is then identified, and the contralateral decompression is then performed. This is done with Kerrison rongeurs and curettes. The ligament, hypertrophied synovium, and bony osteophytes are removed. The contralateral neuroforamen can also be opened. The ipsilateral ligament and medial facet are then removed for ipsilateral decompression. The technique can be performed using either a standard microdiscectomy retractor or a tubular dilator.

Numerous publications have reported excellent results with this technique for treating either lumbar central canal stenosis or a low-grade stable degenerative spondylolisthesis. Rosen et al reviewed 50 cases of patients older than 75 years.[17] They reported excellent results, with a mean drop in Oswestry Disability Index (ODI) scores from 48 to 27. Despite a high baseline level of comorbidities, complications were uncommon, with three durotomies, one pneumonia, and one atrial fibrillation case. Their median length of hospitalization was 29 hours.

Mobbs et al recently reported the results of a randomized prospective trial. In their study, 79 patients were enrolled, with adequate data for 54. The 1:1 randomization resulted in 27 patients in each arm of their study.[18] The mean age was 69.2 years. The results showed that both study groups had significant clinical improvements. However, MIS had a significantly better mean drop in VAS scores for leg pain ($p = 0.013$). MIS patients also had a shorter length of hospitalization (55.1 vs. 100.8 hours, $p = 0.0041$) and time to mobilization (15.6 vs. 33.3 hours, $p < 0.001$). The study had a small cohort with significant patient attrition and limited follow-up. However, despite these concerns, the MIS appeared to trend toward superior early clinical results.

15.3.4 Minimally Invasive Lumbar Fusion

There is a significant body of literature on using minimally invasive transforaminal lumbar interbody fusion (MIS TLIF) to treat various degenerative conditions in the lumbar spine such as spondylolisthesis, stenosis with disc height collapse, and recurrent disc herniation. However, there are no comparative studies that specifically examined the use of MIS versus open TLIF in the elderly patient population per se. However, well-designed comparative studies have been published and are reviewed elsewhere in this textbook (Chapter 4). The major difficulty in analyzing this literature is that the majority of reports did not stratify their patient populations by age, making any post-hoc analysis of age-related effects impossible.

However, there have been case series targeted at examining older patients undergoing MIS TLIF. In a report by Wu et al, a case series of 151 patients were examined, of whom 62 were older than 65 years.[19] The authors did not identify any difference in fusion rates between the age groups, and the overall arthrodesis rate was 88.4%. Similarly, the clinical improvement as measured by ODI and VAS was similar between groups (30.5 point mean ODI decrease for both younger and older patient groups). However, both major and minor complications were more common in the elderly patient group (16.4% overall vs. 6.7%). While this series did not seek to specifically examine the question of whether MIS was more beneficial in elderly patients, it would appear that the well-known surgical risks with spinal fusion in the older patients were not entirely mitigated with the application of a less invasive approach.

In another series by Archavlis et al, patients were excluded if they did not have severe stenosis and spondylolisthesis, thus excluding young patients.[20] A total of 49 patients were treated with either open or MIS TLIF. The mean age was 68 ± 7 years. The authors found similar clinical outcomes with regard to ODI and VAS for pain. There was also no statistical difference in complications, including incidental durotomy, wound-healing problems, new radiculopathy, hardware misplacement, pseudarthrosis, adjacent segment disease, and revision surgery. The overall complication rate was 29 and 28% with MIS and open surgery, respectively. However, meaningful blood loss resulting in the need for transfusion was significantly lower in the MIS group (11 vs. 35%).

With regard to MIS methods for treating more complex pathologies such as spinal deformity or trauma, there still remains little high-quality evidence to demonstrate the advantages of MIS definitively. Certainly, no true comparative studies are available, except those that have attempted to match patients through propensity matching. To this end, some early studies from the International Spine Study Group (ISSG) have suggested that MIS methods may reduce short-term complication rates. In the report by Uribe et al, deformity surgery was divided into a truly MIS approach, a hybrid between MIS and open surgery, and an open group.[21] In that study of propensity-matched patients, there were 20 patients in each subgroup. Intraoperative complications were 0, 5.3, and 25%, respectively. Postoperative complication rates were 30, 47, and 50%, respectively. While the ability to correct a spinal deformity varied between groups, this study did show a trend toward lower complication rates with MIS in complex cases.

15.4 Conclusion

The literature regarding the effects of MIS on the elderly population does not provide any definitive Class I evidence to show superiority when compared to open surgery. However, new techniques such as VBA and interspinous spacers may be superior to alternative traditional open surgeries used to treat the same pathologies. Regarding fusion and more complex surgeries, there is a suggestion that MIS may result in lower complication rates, but higher levels of evidence are needed for definitive recommendations. A Grade 2C recommendation can be made for using MIS to treat geriatric patients.

15.5 Editors' Commentary

15.5.1 Minimally Invasive Surgery

The statement "Less is more" is perhaps more accurate in geriatric surgery than in any other subspecialty area. The goal in geriatric spine surgery should not be to return the spine to the shape it had at age 20 years, but to return maximal function to the individual with the lowest risk and least impact on their life possible. This is exactly what MIS is designed to do. Probably, the most common spine surgical procedure performed in the geriatric population is decompression of stenosis of the lumbar spine. It has now been reported in multiple peer-reviewed publications that MIS decompression can be performed in the geriatric population with less blood loss, less pain, less requirement for pain medication, less hospitalization, less physiologic stress, fewer infections, less overall complications, lower incidence of iatrogenic instability, and less need for inpatient rehabilitation compared to open decompression of stenosis. In short, in virtually every area examined to date, compared to open laminectomy, MIS is a vastly superior technique for decompression of stenosis in the elderly population.

15.5.2 Open Surgery

Techniques such as VBA and the placement of interspinous spacers have never been done through large incisions and, in that sense, cannot really be considered to have been developed out of a drive to minimize procedure invasiveness—they are just smaller surgeries. We agree these procedures can be used to treat elderly patients, the patient population for which they are best suited. These two surgical procedures, incidentally, have very controversial evidentiary support.

While all spine surgeons would prefer to perform less invasive procedures in the elderly, there are characteristics of this patient population which may also unfortunately limit the success of MIS techniques. Nearly all MIS is done using fluoroscopy, a technique which may have limitations in the setting of osteoporosis or osteopenia. The increased incidence of low bone density in the elderly population also can lead to increased rates of subsidence of unilateral pedicle screws and intervertebral cages, a technique that is frequently employed in MIS. Using open techniques, bilateral instrumentation is nearly always placed and provides greater structural support. Although a second surgical site can be utilized during MIS to place bilateral instrumentation, this may compromise some of the purported advantages of MIS such as reduced muscular injury and reduced operating room time. Finally, low bone density occasionally results in intraoperative use of salvage techniques such as hook placement in deformity surgery—this is not possible using MIS approaches.

Optimizing care for the elderly with spinal disease is best done using careful surgical indications and preoperative algorithms to address problematic characteristics of elderly patients. Creating surgical shortcuts to minimize procedure invasiveness may have adverse consequences in this structurally and medically compromised patient population.

References

[1] McGirt MJ, Parker SL, Lerner J, Engelhart L, Knight T, Wang MY. Comparative analysis of perioperative surgical site infection after minimally invasive versus open posterior/transforaminal lumbar interbody fusion: analysis of hospital billing and discharge data from 5170 patients. J Neurosurg Spine. 2011; 14(6):771–778

[2] Wang M, Sherman A, Vanni S, Levi A. Complications associated with lumbar stenosis surgery in patients older than 75 years of age. Neurosurg Focus. 2003; 14(2):1–4

[3] Zheng F, Cammisa FP, Jr, Sandhu HS, Girardi FP, Khan SN. Factors predicting hospital stay, operative time, blood loss, and transfusion in patients undergoing revision posterior lumbar spine decompression, fusion, and segmental instrumentation. Spine. 2002; 27(8):818–824

[4] Raffo CS, Lauerman WC. Predicting morbidity and mortality of lumbar spine arthrodesis in patients in their ninth decade. Spine. 2006; 31(1):99–103

[5] Arts M, Brand R, van der Akker M, Koes B, Bartels R, Preul W. Tubular discectomy vs. conventional microdiscectomy for sciatica: a randomized controlled trial. JAMA. 2009; 302:149–158

[6] Galibert P, Deramond H, Rosat P, Le Gars D. Preliminary note on the treatment of vertebral angioma by percutaneous acrylic vertebroplasty [in French]. Neurochirurgie. 1987; 33(2):166–168

[7] Klazen CA, Lohle PN, de Vries J, et al. Vertebroplasty versus conservative treatment in acute osteoporotic vertebral compression fractures (Vertos II): an open-label randomised trial. Lancet. 2010; 376(9746):1085–1092

[8] Voormolen MH, Mali WP, Lohle PN, et al. Percutaneous vertebroplasty compared with optimal pain medication treatment: short-term clinical outcome of patients with subacute or chronic painful osteoporotic vertebral compression fractures. The VERTOS study. AJNR Am J Neuroradiol. 2007; 28 (3):555–560

[9] Firanescu C, Lohle PN, de Vries J, et al. VERTOS IV study group. A randomised sham controlled trial of vertebroplasty for painful acute osteoporotic vertebral fractures (VERTOS IV). Trials. 2011; 12:93

[10] Blasco J, Martinez-Ferrer A, Macho J, et al. Effect of vertebroplasty on pain relief, quality of life, and the incidence of new vertebral fractures: a 12-month randomized follow-up, controlled trial. J Bone Miner Res. 2012; 27(5): 1159–1166

[11] Kallmes DF, Comstock BA, Heagerty PJ, et al. A randomized trial of vertebroplasty for osteoporotic spinal fractures. N Engl J Med. 2009; 361(6): 569–579

[12] Buchbinder R, Osborne RH, Ebeling PR, et al. A randomized trial of vertebroplasty for painful osteoporotic vertebral fractures. N Engl J Med. 2009; 361(6):557–568

[13] Nandakumar A, Clark NA, Peehal JP, Bilolikar N, Wardlaw D, Smith FW. The increase in dural sac area is maintained at 2 years after X-stop implantation for the treatment of spinal stenosis with no significant alteration in lumbar spine range of movement. Spine J. 2010; 10(9):762–768

[14] Zucherman JF, Hsu KY, Hartjen CA, et al. A multicenter, prospective, randomized trial evaluating the X STOP interspinous process decompression system for the treatment of neurogenic intermittent claudication: two-year follow-up results. Spine. 2005; 30(12):1351–1358

[15] Strömqvist BH, Berg S, Gerdhem P, et al. X-stop versus decompressive surgery for lumbar neurogenic intermittent claudication: randomized controlled trial with 2-year follow-up. Spine. 2013; 38(17):1436–1442

[16] Lee J, Hida K, Seki T, Iwasaki Y, Minoru A. An interspinous process distractor (X STOP) for lumbar spinal stenosis in elderly patients: preliminary experiences in 10 consecutive cases. J Spinal Disord Tech. 2004; 17(1):72–77, discussion 78

[17] Rosen DS, O'Toole JE, Eichholz KM, et al. Minimally invasive lumbar spinal decompression in the elderly: outcomes of 50 patients aged 75 years and older. Neurosurgery. 2007; 60(3):503–509, discussion 509–510

[18] Mobbs RJ, Li J, Sivabalan P, Raley D, Rao PJ. Outcomes after decompressive laminectomy for lumbar spinal stenosis: comparison between minimally invasive unilateral laminectomy for bilateral decompression and open laminectomy: clinical article. J Neurosurg Spine. 2014; 21(2):179–186

[19] Wu WJ, Liang Y, Zhang XK, Cao P, Zheng T. Complications and clinical outcomes of minimally invasive transforaminal lumbar interbody fusion for the treatment of one- or two-level degenerative disc diseases of the lumbar spine in patients older than 65 years. Chin Med J (Engl). 2012; 125(14):2505–2510

[20] Archavlis E, Carvi y Nievas M. Comparison of minimally invasive fusion and instrumentation versus open surgery for severe stenotic spondylolisthesis with high-grade facet joint osteoarthritis. Eur Spine J. 2013; 22(8):1731–1740

[21] Uribe JS, Deukmedjian AR, Mummaneni PV, et al. International Spine Study Group. Complications in adult spinal deformity surgery: an analysis of minimally invasive, hybrid, and open surgical techniques. Neurosurg Focus. 2014; 36(5):E15

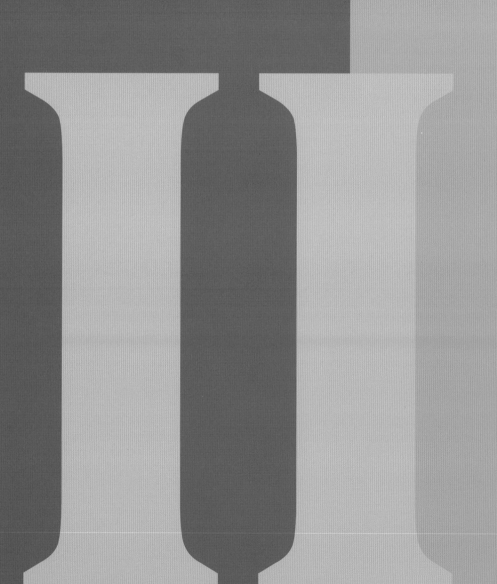

Part II

Trauma

16 Thoracolumbar Burst Fractures: Can Thoracolumbar Burst Fractures Be Effectively Managed Using Minimally Invasive Surgery Techniques?

MIS: Gurpreet S. Gandhoke, David O. Okonkwo, and Adam S. Kanter
Open: Amandeep Bhalla and Kristen E. Radcliff

16.1 Introduction

Indications for surgical management of acute thoracolumbar burst fractures are well described and include decompression of neural elements, restoration of spinal alignment, and promotion of arthrodesis.[1,2,3,4] Patients requiring surgery for thoracolumbar burst fractures may be treated via an anterior approach, posterior approach, or combined anterior–posterior approach. The goals of surgery are neural decompression, stabilization, and correction of an associated deformity when present. Anterior instrumentation has been shown to produce equivalent arthrodesis and correction of kyphotic deformity compared to posterior instrumentation while allowing for direct visualization of the spinal canal and, theoretically, a superior decompression.[5] However, traditional anterior approaches to the thoracolumbar spine carry significant morbidity, including pneumothorax, aortic injury, disruption of the lumbar plexus, retrograde ejaculation, and development of abdominal or diaphragmatic hernia.[6]

To minimize exposure-related morbidity, a number of anterolateral laparoscopic and thoracoscopic approaches for instrumentation at the thoracolumbar junction have been attempted.[7] The minimally invasive extreme lateral approach is a technique that has been previously described for the treatment of spine pathology including degenerative and scoliotic lumbar disease.[8] Its use in trauma, particularly in the treatment of burst fractures, is more limited in the literature. The thoracic spine from T6–T7 level and up to the L4–L5 disc space is accessible to treat pathology utilizing this minimally invasive approach.

16.2 Advantages of Minimally Invasive Surgery

To access the anterior thoracolumbar spine from T12–L2, the conventional open approach consists of a lateral incision over the ribs and dissection of muscular layers until exposure of the peritoneum is achieved, followed by mobilization of the diaphragm and retraction of lung parenchyma to access the retroperitoneal space.[9,10] This approach commonly requires insertion of a chest tube until the pleural effusion resulting from diaphragmatic dissection has drained. Complications specific to anterior spine surgery include aortic laceration (0.08%), pneumothorax (1.8%), and post-thoracotomy pain syndrome persisting for greater than 6 months (9%).[6]

Anterior approaches for vertebrectomy and arthrodesis via laparoscopic and video-assisted thoracoscopic techniques have been well described in the literature.[7,11,12,13,14] These approaches to the anterior thoracolumbar spine have been shown to result in shorter hospitalizations when compared to open approaches.[12,15] Disadvantages of endoscopic approaches include the requirement for single lung intubation, a steep and long learning curve, representation of three-dimensional anatomy in two dimensions, extensive and expensive instrumentation, extended operative times, relative inability to tackle inadvertent complications without having to open exposure, and the difficulty in placement of large reconstructive anterior instrumentation.

The lateral transpsoas approach has been previously described for the treatment of degenerative thoracolumbar disease.[16] It is a minimally invasive approach that utilizes sequential dilation with electromyographic (EMG) neuromonitoring to place an expandable tubular retractor. It provides the additional benefit of minimizing dissection of the great vessels and the sympathetic plexus, thus reducing the risk of vascular injury and retrograde ejaculation.[17] When the approach is retro pleural, there is no violation of the pleural or the peritoneal cavity posing less risk of complications associated with open thoracotomy, including the development of a cerebrospinal pleural fistula.[18] The amount of kyphosis correction achieved is equivalent to that achieved with open anterior procedures.[14,19] Additional benefits include the ability of the approach to be performed without rib resection and lung deflation. This minimally invasive lateral approach to the thoracic spine offers a very good alternative to an open thoracotomy or a video-assisted thoracoscopic corpectomy. Through a small corridor, corpectomy can be performed at most levels from T6 to L4, allowing for decompression, correction of deformity, and fusion.

16.3 Advantages of Open Surgery

Indications for an open anterior approach include burst fracture with incomplete paraplegia, retropulsed fragment with significant canal compromise, significant kyphotic deformity (> 30 degrees), delay from injury rendering ligamentotaxis ineffective, and traumatic disc herniation with flexion–distraction injury.[20] The anterior approach aids in reconstruction of the anterior column with a load-sharing construct, which reduces posterior cantilever loads and the risk of late kyphotic failure. Short segment anterior or posterior fixation may be employed to neutralize the construct and impart additional stability. Anterior-only procedures have the distinct advantage of limiting the levels of fusion necessary. A circumferential fusion is necessary, however, to stabilize three-column spinal injuries in the setting of symptomatic canal occlusion. If the posterior tension band has failed, supplemental posterior stabilization is also recommended.

The anterior approach to the thoracolumbar spine affords the most direct visualization of the spinal cord via corpectomy, which optimizes ability to achieve complete neural decompression. Iatrogenic neurologic injury is not reported in major series, likely because of the safety resulting from direct anterior visualization of the thecal sac.[20] The adequacy of the anterior decompression is of chief importance, and compromise of the surgical exposure through minimally invasive techniques may result in residual compression and subsequent irreversible neurologic injury. The anterior approach is superior to the transpsoas minimally invasive technique in surgical exposure, as the latter was designed to access the midportion of the disc space. With the lateral approach, it is difficult to gain access to the retropulsed fragment in the spinal canal from the lateral aspect of the midportion of the disc space without significant traction across, which risks stretch injury to the lumbar plexus.

Bleeding is a significant risk in the setting of acute fracture, and a very common complication in the surgical management of thoracolumbar burst fractures. With improved visualization, the anterior approach aids in better control of bleeding. The surgical path through the psoas muscle may cause additional bleeding, and the very nature of minimally invasive surgery (MIS) undermines the adequacy of exposure necessary to control it. The open anterior approach also improves visualization both cephalad and caudad to the injured vertebral body, so that adequate discectomies and end plate preparation can be performed.

The posterior transpedicular approach offers distinct advantages including decreased operating time, blood loss, and morbidity.[21,22] The nature of the approach allows for repair of posterior dural tears.[23] Posterior instrumentation assists in applying distractive forces for decompression and graft passage, as well as compressive forces to aid in stabilization.[24] The posterior approach also affords for considerable deformity correction of the kyphosis and collapse inherent in thoracolumbar burst fractures. Posterior approach also allows for additional bone grafting surface across the posterior elements bilaterally. The open approach also allows repair of traumatic durotomies and decompression of nerve root fragments entrapped in the bony fragments. The posterior approach also has fewer complications of hemopneumothorax, abdominal distension, and ileus.

16.4 Case Illustration

A 17-year-old woman was the restrained driver in a high-speed motor vehicle collision. She presented with severe low back pain but remained neurologically intact (American Spinal Injury Association impairment score E [ASIA-E]). Computed tomography (CT) scan demonstrated an L1 burst fracture with 70% loss of height of the vertebral body and retropulsion-causing canal narrowing of 60%, with associated right L1 pedicle and laminar fractures (► Fig. 16.1). Magnetic resonance imaging (MRI; ► Fig. 16.1a, b, e) demonstrated a disrupted posterior ligamentous complex, for a TLICS[25] (Thoracolumbar Injury Classification and Severity) score of 5 (► Fig. 16.1c, f).

16.5 Surgical Technique in Minimally Invasive Surgery

The major anatomic landmarks to consider when preparing for this surgery are the ribs, lung, diaphragm, aorta, and the spinal curvature. The diaphragm will be in the surgical access path when accessing the spine for the levels from T10 to L1. The

diaphragmatic tendinous attachments may be encountered down to the L3 vertebra.

When operating in the pleural cavity with the minimally invasive retractor system, double-lumen intubation and lung deflation is not required. We approach the thoracic spine with retractor placement and expansion in between the ribs, without its resection, thus gaining adequate access to the pleural cavity. Care should be taken to avoid injury to the neurovascular bundle that lies under the inferior aspect of each rib.

Preoperative MRI should be carefully evaluated to examine for the position of the aorta, the sympathetic plexus, and its relation to the psoas muscle and the spinal curvature, which may place the aorta in the path of the lateral surgical corridor.

16.5.1 Position

After induction of general anesthesia, the patient is placed in the lateral decubitus position with the left side up. We prefer to use the left side to access the spine given the aorta and iliac arteries are more pliable and forgiving than the vena cava system and more likely to withstand surgical handling without injury. In patients with scoliosis, the aorta may lie on the lateral aspect of the vertebral bodies and thus would require access from the opposite (right) side.

The patient is positioned on the table such that the table break lies at the midpoint of the iliac crest and the greater trochanter. All pressure points are padded and the patient is secured to the table with tape at the following locations:
• Over the iliac crest below the table break.
• Over the thoracic region above the region of the surgical exposure.
• From the iliac crest inferiorly securing to the foot of the table.

The bed is slightly flexed to expand the costo-pelvic interval and the intercostals. The table (not the C arm) is carefully adjusted to obtain true anteroposterior (AP; the spinous processes should be midline and the pedicles should be equidistant from the spinous processes) and lateral images (crisp end plates should be visualized).

Fluoroscopy is then utilized to mark out the fracture site on the skin, identifying the superior aspect of the disc space above and the inferior aspect of the disc space below the fractured vertebrae.

When operating within the pleural cavity (to access the spinal levels from the L1 body and above), the approach is typically in between the ribs. The incision is again marked utilizing fluoroscopy and will run parallel and in between the ribs, along the superior aspect of the inferior rib, to avoid injury to the neurovascular bundle.

A chlorhexidine wipe and ChloraPrep solution is used to sterilize the surgical site.

16.5.2 Anatomic Considerations during Access to the Retroperitoneum

The main paired abdominal muscles include the external oblique muscles, internal oblique muscles, transversus abdominis muscles, and their respective aponeuroses, which provide core strength and protection to the abdominal wall viscera. The

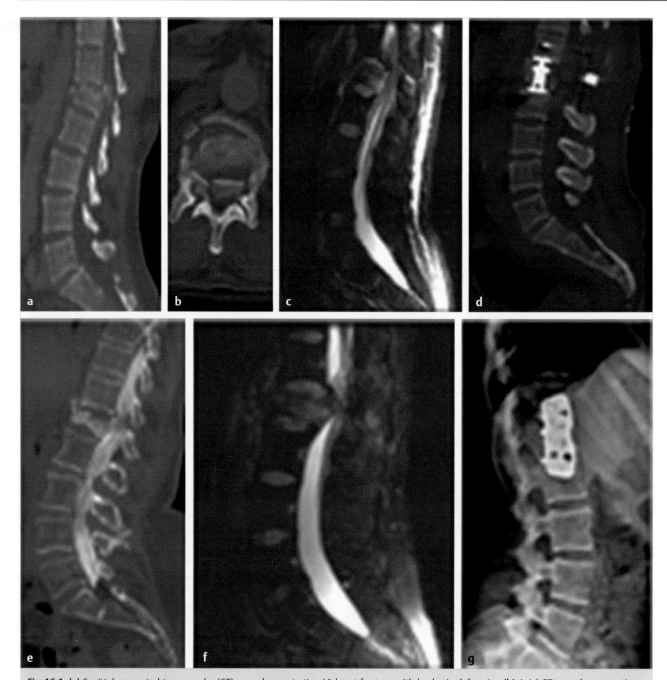

Fig. 16.1 **(a)** Sagittal computed tomography (CT) scan demonstrating L1 burst fracture with kyphotic deformity. **(b)** Axial CT scan demonstrating significant retropulsion of fractured vertebral body. **(c)** Sagittal T2 magnetic resonance imaging (MRI) demonstrating kyphotic injury and associated significant ligamentous injury. **(d)** Postoperative sagittal CT demonstrating corpectomy, cage placement, and correction of kyphotic deformity. **(e)** Sagittal CT myelogram demonstrating L1 burst fracture with kyphotic deformity. **(f)** Sagittal T2 MRI demonstrating kyphotic injury and associated significant ligamentous injury. **(g)** Postoperative lateral radiograph demonstrating corpectomy, cage placement, and correction of kyphotic deformity.

transversalis fascia is one of the main components that maintain structural integrity of the retroperitoneal space. A 4-cm transverse incision is made along the lateral flank at the midline level of the index vertebral body. The incision should be made parallel to the direction of the fibers of the external oblique to minimize the possibility of injury to the motor nerves supplying them. This prevents abdominal wall pseudo-hernia formation from loss of tone to these abdominal wall muscles. Blunt dissection with anterior sweeping movements of the

retroperitoneal contents is then performed to enable palpation of the psoas muscle and the transverse process of the index vertebra.

16.5.3 Thoracic Access

We use the rib-spreading technique to dissect down to the ribs, through the intercostal musculature, down to the pleura. Pleural access is gained by dissection along the superior aspect of the lowest rib. Once within the pleural cavity, finger dissection is utilized to gently palpate the lung, and the initial dilator is then passed into the pleural cavity in a dorsal trajectory following the curvature of the rib until landing at the intersection of the rib head and spine, as confirmed with fluoroscopy. The dilator is then gently positioned in the center of the vertebral body, taking care not to injure the segmental artery. The remaining dilators are then passed over the initial dilator down to the spine, followed by the final retractor system.

16.5.4 Retroperitoneal Access

The T12–L1 level, in our experience, can be accessed both through the transpleural route and through the diaphragm in the retroperitoneal space. The levels below L1 down to the L5 superior end plate require a retroperitoneal access route. A 4-cm flank incision is performed as above to gain access to the retroperitoneal space via blunt finger dissection, carefully sweeping the abdominal contents ventrally as each layer of the lateral musculature and fascia are traversed. Loss of resistance from muscles (external oblique, internal oblique, transversalis muscle and fascia transversalis) indicates that the retroperitoneal space has been reached.

Using a blunt-tipped snap to spread the fibers of the oblique muscles under vision ensures the security of the iliohypogastric and ilioinguinal nerves and thus preventing a lumbar hernia from loss of tone in the muscles of the anterior abdominal wall.

Once the tip of the transverse process is encountered, the finger is directed medially to feel for the psoas muscle, gently sweeping anteriorly and away any fascial adhesions. The first dilator is then passed with the finger as its guide through the oblique muscle layers down to the retroperitoneal space and docked on the psoas muscle in the center of the vertebral body.

16.5.5 Electrophysiological Monitoring

The lumbar plexus tends to lie in the posterior one-third of the psoas muscle. Electrophysiological monitoring is utilized in all cases to enable safe passage of the dilators and retractor system to minimize retraction and damage to these motor nerves. We utilize the Neurovision neuromonitoring, which continuously searches for the stimulus threshold that elicits an EMG response and reports this threshold both audibly and visually. As the stimulus source (the dilators and the retractor system also act as electrodes and are insulated to minimize current shunting) moves closer to the nerve, less stimulus intensity is required to elicit a response, resulting in a lower threshold, which provides an indication of the relative proximity of the dilator to the nerves.

We consider threshold values of 10 mA and greater as a marker of safe distance from the nerves.

Lower thresholds of stimulation of the nerve should be posterior to the working operative field, confirming that the lumbar plexus is behind the retractor and not pushed anteriorly.

16.5.6 Procedure

We utilize the MaXcess retractor system (NuVasive, Inc., San Diego, CA), advancing it over the dilators and minimally expanding it to reveal the inferior aspect of the rostral vertebral

body and the superior aspect of the caudal vertebral body adjacent to the fractured level.

Minimal retraction is key to prevent stretch-related injury and weakness of the psoas muscle. We utilize two-click dilation in the AP plane and six-retractor-click dilation in the craniocaudad plane

The handles of the retractor system are positioned ventrally for intercostal access in the pleural cavity to enable the center blade to retract the lung and/or diaphragm during exposure of the spine. Below L1, the retractor handles are positioned posteriorly. The retractor is gently opened to expose the disc spaces above and below the index level; wanding of the blades is often required to enable full rostral-caudal exposure while limiting superficial skin and rib expansion. Depending upon retractor positioning, either the third blade or a fourth blade can be used to ventrally retract the lung, while additional blade expanders are placed down the blades to further minimize access to visceral and pleural contents into the surgical corridor. An EMG blunt-tip probe is used to locate the laterally traversing nerve root (ideally behind the posterior retractor blade) to ensure that it lies outside the surgical corridor. In the manner described earlier, we have been able to access the spine from T6 to the L5 disc space. Superior to T6, the intercostal spaces become smaller; this along with the presence of the scapula makes access exceedingly difficult.

Once exposed, it is important to safely locate and sacrifice the segmental arterial branch supplying the vertebral body that takes off as a branch of the posterior intercostal artery arising from the aorta. This minimizes nuisance blood loss if it is lacerated inadvertently, but more so prevents possible avulsion of the vessel from the aorta during further dissection.

Total discectomies are then performed above and below the fractured body in routine fashion as previously described.[16]

Using kerrisons, rongeurs, and a high-speed drill, the fractured vertebral body is removed, starting centrally to create a potential space where displaced posterior fragments can be persuaded into and away from the neural elements until the underlying posterior ligament and dura is visualized. The remaining fractured body is further removed from the disc space above to below; the anterior cortical surface does not need to be removed in its entirety, given that complete removal dramatically increases the possibility of a great vessel or visceral injury. The residual anterior bone can further act as a buttress to the cage and aide in surface area for arthrodesis materials. Once the corpectomy is complete, the end plates are prepared, and an expandable titanium cage filled with morselized autograft (collected during the bony removal) is inserted, its positioning confirmed by fluoroscopy in both the AP and lateral planes. The cage is ideally positioned anterior to midline to make use of the greater structural integrity of the apophyseal ring as compared to that of the weaker central body. The lateral bodies of the vertebrae above and below the cage are carefully drilled flush to enable level placement of a lateral plate, which is then secured with four vertebral screws. The posterior screws are placed with bicortical purchase for added construct stability, while the anterior screws utilize unilateral cortical purchase, to minimize contralateral visceral or vascular injury at the point of a cortical breach. Final imaging is performed in the AP and lateral plane to confirm hardware placement

(▶ Fig. 16.1d, g), following which copious irrigation and meticulous hemostasis are performed.

16.5.7 Closure

The retractor is carefully contracted and extracted under direct visualization to confirm that there is no bleeding upon its removal. If pleural opening occurred during surgical access, a red rubber catheter is placed through the defect prior to closure, following which positive pressure ventilation and suction during Valsalva is used to minimize air in the intrapleural cavity. The catheter is removed through a purse-string suture prior to dermal closure. A chest radiograph should be obtained postoperatively to confirm and track pneumothorax.

If concern for an occult bowel injury is raised during the retroperitoneal approach, a duodenal tube is placed and 100 mL of Gastrografin is administered, following which a CT scan of the abdomen and pelvis is performed 8 hours after surgery to confirm bowel integrity and lack of dye extravasation.

16.6 Surgical Technique in Open Surgery

Thoracoabdominal and retroperitoneal approaches are preferred for most thoracolumbar injuries between T10 and L1 and between T12 and L4, respectively. The thoracolumbar spine is typically approached from the left to circumvent the liver and requires less mobilization of the vena cava.[26] Approaches to the thoracolumbar junction may also involve takedown of a portion of the diaphragm. A transperitoneal approach may be utilized in markedly obese patients and in cases where prior retroperitoneal exposure has been performed.[26] The patient is positioned in the lateral decubitus position with the break in the table centered over the fracture to improve exposure. An oblique incision is made under the 12th rib. Rib may be excised to be used as autograft, or the spine can also be approached through the intercostal space. Care is taken to remain extrapleural, and if the diaphragm is incised a cuff of tissue should remain with the chest wall to facilitate later repair. Once exposure of the spine is established, a localizing radiograph can be taken to confirm the level of the fracture. The psoas is then gently elevated from the vertebral body and care is taken to cauterize the segmental arteries. The pedicle is carefully removed revealing the posterior margin of the vertebral wall. Discectomy is done above and below the injured vertebrae, followed by direct decompression across the vertebral body to the contralateral pedicle. A corpectomy is then performed, followed by restoration of alignment and graft placement with instrumentation.

16.7 Discussion of Minimally Invasive Surgery

16.7.1 Level I Evidence in Minimally Invasive Surgery

There is no level I study available.

16.7.2 Level II Evidence in Minimally Invasive Surgery

There are no prospective studies comparing open approaches to MIS lateral approach for management of thoracolumbar burst fractures.

16.7.3 Level III and Level IV Evidence in Minimally Invasive Surgery

There are no level III and IV studies directly comparing MIS approaches to open lateral approach in the management of thoracolumbar burst fractures. There are clinical studies on thoracolumbar burst fractures managed with MIS approaches.

Smith and colleagues[27] in 2010 reported on 52 patients with thoracic and lumbar fractures (mostly T12 and L1), and most of these patients had a spinal cord injury. Of note, they used a transpleural approach in 9 of the patients and were able to avoid chest tube placement in all but 2 of these patients. All patients underwent supplemental internal fixation. In 75% of the cohort they used anterolateral fixation, in 46% of the cohort they used pedicle screw fixation, and in 29% of the cohort they used both anterior and posterior fixations. While 83% of the patients underwent follow-up at 1 year, half of the patients had 2 years of follow-up. None of the patients were reported to have complications requiring surgical revision or re-exploration.

Baaj et al[28] reported on 80 consecutive patients who underwent the mini-open lateral approach with corpectomy and fusion for trauma (71%), tumor (26%), and infection (3%). There were no postoperative neurological complications. They conclude that the mini-open anterolateral approach to the thoracolumbar spine is an appealing alternative to the traditional open approaches. They stress that this approach is technically demanding and requires proficiency in the use of minimally invasive spinal surgery instruments and retractors.

Khan et al[29] reported on 25 consecutive patients with a variety of diagnoses (tumors, $n = 10$; infection, $n = 5$; burst fractures, $n = 9$; disc herniation, $n = 1$) treated by the minimally invasive transpsoas approach for a thoracolumbar corpectomy and reconstruction. They report a significant reduction in surgical time and blood loss in comparison to open techniques. A 62% decrease in self-reported visual analog scale (VAS) scores was observed. No wound complications or radiographic evidence of implant subsidence or failure were observed at a mean follow-up of 5 months.

16.8 Complications in Minimally Invasive Surgery

The lateral transpsoas approach has some unique complications by virtue of its access corridor. These include bowstringing of the psoas and lumbar plexus from applying too much table break in order to splay open the space between the costal angle and the pelvis, injury to the subcostal, iliohypogastric, ilioinguinal, and genitofemoral nerves predisposing to abdominal wall hernias. End plate violation leading to graft subsidence, injury to the great vessels leading to catastrophic blood loss, and a postoperative hip flexor weakness from an increased psoas dilation time and also from injury to the lumbar plexus. Bowel perforation is another potential complication with serious consequences, which has been reported with the lateral approach.[30]

Uribe et al[31] recently report on 13,004 patients who were treated with MIS-LIF (minimally invasive lumbar interbody fusion) by 40 surgeons. Of those patients, 0.08% experienced a visceral complication (bowel injury), 0.10% experienced a vascular injury, 0.27% experienced a superficial wound infection, and 0.14% experienced a deep wound infection.

In their series of treating 52 patients with thoracic and lumbar spine fractures with the minimally invasive lateral transpsoas approach, Smith et al[27] reported that 7 (13.5%) patients experienced eight (15.4%) complications, with two instances each of dural tear, intercostal neuralgia, and deep vein thrombosis, and one instance each of pleural effusion and superficial posterior infection. Radiographic subsidence of the anterior cage occurred in seven patients (13.5%).

Baaj et al[28] reported on 80 consecutive patients who underwent the mini-open lateral approach with corpectomy and fusion. Total complication rate was 12.5% (dural tear 2.5%, intercostal neuralgia 2.5%, deep vein thrombosis 2.5%, pleural effusion 1.3%, wound infection 1.3%, hardware failure 1.3%, and hemothorax 1.3%). Two patients needed a reoperation to address the complication (hardware failure, hemothorax). There were no postoperative neurological complications.

Given the benefits of this MIS approach, including short incision, low blood loss, and short hospital stay, this rate compares favorably to that of published open thoracolumbar approach series. In a recent single-institution series that compared transpedicular to anterior thoracolumbar corpectomies, Lu et al[22] found a 32% overall complication rate with the anterior approach, including an 11% revision rate (three implant failures, one splenic injury, one deep wound infection). In a randomized study that compared anterior to posterior decompression and stabilization for traumatic fractures, Wood et al demonstrated a 14% (3 of 22) complication rate with the anterior thoracolumbar approach.[32]

▶ Table 16.1 shows the aggregate complication rate for each listed complication across the referenced studies in this chapter.

Table 16.1 Breakdown of surgical complications for thoracolumbar burst fractures: aggregate from referenced studies for MIS and open approaches

Complications (%)	MIS	Open
Infection	0.27	0.4
Neurologic deficits	0	0.7
Screw/cage complications	1.3	4
CSF leak	1.2	0
Blood transfusion/ coagulation	0	0
Pleural effusion/ pneumonia	1.3	4.9
Nonunion requiring revision	0.02	2.7
Other	1.3	1.4

Abbreviations: CSF, cerebrospinal fluid; MIS, minimally invasive surgery.

16.9 Conclusion of Minimally Invasive Surgery

Level III and Level IV evidence supports that the minimally invasive lateral approach for decompression and stabilization of acute burst fractures of the thoracolumbar spine provides the benefits of anterior thoracotomy approaches, without their shortcomings, and maintains the biomechanical advantages of anterior instrumentation, which are absent in posterior-only surgery. High-risk patients requiring these complex procedures benefit from hastened improvement in quality of life postoperatively.

The open posterior approach requires disruption of the posterior ligamentous complex and mobilization and devascularization of the paraspinal musculature. The advantage of an anterior or lateral approach to the thoracolumbar junction is that it provides maximum exposure for corpectomy while preserving the posterior ligamentous complex and avoiding disruption of the paraspinal musculature. The lateral approach with a tubular retractor avoids the need for an approach surgeon. It also reduces the morbidity of a transthoracic exposure by decreasing lung trauma, minimizing violation of the pleura, and obviating the need for lung deflation. The anterior approach facilitates a direct decompression of the neural elements and allows reconstruction of the anterior column with a robust construct.

An acceptable complication profile with shortened OR (operating room) times, reduced blood loss, and enabling early return to work with use of standard instrumentation and surgical techniques makes the minimally invasive lateral approach an excellent tool in the armamentarium of the spine surgeon.

A randomized controlled trial comparing traditional open techniques with the lateral transpsoas approach to treat thoracolumbar burst fractures is certainly a worthy endeavor. Based on the available evidence, we assign grade 1C of recommendation for the minimally invasive lateral transpsoas surgical approach in the management of thoracolumbar burst fractures.

16.10 Discussion of Open Surgery

16.10.1 Level I Evidence in Open Surgery

There are no level I studies available.

16.10.2 Level II Evidence in Open Surgery

There are no prospective studies comparing open approaches to MIS lateral approach for management of thoracolumbar burst fractures. There is, however, level II evidence comparing the open anterior approach to the open posterior transpedicular approach in the management of thoracolumbar burst fractures. In a randomized study, Lin et al prospectively examined 64 patients with thoracolumbar burst fractures who were randomized to treatment by anterior approach versus posterior transpedicular approach with subtotal corpectomy, decompression, and reconstruction.[33] At 2-year follow-up, all patients achieved solid fusion, with significant neurological improvement. The study found less intraoperative blood loss, shorter surgical time, and better pulmonary function with posterior surgery. The Frankel scale, ASIA motor scale, and radiologic results were not significantly different.

16.10.3 Level III and Level IV Evidence in Open Surgery

There are no level III and IV studies directly comparing open approaches to MIS lateral approach in the management of thoracolumbar burst fractures. There are clinical studies on thoracolumbar burst fractures managed with open approaches.

Kaneda et al[34] treated 150 patients with burst fractures of the thoracolumbar spine and associated neurological deficits with a single-stage anterior decompression, strut grafting, and Kaneda instrumentation. In all, 95% of patients had an improvement in neurological function. At a mean of 8-year follow-up, the authors reported a 93% fusion rate, and 86% of all patients who had been employed before injury returned to their same jobs.

Sasso et al[35] retrospectively reviewed 40 patients with unstable three-column thoracolumbar burst fractures treated with anterior decompression and two-level anterior instrumentation. There were no cases of neurologic deterioration and 91% of patients with incomplete neurological deficit improved by at least one modified Frankel grade. In all, 95% went on to a stable arthrosis.

Sudo et al[36] performed a retrospective comparative study of anterior decompression and strut grafting versus posterior decompression and pedicle screw fixation with vertebroplasty with osteoporotic thoracolumbar fractures with neurologic deficits. For the posterior group, a direct midline posterior approach was utilized with laminectomies and vertebroplasty using calcium phosphate cement. For patients in the posteriorly treated group with significant vertebral collapse and with neural compression even after the laminectomy, a transpedicular decompression with cement placement and pedicle instrumentation was performed. The authors reported similar operative times and neurologic outcomes with both approaches.

Sasani et al[37] performed a prospective study of 14 patients who sustained thoracolumbar burst fractures and underwent posterior transpedicular decompression and expandable cage placement. They reported statistically significant improvement in VAS scores after surgery, and a mean operating time of 187 minutes.

Dimar et al[38] retrospectively reviewed 69 patients who underwent anterior decompression, strut autografting, and posterior instrumentation with autogenous fusion as either a combined or staged procedure and reported a 96% union rate. Of 22 patients with complete or partial neurologic injury, 12 either partially or totally recovered function.

16.11 Complications in Open Surgery

An open anterior approach may not be the optimal choice for some patients. A patient with thoracolumbar burst fracture who has concomitant chest or abdominal injury may not tolerate an anterior thoracolumbar exposure. Intra-abdominal injury can lead to peritoneal distension, which makes retroperitoneal exposure more challenging. Similarly, preexisting pulmonary disease or morbid obesity may also limit the use of an anterior approach. The anterior approach is difficult for low lumbar fractures, such as L4 and L5, because of the anatomical constraint of the great vessels. Morbid obesity may impair exposure and lead to inadequate visualization for safe decompression. When these conditions are present, the surgeon must balance the relative merits of open anterior and posterior approaches. Rare complications of the open anterior approach include peritoneal entry, damage to the ureter, interruption of lymphatic channels with resulting chylothorax or chylous leak, and splenic rupture. Late complications from the retroperitoneal approach also may include incisional hernia and permanent abdominal swelling on the side of the approach.[20]

Disadvantages to the open posterior approach include the increased difficulty in assessing adequacy of the ventral decompression, increased manipulation of neural elements, and technical challenges with anterior reconstruction from the posterior dissection. Furthermore, there is the potential for iatrogenic destabilization from resection of the posterior spinal elements.

The posterior approach may also be used to indirectly decompress the dura through distraction across segmental spinal instrumentation. The indirect reduction of retropulsed middle column fragments is achieved via the insertion of the posterior annulus fibrosus into the superior vertebral end plate.[39] Disadvantages of the posterior approach without anterior column reconstruction include the risk of the loss of correction, and of a less reliable anterior fusion. Using postoperative CT scanning, Bradford and McBride demonstrated that the average residual stenosis in patients treated with posterior reduction was 26%.[40] Posterior instrumentation alone, particularly when instrumenting fewer segments, carries the risk of hardware failure and recurrence of deformity.[5,41]

16.12 Conclusion of Open Surgery

While the minimally invasive lateral transpsoas technique has been utilized for anterior lumbar interbody fusion in the management of degenerative diseases and scoliosis, there are significant risks of damage to the genitofemoral nerve and lumbar plexus, which are not well visualized during this procedure. The lumbar plexus is located on the posterior abdominal wall in the substance of the psoas muscle and is composed of the anterior rami of the L1, L2, and L3 nerve roots and part of the anterior ramus of L4 nerve root.[42] Although EMG is used as sequential dilators are inserted through the psoas muscle, nerve and groin paresthesias have been reported after surgery.[16] Anatomic studies have demonstrated that there is no clearly safe portion of the psoas to transverse, as the lumbar plexus and nerve roots are contained throughout the psoas muscle.[42,43] Injury to nerves can occur through direct trauma, prolonged retraction, or postoperative hematoma. There is a paucity of literature pertaining to the use of intraoperative EMG neuromonitoring and minimally invasive spine surgery. Although improvements in electromyography systems with hunting algorithms, discrete threshold results, and directional orientations have led to a decrease in incidents of neurologic complications over the past decade,[44] they have not yet been published and validated in a peer-reviewed format compared to other neuromonitoring techniques.

Open surgical approaches offer superior visualization for neurologic decompression, maintenance of hemostasis, and preparation of surfaces for bony fusion. The broader exposure also facilitates bony and soft-tissue releases needed for adequate deformity correction. Significant clinical data support the efficacy of open approaches for treating these injuries. Based on the available evidence, we assign a 1C grade of recommendation for open surgical approaches in the management of thoracolumbar burst fractures. Future studies directly comparing the MIS lateral approach to open surgical approaches are warranted.

16.13 Editors' Commentary

16.13.1 Minimally Invasive Surgery

Treating thoracolumbar burst fractures using MIS technique requires a concept change regarding what is required to treat an unstable burst. The first question that must be asked is, "Can the neural elements be decompressed using MIS technique?" The answer is, "Yes." Using either a unilateral or a bilateral tubular approach gives adequate exposure to push the dorsally displaced disc and vertebral elements ventrally. The second question is, "Is there enough exposure to perform a vertebrectomy and anterior reconstruction?" The answer to this is, "with appropriate retraction, there can be." Numerous examples are in the literature now of vertebrectomy and anterior reconstruction. This usually combines an expandable tubular retractor and an expandable cage. This has not only been demonstrated for trauma, but for tumors and infections as well. However, the third question that must be asked is, "Does every burst fracture require anterior reconstruction?" And the answer to this question is, "Probably not." Depending on the extent of the burst, some (perhaps many) fractures can be successfully treated using posterior instrumentation alone. The advantage of this approach is a much smaller operation, faster recovery, fewer complications, and the maintenance of completely vascularized and innervated anatomy around the burst predisposes to faster healing. Although one might make the argument that less correction of the sagittal deformity will lead to chronic back pain, this has never been supported by the literature. Furthermore, since we lose roughly 50% of our correction with traditional open techniques, the faster healing seen in the MIS-treated patients might actually result in similar ultimate corrections. Thus, for many burst fractures, MIS treatment might be the optimal technique.

16.13.2 Open Surgery

Treatment of burst fractures without neurologic deficits typically involves nonsurgical approaches including bracing and early mobilization. Assuming that patients who suffer burst fractures are usually undergoing surgical intervention in the setting of neurologic deficits that require direct decompression of the spinal cord or cauda equina, optimal visualization of the neural elements is necessary. Application of a technique such as a transpsoas approach, which was developed to access the middle of the disc space in the AP axis for placement of an interbody cage, is poorly suited to decompress the spinal canal. Additionally, moving the operative corridor further posteriorly in order to gain access to the spinal canal increases the risk of lumbar plexus injury during passage through the psoas since the plexus tends to be located in the posterior aspect of the muscle.

The surgical corridor provided by an expandable retractor also limits the ability to place the large allograft bone struts or cages, which are often required to reconstruct the injured vertebrae compared to a larger open incision. Regardless of the use of anterior reconstruction and plating, patients often require supplemental posterior instrumentation. This raises questions about the need for anterior surgery in the first place given a thorough decompression and stabilization procedure can typically be accomplished using a posterior approach alone. Lastly, the use of anterior-only approaches is less versatile for treatment of injuries with posterior tension band injuries that would benefit from posterior stabilization to restore the tension band and prevent delayed development of kyphosis. Multiple studies have demonstrated the poor inter- and intraobserver reliability in assessment of the posterior ligamentous complex. Burst fractures with posterior ligamentous injuries cannot be treated intraoperatively when only an anterior approach is performed and therefore the fracture may be insufficiently stabilized.

References

[1] Aebi M, Etter C, Kehl T, Thalgott J. Stabilization of the lower thoracic and lumbar spine with the internal spinal skeletal fixation system. Indications, techniques, and first results of treatment. Spine. 1987; 12(6):544–551

[2] Clohisy JC, Akbarnia BA, Bucholz RD, Burkus JK, Backer RJ. Neurologic recovery associated with anterior decompression of spine fractures at the thoracolumbar junction (T12–L1). Spine. 1992; 17(8) Suppl:S325–S330

[3] Dai LY, Jiang SD, Wang XY, Jiang LS. A review of the management of thoracolumbar burst fractures. Surg Neurol. 2007; 67(3):221–231, discussion 231

[4] Denis F. The three column spine and its significance in the classification of acute thoracolumbar spinal injuries. Spine. 1983; 8(8):817–831

[5] McDonough PW, Davis R, Tribus C, Zdeblick TA. The management of acute thoracolumbar burst fractures with anterior corpectomy and Z-plate fixation. Spine. 2004; 29(17):1901–1908, discussion 1909

[6] Faciszewski T, Winter RB, Lonstein JE, Denis F, Johnson L. The surgical and medical perioperative complications of anterior spinal fusion surgery in the thoracic and lumbar spine in adults. A review of 1223 procedures. Spine. 1995; 20(14):1592–1599

[7] Kim DH, Jaikumar S, Kam AC. Minimally invasive spine instrumentation. Neurosurgery. 2002; 51(5) Suppl:S15–S25

[8] Bergey DL, Villavicencio AT, Goldstein T, Regan JJ. Endoscopic lateral transpsoas approach to the lumbar spine. Spine. 2004; 29(15):1681–1688

[9] Gumbs AA, Bloom ND, Bitan FD, Hanan SH. Open anterior approaches for lumbar spine procedures. Am J Surg. 2007; 194(1):98–102

[10] Westfall SH, Akbarnia BA, Merenda JT, et al. Exposure of the anterior spine. Technique, complications, and results in 85 patients. Am J Surg. 1987; 154 (6):700–704

[11] Anand N, Regan JJ. Video-assisted thoracoscopic surgery for thoracic disc disease: Classification and outcome study of 100 consecutive cases with a 2-year minimum follow-up period. Spine. 2002; 27(8):871–879

[12] Cunningham BW, Kotani Y, McNulty PS, et al. Video-assisted thoracoscopic surgery versus open thoracotomy for anterior thoracic spinal fusion. A comparative radiographic, biomechanical, and histologic analysis in a sheep model. Spine. 1998; 23(12):1333–1340

[13] Escobar E, Transfeldt E, Garvey T, Ogilvie J, Graber J, Schultz L. Video-assisted versus open anterior lumbar spine fusion surgery: a comparison of four techniques and complications in 135 patients. Spine. 2003; 28(7):729–732

[14] Scheufler KM. Technique and clinical results of minimally invasive reconstruction and stabilization of the thoracic and thoracolumbar spine with expandable cages and ventrolateral plate fixation. Neurosurgery. 2007; 61(4):798–808, discussion 808–809

[15] McAfee PC, Regan JR, Zdeblick T, et al. The incidence of complications in endoscopic anterior thoracolumbar spinal reconstructive surgery. A prospective multicenter study comprising the first 100 consecutive cases. Spine. 1995; 20(14):1624–1632

[16] Ozgur BM, Aryan HE, Pimenta L, Taylor WR. Extreme Lateral Interbody Fusion (XLIF): a novel surgical technique for anterior lumbar interbody fusion. Spine J. 2006; 6(4):435–443

[17] Bohlman HH, Freehafer A, Dejase J. Late anterior decompression for spinal cord injuries. J Bone Joint Surg Am 1975(57A):1025

[18] Bohlman HH, Zdeblick TA. Anterior excision of herniated thoracic discs. J Bone Joint Surg Am. 1988; 70(7):1038–1047

[19] McCormick PC. Retropleural approach to the thoracic and thoracolumbar spine. Neurosurgery. 1995; 37(5):908–914

[20] Kirkpatrick JS. Thoracolumbar fracture management: anterior approach. J Am Acad Orthop Surg. 2003; 11(5):355–363

[21] Viale GL, Silvestro C, Francaviglia N, et al. Transpedicular decompression and stabilization of burst fractures of the lumbar spine. Surg Neurol. 1993; 40(2): 104–111

[22] Lu DC, Lau D, Lee JG, Chou D. The transpedicular approach compared with the anterior approach: an analysis of 80 thoracolumbar corpectomies. J Neurosurg Spine. 2010; 12(6):583–591

[23] Pickett J, Blumenkopf B. Dural lacerations and thoracolumbar fractures. J Spinal Disord. 1989; 2(2):99–103

[24] Ayberk G, Ozveren MF, Altundal N, et al. Three column stabilization through posterior approach alone: transpedicular placement of distractable cage with transpedicular screw fixation. Neurol Med Chir (Tokyo). 2008; 48(1):8–14, discussion 14

[25] Vaccaro AR, Lehman RA, Jr, Hurlbert RJ, et al. A new classification of thoracolumbar injuries: the importance of injury morphology, the integrity of the posterior ligamentous complex, and neurologic status. Spine. 2005; 30 (20):2325–2333

[26] Whang PG, Vaccaro AR. Thoracolumbar fractures: anterior decompression and interbody fusion. J Am Acad Orthop Surg. 2008; 16(7):424–431

[27] Smith WD, Dakwar E, Le TV, Christian G, Serrano S, Uribe JS. Minimally invasive surgery for traumatic spinal pathologies: a mini-open, lateral approach in the thoracic and lumbar spine. Spine. 2010; 35(26) Suppl:S338–S346

[28] Baaj AA, Dakwar E, Le TV, et al. Complications of the mini-open anterolateral approach to the thoracolumbar spine. J Clin Neurosci. 2012; 19(9):1265–1267

[29] Khan SN, Cha T, Hoskins JA, Pelton M, Singh K. Minimally invasive thoracolumbar corpectomy and reconstruction. Orthopedics. 2012; 35(1): e74–e79

[30] Tormenti MJ, Maserati MB, Bonfield CM, Okonkwo DO, Kanter AS. Complications and radiographic correction in adult scoliosis following combined transpsoas extreme lateral interbody fusion and posterior pedicle screw instrumentation. Neurosurg Focus. 2010; 28(3):E7

[31] Uribe JS, Deukmedjian AR. Visceral, vascular, and wound complications following over 13,000 lateral interbody fusions: a survey study and literature review. Eur Spine J. 2015; 24 Suppl 3:386–396

[32] Wood KB, Bohn D, Mehbod A. Anterior versus posterior treatment of stable thoracolumbar burst fractures without neurologic deficit: a prospective, randomized study. J Spinal Disord Tech 2005;18(Suppl):S15-S23

[33] Lin B, Chen ZW, Guo ZM, Liu H, Yi ZK. Anterior approach versus posterior approach with subtotal corpectomy, decompression, and reconstruction of spine in the treatment of thoracolumbar burst fractures: a prospective randomized controlled study. J Spinal Disord Tech 2011 Jun [doi: 10.1097/ BSD.0b013e3182204c53][Epub]

[34] Kaneda K, Taneichi H, Abumi K, Hashimoto T, Satoh S, Fujiya M. Anterior decompression and stabilization with the Kaneda device for thoracolumbar burst fractures associated with neurological deficits. J Bone Joint Surg Am. 1997; 79(1):69–83

[35] Sasso RC, Best NM, Reilly TM, McGuire RA, Jr. Anterior-only stabilization of three-column thoracolumbar injuries. J Spinal Disord Tech. 2005; 18 Suppl: S7–S14

[36] Sudo H, Ito M, Kaneda K, et al. Anterior decompression and strut graft versus posterior decompression and pedicle screw fixation with vertebroplasty for osteoporotic thoracolumbar vertebral collapse with neurologic deficits. Spine J. 2013; 13(12):1726–1732

[37] Sasani M, Ozer AF. Single-stage posterior corpectomy and expandable cage placement for treatment of thoracic or lumbar burst fractures. Spine. 2009; 34(1):E33–E40

[38] Dimar JR, II, Wilde PH, Glassman SD, Puno RM, Johnson JR. Thoracolumbar burst fractures treated with combined anterior and posterior surgery. Am J Orthop. 1996; 25(2):159–165

[39] Edwards WT, Zheng Y, Ferrara LA, Yuan HA. Structural features and thickness of the vertebral cortex in the thoracolumbar spine. Spine. 2001; 26(2):218–225

[40] Bradford DS, McBride GG. Surgical management of thoracolumbar spine fractures with incomplete neurologic deficits. Clin Orthop Relat Res. 1987 (218):201–216

[41] Ebelke DK, Asher MA, Neff JR, Kraker DP. Survivorship analysis of VSP spine instrumentation in the treatment of thoracolumbar and lumbar burst fractures. Spine. 1991; 16(8) Suppl:S428–S432

[42] Moro T, Kikuchi S, Konno S, Yaginuma H. An anatomic study of the lumbar plexus with respect to retroperitoneal endoscopic surgery. Spine. 2003; 28 (5):423–428, discussion 427–428

[43] Banagan K, Gelb D, Poelstra K, Ludwig S. Anatomic mapping of lumbar nerve roots during a direct lateral transpsoas approach to the spine: a cadaveric study. Spine. 2011; 36(11):E687–E691

[44] Uribe JS, Vale FL, Dakwar E. Electromyographic monitoring and its anatomical implications in minimally invasive spine surgery. Spine. 2010; 35(26) Suppl: S368–S374

17 Open and Minimally Invasive Treatment of Cervical Spine Fractures

MIS: Michael Y. Wang and Joanna Gernsback
Open: S. Babak Kalantar and Joseph Paul Letzelter III

17.1 Introduction

Cervical spine trauma is a morbid problem causing potentially debilitating injuries in young patients and the elderly. Cervical spine trauma is associated with high-impact injuries in young patients and low-impact mechanisms in the elderly; hence, it usually occurs in a bimodal distribution. Common causes include motor vehicle accidents, falls, violence, and sports. C1 and C2 fractures are distinct from the fractures that occur in the subaxial spine, and account for 70% of all cervical fractures.[1] Gallie described C1–C2 wiring for fractures in 1939,[2] and the occipitocervical fusion was described in 1969 by Newman and Sweetnam[3] as an option for dens fractures. The odontoid screw was described by Böhler[4] in 1982, as another option for odontoid fractures. C1 lateral mass screws were described in 1994 by Goel and Laheri, for atlantoaxial dislocation,[5] and in 2001 Harms and Melcher added C2 pars screws.[6] Transarticular screws were described in 1987 by Grob and Magerl.[7] In the subaxial cervical spine, unstable fractures include teardrop fractures, jumped facets, and burst fractures associated with significant retropulsion. Treatment of subaxial cervical fractures began with Horlsey[8] and the simple laminectomy in 1895. Rogers presented spinous process wiring for trauma in 1942.[9] The anterior cervical discectomy and fusion was presented in 1955 by Smith and Robinson, and Cloward,[9] with the plate being added in the 1980s. Posterior lateral mass screws were described by Roy-Camille in 1980.[9] The focus of this chapter is unstable fractures, namely, those that require operative intervention for either internal fixation or decompression of neural elements. Although minimally invasive surgery (MIS) techniques for cervical spine fractures are in their infancy, several have been described. We will present an evidence-based discussion comparing the traditional treatment or "open" surgery for cervical spine fractures with MIS techniques.

17.2 Advantages of Minimally Invasive Surgery

MIS offers decreased operative time and blood loss, which are both beneficial in polytrauma and elderly patients, who may not tolerate longer procedures with significant blood loss. It avoids the necessity of significant muscle dissection, which may decrease postoperative neck pain. It eliminates the need for halos in some trauma patients. The incisions are smaller, meaning lower rates of wound problems and better cosmetic results.

17.3 Advantages of Open Surgery

Open treatment for cervical spine fractures has many potential advantages, which may not only affect the technical ease of performing the procedure but also can potentially result in improved outcomes. The most obvious benefit of open treatment is visualization. Open treatment provides the surgeon with better visualization of the fracture and neural elements not relying on fluoroscopic or indirect visualization of the traumatized segment. This is most important in cases where a discectomy is being performed and visualization of the spinal cord and canal is necessary. Open treatment also carries the benefit of increased fusion rates, which have been reported as high as 100%. Direct access and exposure to potential fusion surfaces both anteriorly and/or posteriorly can allow for more thorough decortication and more volume of bone graft material. Open treatment has also been shown to have high rates of increased stability due to fixation techniques, which add to increasing the likelihood of fusion.

In cases of traumatic spondylolisthesis in the subaxial spine, open treatment provides the benefit of improved access to the disc space in the case of a disc herniation. Access to the disc space also provides visualization of the neural elements, which aids the surgeon in decompression. Flexion-compression injuries approached anteriorly have been shown to restore the canal diameter by 60% compared to only 6% posteriorly. In summary, open treatment of cervical fractures provides better visualization, increased stability, and higher union rates.

17.4 Case Illustration

A 53-year-old homeless man, with a history of diabetes and glaucoma, was brought to the trauma center after falling off a balcony, approximately 8 ft. He was hypotensive and not moving his extremities. He was awake and mildly confused. He had no motor movement or sensation in his extremities. He had weak rectal tone and priapism. A computed tomography (CT) scan of the cervical spine demonstrated a comminuted fracture of the C4 vertebral body, involving the right transverse foramen, jumped facets at C4–C5, and anterolisthesis of C4 on C5 (▶ Fig. 17.1). The V2 segment was not visualized, suggestive of a vertebral artery injury. Emergent surgical intervention was recommended.

17.5 Surgical Technique in Minimally Invasive Surgery

The patient is brought to the operating room where general endotracheal anesthesia is administered. The patient should be intubated using a fiber optic system. A Foley catheter is inserted, pneumatic compression devices and neurophysiological monitoring leads placed, and an arterial line may be used if indicated. The Mayfield head holder is positioned, and the patient is carefully flipped onto a four-post operating table. All pressure points are padded. Preoperative antibiotics are then

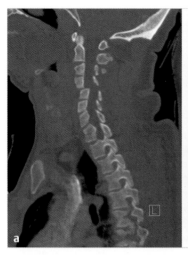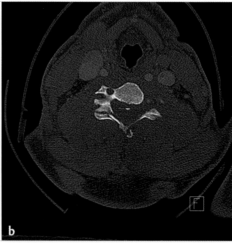

Fig. 17.1 (a) Sagittal and (b) axial initial computed tomography images demonstrating comminuted fractures of the C4 vertebral body, involving the right transverse foramen, jumped facets at C4–C5, and anterolisthesis of C4 on C5.

administered. The fluoroscopic C-arm is then positioned for lateral fluoroscopy.

A Steinman pin is inserted through the skin under fluoroscopy to reach the lateral mass. The pin trajectory should be parallel to the facet joint in the sagittal plane, making the skin entry point about three spinal segments below the dislocation. The entry point is midline in the axial plane, so the pin trajectory is in a superolateral direction. A 1.5-cm skin incision is made at the pin entry point. Serial METRx MD tubular dilators (Medtronic, Minneapolis, MN) are inserted to a final diameter of 18 or 22 mm. An 11-blade scalpel can be used to incise the nuchal fascia to facilitate tube placement. A headlight and surgical loupes improve visualization; an operating microscope would be a more cumbersome option.

The lateral mass surface is exposed using monopolar cautery and pituitary rongeurs to remove intervening soft tissue. A curette is used to remove the synovium of the facet joint to be fused, and the facet is packed with autograft bone.

A 14-mm-deep pilot hole is drilled with a 2.4-mm-diameter cancellous drill. The starting point is 1 mm medial to the midpoint of the lateral mass. The trajectory parallels the facet joint, at 20 degrees lateral. The pilot hole is tapped using a 2.43-mm-diameter cancellous tap. The depth is measured, and an appropriate length 3.5-mm-diameter polyaxial screw (Vertex; Medtronic) is placed. A second screw is placed in the adjacent lateral mass. A 3.2-mm-diameter top-loading connecting rod is attached. The rod should be inserted lengthwise into the tubular dilator and advanced superiorly into the upper polyaxial screw head. The tubular retractor is then slightly elevated to allow the inferior aspect of the rod to be inserted into the lower polyaxial screw head. Setscrews are placed to rigidly fix the construct. If a bilateral construct is desired, the process is repeated on the contralateral side. Proper screw placement is confirmed by anteroposterior fluoroscopy prior to skin closure.

17.6 Surgical Technique in Open Surgery

The patient is brought to the operating room and undergoes general endotracheal intubation with fiber optic assistance to avoid excessive cervical extension. Neurophysiologic leads are placed and baselines are recorded after the administration of anesthesia and then again after positioning. A Foley catheter is placed and anesthesia is administered at an arterial line to monitor blood pressure. A Mayfield head holder is applied and the patient is rotated into the prone position on a Stryker frame table. During rotation, light traction should be applied to increase stability.

After prone positioning and establishing neurophysiology baselines, the large C-arm is brought in and a lateral radiograph is obtained to ensure the dissection is carried down at the correct levels. A standard subperiosteal dissection of the posterior cervical spine is then performed down to the C4–C5 vertebrae. Once down to the desired levels, another radiograph is obtained to ensure the correct levels are in view. The lateral masses are then exposed on both vertebrae.

The dislocation is then reduced by grasping the involved spinous processes from C4 and C5 with a towel clip or tenaculum at the spinolaminar junction. The tenaculum or towel clip can be used to apply gentle traction to the caudal vertebrae while at the same time gentle distraction and a kyphotic moment is applied to the cephalad vertebra to disengage the dislocated facets. After the facets are unlocked, axial traction and reduction are performed to reduce the inferior articular processes posterior to the superior articular processes. During the reduction, it is important to have the neurophysiologist be alert for any acute signal changes. If there is an acute signal change, the procedure should be halted.

After the reduction is performed, the quadrilateral posterior surface of the lateral mass is exposed. A high-speed 2-mm burr is used to penetrate the outer cortex of the lateral mass at an entry point 1 mm medial to the center of the posterior surface of the lateral mass. A tap is then used and aimed parallel to the place of the facet joint with 25 degrees of lateral angulation in the axial plane. Prior to placement of screws, a C4 and C5 laminectomy is performed to adequately decompress the spinal cord. Using a high-speed burr, troughs are created at the junction of the lateral mass and lamina bilaterally. Bony resection can be completed with the burr or small Kerrison rongeur. The interspinous ligament and ligamentum flavum at C3–C4 and C5–C6 are resected and the laminae are lifted off and removed. This bone can be morselized and used for bone graft. A polyaxial unicortical screw is then placed into the lateral masses at

Table 17.1 Literature on MIS versus open cervical spine fractures treatment and MIS alone

Author (year)	Level	Study	Type	Pts	OR time	EBL	LOS	Findings
Wang et al (2011)[11]	III	Prosp	MIS vs. open	19 23	36 57	21 65		Percutaneous odontoid screw is faster with less blood loss, similar outcomes to open
Wang and Levi (2006)[20]	IV	Retro	MIS	20 (10 trauma)		127	3.9	Up to two levels of subaxial lateral mass screws can be placed through a tubular retractor, assuming intraoperative imaging is adequate
Wang et al (2012)[12]	IV	Retro	MIS	7	56			Direct repair of atlas displaced anterior arch fractures with microendoscopy improves bony union
Yoshida et al (2012)[18]	IV	Retro	MIS	1				O-arm navigation can be used for percutaneous pedicle screw fixation of a Hangman's fracture
Wu et al (2013)[17]	IV	Retro	MIS	10	98	25		Percutaneous C2 transpedicular screws can be used for Hangman's fracture
Holly et al (2010)[15]	IV	Retro	MIS	6		100		MIS C1–C2 fusion is technically feasible
Hashizume et al (2003)[16]	IV	Retro	MIS	1	110	30		Anterior odontoid screw fixation can be approached via endoscopy
Wu et al (2012)[13]	IV	Retro	MIS	7	56	<50		Percutaneous anterior triple screw fixation can be used for combined atlas–axis fractures
Dean et al (2010)[14]	IV	Retro	MIS	1			4	Percutaneous anterior triple screw fixation can be used for combined atlas–axis fractures
Fong and Duplessis (2005)[21]	IV	Retro	MIS	2			3	Lateral mass screw and plate constructs can be placed through tubular dilators
Tan et al (2008)[22]	IV	Retro	MIS	36 (6 trauma)	120	55	4.5	Endoscopic ACDF, particularly at C4–C5 and C5-C6, can produce satisfactory results with significant advantages over an open approach
Yao et al (2011)[10]	IV	Retro	MIS	67	107			Endoscopic ACDF can obtain satisfactory results with less morbidity

Abbreviations: ACDF, anterior cervical decompression and fusion; EBL, estimated blood loss; LOS, length of stay; MIS, minimally invasive surgery; OR time, operative time; Prosp, prospective; Pts, patients; Retro, retrospective.

C4 and C5. If facet or lateral mass fracture is encountered, further fixation points can be obtained at C3 and C6 to enhance stability. Prior to rod placement, the lateral portions of the lateral mass as well as the facet joints are decorticated using a small high-speed burr. Bone graft harvested from the laminectomy and/or iliac crest is morselized and placed posterolaterally. The screw heads are lined up and the rods are inserted and gentle compression across the construct is applied and set screws are placed. Screws are placed in standard fashion at C4 and C5. If there is no soft-tissue injury at the adjacent levels, and adequate biomechanical fixation is obtained, then a one-level fusion can be performed. Compression can be applied across the lateral mass screws to achieve alignment. Proper screw placement is confirmed by anteroposterior fluoroscopy prior to skin closure. The paraspinal muscles are approximated with a loose Vicryl stitch and the fascia is then sutured in watertight fashion using no. 1 or 0 Vicryl suture. A layered closure is completed with skin typically closed with a subcuticular Monocryl suture.

17.7 Discussion of Minimally Invasive Surgery

MIS procedures for the cervical spine are still in their infancy and are associated with a steep learning curve. This means there are not yet many studies in the literature (▶ Table 17.1 and ▶ Table 17.2). With one exception, all data for MIS treatment of cervical spine fractures are level IV; that is, it comes from case reviews or case series. Most of these include fewer than 10 patients, though the endoscopic anterior cervical decompression and fusion (ACDF) series[10] includes 67 patients. As more surgeons begin performing and reporting these procedures, the level of evidence will likely improve.

17.7.1 Level I Evidence in Minimally Invasive Surgery

There are no level I studies available.

Table 17.2 Literature on MIS versus open cervical spine fractures treatment and open alone

Author (year)	Level	Study	Type	Pts	OR time	Fusion	LOS	Findings
Kwon et al (2007)[23]	I	RCT	Ant vs. post	20 22	36 57	18/18 19/22	2.75 3.5	Both anterior and posterior fixation approaches are valid treatment options for unilateral facet injuries of the cervical spine
Tan et al (2009)[25]	III	Retro	Open	11	124	100%		Osteosynthesis of the atlas by C1 lateral mass screws C2 pedicle screws and crosslink compression fixation is an ideal option for C1 burst fracture
Aronson et al (1968)[27]	III	Retro	Open	86				Smith–Robinson approach is a valid surgical approach for anterior cervical discectomy and fusion.
Toh et al (2006)[29]	III	Retro	Ant vs. comb/post	24 7				Anterior decompression can restore the spinal canal diameter by 60% compared to only 6% with posterior stabilization alone.
Park et al (2015)[30]	III	Retro	Open	21	133.3			Open reduction with pedicle screw fixation or posterolateral removal of herniated disc fragments is a good treatment option for cervical facet dislocations.
Tokuku et al (2013)[31]	III	Retro	Post vs. comb	26 24	163.3 295.4		313.7g 689.1g	Patients with distractive flexion injuries of the cervical spine treated with posterior pedicle screws were found to have significantly shorter operative times, lower blood loss, and loss of kyphotic correction compared to combination approach.
Esses and Bednar (1991)[32]	IV	Retro	Open	10				Open screw fixation for odontoid fractures is a successful treatment option and can be used for fractures or nonunions.
Geisler et al (1989)[33]	IV	Retro	Open	9		100%		Anterior screw fixation for posteriorly displaced type 2 odontoid fractures shows significant advantages with 100% fusion
Harms and Melcher (2001)[6]	IV	Retro	Open	37		100%		Atlantoaxial instability can be treated with an open approach and polyaxial screws at C1–C2 with no neural or vascular damage and with solid fusion.
Dickman and Sonntag (1998)[35]	IV	Retro	Open	121		98%		Rigidly fixating C1–C2 instability with transarticular screws was associated with a significantly higher fusion rate than that achieved using wired grafts alone.

Abbreviations: Ant, anterior; Comb, combined; EBL, estimated blood loss; LOS, length of stay; MIS, minimally invasive surgery; OR time, operative time; Post, posterior; Pts, patients; RCT, randomized controlled trial; Retro, retrospective study.

17.7.2 Level II Evidence in Minimally Invasive Surgery

There are no level II studies available.

17.7.3 Level III Evidence in Minimally Invasive Surgery

Wang et al studied type II and rostral III odontoid fractures treated with anterior screw fixation. They treated 42 patients with either an open or a percutaneous anterior procedure. They found that the percutaneous group had significantly shorter operating times and less blood loss. There was no difference in clinical outcomes or radiation times between the two groups. They concluded that percutaneous anterior screw fixation is a safe and reliable procedure for type II and rostral III odontoid

fractures.[11] This is the only level III evidence available for MIS management of cervical spine fractures.

17.7.4 Level IV Evidence in Minimally Invasive Surgery

Wang et al[12] treated seven anterior atlas arch fractures using a direct C1 repair performed via a tubular retractor system and endoscopy. Operative time ranged from 45 to 75 minutes. Two of the seven patients had transient dysphagia. All but one had evidence of a bony fusion on follow-up imaging.

There have been descriptions of minimally invasive triple anterior screw fixation,[13,14] for combined C1–C2 fractures, which consists of an odontoid screw and bilateral C1–C2 transarticular screws. Surgical time ranged from 36 to 78 minutes, and blood loss ranged from 10 to 50 mL. At follow-up, all eight patients had odontoid union, stability of C1–C2, and no screw failure. This procedure is recommended by the study authors for atlas fracture with transverse ligament rupture and odontoid fracture, particularly in elderly patients and those with multiple injuries who would not tolerate a halo or a longer traditional surgery.

Level IV evidence for MIS treatment of odontoid fractures includes C1–C2 fusion[15] and an endoscopically assisted anterior odontoid screw.[16] The C1–C2 fusion, using a tubular retractor and the Harms and Melcher technique,[6] was reported by Holly et al in six patients. Average blood loss was 100 mL and all six patients achieved bony fusion without postoperative complications. Hashizume et al treated one patient with an endoscopic anterior screw, with 30 mL of blood loss in 110 minutes. The result was an asymptomatic nonunion.

There have been descriptions of percutaneous C2 pedicle screws for Hangman's fractures,[17,18] without the associated large incision or blood loss of an open procedure. A series of 10 patients[17] undergoing bilateral C2 transpedicular screw placement had operative times from 60 to 130 minutes, and all had less than 50 mL of blood loss. Three of the 20 screws breached the pedicle wall, but without causing symptoms or requiring additional surgery. The use of O-arm navigation[18] may prevent pedicle breaches. All 10 patients had bony fusion on follow-up imaging and full range of neck motion on clinical exam. This procedure is only appropriate for some types of Hangman's fractures.

Minimally invasive cervical lateral mass screws have been described in case series of trauma patients using both rods[19,20] and plates.[21] The procedure can be performed unilaterally or bilaterally, and has been described for one- and two-level constructs, from C3 to C7. This procedure is highly dependent on fluoroscopic guidance; thus, it is more suitable for higher levels and patients with longer necks. Use of the O-arm could theoretically overcome this obstacle. The minimally invasive technique avoids the significant muscle dissection associated with an open approach, which may decrease postoperative neck pain by maintaining the integrity of the posterior tension band.

Endoscopic ACDFs for one or two levels have been described,[10,22] ideally for C4–C5 and C5–C6, but also for C3–C4 and C6–C7. Two case series, with 103 patients, had a mean operating time of 112 minutes. Most patients had good outcomes. Of note, only 6 of the patients included in the two studies using this technique were trauma patients; however, since an ACDF is essentially the same surgery, regardless of indication, it is likely that this approach could be used for cervical fractures, though it has not yet been described in the trauma population.

17.8 Complications in Minimally Invasive Surgery

MIS surgery is at risk for the same complications as open surgery. Intraoperative complications such as injury to vasculature, nerves, or the esophagus are uncommon, but may not be recognized at the time of surgery due to the limited visualization. Screw malposition likely occurs at similar rates as in open surgery, since screws are typically placed primarily using fluoroscopy. A small number of MIS cases have to be converted to

Table 17.3 Breakdown of complications: aggregate from studies comparing minimally invasive surgery (MIS) versus open repair of cervical spine fractures with reported complication data[10,11,12,13,14,15,16,17,18,19,20,21,22]

Complication (%)	MIS	Open
Infection	1.7	0
New neurologic deficit	0	0
Hardware complication	5	2
Nonunion	5	4.3
Convert to open	3.3	NA
Other	3.3	8.7

Abbreviations: MIS, minimally invasive surgery; NA, not available.

open cases due to patient anatomy and insufficient visualization, typically in lower cervical levels. Postoperative dysphagia has been noted in several cervical MIS procedures, but it is uncommon and resolves spontaneously. Wound infections likely occur at lower rates than in open surgeries, due to smaller incisions and decreased operating time. Long-term complications, such as adjacent level disease and pseudoarthrosis, have been documented. Overall, complication rates are low for cervical MIS procedures, but the total number of procedures performed to date is small, making it difficult to compare it with open surgery (▶ Table 17.3).

17.9 Conclusion of Minimally Invasive Surgery

Minimally invasive techniques have been gaining popularity in all regions of the spine, due to decreased muscle dissection, meaning decreased pain and blood loss, and often, decreased operating time. These benefits are most important in elderly patients and patients with polytrauma, who will not tolerate a traditional surgery. They also offer smaller incisions, leading to a lower risk of wound breakdown or infection, and better cosmetic results. In cases of cervical spine trauma, they allow a patient to forgo a long immobilization in a halo brace, which may also not be tolerated in these target populations. The downsides are the significant learning curve associated with these techniques and their limited working room. Accessibility and visibility on fluoroscopy also limit the possible approaches. All of the minimally invasive techniques are relatively new and not in widespread use; additional follow-up and studies will be required to evaluate them fully. Currently, only a grade 2C recommendation can be made for using minimally invasive techniques to treat cervical fractures.

17.10 Discussion of Open Surgery

Open treatment of cervical fractures ranges from level II to level IV evidence depending on the fracture type investigated. Many of these fractures are not very common; thus, a large population study proves difficult. However, there are some studies, especially concerning posterior fusion with lateral mass screws for subaxial fractures, that have accumulated larger study populations and have a higher level of evidence.

17.10.1 Level I Evidence in Open Surgery

Kwon et al studied unilateral facet injuries treated with anterior versus posterior fixation.[23] They randomized 42 patients to undergo either anterior cervical discectomy and fusion or posterior fixation. They found no significant difference in regard to time to achieving discharge criteria, postoperative pain, infection, radiographic union, or alignment. They found that patients who had undergone the anterior approach had a higher rate of swallowing difficulty, which did not reach statistical significance. Conversely, the anterior approach, when compared to the posterior approach, carried a higher rate of union, lower rate of wound infection, and better radiographic alignment. However, none of these were found to be of statistical significance. They concluded that both open anterior and open posterior fixation approaches are valid treatment options.

17.10.2 Level II Evidence in Open Surgery

There are no level II studies available.

17.10.3 Level III Evidence in Open Surgery

Magerl's technique for treating atlas fractures has been shown to be an effective means of arthrodesis.[24] Tan et al also studied C1 lateral mass and C2 pedicle screws with crosslink compression fixation for unstable atlas fractures.[25] They found among the 11 patients studied that there were no neurologic deficits postoperatively, no vertebral artery complications, or other complications. Radiographic studies at 3 months showed bone fusion with stability in all patients. This technique also carried the advantage of direct visualization of the fracture and a decreased risk of injury to the vertebral arteries.

Hangman's fractures can be treated anteriorly or posteriorly.[26] Anterior treatment is necessary in the case of a traumatic disc herniation causing canal compromise. This approach puts the superior laryngeal nerve at risk.[27] The posterior approach on the other hand, by level III evidence, is the most effective method for stabilization. Screws are placed along the C2 pars interarticularis for osteosynthesis. Roy-Camille et al first described this procedure.[28] The screws are placed across the fracture line lagging the anterior fragment to the posterior fragment creating interfragmentary compression. In type III fractures, the C2 screws can be coupled to lateral mass screws at C3 for C2–C3 fusion.

Toh et al studied the anterior approach for decompression and fusion in the subaxial spine for patients with burst fractures or teardrop dislocation fractures. They found anterior decompression has been shown to restore the spinal canal diameter by 60% compared to only 6% with posterior stabilization alone.[29] Posterior fusion with cervical pedicle screws for subaxial cervical fractures has been shown to decrease subluxation in flexion-distraction subaxial cervical injuries. Park et al studied 21 patients with cervical subaxial facet dislocations,[30] 6 of whom also had disc herniations and all of whom had neurological symptoms. All patients underwent posterior open reduction and cervical pedicle screws. In cases with traumatic disc herniation, the herniated disc fragments were excised through a posterolateral approach. All patients improved neurologically. The mean segmental angles improved from 7.3 to – 5.9 degrees. The mean subluxation improved from 23.4 to 2.6%. Magnetic resonance imaging (MRI) confirmed that all disc fragments were successfully removed.

Tofuku et al studied subaxial cervical distraction flexion injuries treated with either posterior cervical screws or combined anterior–posterior approach. They retrospectively followed 50 patients, 24 of which underwent posterior wiring and fusion along with anterior decompression and fusion, while 26 of the patients underwent decompression and fusion with cervical pedicle screws. Patients treated with posterior pedicle screws only were found to have significantly shorter operative times, lower blood loss, and loss of kyphotic correction. Thus, they concluded posterior cervical pedicle screws were a reasonable treatment alternative for cervical distractive flexion injuries.[31] The combined posterior and anterior approach can be used in the presence of severe posterior ligamentous disruption.

17.10.4 Level IV Evidence in Open Surgery

Odontoid fractures treated with an odontoid screw have been shown to have level IV evidence. This technique, popularized by Bohler, has been shown to have a high fracture union rate.[32,33] One study found that out of 10 patients, 9 achieved fusion. The one that did not was lost to follow-up secondary to death from other injuries.[32] There was also no difference in cervical range of motion in elderly patients undergoing anterior screw fixation versus posterior fusion.[34] Posterior fusion for odontoid fractures is another option, but carries only level IV evidence. This technique can be performed with sublaminar wires, Magerl's screw technique or with C1 lateral mass and C2 pars screw fixation.[6] Harms et al studied 37 patients who underwent C1–C2 fusion with polyaxial screws into the lateral mass of C1 and the pars interarticularis of C2 with rod fixation. They found no neural or vascular damage in any patients, and early follow-up indicated fusion in all patients.

Dickman et al also studied posterior C1–C2 transarticular screw fixation for atlantoaxial arthrodesis. In their study, 121 patients underwent C1–C2 transarticular screws. At radiographic follow-up, 98% of the screws were in satisfactory position, while 2% were not, but this did not cause any clinical sequelae. Long-term follow-up at an average of 22 months found a 98% fusion rate. There were no neurologic sequelae.[35] This technique has also been shown to be comparable to the Magerl technique with minimal complications.[36]

17.11 Complications in Open Surgery

Complications of open treatment of cervical fractures and injuries can occur as a result of surgical approach, perioperatively, or late complications. Anterior approaches to the cervical spine are at risk for injury to the recurrent laryngeal nerve, superior laryngeal nerve, cervical sympathetic chain, esophagus, spinal cord, carotid, and vertebral arteries. Varying symptoms can result, including dysphonia, hoarseness, dysphagia, or more serious vascular or neurologic injury. Posterior approaches are at risk for spinal cord, nerve root, and vertebral artery injuries. Both approaches can be at risk for epidural hematoma, cerebrospinal fluid leakage, and wound infections. Late complications include progressive adjacent segment degeneration, neck pain, loss of range of motion, late instability, and late kyphotic deformity.

17.12 Conclusion of Open Surgery

Cervical spine fractures are common injuries in the elderly and in high-energy mechanisms in the younger population. Advanced imaging is important to characterize the extent of these fractures and help plan treatment. If stable, most fractures can successfully be treated conservatively. However, if unstable, surgical intervention may be necessary. There are a variety of options when choosing surgical approaches, and each approach and fixation method should be carefully chosen based on the injury, patient, and surgeon experience. Current open techniques have been utilized and improved upon for years. A grade 1C recommendation can be made for the use of open techniques in the treatment of cervical fractures. The majority of the literature supports open surgery, as there has not been a significant number of evidence-based research evaluating MIS.

17.13 Editors' Commentary

17.13.1 Minimally Invasive Surgery

So far, MIS applications to cervical trauma are limited. This is a combined result of several factors. First, anterior cervical surgery requires minimal muscle dissection and the anterior cervical structures are easily retracted out of the surgical corridor; thus, many of the advantages of MIS surgery have already been eliminated. Second, cervical fractures can be remarkably complex and require equally complex solutions. MIS technology has not yet reached the level of development to confidently attack these complexities. Third, the directional orthogonality of the multiple cervical muscle planes makes "dilation" over multiple levels difficult. Fourth, because of the close proximity of the cervical spinal cord to the surgical manipulations and the devastating consequences that can occur in the event of a mishap, development in this area has not been "high priority." Finally, because much cervical trauma surgery occurs in the middle of the night, conditions necessary for new technique/technology development are rarely available.

Perhaps, the exception to these barriers is the technique of posterior facet screw placement. This has been previously reported, but is mostly limited to one- or at most two-level stabilization of relatively straightforward traumatic conditions such as jumped or locked facets. In fact, this is an excellent example of where MIS techniques can be applied, but these isolated events may not be sufficient to lure surgeons to learn the skills necessary to perform the operation. Until our technology makes further advancements, this is an area of MIS surgery that we do not see advancing rapidly.

17.13.2 Open Surgery

The treatment of cervical injuries associated with trauma presents a set of unique circumstances that surgeons contemplating the use of MIS techniques must consider. More than any degenerative condition, traumatic injuries are associated with changes in bony architecture that may be poorly represented by preoperative imaging due to poorly visualized or unvisualized fracture lines or dynamic anatomic relationships due to secondary fracture displacement. Both underrepresented fracture complexity and postimaging displacement create a potentially dangerous surgical environment. This is true when surgeries are done using open techniques and even more so when the surgical techniques rely heavily on fluoroscopy, an imaging modality that lends itself more to landmark identification than demonstration of anatomic detail. Open surgery is more flexible with respect to seeking alternative fixation strategies when the planned screw trajectory or anatomic structure is unexpectedly compromised by instability or insufficient bone stock. Finally, one- or two-level constructs are exceptions rather than rules for traumatic injury in the cervical spine aside from the posterior treatment of odontoid fractures (in which bone grafting technique is critical due to the challenging fusion environment). In summary, while there is scant experience in the literature with which to evaluate MIS applications in the treatment of cervical trauma, the principles of trauma surgery ensure that these techniques will be unlikely to achieve even modest adoption because of the associated unnecessary risk and potential for adverse events.

References

[1] Spivak JM, Weiss MA, Cotler JM, Call M. Cervical spine injuries in patients 65 and older. Spine. 1994; 19(20):2302–2306
[2] Gallie W. Fractures and dislocations of the cervical spine. Am J Surg. 1939; 46(3):495–499
[3] Newman P, Sweetnam R. Occipito-cervical fusion. An operative technique and its indications. J Bone Joint Surg Br. 1969; 51(3):423–431
[4] Böhler J. Anterior stabilization for acute fractures and non-unions of the dens. J Bone Joint Surg Am. 1982; 64(1):18–27
[5] Goel A, Laheri V. Plate and screw fixation for atlanto-axial subluxation. Acta Neurochir (Wien). 1994; 129(1–2):47–53
[6] Harms J, Melcher RP. Posterior C1-C2 fusion with polyaxial screw and rod fixation. Spine. 2001; 26(22):2467–2471
[7] Grob D, Magerl F. Surgical stabilization of C1 and C2 fractures. Orthopade. 1987; 16(1):46–54
[8] Keller T. Victor Horsley's surgery for cervical caries and fracture. The Centennial Anniversary. Spine. 1996; 21(3):398–401
[9] Omeis I, DeMattia JA, Hillard VH, Murali R, Das K. History of instrumentation for stabilization of the subaxial cervical spine. Neurosurg Focus. 2004; 16(1): E10
[10] Yao N, Wang C, Wang W, Wang L. Full-endoscopic technique for anterior cervical discectomy and interbody fusion: 5-year follow-up results of 67 cases. Eur Spine J. 2011; 20(6):899–904
[11] Wang J, Zhou Y, Zhang ZF, Li CQ, Zheng WJ, Liu J. Comparison of percutaneous and open anterior screw fixation in the treatment of type II and rostral type III odontoid fractures. Spine. 2011; 36(18):1459–1463
[12] Wang J, Zhou Y, Zhang ZF, et al. Direct repair of displaced anterior arch fracture of the atlas under microendoscopy: experience with seven patients. Eur Spine J. 2012; 21(2):347–351
[13] Wu AM, Wang XY, Chi YL, et al. Management of acute combination atlas-axis fractures with percutaneous triple anterior screw fixation in elderly patients. Orthop Traumatol Surg Res. 2012; 98(8):894–899
[14] Dean Q, Jiefu S, Jie W, Yunxing S. Minimally invasive technique of triple anterior screw fixation for an acute combination atlas-axis fracture: case report and literature review. Spinal Cord. 2010; 48(2):174–177

[15] Holly LT, Isaacs RE, Frempong-Boadu AK. Minimally invasive atlantoaxial fusion. Neurosurgery. 2010; 66(3) Suppl:193–197

[16] Hashizume H, Kawakami M, Kawai M, Tamaki T. A clinical case of endoscopically assisted anterior screw fixation for the type II odontoid fracture. Spine. 2003; 28(5):E102–E105

[17] Wu YS, Lin Y, Zhang XL, et al. Management of Hangman's fracture with percutaneous transpedicular screw fixation. Eur Spine J. 2013; 22(1):79–86

[18] Yoshida G, Kanemura T, Ishikawa Y. Percutaneous pedicle screw fixation of a Hangman's's fracture using intraoperative, full rotation, three-dimensional image (O-arm)-based navigation: a technical case report. Asian Spine J. 2012; 6(3):194–198

[19] Wang MY, Prusmack CJ, Green BA, Gruen JP, Levi AD. Minimally invasive lateral mass screws in the treatment of cervical facet dislocations: technical note. Neurosurgery. 2003; 52(2):444–447, discussion 447–448

[20] Wang MY, Levi AD. Minimally invasive lateral mass screw fixation in the cervical spine: initial clinical experience with long-term follow-up. Neurosurgery. 2006; 58(5):907–912, discussion 907–912

[21] Fong S, Duplessis S. Minimally invasive lateral mass plating in the treatment of posterior cervical trauma: surgical technique. J Spinal Disord Tech. 2005; 18(3):224–228

[22] Tan J, Zheng Y, Gong L, Liu X, Li J, Du W. Anterior cervical discectomy and interbody fusion by endoscopic approach: a preliminary report. J Neurosurg Spine. 2008; 8(1):17–21

[23] Kwon BK, Fisher CG, Boyd MC, et al. A prospective randomized controlled trial of anterior compared with posterior stabilization for unilateral facet injuries of the cervical spine. J Neurosurg Spine. 2007; 7(1):1–12

[24] McGuire RA, Jr, Harkey HL. Primary treatment of unstable Jefferson's fractures. J Spinal Disord. 1995; 8(3):233–236

[25] Tan J, Li L, Sun G, et al. C1 lateral mass-C2 pedicle screws and crosslink compression fixation for unstable atlas fracture. Spine. 2009; 34(23):2505–2509

[26] Schneider RC, Livingston KE, Cave AJ, Hamilton G. "Hangman's fracture" of the cervical spine. J Neurosurg. 1965; 22:141–154

[27] Aronson N, Filtzer DL, Bagan M. Anterior cervical fusion by the Smith-Robinson approach. J Neurosurg. 1968; 29(4):396–404

[28] Roy-Camille R, Saillant G, Mazel C. Internal fixation of the unstable cervical spine by a posterior osteosynthesis with plats and screws. In: The Cervical Spine Research Society, ed. The Cervical Spine. 2nd ed. Philadelphia, PA: Lippincott Williams & Wilkins; 1989:390–403

[29] Toh E, Nomura T, Watanabe M, Mochida J. Surgical treatment for injuries of the middle and lower cervical spine. Int Orthop. 2006; 30(1):54–58

[30] Park JH, Roh SW, Rhim SC. A single-stage posterior approach with open reduction and pedicle screw fixation in subaxial cervical facet dislocations. J Neurosurg Spine. 2015; 23(1):35–41

[31] Tofuku K, Koga H, Yone K, Komiya S. Distractive flexion injuries of the subaxial cervical spine treated with a posterior procedure using cervical pedicle screws or a combined anterior and posterior procedure. J Clin Neurosci. 2013; 20(5):697–701

[32] Esses SI, Bednar DA. Screw fixation of odontoid fractures and nonunions. Spine. 1991; 16(10) Suppl:S483–S485

[33] Geisler FH, Cheng C, Poka A, Brumback RJ. Anterior screw fixation of posteriorly displaced type II odontoid fractures. Neurosurgery. 1989; 25(1):30–37, discussion 37–38

[34] Stulík J, Suchomel P, Lukás R, et al. Primary osteosynthesis of the odontoid process: a multicenter study. Acta Chir Orthop Traumatol Cech. 2002; 69(3):141–148

[35] Dickman CA, Sonntag VK. Posterior C1-C2 transarticular screw fixation for atlantoaxial arthrodesis. Neurosurgery. 1998; 43(2):275–280, discussion 280–281

[36] Melcher RP, Puttlitz CM, Kleinstueck FS, Lotz JC, Harms J, Bradford DS. Biomechanical testing of posterior atlantoaxial fixation techniques. Spine. 2002; 27(22):2435–2440

18 Thoracolumbar Metastatic Tumors: Comparison of Minimally Invasive Surgery versus Open Techniques for Addressing Thoracolumbar Metastatic Tumor Resection and Stabilization

MIS: Prashanth J. Rao and Ralph J. Mobbs
Open: Peter S. Rose and Michelle J. Clarke

18.1 Introduction

Cancer is currently the second leading cause of death in the United States, Australia, and most western nations; it is already the leading cause of death in some developed countries. The majority of patients with cancer have spinal metastases present at autopsy,[1,2] with around 30% of them exhibiting symptomatic metastatic spinal disease.[3] While only a minority (10%) of these progress to epidural spinal cord, conus medullaris, or cauda equina compression, because of the large numbers involved, metastatic compression of the neural elements is a common occurrence in clinical practice.[3] In most estimates, oncologic neurologic compression along the spinal axis is approximately twice as common as traumatic spinal cord injuries.

Radiotherapy is used in the treatment of almost all patients with symptomatic spinal metastases. While the response of any given lesion to radiotherapy is not known, estimates of radiosensitivity can be made based on histology (▶ Table 18.1). However, radiation therapy is not able to restore mechanical integrity to a spine compromised by pathologic fracture or impending instability. As well, once neurologic signs are present, level I evidence has demonstrated the superiority of direct decompressive surgery followed by radiotherapy to radiotherapy alone in the care of patients with common metastatic histologies.[4] Clinical experience and published data have shown a benefit for direct decompressive treatment of the spinal cord rather than stabilization alone and/or indirect decompression by laminectomy.

Patients undergoing decompression and stabilization procedures for metastatic spinal cord compression have traditionally been approached in an open manner. However, advances in instrumentation, imaging, and navigation now make minimally invasive approaches possible. These techniques most commonly involve the use of percutaneously placed pedicle screw instrumentation along with decompression through a limited open or tubular retractor system.[5]

18.2 Indications for Surgery for Metastatic Epidural Neurologic Compression

Patients who present with or have impending spinal instability and/or neurologic deficit from typical solid organ metastases are considered for surgical treatment. Patients with hematopoietic malignancies and certain highly chemo- or radiosensitive solid organ metastases (e.g., lymphoma, germ cell tumors) can often be managed without surgical intervention because of

the ability to achieve rapid disease regression and decompression of neural elements with these modalities. Patients who have widely disseminated disease with an anticipated life expectancy less than 3 months or multiple sites of spinal involvement seldom benefit from aggressive surgical intervention. Additionally, once a dense neurologic deficit is present, particularly for greater than 48 hours, the likelihood of meaningful recovery is low and surgery is generally not indicated. Surgeons must also evaluate potential surgical patients for their

Table 18.1 Radiosensitivity of common metastatic histologies

	Histology	Value of radiation as sole treatment
Highly radiosensitive	Myeloma	Effective treatment
	Lymphoma	
	Germ cell tumors	
Moderately radiosensitive	Breast cancer	
	Small cell lung cancer	
Moderately radioresistant	Colon cancer	
	Non–small cell lung cancer	
Highly radioresistant	Renal cell carcinoma	
	Thyroid carcinoma	Suboptimal/Unreliable treatment
	Sarcoma	
	Melanoma	

fitness to undergo surgical procedures (particularly if a patient is in the process of receiving chemotherapy at the time of presentation).

Several clinical scales have been introduced to guide the treatment of patients with metastatic disease to the spine. The Spinal Instability Neoplastic Score (SINS) from the Spine Oncology Study Group is the most contemporary method to evaluate for present or potential spinal instability from neoplastic processes.[6] While a number of clinical scoring systems exist to stratify patients for aggressive, palliative, or nonoperative treatment, the modified Tokuhashi score is currently the most widely accepted treatment framework in clinical practice.[7] It assesses the patient's spinal and extraspinal disease burden, histology, neurologic status, and performance status to guide treatment recommendations.

18.3 Advantages of Minimally Invasive Surgery

The surgical treatment for the majority of patients with metastatic epidural neurologic compression is palliative, while a cure can be achieved in only a minority of select patients with surgically resectable or chemoradiotherapy sensitive disease.[8,9] Due to the poor general condition of these patients, open spinal decompression with stabilization surgery may be associated with high morbidity rates.[8,10,11] Basic principles of a minimally invasive surgery (MIS) approach in spine surgery include the following: (1) avoid iatrogenic muscle injury by self-retaining retractors; (2) do not disrupt tendon attachment sites of key muscles, particularly the origin of the multifidus muscle on the spinous process; (3) use known anatomic neurovascular and muscle compartment planes; and (4) minimize collateral soft-tissue injury by limiting the width of the surgical corridor.[12]

There are several important advantages of MIS techniques for spinal decompression and stabilization in metastatic spine disease. Although complete tumor resection through an MIS access could be a limitation, the goal of surgery (open or MIS) in these cases is tumor debulking, neuronal decompression, and mechanical stabilization, which can be achieved readily via an MIS technique. Definitive treatment in such cases is in fact chemoradiotherapy, which can be started earlier in MIS patients given that wound and general recovery are quicker. Although circumferential compression is common, the majority of the metastatic disease is in the vertebral body. A common MIS approach is posterior for spinal metastatic disease; however, anterior or lateral approaches are available to be utilized as either a stand-alone or combined with percutaneous posterior pedicle screw stabilization. Another advantage of the MIS technique is faster wound healing, which lessens the risk of wound dehiscence following radiotherapy. It is common knowledge that prolonged operative time is associated with increased infection rates and elevated blood loss, and blood transfusion is associated with risk of systemic infection, gastrointestinal complaints, and hemolytic reactions.[13] Due to the minimization of surgical exposure, MIS techniques result in reduced blood loss. Although the criticism of MIS technique is longer operative times, as a result of minimal wound exposure, the operative time is in fact reduced.[14,15] The morbidity of spine surgery in patients with neuronal compression from metastatic tumor can be minimized with MIS techniques by reducing operative time, blood loss, and iatrogenic muscle injury, and decreasing the need for blood transfusions.

18.4 Advantages of Open Surgery

Although some cases are selected for an anterior approach, the majority of patients are approached with a midline posterior approach using pedicle screw stabilization above and below the level of the pathology and a transpedicular or limited costotransversectomy for decompression of the neural elements. When possible, a cage or methylmethacrylate is used to reconstruct the anterior column.

The open technique for stabilization and decompression has several advantages. It is the only technique for which level I evidence supports the surgical treatment of patients with metastatic epidural spinal cord compression. A key aspect in studies that have demonstrated a benefit to surgery in these patients has been the ability to perform a direct decompression of the neural elements. Metastatic tumors leading to cord compression arise in the vertebral body in approximately 85% of cases but commonly demonstrate near circumferential involvement of the spinal canal. Depending on the local anatomy of the tumor, it can be difficult for surgeons to fully access the spinal canal and perform a true direct decompression of the neural elements with MIS techniques. The majority of tumors leading to metastatic spinal cord compression are lytic; an open technique affords the surgeon the widest array of options for reconstruction of the anterior column through a transpedicular or limited costotransversectomy approach. These cases often present in an urgent clinical fashion, and open techniques employ standard spinal instruments, instrumentation, and imaging capabilities that are readily available even when cases are performed on an unscheduled or "add-on" basis.

The techniques of the open approach are an adaptation of techniques known to qualified spine surgeons and do not require any steep learning curves that MIS techniques may have; they are readily "scalable" to apply to lesions that involve more than a single level of compression and are also applicable along the entire length of the spinal axis. While MIS techniques hold the potential for lower complications and more rapid institution of adjuvant treatments, no high-level evidence demonstrates this to be the case. Even if radiotherapy can theoretically be administered 7 to 10 days earlier with MIS techniques, there is no established clinical benefit to this. The net length of surgical incision used in standard surgeries is often substantially less than the sum of incisions used in an MIS procedure given the need for separate incisions for decompression, placement of each screw, and rod placement.

18.5 Case Illustration

A 58-year-old female patient presented with a 2-month history of back pain. She was a heavy smoker but otherwise had no significant past medical history. X-ray of the chest revealed a lung lesion on the right that on computed tomography (CT) guided biopsy was diagnosed as a large cell carcinoma of the lung. Also on the CT scan, a single metastatic lesion was found at the T9 level. She underwent radiation to the spinal lesion for 2 days

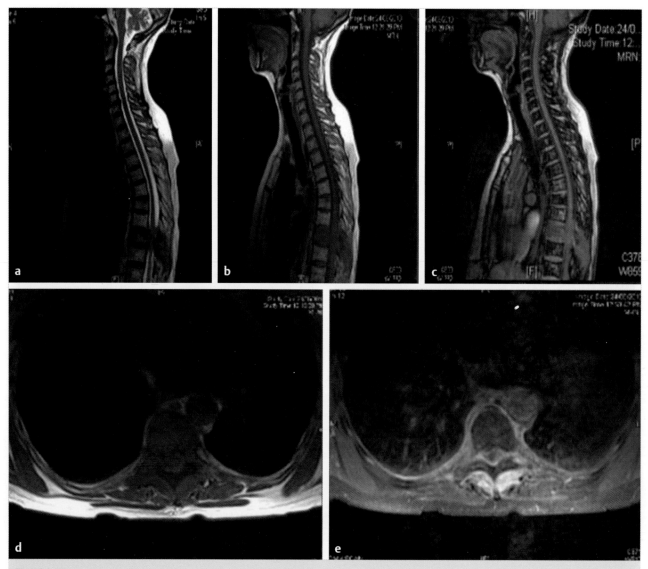

Fig. 18.1 Preoperative magnetic resonance imaging scan. **(a)** Sagittal T2-weighted image of cervicothoracic region demonstrating circumferential spinal cord compression by metastatic tumor at T9 level. **(b)** Sagittal T1-weighted image of cervicothoracic region. **(c)** Contrast-enhanced sagittal image of cervicothoracic region. **(d)** Axial T2-weighted image at T9 level demonstrating spinal cord compression. **(e)** Axial contrast-enhancing image.

and then developed rapidly progressive paraplegia (T10 sensory level, 1/5 MRC [Medical Research Council] grade power in lower limbs). On MRI (whole spine) scan (▶ Fig. 18.1), circumferential spinal cord compression was identified at the T9 vertebral level due to tumor involving all the three columns. On T2-weighted images (▶ Fig. 18.1a, d), there was no cerebrospinal fluid evident around the spinal cord at that level. With the administration of contrast (▶ Fig. 18.1c, e), the tumor was enhancing and involved all the spinal columns including the prevertebral soft tissue.

Median survival was estimated to be between 6 to 9 months after a discussion with her oncologist. After thorough discussion with the patient, it was decided to proceed with surgery within 12 hours after the onset of paraplegia.

18.6 Surgical Technique in Minimally Invasive Surgery

18.6.1 Step 1: Decompression

After induction of general endotracheal anesthesia patient was positioned prone on a Jackson table with Harbor Bridge. Suitable padding of all pressure areas was done. Image intensifier confirmation of the index level was performed prior to prepping and draping. Local anesthetic 0.25% Marcaine with adrenaline was infiltrated along the incision line. A small 4-cm midline incision was placed at the index level. Subperiosteal muscle dissection was performed to expose the T9 lamina, and facet joints (T8/T9) and Versatrac retractors were placed. A T9 laminectomy

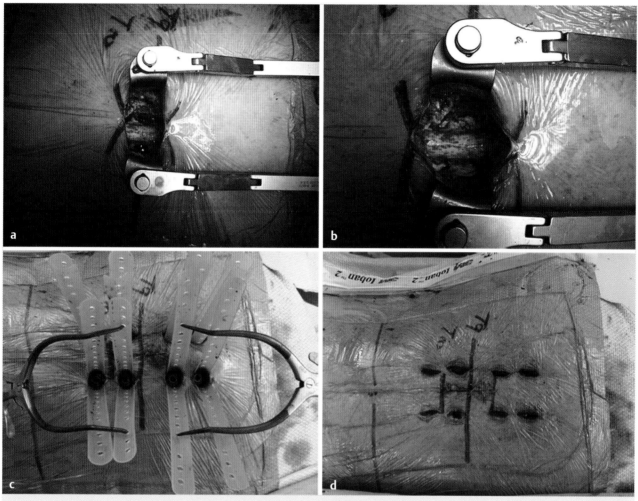

Fig. 18.2 Minimally invasive surgery technique (decompression). **(a)** Laminectomy and posterior spinal cord decompression. **(b)** Transpedicular anterior spinal cord decompression and methylmethacrylate augmented reconstruction. **(c)** Stabilization with percutaneously inserted pedicle screws and rods. **(d)** Demonstration of midline and percutaneous pedicle screw wounds.

was performed with high-speed burr and Kerrison rongeurs. Extradural tumor with ligamentum flavum was removed with pituitary rongeurs to decompress the spinal cord posteriorly (▸ Fig. 18.2a). Bilateral pediculotomies were performed, and tumor involving the pedicles was removed and the posterior part of the vertebral body reached. Extradural tumor compressing the spinal cord anteriorly and involving the posterior half of the vertebral body was removed with pituitary rongeurs resulting in 360-degree decompression of the spinal cord. Vertebroplasty was performed with methylmethacrylate (▸ Fig. 18.2b) and after hemostasis the wound was closed in layers.

18.6.2 Step 2: Stabilization

Percutaneous pedicle screws (T7, T8, T10, and T11) were placed under image intensifier guidance. Suitable sized rods were threaded onto screw heads and secured with set screws. (▸ Fig. 18.2c,d; ▸ Fig. 18.3; and ▸ Fig. 18.4)

18.7 Surgical Technique in Open Surgery

The patient is positioned prone on a radiolucent frame with fluoroscopy used for initial localization and to verify implant position. A midline incision is used to expose to the transverse processes from T7 to T11 and pedicle screws are placed using the surgeon's technique of choice (anatomic landmarks are the preference of the author) typically two levels above and two levels below the tumor.

A holding rod is maintained on one side at all times to guard against subluxation. A laminectomy is performed from the pedicles of T8 to the pedicles of T10, and the dural plane is accessed above the level of tumor. Once all dorsal tumor is removed, the pedicle on one side is removed and the plane between the posterior longitudinal ligament (PLL) and the dura is identified (the PLL is a natural anatomic barrier to tumor extension and a reliable landmark in cases not previously

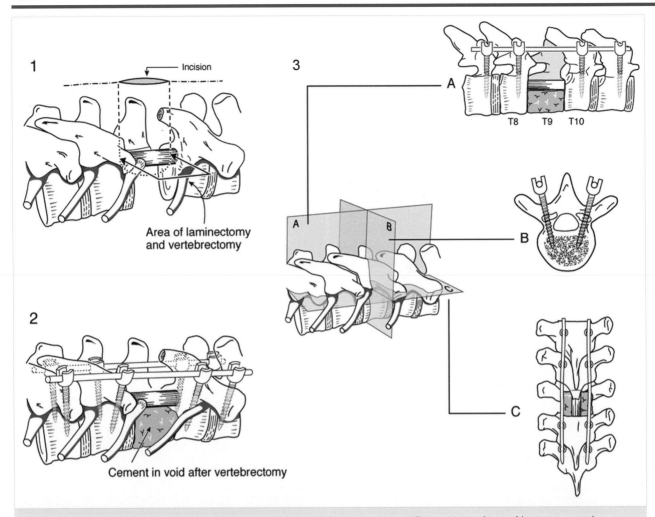

Fig. 18.3 Line illustrations of the minimally invasive surgery technique. **(1)** Demonstrating midline incision and area of laminectomy and vertebrectomy. **(2)** Vertebral body reconstruction with methylmethacrylate. **(3)** Percutaneous pedicle screw fixation and stabilization. (Reproduced with permission of John Wiley and Sons.)

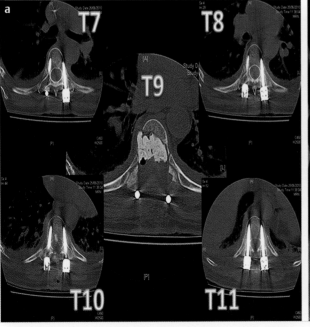

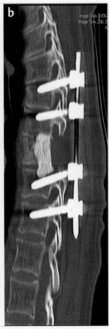

Fig. 18.4 (a) Axial and **(b)** sagittal postoperative computed tomography scan demonstrating decompression, reconstruction with methylmethacrylate, and stabilization.

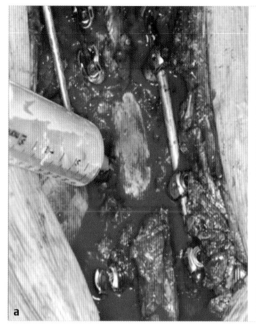
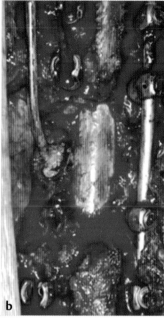

Fig. 18.5 (a) Insertion of methylmethacrylate (dyed blue) into lytic defect following decompression and instrumentation. **(b)** View following decompression and stabilization.

manipulated). Tumor coming out of the vertebral body is removed using curettes, rongeurs, and suction curettage. The PLL is sectioned with tenotomy scissors and removed to avoid leaving tumor remnants in close proximity to the neural elements.

A second holding rod is placed on the decompressed side and then the initial rod is removed from the side not yet decompressed. If necessary to achieve complete decompression, a second transpedicular decompression is performed on this side to remove any residual tumor. Decompression is verified by passing a curved instrument underneath the spinal cord to verify a free plane; if necessary, an intraoperative ultrasound may be performed to verify decompression.

Once decompression is performed, the lytic defect in the anterior column is reconstructed; the author's preferred technique is to use methylmethacrylate although static and expandable cages may be used as well (▶ Fig. 18.5). In most cases, a rigorous decortication and fusion is not attempted. Decortication removes natural anatomic barriers to tumor extension at adjacent levels, and fusion is unlikely to occur in the face of radiotherapy and chemotherapy. Closure is in anatomic layers with a suction drain used only if bleeding is significant.

18.8 Discussion of Minimally Invasive Surgery

18.8.1 Level I Evidence in Minimally Invasive Surgery

No level I evidence is available in the literature.

18.8.2 Level II Evidence in Minimally Invasive Surgery

There are two level II evidence studies in literature. In a prospective study of 25 patients, Tancioni et al[16] performed posterior decompression, anterior column reconstruction using transpedicular balloon kyphoplasty with polymethyl-methacrylate augmentation, and percutaneous pedicle screw fixation utilizing MIS technique. In all, 88% of the patients improved neurologically and 96% improved with respect to pain scores. These results persisted until death or disease progression elsewhere in a majority of patients. Radiotherapy was initiated 2 weeks after surgery in all patients.

Zairi[17] et al prospectively evaluated 10 patients with palliative spinal metastatic disease who underwent MIS decompression and stabilization using tubular retractors for decompression without anterior column reconstruction. Postoperatively 80% of patients improved by at least 1 Frankel grade, 71% of preoperatively nonambulatory patients were ambulatory post operation, and pain improved in all patients. Seven of the 10 patients were discharged home, while 3/10 were transferred to oncology unit. Mean length of stay (MLOS) was 6 days, mean operative time (MOT) was 170 minutes, and mean blood loss (MBL) was 400 mL. No blood transfusion was required.

18.8.3 Level III and IV Evidence in Minimally Invasive Surgery

There are multiple heterogeneous studies as detailed in ▶ Table 18.2 demonstrating similar results as the previously mentioned level II studies. Mclain used an endoscopic-assisted transpedicular approach for anterior decompression with titanium cage placement in nine patients with metastases to the thoracic spine. All nine patients avoided lengthy ICU (intensive care unit) admissions (average: 1.4 days) typically seen after undergoing thoracotomy for upper thoracic spine metastases. Six of the nine patients with neurologic deficit preoperatively showed improvement in their deficit following surgery.[18] Huang et al performed a retrospective analysis comparing 29 patients undergoing "minimal-access spine surgery" versus 17 patients undergoing standard thoracotomy (ST) for metastatic lesions between T3 and T12. Both groups were comparable for mean blood loss, complication rate, and return to ambulation

Table 18.2 Studies on MIS technique for spinal metastatic disease: operative data, outcomes, and complication rate

Author	No. of patients	MBL (mL)	MOT (min)	LOS (d)	MNI (%)	MPA (%)	MCR (%)
Lin et al[27]	25	1,047	324	N/A	76	68	4
Tancioni et al[16] (prospective)	25	N/A	N/A	6	88	96	12
Zairi et al[17] (prospective)	10	400	170	6	100	100	10
Rosenthal et al[26]	4	1,450	390	7.5	100	100	0
Huang et al[28]	41 (VATS)	775	190	N/A	N/A	N/A	54
Huang et al[19]	29 (MASS)	1,100	179		70.8		24
Le Huec et al[31]	2	350	156	N/A	100	100	50
McLain[18]	8	1,677	360	6.5	100	100	0
Mobbs et al[29]	1				100	100	0
Deutsch et al[15]	8	227	132	4	62.5	62.5	0
Mühlbauer et al[32]	5	1,120	360	N/A	100	100	0
Kan and Schmidt[30]	5	610	258	6.25	100	100	0
Payer and Sottas[33]	11	711	N/A		91	N/A	18
Taghva et al[34]	1	1,200	420	5	100	100	0

Abbreviations: LOS, length of stay; MASS: minimal access spine surgery; MBL, mean blood loss; MCR, mean complication rate; MNI, median neurologic improvement; MOT, mean operative time; MPA, median pain alleviation; N/A, not available; VATS, video-assisted thoracoscopic surgery.

following surgery (MASS [minimal access spine surgery] 70.8% vs. ST 69.2%), with the MASS group exhibiting significantly shorter ICU admissions.[19] These studies are similar to the surgery plus radiotherapy treatment outcomes in the level I study of Patchell et al[4] emphasizing the equipoise of MIS technique to open technique with respect to clinical effectiveness.

One level III study by Lau and Chou[20] retrospectively studied open versus "mini-open" posterior corpectomy with cage reconstruction in 49 patients with thoracic spine metastases. Twenty-eight patients underwent an open approach, whereas 21 patients underwent a mini-open approach with fascial and muscle dissection limited to the level of metastasis, and pedicle screws inserted percutaneously. All patients underwent anterior column reconstruction via an expandable titanium cage. Patients in the mini-open group showed significantly less blood loss and shorter hospital stays (7.4 vs. 11.4 d) when compared with patients in the open group. Patients in the mini-open group also trended toward lower perioperative complications and infection rates, while maintaining similar rates of 30-day complications, need for reoperations, and postoperative ASIA grade changes when compared to the open group. The study, however, did not extend into analysis of quality of life measures or timing of adjuvant chemoradiation.

18.9 Complications in Minimally Invasive Surgery

Zairi et al reported only one benign complication (UTI [urinary tract infection]),[17] while Tancioni found a 12% complication rate,[16] one wound infection and two medical complications (pneumonia and DVT [deep vein thrombosis]). In the review by Molina, the median complication rates for video-assisted thoracoscopic surgery (VATS) were 0% (0-54%), for MASS were 9% (0-24%), and for open thoracotomy were 30.5% (15-94.4%).[9] In Huang et al's series of VATS, complications included severe

bleeding in five cases, two deaths, one pericardial penetration, one case of implant failure, and one superficial wound infection. The majority of the other studies report a low rate of complications. In another VATS study, Le Huec et al found a regressive, incomplete recurrent laryngeal nerve palsy in a patient after resection of a metastatic lesion in the T1–T2 vertebral bodies. Apart from the study of Huang and colleagues, there are no cases of mortality related to surgery as opposed to 4 to 8% in open surgery group.[8,10,11]

Recurrence during follow-up period is infrequently reported. There were no recurrences in the study of Zairi et al, while Tancioni found 8% recurrence associated with disease progression and Huang et al found one recurrence in a cohort of 29 patients.

18.10 Conclusion of Minimally Invasive Surgery

There is evidence of similar effectiveness with regard to neurological recovery and pain alleviation when comparing MIS to open techniques based on literature review. This demonstrates the basic principle of metastatic spine disease management that en bloc spondylectomy is not necessary and the goals are surgical decompression and stabilization to relieve pain and improve neurological function. MIS technique, more importantly, is associated with reduced operative time, blood loss, length of hospital stay, and complication rate that results in lower morbidity rates in a patient with poor general condition.

There are, however, minimal direct comparison studies available between the two techniques. Research that does compare these open versus MIS techniques suggests similar neurologic outcomes and pain relief, with lower blood loss, shorter hospital stays, and lower complication rates for patients undergoing a minimally invasive procedure. Due to this lack of support, only a grade 2B recommendation using the grading scale of Guyatt et al may be given to the evidence supporting the potential superiority of minimally invasive over open techniques in the management of thoracolumbar metastatic lesions. However, with the evidence from multiple level II and III studies, a grade 1C recommendation may be assigned supporting improved pain scores and neurologic outcomes in patients undergoing MIS decompression and stabilization, on par with historical data from numerous open studies. The issue of steep learning curve for MIS technique needs to be addressed. Having said that, as the proficiency of MIS techniques among spine surgeons is improving, it is prudent to assume that the effectiveness will be enhanced and morbidity will be reduced in future studies than currently available.

18.11 Discussion of Open Surgery

18.11.1 Level I Evidence in Open Surgery

Level I evidence in favor of direct decompression is found in the study by Patchell et al.[4] This prospective randomized trial was stopped early by a data safety monitoring committee because of the significant benefits recognized by the surgery group. In this multi-institutional trial, patients presenting with metastatic spinal cord compression were randomized to radiotherapy alone or direct surgical decompression followed by radiotherapy. Patients treated surgically were significantly more likely to remain ambulatory (84% compared to 57%, $p = 0.001$). Patients also retained the ability to walk significantly longer (median: 122 vs. 13 days, $p = 0.003$). In nonambulatory patients, significantly higher number of patients treated surgically regained the ability to walk than those treated with radiation alone (62 vs. 19%, $p = 0.01$). Similar results were seen for secondary endpoints of continence and neurologic function.

18.11.2 Level II Evidence in Open Surgery

Quan and colleagues[8] and Ibrahim et al[10] in separate studies have reported prospective outcomes for patients treated surgically using a treatment framework very similar to that of Patchell et al using open surgery. Both trials found results similar to those of Patchell et al., and both demonstrated significant improvements in quality of life with surgical intervention. In a prospective study by Quan et al, 118 patients with a histologic variety of spinal column metastases were followed up over 1 year after surgery. Surgery varied between anterior, posterior, and combination approaches. Following decompression and stabilization, 68% of patients who were nonambulatory before surgery regained mobility. A statistically significant improvement in quality of life and physical functioning was maintained throughout the 12-month follow-up. In a multicenter, prospective study of 223 patients by Ibrahim et al, the authors showed a similar improvement in postoperative pain and radiculopathy, with 47% of patients improving by greater than 1 KPS (Karnofsky performance scale) score and 39% of patients regaining urinary sphincter control.

Klimo and colleagues[21] performed a meta-analysis of published articles analyzing modern surgical techniques compared with radiotherapy alone based on published reports of 24 surgical studies (999 patients) and 4 radiotherapy studies (543 patients). The results showed that patients treated surgically were 1.3 times more likely to be ambulatory after treatment and twice as likely to regain ambulation if not ambulatory at the start of treatment for metastatic epidural spinal cord compression.

Thomas[22] analyzed the data in Patchell et al's study from a cost-effectiveness standpoint. His team performed an incremental cost-effectiveness analysis and demonstrated strong evidence that direct surgical decompression combined with radiation therapy is cost-effective in terms of cost per additional day of ambulation (~$60) and cost per life year gained (~$31,000).

18.11.3 Level III and IV Evidence in Open Surgery

Dozens of level III and IV evidence articles report the use of open surgical techniques in the treatment of metastatic epidural spinal cord compression (▶ Table 18.3). The 2004 article by Wang and colleagues[11] detailing the results of 140 patients treated with posterior stabilization and direct decompression via transpedicular approaches provides a good example of uncontrolled evidence in favor of open surgical intervention. The authors reported 96% of patients experiencing improved pain and stable or improved neurologic status. Seventy-five percent of nonambulatory patients regained the ability to walk; 90% of patients had good or better performance scores by 1 month following surgery.

A similar large single-institution series was reported by Tancioni and colleagues.[23] Their analysis of 151 consecutive patients treated with surgery and radiotherapy for metastatic epidural spinal cord compression demonstrated alleviation of pain in 91% of patients and recovery of neurologic function in 62.5%. Median survival was 14 months and was dictated by the primary histology.

A more modern but well-performed retrospective series couples the use of direct surgical decompression with postoperative stereotactic radiosurgery to enhance local disease control (often referred to as "separation surgery"). Laufer and colleagues[24] reported the results of 186 patients treated in this manner with a very impressive 84% local control at 1 year (detecting both clinical and radiographic disease progression).

18.12 Complications in Open Surgery

Aggressive surgery for spinal metastases does pose a risk of mortality. In Patchell et al's randomized trial,[4] the 30-day mortality in the surgery group was 6% (compared to 14% in patients randomized to radiation alone). Quan et al[8] reported a similar rate (7.6%), as did Ibrahim et al[10] (5.8%) and Wang et al[11] (4.3%).

Total surgical morbidity is reported as approximately 20 to 25% across several rigorous studies (Quan et al[8] 26%; Ibrahim et al[10] 21%; Wang et al[11] 19.3%). Wound complications are the most common direct surgical complication seen in open surgery for metastatic spinal cord compression. Wang and colleagues reported wound complications in 16/140 patients in their series (11.4%) in a large, well-documented level III study.[11]

Table 18.3 Studies on open surgery for thoracolumbar metastatic disease[21]

Author	No. of pts	EBL	MLOS	MOR	Neuro-recovery (%)	Pain improvement (%)	CR	Miscellaneous
Patchell et al[4]	101	N/A	10 d (equal for surg + rads group)	N/A	Maint. of Frankel score at 30 d: Rads: 61% Surg: 91%	N/A	N/A	–30-d mortality rate: Surgery group: 6% Rad group: 14% –20% crossover from rads group to surgery group
Quan et al[8]	118	718 mL	9.7 d	53%: <2 h 42%: 2–3 h 5%: 3–4 h	45% of pts with full recovery of neurologic deficit	83% resolution of radicular symptoms	45 total 2 dural tear 8 wound infections	48% mortality rate at 1 y 7% mortality rate at 30 d
Ibrahim et al[10]	223	N/A	N/A	N/A	47% improved > 1 KPS 53% pts regained mobility	60% w/ complete resolution back/radicular pain	Implant failure: 2.2% Wound comp: 4% OR (CSF leak, thoracic duct injury): 7.2%	Peri-op mortality rate: 5.8% Morbidity: 21% 39% regaining urinary sphincter control
Wang et al[11]	140	15,00 mL	9 d	5.1 h	52% of ASIA grade D pts improving to grade E. 75% of pts with poor pre-op ECOG scores improved and became ambulatory	96% improved back/leg pain after surgery	20 pts 4 pts with wound dehiscence	Overall median survival: 7.7 mo
Tancioni et al[23]	151	N/A	N/A	N/A	94% recovery of neurologic deficit	91% remission of pain	N/A	Median survival of 14 mo
Weigel et al[25]	76	N/A	N/A	N/A	58% improving one Frankel grade 70% becoming ambulatory	89% with moderate to complete resolution of pain	16 pts 4 pts: neurologic deterioration 2 pts: hardware failure	Paraplegia developed in 18% during follow-up associated with mean survival of 3.4 mo

Abbreviations: ASIA, American Spinal Injury Association; CR, complication rate; CSF, cerebrospinal fluid; EBL, estimated blood loss; ECOG, Eastern Cooperative Oncology Group; KPS, Karnofsky performance scale; Maint, maintenance; MLOS, mean length of stay; MOR, mean operative time; N/A, not available; pts, patients; rads, radiotherapy; surg, surgery.

The studies by Quan et al[8] and Ibrahim et al[10] reported lower morbidity rates (6.8 and 4%, respectively). Patchell et al's study did not directly report this.

Relatively few studies report symptomatic local recurrence rates for repeated metastatic compression. Quan et al reported this rate as 8.5%, with 30% of patients with recurrence progressing to paraplegia.[8] Weigel et al reported this rate to be as high as 22% in an admittedly older study; most patients with local recurrence did not receive radiotherapy.[25]

18.13 Conclusion of Open Surgery

The value of direct surgical decompression for metastatic spinal cord compression has been demonstrated in a prospective randomized study (one of the few areas in spine surgery where level I evidence exists to support surgical intervention). Surgery has been shown to have clinically relevant benefit over radiotherapy alone that remains cost-effective even in the current era of scrutiny of aggressive treatments. These results have been replicated in prospective observational studies (level II evidence) as reproducible in clinical practice outside of the confines of a strict study protocol. Additional evidence from meta-analysis similarly supports the value of open treatment. Given the amount of level I and II evidence, a grade 1A recommendation may be given to the clinical benefit of surgical decompression with or without adjuvant therapy over radiotherapy alone in the treatment of thoracolumbar metastases.

While the complication rate of complex surgery in medically frail patients is substantial and approaches 25%, clinical experience demonstrates that it is manageable. Wound complications comprise only a minority of complications that are seen. The MIS literature is evolving and less mature than that of the literature on open surgery. Additionally, it reflects the experience of highly skilled surgeons treating carefully selected patients. As such, it is not clear whether the complication rate of patients treated with these techniques is different or whether the intermediate to long-term outcome is the same.

Clearly the treatment for any patient must be individualized based on their clinical presentation and the experience and preferences of the treating surgeon (the authors of this chapter all perform both open and MIS treatments for metastatic disease of the spine). Given the lack of any evidence directly comparing minimally invasive versus open approaches to thoracolumbar metastases, only a grade 2C recommendation using the *Guyatt et al* grading scale may be assigned to the theory that MIS offers equal or improved morbidity/mortality rates, complication rates, neurologic improvement, and pain scores over open therapy. Open surgical treatment of metastatic spine disease remains an approach that is accessible to all surgeons trained in basic techniques and available at any institution performing spine surgery with standard equipment. It is robustly applicable to a wide variety of clinical presentations and anatomy and can provide the surgeon with direct visualization of tumor decompression. Finally, in an era of uncertain cost constraints, open surgical decompression relies on standard implants and instruments and is a proven, cost-effective intervention.

18.14 Editors' Commentary

18.14.1 Minimally Invasive Surgery

The authors minutely review the literature supporting circumferential spinal cord decompression with spinal stabilization and adjuvant radiotherapy over to radiotherapy alone for patients with metastatic epidural spinal cord compression. Not covered in this chapter is the role that stereotactic body radiotherapy (SBRT) has played in altering the extent of surgery required to treat these patients, namely, moving away from complete vertebrectomies and toward "separation surgery" with reductions in operative times, blood loss, and need for anterior column reconstructions.

The use of MIS techniques in the surgical management of metastatic spine disease draws on the principles applied in using MIS techniques for degenerative and traumatic disorders. And in so doing, it offers lower rates of recovery time, blood loss, operative times, length of stay, opioid use, and wound healing issues including surgical site infections. A variety of MIS techniques are available for use in the metastatic spine tumor patient population, some of which are as follows: stand-alone percutaneous instrumentation, image-guided navigation, vertebral augmentation, radiofrequency ablation, and laser interstitial thermal therapy in addition to the tubular circumferential decompression plus percutaneous instrumentation described by the authors. This latter "MIS separation surgery" followed by SBRT represents the evolution of treatment from the level I data establishing the role of surgery in metastatic disease of the spine. The same goals of treatment are accomplished but with the added benefit over typical open techniques of reduced surgical morbidity—an optimal combination in these patients who have a pressing need for prompt initiation of additional therapies and/or face a short life expectancy.

18.14.2 Open Surgery

Surgery to treat metastatic disease that has spread to the spine is often unpredictable due to features such as tumor vascularity, bone quality, adherence of tumor tissue to neural elements, and extension of bony involvement beyond what is appreciated on preoperative imaging often leading to the need for extensive reconstruction during surgical decompression. Each of these features frequently encountered in surgical procedures in the setting of metastatic disease poses significant difficulties when performing MIS surgeries, though they are less problematic in the setting of open surgery. Open surgery allows better direct visualization of bleeding tumor tissue and feeding vessels, and access to neural elements from a variety of angles to facilitate safe decompression when tumor tissue is adherent. Additionally, the extensile nature of open surgery allows the surgeon to include spinal segments above or below those identified on preoperative planning if bone quality demands greater fixation or if there is in actuality a greater vertebral destruction by the tumor realized at the time of surgery.

Patients with intractable axial pain may benefit from stabilization procedures without the need for decompression or realistic hope of achieving fusion due to short life expectancy and poor host features that prevent bone formation. This population of patients may present a unique opportunity for MIS surgery to provide a similar benefit to these patients through utilization of smaller incisions, less time away from chemotherapy/radiotherapy while incisions heal in the setting of poor fusion potential regardless of technique. This small subset of patients is far exceeded by those who present with epidural tumor extension who are indicated for surgery by neurologic deficits associated with spinal cord or neural element compression. Despite some theoretical potential benefits of MIS in this challenging patient population, most cases may benefit from open techniques to optimize outcome and minimize complication rates.

References

[1] Wong DA, Fornasier VL, MacNab I. Spinal metastases: the obvious, the occult, and the impostors. Spine. 1990; 15(1):1–4

[2] Lenz M, Freid JR. Metastases to the skeleton, brain and spinal cord from cancer of the breast and the effect of radiotherapy. Ann Surg. 1931; 93(1):278–293

[3] Sciubba DM, Gokaslan ZL. Diagnosis and management of metastatic spine disease. Surg Oncol. 2006; 15(3):141–151

[4] Patchell RA, Tibbs PA, Regine WF, et al. Direct decompressive surgical resection in the treatment of spinal cord compression caused by metastatic cancer: a randomised trial. Lancet. 2005; 366(9486):643–648

[5] Rose PS, Clarke MJ, Dekutoski MB. Minimally invasive treatment of spinal metastases: techniques. Int J Surg Oncol. 2011; 2011:494381

[6] Fisher CG, DiPaola CP, Ryken TC, et al. A novel classification system for spinal instability in neoplastic disease: an evidence-based approach and expert consensus from the Spine Oncology Study Group. Spine. 2010; 35(22):E1221–E1229

[7] Tokuhashi Y, Matsuzaki H, Oda H, Oshima M, Ryu J. A revised scoring system for preoperative evaluation of metastatic spine tumor prognosis. Spine. 2005; 30(19):2186–2191

[8] Quan GM, Vital JM, Aurouer N, et al. Surgery improves pain, function and quality of life in patients with spinal metastases: a prospective study on 118 patients. Eur Spine J. 2011; 20(11):1970–1978

[9] Molina CA, Gokaslan ZL, Sciubba DM. A systematic review of the current role of minimally invasive spine surgery in the management of metastatic spine disease. Int J Surg Oncol. 2011; 2011:598148

[10] Ibrahim A, Crockard A, Antonietti P, et al. Does spinal surgery improve the quality of life for those with extradural (spinal) osseous metastases? An international multicenter prospective observational study of 223 patients. Invited submission from the Joint Section Meeting on Disorders of the Spine and Peripheral Nerves, March 2007. J Neurosurg Spine. 2008; 8(3):271–278

[11] Wang JC, Boland P, Mitra N, et al. Single-stage posterolateral transpedicular approach for resection of epidural metastatic spine tumors involving the vertebral body with circumferential reconstruction: results in 140 patients. Invited submission from the Joint Section Meeting on Disorders of the Spine and Peripheral Nerves, March 2004. J Neurosurg Spine. 2004; 1(3):287–298

[12] Kim CW. Scientific basis of minimally invasive spine surgery: prevention of multifidus muscle injury during posterior lumbar surgery. Spine. 2010; 35(26) Suppl:S281–S286

[13] Pull ter Gunne AF, Skolasky RL, Ross H, van Laarhoven CJ, Cohen DB. Influence of perioperative resuscitation status on postoperative spine surgery complications. Spine J. 2010; 10(2):129–135

[14] Schwab JH, Gasbarrini A, Cappuccio M, et al. Minimally invasive posterior stabilization improved ambulation and pain scores in patients with plasmacytomas and/or metastases of the spine. Int J Surg Oncol. 2011; 2011:239230

[15] Deutsch H, Boco T, Lobel J. Minimally invasive transpedicular vertebrectomy for metastatic disease to the thoracic spine. J Spinal Disord Tech. 2008; 21(2):101–105

[16] Tancioni F, Navarria P, Pessina F, et al. Early surgical experience with minimally invasive percutaneous approach for patients with metastatic epidural spinal cord compression (MESCC) to poor prognoses. Ann Surg Oncol. 2012; 19(1):294–300

[17] Zairi F, Arikat A, Allaoui M, Marinho P, Assaker R. Minimally invasive decompression and stabilization for the management of thoracolumbar spine metastasis. J Neurosurg Spine. 2012; 17(1):19–23

[18] McLain RF. Spinal cord decompression: an endoscopically assisted approach for metastatic tumors. Spinal Cord. 2001; 39(9):482–487

[19] Huang TJ, Hsu RW, Li YY, Cheng CC. Minimal access spinal surgery (MASS) in treating thoracic spine metastasis. Spine. 2006; 31(16):1860–1863

[20] Lau D, Chou D. Posterior thoracic corpectomy with cage reconstruction for metastatic spinal tumors: comparing the mini-open approach to the open approach. J Neurosurg Spine. 2015; 23(2):217–227

[21] Klimo P, Jr, Thompson CJ, Kestle JR, Schmidt MH. A meta-analysis of surgery versus conventional radiotherapy for the treatment of metastatic spinal epidural disease. Neuro Oncol. 2005; 7(1):64–76

[22] Thomas KC, Nosyk B, Fisher CG, et al. Cost-effectiveness of surgery plus radiotherapy versus radiotherapy alone for metastatic epidural spinal cord compression. Int J Radiat Oncol Biol Phys. 2006; 66(4):1212–1218

[23] Tancioni F, Navarria P, Pessina F, et al. Assessment of prognostic factors in patients with metastatic epidural spinal cord compression (MESCC) from solid tumor after surgery plus radiotherapy: a single institution experience. Eur Spine J. 2012; 21 Suppl 1:S146–S148

[24] Laufer I, Iorgulescu JB, Chapman T, et al. Local disease control for spinal metastases following "separation surgery" and adjuvant hypofractionated or high-dose single-fraction stereotactic radiosurgery: outcome analysis in 186 patients. J Neurosurg Spine. 2013; 18(3):207–214

[25] Weigel B, Maghsudi M, Neumann C, Kretschmer R, Müller FJ, Nerlich M. Surgical management of symptomatic spinal metastases. Postoperative outcome and quality of life. Spine. 1999; 24(21):2240–2246

[26] Rosenthal D, Marquardt G, Lorenz R, Nichtweiss M. Anterior decompression and stabilization using a microsurgical endoscopic technique for metastatic tumors of the thoracic spine. J Neurosurg. 1996; 84(4):565–572

[27] Lin F, Yamaguchi U, Matsunobu T, et al. Minimally invasive solid long segmental fixation combined with direct decompression in patients with spinal metastatic disease. Int J Surg. 2013; 11(2):173–177

[28] Huang TJ, Hsu RW, Sum CW, Liu HP. Complications in thoracoscopic spinal surgery: a study of 90 consecutive patients. Surg Endosc. 1999; 13(4):346–350

[29] Mobbs RJ, Nakaji P, Szkandera BJ, Teo C. Endoscopic assisted posterior decompression for spinal neoplasms. J Clin Neurosci. 2002; 9(4):437–439

[30] Kan P, Schmidt MH. Minimally invasive thoracoscopic approach for anterior decompression and stabilization of metastatic spine disease. Neurosurg Focus. 2008; 25(2):E8

[31] Le Huec JC, Lesprit E, Guibaud JP, Gangnet N, Aunoble S. Minimally invasive endoscopic approach to the cervicothoracic junction for vertebral metastases: report of two cases. Eur Spine J. 2001; 10(5):421–426

[32] Mühlbauer M, Pfisterer W, Eyb R, Knosp E. Minimally invasive retroperitoneal approach for lumbar corpectomy and anterior reconstruction. Technical note. J Neurosurg. 2000; 93(1) Suppl:161–167

[33] Payer M, Sottas C. Mini-open anterior approach for corpectomy in the thoracolumbar spine. Surg Neurol. 2008; 69(1):25–31, discussion 31–32

[34] Taghva A, Li KW, Liu JC, Gokaslan ZL, Hsieh PC. Minimally invasive circumferential spinal decompression and stabilization for symptomatic metastatic spine tumor: technical case report. Neurosurgery. 2010; 66(3):E620–E622

19 Intradural Spine Tumors: Is There an Advantage to Removing Intradural Spine Tumors Using an MIS Approach?

MIS: Anthony Conte and Trent L. Tredway
Open: Jeremy Fogelson and Michelle J. Clarke

19.1 Introduction

Intradural extramedullary spinal cord tumors (IDEM) are rare but surgically challenging lesions. Intradural spinal cord tumors make up over two-thirds of all spinal cord tumors, occurring with an incidence of 1 to 10 per 100,000 people.[1,2,3,4,5,6,7] Intradural tumors exhibit a slight male predominance and most commonly present in the sixth to seventh decades of life.[7] The majority of intradural tumors are schwannomas, comprising between 55 and 65% of IDEMs. Approximately 10 to 25% of IDEMs are meningiomas, most commonly found in the thoracic spine. Neurofibromas are also frequently seen. Additionally, intradural ependymomas, hemangioblastomas, paragangliomas, cavernomas, sarcomas, and epidermoid cysts have been reported in the literature.[1,2,3,4,5,6,7] The most common presentation of IDEMs is localized back/leg pain, with 40 to 50% of patients also exhibiting sensory or motor symptoms.[8,9] Approximately one-fourth of patients will present with symptoms of bowel/bladder incontinence or retention.

Intramedullary spinal cord tumors make up approximately 2% of all central nervous system tumors and 5 to 10% of all spinal tumors.[10,11,12,13,14,15,16,17] Ependymomas are the most common intramedullary tumor type in adults, accounting for 60% of lesions. Approximately 40% of ependymomas originate from the filum terminale, the majority of which are myxopapillary ependymomas.[14,17,18] Astrocytomas make up 90% of intramedullary spinal cord tumors (IMSCT) in patients younger than 10 years but decrease in frequency with age to become the second most common intramedullary tumor in adults.[14,17,18] Hemangioblastomas are the third most frequent IMSCT encountered in the adult population comprising 2 to 5% of all IMSCT[19] with 25% of lesions occurring in patients with von Hippel–Lindau (VHL) disease.[20,21] Other neoplastic lesions including gangliogliomas, metastases, lipomas, and lymphomas and nonneoplastic lesions such as cavernomas, cysts, and dysembryogenic lesions may also be observed as are intramedullary spinal cord masses.

Surgical treatment of IMSCT is pathology dependent, yet maximizing treatment while preserving neurologic function is the common primary aim. Gross total resection is the primary treatment for an ependymoma to achieve cure or long-term tumor control.[15,22,23,24] Often these lesions have a reasonable surgical plane and smaller lesions can be removed en bloc. Occasionally, internal debulking to lessen the traction on the spinal cord is performed. This allows the surgeon to confirm pathology, given the goals for the surgical treatment of astrocytomas are different. The main surgical goal in treating astrocytomas is to obtain tissue for histopathologic diagnosis, given that many of these lesions are unresectable. Unlike ependymomas, astrocytomas are infiltrative, and the risk of neurologic injury must be balanced with the desire for a subtotal debulking or gross total resection. Although extent of resection may correlate with outcome, usually intraoperative pathologic confirmation of high-grade astrocytomas dampens the enthusiasm for

further resection.[15,25,26,27] Dural tube expansion through patch grafting may be employed to provide space for tumor growth and delay neurologic deficit.

Hemangioblastomas are well circumscribed, highly vascular lesions. Due to their vascularity, dissecting around the tumor capsule, cauterizing feeding vessels, and removing the mass without disruption of the capsule are preferred.[19,28,29,30]

Intradural tumors of 2 to 3 cm in size have been reported (range: 1–6 cm).[1,2] Often these tumors span multiple vertebral levels. Depending on tumor size, internal debulking with ultrasonic aspiration may need to be employed prior to resection. However, most intradural extramedullary tumors can often be readily dissected from the neural elements with minimal risk of cord or nerve root injury. This chapter explores the ability of a surgeon to achieve these major surgical goals through minimally invasive surgical (MIS) techniques versus the more traditional open surgical approaches.

19.2 Advantages of Minimally Invasive Surgery

Since intradural spinal cord tumors are quite rare, there is a paucity in the literature regarding MIS techniques for tumor resection. In fact, to the authors' knowledge, there have been only three published reports. However, extrapolating from the literature in regard to minimally invasive treatment of various types of spinal pathology, the potential advantages may include decreased perioperative pain, lower blood loss, lower infection rate, decreased risk of dead space leading to pseudomeningocele formation, as well as decreased bone removal and tissue destruction which theoretically will decrease the rate of postoperative deformity.

19.3 Advantages of Open Surgery

Open techniques allow a wider exposure of the surgical field and familiar techniques can be employed by the neurosurgeon. The traditional midline laminectomy approach is common and does not require special retractors or suturing tools.

19.4 Case Illustration

A 32-year-old woman with a history of neurofibromatosis type 2 presented to the neurosurgical clinic with worsening back pain. The patient stated that this pain has increased in severity over the past 3 months, without radiation into the lower extremities, preventing her from participating in running and other fitness classes. Over the past 3 weeks, she has complained of a generalized numbness sensation throughout bilateral feet. She states that during this time period, she had stumbled a number of times and even fallen to the ground twice. Patient

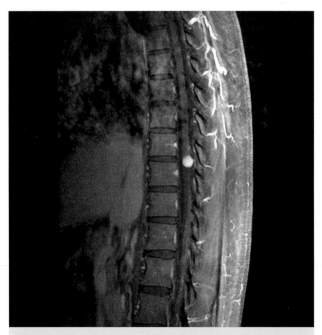

Fig. 19.1 Sagittal MRI with contrast demonstrating an intradural extramedullary as well as an intramedullary lesion.

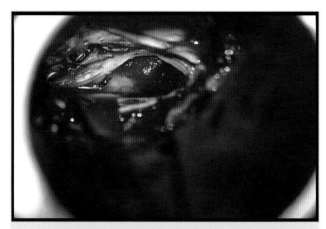

Fig. 19.3 Intraoperative photograph demonstrating resection cavity after removing the intramedullary tumor (ependymoma).

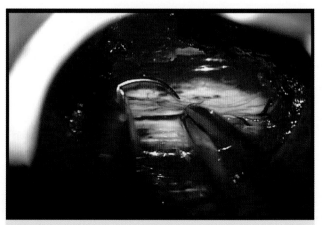

Fig. 19.4 Intraoperative photograph depicting dural closure.

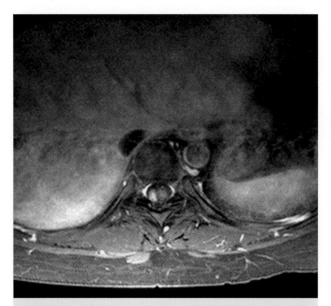

Fig. 19.2 Axial MRI with contrast demonstrating both an intradural extramedullary tumor and an intramedullary tumor.

19.5 Surgical Technique in Minimally Invasive Surgery

After obtaining consent, the patient underwent a minimally invasive approach using a tubular retractor and microscope. The patient was placed prone on a Jackson's table with Wilson's frame. A 2-cm right paramedian incision, 1.5-cm off midline, was made. Employing a muscle-splitting approach, serial dilators were used to aid in the docking of an expandable tubular retractor on the right T7 lamina and base of the spinous process. A hemilaminectomy with undercutting of the spinous process was performed to gain exposure for the intradural exploration. Upon midline opening the dura, the extramedullary tumor was internally debulked with an ultrasonic aspirator and meticulously resected off the spinal cord (▶ Fig. 19.3). After resection of the tumor, the dura was closed using a Castro-Viejo needle driver, knot pusher, and bayoneted forceps (▶ Fig. 19.4). The dura closure was reinforced with a dural substitute and dural sealant.

currently denies bowel or bladder incontinence, retention, or saddle anesthesia. Preoperative exam is significant for 4 + /5 strength in the right quadriceps muscle and 4 + /5 strength with dorsiflexion and plantarflexion bilaterally. There is no Hoffman's reflex, but patient does exhibit clonus and 3 + patellar reflexes bilaterally. Rectal tone and sensation are normal. Imaging studies included an MRI with and without contrast and revealed an intradural extramedullary tumor at the level of T7 (▶ Fig. 19.1 and ▶ Fig. 19.2).

19.6 Surgical Technique in Open Surgery

The patient is taken to the operating room, placed under general anesthesia, and carefully positioned. Somatosensory-evoked potential and motor-evoked potential monitoring is used throughout the case. Standard open complete laminectomy (T6–T9) and medial facetectomy through a midline bilateral exposure is performed. Ultrasound is brought in to verify that the bone work provides adequate exposure for the tumor resection. A midline durotomy is completed just beyond the suspected margins of the tumor, tacking the dural leaves to the paraspinal muscles to maximize exposure and prevent blood from obscuring the field.

Attention is then turned to obtaining a pathologic diagnosis and maximizing tumor resection. Under the operating microscope, the arachnoid layer is sharply dissected off the tumor surface. The tumor capsule is then entered, and the tumor is internally debulked using an ultrasonic aspirator, allowing further delivery of tumor margins into the surgical bed. Once margins are clearly identified, the tumor is carefully dissected off the spinal cord. The subarachnoid space is then irrigated, hemostasis is achieved, and the dura is closed with 4–0 Nurolon sutures. A Valsalva maneuver is used to confirm watertight closure. The patient is kept on bedrest with head of bed flat for the next 48 hours. Consideration for an instrumented fusion is given in a delayed manner after confirming a gross total resection on postoperative MRI.

19.7 Discussion of Minimally Invasive Surgery

19.7.1 Level I/II Evidence in Minimally Invasive Surgery

There is no level I or level II evidence available.

19.7.2 Level III/IV Evidence in Minimally Invasive Surgery

To the author's knowledge, there are five patients (▶ Table 19.1) reported in the neurosurgical literature who received minimally invasive resection of intramedullary spinal cord tumors.[31,32,33]

In the case report by Ogden and Fessler,[31] a tubular muscle-splitting retractor system was used to limit trauma to the ipsilateral paraspinal muscles and their insertions. The

decreased trauma to the paraspinal muscles may reduce the risk of late postoperative kyphotic deformity. In some series of conventional open approaches to IMSCTs, the rate of postoperative kyphotic deformity varies from 10 to 100%,[34,35,36] but this is more common in the pediatric population compared to adults. It is notable that pediatric IMSCT patients are at higher risk of deformity as evidenced by the literature demonstrating deformity as a presenting feature of IMSCT in children.[37] Thus, sparing the paraspinal muscle's further trauma may be advantageous. The second major difference in exposure in this case report is the use of a modified hemilaminar approach. Exposure was increased through the resection of the ventral spinous process and contralateral lamina which provided a view of the entire dorsal surface of the spinal cord. The disadvantage to this is a "slightly oblique working angle and a deeper operating field."[31] Additionally, Ogden and Fessler noted that the additional bone work required to extend the hemilaminar approach for adequate visualization is not biomechanically detrimental. This assertion may be supported by the study conducted by Lee et al that compared traditional open versus muscle-sparing hemilaminotomies in a biomechanical cadaveric dissection model. This study demonstrated a significantly more stable spine when hemilaminotomies were employed.[38] It should be noted that this study was performed on the lumbar spine and not on the more rigid thoracic spine.

Because this is a relatively new extension of the MIS technique, it is unclear what the surgical limitations are in regard to location, size, and characteristics of candidate lesions. Ogden and Fessler noted that large tumors more than two spinal segments, or those with difficult dissection planes, may best be approached through a traditional open approach. It is also notable in this case that a small area of enhancement was seen in the resection cavity on the postoperative MRI. Most likely this is granulation tissue, although residual tumor is a possibility.

The case series published by Haji et al included 20 patients with spinal tumors, 2 of which were intramedullary.[32] One was a conus teratoma, and the other an intramedullary inclusion tumor. The patient with the teratoma developed recurrent symptoms and was found to have 75% residual tumor which required an open revision surgery. The other case was also noted to have residual tumor, although no complications were reported.

The series by Gandhi et al included two hemangioblastoma patients who underwent MIS resection through a tubular retractor, without any complications.[33] The procedures were performed with similar techniques to those employed by Ogden and Fessler.

There are other reports of MIS techniques used in the resection of intradural extramedullary pathology.[32,33,39] Given that

Table 19.1 MIS tubular retractor, published cases

Case	Series	Pathology	Complications	Gross total resection
1	Ogden and Fessler[31]	Ependymoma	None	Yes
2	Haji et al[32]	Teratoma	Yes[a]	No
3	Haji et al[32]	Inclusion tumor	None	No
4	Gandhi et al[33]	Hemangioblastoma	None	Yes
5	Gandhi et al[33]	Hemangioblastoma	None	Yes

Note: Table created based on compiling these case series.

[a]Revision open surgery required within 18 months due to recurrent symptoms and 75% residual tumor noted on MRI.

this is a similar approach and exposure to intramedullary surgery, these studies may lend some insight to MIS IMSCT resection as well. The major limitation in comparison is the simple fact that resecting an extramedullary tumor has much less neurologic risk than an intramedullary tumor. However, the wound and spinal fluid issues should be relatively similar. All of these reports are level III/IV evidence and consist of case reports and retrospective case series.

Raygor et al[1] retrospectively examined 51 patients with a thoracolumbar intradural extramedullary tumor undergoing resection via a minimally invasive transspinous or open approach (25 in MIS group vs. 26 in open group). Mean estimated blood loss was found to be significantly lower in the minimally invasive group, with no statistically significant difference in extent of resection, postoperative improvement in ASIA scores, recurrence rate, or length of hospitalization. Open surgery trended toward a higher rate of complications, with three cases of persistent cerebrospinal fluid (CSF) leak requiring lumbar drain placement. Additionally, there was one subfascial wound infection and one epidural hematoma, both requiring reoperation. The MIS group trended toward a lower complication rate, with one pulmonary embolism and one pseudomeningocele treated conservatively.

Haji et al in the same series noted above also described MIS removal of extramedullary tumors. Eleven of the 20 patients in the series were intradural extramedullary, 2 were intramedullary, and 7 were extradural tumors. The extradural tumors are likely not as applicable, given the CSF issues related to intentional durotomy. Thus, of 13 intradural cases, there was one CSF leak reported, with a rate of 8%. That particular patient required two returns to the operating room to resolve the CSF leak. Furthermore, 5 of these 13 (38%) intradural tumors received a subtotal resection, although only 1 of the 5 required revision tumor removal with a standard open approach. The length of follow-up time was not noted in the study.[32]

In the case series published by Nzokou et al, four patients had intradural tumors removed with a tubular MIS technique, achieving gross total resection.[39] Three of these four patients had myelopathy preoperatively. It was noted that there were no complications, although a case illustration mentioned temporary weakness postoperatively.

The subset of patients from the publication by Gandhi and German included 14 patients with resection of intradural tumors, 2 of which were intramedullary (hemangioblastomas). There were no unplanned subtotal resections, with two patients undergoing a planned biopsy, and a third who had complete resection of the intended lesion with planned residual multiple other lesions. There were no CSF leaks noted. Wound dehiscence occurred in a patient after meningioma resection, but the dura was noted to be intact and not leaking. Another patient underwent anterior cervical diskectomy and fusion at an adjacent level, probably related to preexisting spondylosis.[33]

Park et al published on two patients with intradural extramedullary tumors removed through a tubular retractor. They described utilizing a special U-clip for dural closure, which was originally intended for vascular anastomosis. Both tumors were completely resected without any reported complications.[40] Tredway et al reported on six patients who underwent intradural extramedullary tumor removal through a tubular retractor. Five cases were schwannomas, and one was a myxopapillary ependymoma. All cases received gross total resection without any reported complications.[41]

The hemilaminar approach has been described using a standard open incision as a way to resect intra- and extramedullary tumors while eliminating the need to resect the spinous process or perform an extracavitary approach.[42,43,44,45,46,47,48,49,50] Similar to cases discussed earlier, the reduced bone work not only lessens the extent of surgical exposure but may prevent late deformity by preserving bone, ligament, and muscular attachments. However, compared to the tubular retractor, the open exposure with the open hemilaminar approach may allow easier instrument access.

19.8 Complications in Minimally Invasive Surgery

As noted earlier, there is a paucity of published reports regarding this technique. Of the five patients whom the authors are aware, at least two received subtotal resections, one of who required early return to the operating room. The rate of CSF leak may be lower with MIS techniques, but without better head-to-head comparisons, that conclusion is unclear.

19.9 Conclusion of Minimally Invasive Surgery

Given the abundance of level III/IV evidence, with a number of retrospective cohort studies already published, a grade 1C recommendation may be assigned to the evidence that minimally invasive intradural extramedullary tumor resection affords similar efficacy, resection rates, and neurologic improvement compared with open resection, with the potential to decrease operative blood loss and complication rates. However, due to the limited investigation into the use of minimally invasive techniques for the removal for intramedullary spine tumors, and a small patient population, conclusions on the efficacy of this method are not yet well founded. Only a grade 2C may be assigned to the evidence supporting MIS approach as a safe alternative for intramedullary tumor resection. In centers where a number of intradural tumor resections are performed, experienced surgeons may be able to develop the surgical technique and improve the instruments to allow more widespread and safe use.

19.10 Discussion of Open Surgery

19.10.1 Level I/II Evidence in Open Surgery

There is no level I or level II evidence available.

19.10.2 Level III/IV Evidence in Open Surgery

The main advantage to any open procedure is a large working channel and excellent exposure of the neural elements. Maximal anatomical awareness is a necessity to protect the patient against iatrogenic neurologic deficit. The majority of IMSCTs are approached through a posterior midline myelotomy. This direct midline approach splits the posterior columns, and the most likely iatrogenic complaint is sensory disturbances and proprioceptive dysfunction of the lower extremities, which worsens with laterality. One of the most challenging aspects of the case is determining the anatomic midline, which is aided by the unobstructed open approach. Vascular structures on the surface of the cord, natural sulci, and the location of the dentate ligaments and dorsal nerve roots provide information to the surgeon for this determination. Only facile MIS surgeons with a comprehensive, open IMSCT experience should attempt this challenging approach. There are no studies directly determining the experience level needed to tackle IMSCTs; however, there are many studies supporting improved surgical outcomes with greater surgery-specific experience.[51]

A wealth of knowledge on intramedullary spinal cord tumors comes from the pediatric population. Numerous case series and retrospective case review studies have shown that a gross-total or subtotal resection may be achieved via an open approach with minimal risk of neurologic deterioration. A study by Constantini et al reviewed 164 patients undergoing intramedullary tumor resections over a 21-year span. Most of these patients had low-grade gliomatous lesions. Using an open midline approach, a gross-total or subtotal resection (>80% resection) was achieved in more than 88% of patients, with 76% of all patients staying at or improving upon their neurologic baseline.[12] These data are on par with a number of other similar retrospective studies, showing an open approach provides the exposure and comfort to offer maximal resection, while reducing need for postoperative radiation.

As resection of an IMSCT necessitates a durotomy, a solid surgical strategy is required for dural closure. There are two components to the closure. First, obtaining a watertight closure to prevent ongoing CSF egress and associated complications. Second, consideration can be given to expanding the dural tube through patch grafting to allow tumor expansion with less cord trauma in certain cases, such as incompletely resected astrocytomas or ependymomas. Obviously, a wide working channel and excellent visualization of the durotomy will help facilitate a tight dural closure. While the MIS literature is filled with studies demonstrating the low complication rate with unrepaired incidental durotomies, these are in elective degenerative cases usually involving small tears simply treated by packing and sealant, and eliminating dead space with tubular retractor removal.[52,53] The intended durotomy required for IMSCT surgery is much larger and some of these patients will undergo radiation therapy; thus, superb wound closure should be a priority and is more easily facilitated through the open incision. That said, it is noted that McGirt et al saw a decreased rate of CSF leaks in patients with laminoplasty versus laminectomy in a series of IMSCTs[34]; so, dead-space reduction is valuable, and the retention of posterior spinal elements as promoted by advocates of MIS may be of value.

Surgical treatments of IMSCTs have been associated with spinal deformity, but the cause is actually unknown. It has been theorized that it may be secondary to the wide exposure and resection of the facet joint complexes or may actually be related to the decreased proprioception and injury to the paraspinal muscle function that can lead to kyphosis in the cervical and thoracic spine. In children, IMSCT is on the differential for scoliosis.[37] Specifically, it is theorized that the spinal cord damage results in asymmetric weakness of the paraspinal/core musculature. Following surgical removal of IMSCTs, risk factors for deformity include young age, location, radiation therapy, and surgical extent of exposure.[34,36,54,55] For instance, following surgery, late deformity requiring fusion in pediatric patients was reported to range from 27 to 88% in those who underwent radiation therapy, further emphasizing local muscle factors in deformity development.[36,54] However, it should be noted that in skeletally mature patients, the progression of deformity from performing laminectomies is theoretically less. Thus, MIS surgery may offer an advantage in protecting these muscles as noted earlier. That said, when studied specifically, it would be assumed that laminectomy (with the greatest muscular disruption and total lack of posterior element lever arms) would have a greater rate of late deformity than laminoplasty (retention of the posterior lever arms), yet that has not been shown in IMSCT surgery.[34] In the study of late deformity performed by McGirt and colleagues, laminectomy and laminoplasty patients had the same incidence of late deformity; thus, it is unknown if the decrease in muscle trauma offered by MIS surgery would be protective, or if these patients are simply at higher risk due to sequela of harboring an IMSCT.

The most obvious advantage of the open procedure is the lack of limitations with regard to size, location, and tumor characteristics. MIS surgery is limited by retractor size and angles; thus, exposure may be limited. Traditional open surgery allows multilevel exposure, albeit potentially necessitating near-simultaneous arthrodesis. For instance, ▸ Fig. 19.3 demonstrates a patient who underwent a C2–T4 ependymoma resection and cervical fusion in staged fashion. Another benefit of the open procedure is the opportunity to perform a fusion, if necessary, in the same sitting (▸ Fig. 19.3 and ▸ Fig. 19.4) or, in many of our cases, following a short staged delay to allow an unaffected postoperative MRI. In a study by Raygor et al[1] examining minimally invasive versus open resection in 51 patients with thoracolumbar intradural extramedullary tumors, investigators found a greater mean tumor size in patients undergoing open resection (3 vs. 1.9 cm in MIS). Four of the 26 patients undergoing open tumor resection required instrumentation (3 pedicle screw fixation, 1 laminoplasty) necessitated from either the degree of bony erosion, preexisting spondylosis, or iatrogenic instability created via decompression. Though postoperative clinical results were similar between the two groups, researchers concluded that given the limited surgical corridor using an MIS approach, intradural tumors spanning two or more levels with or without extraforaminal/lateral extension and bony erosion should be managed via an open approach.

19.11 Complications in Open Surgery

The complications typically attributed to the open technique include development of deformity or delayed instability, increased infection rate, pseudomeningocele, and increased pain. Given there are no direct, comparative studies between open and minimally invasive resection of IMSCTs, it is unclear that the open approach would afford a higher complication rate for this pathology.

19.12 Conclusion of Open Surgery

Owing to the complexity of these cases, and the general rarity of intramedullary and intradural spinal cord tumors, we feel that the MIS approach has limited utility based on the small number of cases which could be safely and adequately treated, and the reduced experience and familiarity of approaching an intramedullary tumor at an oblique angle. Based on the lack of scientific literature, a grade 2C recommendation is assigned to the evidence supporting MIS over open resection for IMSCT. A grade 2A recommendation may be given to the support for open resection of intradural extramedullary tumors spanning two or more levels, given the benefit of added visualization and lower technical difficulty.

Given the rarity of intramedullary spinal cord tumors, and the variety of pathologies and conditions from which it presents, each approach may hold unique risks and benefits for resection. Currently, the open approach is considered the standard treatment for IMSCTs. Perhaps, we should conclude that in some cases, MIS may offer an advantage, that is, in patients with VHL disease or neurofibromatosis harboring numerous tumors. A grade 2B may be assigned to the evidence supporting adequate resections of IMSCT, with an increased risk of subsequent kyphotic spinal deformity in postoperative patients. At this point, the traditional open approach is recommended for resection of the majority of intramedullary spinal cord tumors. However, in the hands of experienced, minimally invasive spinal neurosurgeons, some intramedullary spinal cord tumors may be treated safely and effectively.

19.13 Editors' Commentary

19.13.1 Minimally Invasive Surgery

Intradural extramedullary tumors, in particular, are ideal for MIS resection. They literally are "cherries" waiting to be picked from the tree. The question is obvious: Do you need to cut down the tree to get the cherry (laminectomy), or can you simply pick it off the tree with your fingers (MIS)? Using an incision only 1.5 cm off the midline, and performing a hemilaminectomy and removal of the ventral surface of the spinous process and contralateral ventral lamina (similar to that for decompression of stenosis), provides a midline exposure for durotomy and exposure of the tumor that is equivalent to open laminectomy. Because of the isolated nature of schwannomas and neurofibromas, and most meningiomas, complete resection is then an easy technical procedure. Reconstruction and stabilization are rarely required, and all the other well-known advantages of MIS surgery then come into play. The end result is that what was a scary "major" operation with potential long-term stabilization consequences becomes a short hospitalization with minimal potential delayed instability sequelae.

19.13.2 Open Surgery

In surgical treatment of these relatively rare tumors, it is difficult to construct a set of circumstances whereby the advantages imparted by MIS techniques can overcome the difficulty such techniques present in terms of identifying midline structures to appropriately divide the spinal cord, completing a watertight dural repair and resecting the tumor. It is well recognized that the learning curve associated with MIS provides the major stumbling block to widespread adoption of these techniques; very few surgical practices include sufficient volume of intradural spinal cord tumors to justify the prolonged learning curve during which more case-to-case technical backslide may occur because of the relatively paucity of these surgeries. There is little available literature to argue against the use of a MIS technique in the treatment of intradural tumors as it has been so uncommonly described. For all but the most experienced MIS surgeons, the treatment of metastatic spinal lesions with MIS techniques should not be attempted due to the potential for magnification of intraoperative complications including an increased risk of spinal cord injury and persistent CSF leak.

References

[1] Raygor KP, Than KD, Chou D, Mummaneni PV. Comparison of minimally invasive transspinous and open approaches for thoracolumbar intradural-extramedullary spinal tumors. Neurosurg Focus. 2015; 39(2):E12

[2] Turel MK, D'Souza WP, Rajshekhar V. Hemilaminectomy approach for intradural extramedullary spinal tumors: an analysis of 164 patients. Neurosurg Focus. 2015; 39(2):E9

[3] Mehta AI, Adogwa O, Karikari IO, et al. Anatomical location dictating major surgical complications for intradural extramedullary spinal tumors: a 10-year single-institutional experience. J Neurosurg Spine. 2013; 19(6):701–707

[4] Ahn DK, Park HS, Choi DJ, Kim KS, Kim TW, Park SY. The surgical treatment for spinal intradural extramedullary tumors. Clin Orthop Surg. 2009; 1(3): 165–172

[5] Song KW, Shin SI, Lee JY, Kim GL, Hyun YS, Park DY. Surgical results of intradural extramedullary tumors. Clin Orthop Surg. 2009; 1(2):74–80

[6] Cohen-Gadol AA, Zikel OM, Koch CA, Scheithauer BW, Krauss WE. Spinal meningiomas in patients younger than 50 years of age: a 21-year experience. J Neurosurg. 2003; 98(3) Suppl:258–263

[7] Hirano K, Imagama S, Sato K, et al. Primary spinal cord tumors: review of 678 surgically treated patients in Japan. A multicenter study. Eur Spine J. 2012; 21 (10):2019–2026

[8] Raco A, Esposito V, Lenzi J, Piccirilli M, Delfini R, Cantore G. Long-term follow-up of intramedullary spinal cord tumors: a series of 202 cases. Neurosurgery. 2005; 56(5):972–981, discussion 972–981

[9] Levy WJ, Latchaw J, Hahn JF, Sawhny B, Bay J, Dohn DF. Spinal neurofibromas: a report of 66 cases and a comparison with meningiomas. Neurosurgery. 1986; 18(3):331–334

[10] Brotchi J, Dewitte O, Levivier M, et al. A survey of 65 tumors within the spinal cord: surgical results and the importance of preoperative magnetic resonance imaging. Neurosurgery. 1991; 29(5):651–656, discussion 656–657

[11] Brotchi J. Intrinsic spinal cord tumor resection. Neurosurgery. 2002; 50(5): 1059–1063

[12] Constantini S, Miller DC, Allen JC, Rorke LB, Freed D, Epstein FJ. Radical excision of intramedullary spinal cord tumors: surgical morbidity and long-term follow-up evaluation in 164 children and young adults. J Neurosurg. 2000; 93(2) Suppl:183–193

[13] Epstein FJ, Farmer JP, Freed D. Adult intramedullary astrocytomas of the spinal cord. J Neurosurg. 1992; 77(3):355–359

[14] McCormick PC, Torres R, Post KD, Stein BM. Intramedullary ependymoma of the spinal cord. J Neurosurg. 1990; 72(4):523–532

[15] Sandalcioglu IE, Gasser T, Asgari S, et al. Functional outcome after surgical treatment of intramedullary spinal cord tumors: experience with 78 patients. Spinal Cord. 2005; 43(1):34–41

[16] Tihan T, Chi JH, McCormick PC, Ames CP, Parsa AT. Pathologic and epidemiologic findings of intramedullary spinal cord tumors. Neurosurg Clin N Am. 2006; 17(1):7–11

[17] Yang S, Yang X, Hong G. Surgical treatment of one hundred seventy-four intramedullary spinal cord tumors. Spine. 2009; 34(24):2705–2710

[18] Innocenzi G, Raco A, Cantore G, Raimondi AJ. Intramedullary astrocytomas and ependymomas in the pediatric age group: a retrospective study. Childs Nerv Syst. 1996; 12(12):776–780

[19] Lonser RR, Oldfield EH. Spinal cord hemangioblastomas. Neurosurg Clin N Am. 2006; 17(1):37–44

[20] Couch V, Lindor NM, Karnes PS, Michels VV. von Hippel-Lindau disease. Mayo Clin Proc. 2000; 75(3):265–272

[21] Neumann HP, Lips CJ, Hsia YE, Zbar B. Von Hippel-Lindau syndrome. Brain Pathol. 1995; 5(2):181–193

[22] Chang UK, Choe WJ, Chung SK, Chung CK, Kim HJ. Surgical outcome and prognostic factors of spinal intramedullary ependymomas in adults. J Neurooncol. 2002; 57(2):133–139

[23] Hanbali F, Fourney DR, Marmor E, et al. Spinal cord ependymoma: radical surgical resection and outcome. Neurosurgery. 2002; 51(5):1162–1172, discussion 1172–1174

[24] Lee J, Parsa AT, Ames CP, McCormick PC. Clinical management of intramedullary spinal ependymomas in adults. Neurosurg Clin N Am. 2006; 17(1):21–27

[25] Roonprapunt C, Houten JK. Spinal cord astrocytomas: presentation, management, and outcome. Neurosurg Clin N Am. 2006; 17(1):29–36

[26] Jallo GI, Danish S, Velasquez L, Epstein F. Intramedullary low-grade astrocytomas: long-term outcome following radical surgery. J Neurooncol. 2001; 53(1):61–66

[27] Constantini S, Miller DC, Allen JC, et al. Radical excision of intramedullary spinal cord tumors: surgical morbidity and long-term follow-up evaluation in 164 children and young adults. J Neurosurg. 2000; 93(2) Suppl:183–193

[28] Lonser RR, Weil RJ, Wanebo JE, DeVroom HL, Oldfield EH. Surgical management of spinal cord hemangioblastomas in patients with von Hippel-Lindau disease. J Neurosurg. 2003; 98(1):106–116

[29] Roonprapunt C, Silvera VM, Setton A, Freed D, Epstein FJ, Jallo GI. Surgical management of isolated hemangioblastomas of the spinal cord. Neurosurgery. 2001; 49(2):321–327, discussion 327–328

[30] Pluta R, Iluiano B, DeVroom H, et al. Anterior vs posterior surgical approach for ventral spinal hemangioblastomas in con Hippel-Lindau disease. J Neurosurg. 2003; 98:117–124

[31] Ogden AT, Fessler RG. Minimally invasive resection of intramedullary ependymoma: case report. Neurosurgery. 2009; 65(6):E1203–E1204, discussion E1204

[32] Haji FA, Cenic A, Crevier L, Murty N, Reddy K. Minimally invasive approach for the resection of spinal neoplasm. Spine. 2011; 36(15):E1018–E1026

[33] Gandhi RH, German JW. Minimally invasive approach for the treatment of intradural spinal pathology. Neurosurg Focus. 2013; 35(2):E5

[34] McGirt MJ, Garcés-Ambrossi GL, Parker SL, et al. Short-term progressive spinal deformity following laminoplasty versus laminectomy for resection of intradural spinal tumors: analysis of 238 patients. Neurosurgery. 2010; 66(5):1005–1012

[35] Yeh JS, Sgouros S, Walsh AR, Hockley AD. Spinal sagittal malalignment following surgery for primary intramedullary tumours in children. Pediatr Neurosurg. 2001; 35(6):318–324

[36] Jonge TD, Slullitel H, Dubouseset J, Miladi L, Wicart P, Illes T. Late-onset spinal deformities in children treated with laminectomy and radiation therapy for malignant tumors. Eur J Spine.. 2005; 14(8):765–771

[37] Banna M, Pearce GW, Uldall R. Scoliosis: a rare manifestation of intrinsic tumours of the spinal cord in children. J Neurol Neurosurg Psychiatry. 1971; 34(5):637–641

[38] Lee MJ, Bransford RJ, Bellabarba C, et al. The effect of bilateral laminotomy versus laminectomy on the motion and stiffness of the human lumbar spine: a biomechanical comparison. Spine. 2010; 35(19):1789–1793

[39] Nzokou A, Weil AG, Shedid D. Minimally invasive removal of thoracic and lumbar spinal tumors using a nonexpandable tubular retractor. J Neurosurg Spine. 2013; 19(6):708–715

[40] Park P, Leveque JC, La Marca F, Sullivan SE. Dural closure using the U-clip in minimally invasive spinal tumor resection. J Spinal Disord Tech. 2010; 23(7):486–489

[41] Tredway TL, Hrubes MR, Song JK, Christie SD, Fessler RG. Minimally invasive resection of intradural-extramedullary neoplasms. Neurosurgery. 2006; 58

[42] Balak N. Unilateral partial hemilaminectomy in the removal of a large spinal ependymoma. Spine J. 2008; 8(6):1030–1036

[43] Bertalanffy H, Mitani S, Otani M, Ichikizaki K, Toya S. Usefulness of hemilaminectomy for microsurgical management of intraspinal lesions. Keio J Med. 1992; 41(2):76–79

[44] Kanemoto Y, Ohnishi H, Koshimae N, et al. Ventral T-1 neurinoma removed via hemilaminectomy without costotransversectomy–case report. Neurol Med Chir (Tokyo). 1999; 39(9):685–688

[45] Koch-Wiewrodt D, Wagner W, Perneczky A. Unilateral multilevel interlaminar fenestration instead of laminectomy or hemilaminectomy: an alternative surgical approach to intraspinal space-occupying lesions. Technical note. J Neurosurg Spine. 2007; 6(5):485–492

[46] Oktem IS, Akdemir H, Kurtsoy A, Koç RK, Menkü A, Tucer B. Hemilaminectomy for the removal of the spinal lesions. Spinal Cord. 2000; 38(2):92–96

[47] Pompili A, Caroli F, Cattani F, et al. Unilateral limited laminectomy as the approach of choice for the removal of thoracolumbar neurofibromas. Spine. 2004; 29(15):1698–1702

[48] Sario-glu AC, Hanci M, Bozkuş H, Kaynar MY, Kafadar A. Unilateral hemilaminectomy for the removal of the spinal space-occupying lesions. Minim Invasive Neurosurg. 1997; 40(2):74–77

[49] Sridhar K, Ramamurthi R, Vasudevan MC, Ramamurthi B. Limited unilateral approach for extramedullary spinal tumours. Br J Neurosurg. 1998; 12(5):430–433

[50] Iacoangeli M, Gladi M, Di Rienzo A, et al. Minimally invasive surgery for benign intradural extramedullary spinal meningiomas: experience of a single institution in a cohort of elderly patients and review of the literature. Clin Interv Aging. 2012; 7:557–564

[51] Dasenbrock HH, Clarke MJ, Witham TF, Sciubba DM, Gokaslan ZL, Bydon A. The impact of provider volume on the outcomes after surgery for lumbar spinal stenosis. Neurosurgery. 2012; 70(6):1346–1353, discussion 1353–1354

[52] Wong AP, Shih P, Smith TR, et al. Comparison of symptomatic cerebral spinal fluid leak between patients undergoing minimally invasive versus open lumbar foraminotomy, discectomy, or laminectomy. World Neurosurg. 2014; 81(3–4):634–640

[53] Ruban D, O'Toole JE. Management of incidental durotomy in minimally invasive spine surgery. Neurosurg Focus. 2011; 31(4):E15

[54] Yao KC, McGirt MJ, Chaichana KL, Constantini S, Jallo GI. Risk factors for progressive spinal deformity following resection of intramedullary spinal cord tumors in children: an analysis of 161 consecutive cases. J Neurosurg. 2007; 107(6) Suppl:463–468

[55] Fassett DR, Clark R, Brockmeyer DL, Schmidt MH. Cervical spine deformity associated with resection of spinal cord tumors. Neurosurg Focus. 2006; 20(2):E2

20 Quality of Life in Advanced Tumors: Can Minimally Invasive Surgery Techniques Improve the Quality of Life of Patients with Advanced Oncologic Disease to Allow for Decreased Pain or Should Traditional Techniques of Palliation Be Used?

MIS: Ankit I. Mehta
Open: Alp Yurter and Daniel M. Sciubba

20.1 Introduction

Metastatic cancer causes approximately 500,000 deaths every year.[1] Moreover, metastatic epidural spinal cord compression (MESCC) is an increasingly common and debilitating process associated with cancer where compression of the spinal cord causes neurological deficit.[1,2] There were a projected 1.5 million new cases of cancer in the United States in 2010,[3] with MESCC occurring in 5 to 10% of patients with cancer. The most common primary tumors that metastasize to the spine consist of lung, breast, prostate, melanoma, gastrointestinal (GI), and kidney.[4,5] The prognosis of these individual metastatic cancers is variable. In a retrospective review of MESCC at Johns Hopkins University from 1996 to 2006, the mean survival after surgery was 10.8 months with the median survivals at the following: lung (4.3 months), breast (21 months), prostate (3.8 months), melanoma (40.9 months), GI (5.1 months), and kidney (19.8 months).[6]

Management of spinal metastases is undergoing an exciting transition given patients are living longer with improved medical therapies and the operative management is transitioning toward minimally invasive approaches. As with every paradigm shift, a critical view of this transition must be taken to weigh the advantages and disadvantages for patients. Minimally invasive surgery (MIS) aims to decrease the morbidities associated with open surgeries by reducing tissue damage. In the context of spinal metastases, MIS encompasses a variety of techniques, such as endoscopy video-assisted thoracoscopic surgery (VATS),[7] mini-open decompression,[8] minimal access spine surgery (MASS),[9] and percutaneous pedicle screw placement.[10] Vertebral augmentation procedures such as vertebroplasty and kyphoplasty are also considered "minimally invasive," albeit not surgical.[10] In order to keep our discussion focused, we hereby constrain MIS studies for spinal metastases to those involving minimally invasive retractors and/or the mini-open technique. We compare MIS to open surgeries, which consist of corpectomies utilizing posterior, anterior, or mixed approaches, followed by stabilization. The evidence we provide is restricted to studies that provide statistical outcomes specific to patients with spinal metastases.

20.2 Indications of Minimally Invasive Surgery

In general, patients with metastatic spine disease presenting with mechanical instability, radioresistant tumors, medically intractable pain, and/or progressive neurological deficits resulting from spinal cord compression are candidates for surgery, given that they have sufficient life expectancy and health status.[11,12,13] With regard to the life expectancy, the literature suggests a predicted survival of at least 3 months from open surgeries.[8] MIS is suitable for candidates with less favorable characteristics, such as high systemic tumor burden, aggressive tumor pathology, shorter expected survival (less than 6–12 months), and old age.[14,15,16] Because MIS in the field of spinal metastases has expanded significantly only in the past decade, various exclusion guidelines for MIS are accruing based on the approach used.[17]

20.3 Advantages of Minimally Invasive Surgery

MIS is becoming increasingly popular because it provides patients with the desired outcomes associated with open surgery (▶ Table 20.1), but with less medical comorbidities.[18] Since operative management of spinal metastases functions as a palliative measure as opposed to a curative one, MIS may provide a more advantageous approach in the patient's and surgeon's perspective. With an experienced surgical team, MIS can compare favorably to open surgery with regard to operative time.[16,19] More significantly, muscle-splitting retractor technology causes less muscle damage, and consequently reduces the duration of postoperative back pain and axial instability.[20,21] Secondary to reduced soft-tissue trauma are the potential advantages of decreased blood loss, shorter hospitalization stay, and earlier mobilization. The ability to engender faster wound healing rates is critical to the survival of the patient given that it allows for a shorter delay between surgery and an adjuvant therapy regimen.[21,22,23] Because of these advantages, MIS has the potential to treat a wider range of patients with metastatic disease, especially those who were not previously qualified for surgery.[21]

From a financial perspective, a relatively recent study suggests that newer MIS and mini-open techniques significantly lower acute and subacute costs relative to open techniques due to potential decreased complication rates, length of stay (LOS), and blood loss, as well as fewer discharges to rehab. However, these results are based on low-class evidence that does not have long follow-up periods and includes patients of pathologies other than metastasis.[24]

20.4 Advantages of Open Technique

Open surgical techniques are more familiar to spine surgeons and are not associated with as many inherent limitations of

Table 20.1 Literature on minimally invasive surgery (MIS) versus open tumor resection and MIS resection alone

Author (year)	Level	Study	Type	Pts	OR time (min)	EBL (mL)	LOS (d)	Complication rate (%)	Findings[a]
Chou and Lu[28] (2011)	III	Retro	MIS vs. open	M: 5 O: 5	M: 468 O: 408	M: 1,320 O: 3,120	–	M: 20 (wound inf.) O: 20 (epidural hematoma)	Similar neurological improvement
Fang et al[8] (2012)	III	Retro	MIS vs. open	M: 24 O: 17	M: 175 O: 403	M: 1,058 O: 1,721	–	M: 29.2 O: 11.8	• Less blood loss and operative time for MIS • Better local tumor control for open • Similar pain and neurological improvement, survival, complication rate
Mühlbauer et al[29] (2000)	IV	Retro	MIS	1	–	–	–	0	• MIS results in pain and neurological improvements • Stable compound union at 1-y follow-up
Deutsch et al[16] (2008)	IV	Retro	MIS	8	132	227	4	0	• 62.5% rate of pain and neurological improvement • 37.5% survival at 1 y • No tumor recurrence
Taghva et al[14] (2010)	IV	Retro	MIS	1	420	1,200	5	0	• First multilevel MIS vertebrectomy • At 9-mo post-op (last follow-up) patient was neurologically intact and pain free
Lu et al[30] (2011)	IV	Retro	MIS	1	540	150	4	0	• MIS results in pain and neurological improvements
Jandial and Chen[31] (2012)	IV	Retro	MIS	1	210	400	–	–	• MIS results in pain and neurological improvements–dual cage reconstruction is technically easier
Massicotte et al[18] (2012)	IV	Retro	MIS	10	–	335	<1	20% short term: transient pain flares 30% long term (>1 mo post-op): asymptomatic vertebral compression fractures	• MASS results in improvements in VAS, ODI, and QOL • Local control rate was 70%
Zairi et al[19] (2012)	IV	Retro	MIS	10	170	400	6	10%: transient urinary tract infection	• MIS results in pain, decreased opioid usage, and neurological improvements
Kimball et al[15] (2013)	IV	Retro	MIS	2	78	20	5	0	• MIS improves pain and neurological function
Nzokou et al[33] (2013)	IV	Retro	MIS	1	150	25	2	0	• MIS significantly improves pain • This approach may be less invasive than mini-open technique

Abbreviations: EBL, estimated blood loss; LOS, length of stay; MASS, minimal access spine surgery; ODI, Oswestry disability Index; OR, operation room; Pts, patients; QOL, quality of life; Retro, retrospective; VAS, visual analog scale.

[a]Not statistically significant (p > 0.05).

MIS. For example, the restricted operating view in MIS can impede upon the ability to effectively identify anatomical structures and resect tumor; surgeons must be careful not to overuse cauterizing tools when clearing their working window, which can inadvertently lead to muscle and ligament damage.[20] Furthermore, multiple-level lesions and kyphotic deformities are more effectively treated using open surgery, as certain MIS techniques using tubular retractors expose only one vertebral body level.[16] With regard to cost, equipment for open surgeries is cheaper than that needed for thoracoscopic or laparoscopic MIS procedures.[8] Finally, open surgeries are generally reported to have an easier learning curve.[14,25]

One needs to decide between the cases and present only one and describe the MIS and open surgical approaches. There is no need for postoperative figures or outcomes.

20.5 Case Illustration

20.5.1 Minimally Invasive Surgery

A 75-year-old male patient with a history of colon cancer complained of upper back pain beginning weeks before his recent admission. Magnetic resonance imaging (MRI) demonstrated a metastatic lesion at T3, with epidural spinal cord compression (▶ Fig. 20.1). The patient developed some slight paresthesias in his lower extremities and on neurological examination he demonstrated full strength on his motor exam. A costotransvsectomy approach with transpedicular vertebrectomy of T3 for the tumor resection was done with posterior stabilization with

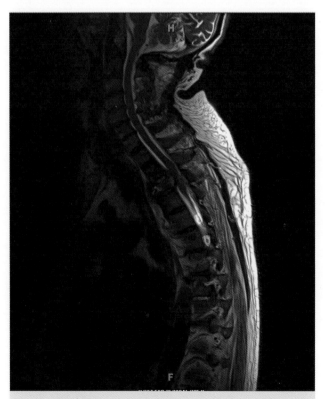

Fig. 20.1 Preoperative T2-weighted sagittal magnetic resonance imaging demonstrates cord-compressing metastatic lesion at the T3 vertebral body with compromised integrity.

percutaneous screws. Especially considering the patient's age, an MIS approach was chosen to expedite healing and reduce time until radiation therapy.

20.6 Surgical Technique in Minimally Invasive Surgery

The patient was brought to the operating table and intubated after induction. The patient was then placed prone on a Jackson table; the head is fixed into a Mayfield head holder. Antiseptics were then applied to the patient's lower neck and upper back. The surgeon was standing on the left of the patient. A line was drawn along the midline of the patient's back. The level of operation was located by counting the number of ribs down from the cephalad, as well as by checking aspects of the pedicles, which appear loose or absent on the AP (anteroposterior) projection. Upon identifying the tumorous vertebral level, small 3-cm incisions are made off the midline to allow for a trajectory conducive to a bilateral costotransversectomy. These areas are infiltrated with about 10 mL of lidocaine each. DuraPrep was applied in two applications over the patient's back and a time-out is done. The patient is then draped in a sterile fashion and the fluoroscope was brought in and draped sterilely as well

At this point, two surgeons began operating in tandem; the dermis was cut through using bipolar and unipolar cautery, and the trapezius and paraspinal muscles are separated using a muscle-splitting approach until the transverse process of the metas⁺atic level was reached. Another X-ray was taken to confirm the level. Bilateral pipeline distractible tubular retractors are positioned to dock upon the transverse processes. Using subperiosteal dissection, the entirety of the affected level, as well as top of the level below and the bottom of the level above, is exposed. With high-speed drill, rongeurs, and curettes, bilateral laminectomy is performed at the affected level, and partial laminectomies are performed at the level above and the level below. Then, a bilateral costotransversectomy was conducted by taking the transverse process and rib off at the affected level and the one above it, allowing for a transpedicular vertebrectomy at the affected level. The cord was completely decompressed from any tumor or bone. Nerve roots (in our case, T2 and T3) are tied using double ligature ties, bipolared, and cut lateral to the ties. Using high-speed drill, curettes, and Kerrison punches, the entirety of the affected vertebral body was removed, as well as the discs above and below. Throughout this time, the patient's evoked potentials are monitored, as motor evoked potentials may return following decompression (in our case, they did not).

A mesh titanium cage filled with allograft bone (to facilitate arthrodesis) was placed in the vertebral body defect and checked for correct alignment via fluoroscopy. Small incisions are made through skin and fascia, so that Jamshidi needles can be placed in alignment with the pedicles at two levels above and below the resected vertebral body. Once placement was confirmed with fluoroscopy, Kirschner's wires are inserted into each of the areas. The patient underwent serial tapping and placement of mesh premeasured screws. Then, a minimally invasive rod was anchored and clamped down into all screws. Fluoroscopic shots are taken again to confirm adequate placement. The fascia and skin are then closed, with a drain inserted into one of the larger incisions.

20.7 Surgical Technique in Open Surgery

The patient was brought to the operating table and intubated after induction. The patient was then placed prone and all pressure points were padded. The patient's back was scrubbed down to sterilize, and an incision was planned at the site of the lesion using external landmarks on the skin. Needles for electrophysiologic monitoring were placed, a time-out was done, and antibiotics were administered.

After marking the patient's back, an incision was made with subperiosteal dissection from two levels above to two levels below the site of metastasis. The pedicles at the two levels above and below the site of tumor were cannulated using a pedicle finder and a ball pit sound. An X-ray is taken to ensure that the markers in the pedicles show adequate placement. Pedicle screws are inserted appropriately to ensure stability during the vertebrectomy. Laminectomies are done from one level above to one level below the metastatic site. The ribs are removed bilaterally with careful dissection of the pleural cavity using subperiosteal dissection. Afterward, a bilateral costotransversectomy is conducted, followed by vertebrectomy of the affected level, as well as removal of adjacent discs. To complete the vertebrectomy, the right-sided T3 nerve root was double ligated and cut. At this point, a distractible cage packed with allograft was inserted into the void. The cage was distracted and the rods and screws were retightened. Then, allograft was packed along the edges of the decorticated posterolateral compartments to facilitate arthrodesis. Once hemostasis was obtained, the layers of tissue were closed to ensure there was no tension on the wound. Additionally, drains are placed subfascially and superficially.

20.8 Discussion of Minimally Invasive Surgery

Though decompressive surgery for metastatic spinal tumors has been conducted since the early 1900s,[26] it was not until 2005 that a randomized, multicenter study demonstrated a significant superiority of direct decompressive surgery with radiation over radiation alone.[27] Now that surgery is a clearly accepted treatment modality, efforts are being made to minimize incidental damage on paraspinal muscles and joints inherent to open approaches, which as aforementioned, yield many advantages. Therefore, MIS is a promising field for those with spinal metastases. Unfortunately, due to the relative novelty of the field, there are only a handful of studies with a low level of evidence.

20.8.1 Level I Evidence in Minimally Invasive Surgery

There are no level I studies available.

20.8.2 Level II Evidence in Minimally Invasive Surgery

There are no level II studies available.

20.8.3 Level III Evidence in Minimally Invasive Surgery

In 2011, Chou et al retrospectively compared the results of five patients treated with mini-open transpedicular corpectomy, circumferential decompression, and expandable cage reconstruction with percutaneous screws to five patients treated with an open approach. The MIS cohort had a mean blood loss (MBL) of 1,320 mL and operative time of 7.8 hours, while the open cohort had an MBL of 3,120 mL and operative time of 6.8 hours. Partial and full neurological recovery was noted in three of three MIS patients with preoperative deficit, while full neurological recovery was observed in three of three open patients with preoperative deficit. No instrumentation failure was noted in either group. The authors reported no statistically significant differences with respect to blood loss, operative time, or complication rate, though this analysis included three other patients with traumatic and primary spinal tumors per surgical cohort.[28]

In 2012, Fang et al retrospectively compared the results of 24 mini-open anterior corpectomy patients to those of 17 posterior total en bloc spondylectomy (TES) patients operated in between 2004 and 2010 for solitary metastases of the thoracolumbar spine. MBL and mean operative time were significantly less for the MIS cohort ($p < 0.05$). Improvements in visual analog scale (VAS) scores were comparable, as were neurological improvement rate, 2-year survival rate, and complication rate ($p > 0.05$). Neither group had hardware failure or loss of sagittal Cobb angle. Slight subsidence (< 3 mm) of the mesh cage was observed in 17.6% of the TES group, while no subsidence of the polymethyl methacrylate block/autograft was observed in the MIS group.[8]

20.8.4 Level IV Evidence in Minimally Invasive Surgery

An overwhelming majority of the current literature regarding MIS techniques for spinal metastases presents a patient or series of patients treated with a certain approach. As a result, a direct comparison to a cohort treated with an open technique cannot be made.

In 2000, Mühlbauer et al treated one patient with metastatic disease using a minimally invasive retroperitoneal approach for lumbar corpectomy and reconstruction, consisting of methylmethacrylate (MMA) packed Harms' cage, modular segmental spinal system (MOSS) screws, and variable screw placement (VSP) plates. At 1-year follow-up, the 59-year-old patient improved from having pain and bilateral sensorimotor deficit, as well as being ambulatory with assistance to requiring no analgesics and being ambulatory without assistance. Radiographs at this time point also demonstrated a stable compound union. There were no complications.[29]

In 2008, Deutsch et al treated eight patients with thoracic metastatic disease and acute neurologic compromise using minimally invasive transpedicular vertebrectomy from 2004 to 2005. MBL was 227 mL, operative time was 2.2 hours, and mean LOS was 4 days. Neurological function and pain improved in 62.5% of patients. Survival was 37.5% at 1 year. The authors reported that the trajectory set by the MIS tubular retractor is superior to that obtained via midline incision in an open procedure; the former allows for direct visualization of the lateral 25% of the ventral spinal canal and indirect access to up to 75% of the ventral spinal canal.[16]

In 2010, Taghva et al treated one patient with MESCC, back pain, and neurological deficits using an MIS circumferential decompression of two thoracic vertebrae, followed by reconstruction with an expandable cage and percutaneous posterolateral instrumentation. This was the first MIS multilevel procedure. Estimated blood loss was 1,200 mL, operative time was 420 min, and LOS was 5 days. The operation occurred without any intraoperative or postoperative complications. By 5 days postoperation, the patient improved from being ambulatory with assistance to ambulatory without assistance, and neurological scores improved from 4 + /5 to 5/5. By 9 months postoperation (the last available follow-up), the patient remained neurologically intact, had no significant back pain, and was not on pain medications. Additionally, the instrumentation was intact and demonstrated no evidence of failure.[14]

In 2011, Lu et al compared the results of the mini-open approach to the open for intradural spinal tumors. Although this was a cohort study, for our discussion of metastases, the result of only one patient who underwent gross tumor resection via mini-open approach was relevant. Blood loss was 150 mL, operative time was 540 min, and LOS was 4 days. No complications occurred. American Spinal Injury Association (ASIA) score improved by 1 grade and pain improved by 2 points on the VAS scale. This technique allowed for complete dorsal access to the spinal canal, with minimal tissue damage compared to the standard midline, open procedure. As a result, there were reduced blood loss and LOS.[30]

In 2012, Jandial et al performed mini-open bilateral transpedicular lumbar vertebrectomy reconstructed with dual expandable cages and short segment fixation on one patient. Blood loss was 400 mL and operative time was 3.5 hours. The patient had an immediate improvement in leg strength and pain significantly improved within 1 week postoperation. Radiographs showed an intact construct immediately and 3 months postoperation. The transpedicular corridors made by the surgeon facilitate the placement of the cages and reduce the need to manipulate the thecal sac. The authors concluded that for select patients requiring circumferential decompression of the lumbar spine, dual-cage reconstruction reduces the technical difficulty of the operation and is a potential alternative to single-cage surgeries. However, biomechanical testing has yet to be conducted to rigorously confirm mechanical stability.[31]

In 2012, Massicotte et al retrospectively reviewed a novel technique in which 10 patients with metastases were treated with the minimal access spinal surgery (MASS) with MMA reconstruction followed by stereotactic body radiotherapy (SBRT). Notably, all patients were treated in an outpatient facility, and nearly all patients were discharged on the same day of admission. MBL was 335 mL. Patients received SBRT 1 to 18 days after MASS; median total dose was 24 Gy consisting of three fractions, with a dose to 90% of the clinical target volume of 22.6 Gy. (As a comparison, Jandial et al performed open surgery using posterolateral transpedicular vertebrectomy with reconstruction on 11 patients with metastatic disease; to allow for adequate wound healing, radiotherapy was not administered until at least 21 days postoperatively.[32]) For the 8 symptomatic patients, median VAS improved only 1 point 1 month postoperation; however, by 5 months postoperation, median improvement was 6 points. Similarly, with respect to the Oswestry Disability Index (ODI), a 30% improvement was seen at 1 month and a 50% at 5 months. These results were maintained at last follow-up. Improvements in global quality of life (QOL) were also sustained. Local tumor recurrence rate was reported to be 30%.[18]

In 2012, Zairi et al operated on 10 patients with thoracolumbar metastases and neurological compromise. These patients were treated using minimally invasive transpedicular vertebrectomy and decompression through a tubular expandable retractor, as well as percutaneous stabilization. MBL was 400 mL, operative time was 170 min, and LOS was 6 days. All patients improved VAS scores, with a mean improvement of 3.5 points, and 80% improved neurological function. Disease progression in 4 patients (40%) resulted in death at a median of 4 months postoperation.[19]

In 2013, Kimball et al treated two consecutive patients with severe neurological compromise resulting from lumbar epidural metastases that underwent MIS decompression through a tubular retractor without stabilization. MBL was 20 mL, operative time was 78 min, while LOS was 5 days. These patients experienced immediate improvements in function and pain, with reduced dependence on opiates; motor scores improved from 2/5 in both patients to 3/5 and 4 + /5, while pain levels decreased from 9/10 and 8/10 to 2/10 in both patients. Within the follow-up period, no complications were noted. One patient succumbed to the disease 4 months postoperation, while another died from myocardial infarction resulting from a history of coronary artery disease 2 weeks postoperation.[15]

In 2013, Nzokou et al reported the results of one patient with metastatic disease treated with gross total resection via nonexpandable tubular retractor without stabilization. Operative time was 150 min, blood loss was 25 mL, and LOS was 2 days. The patient was neurologically unaffected both pre- and postoperation but experience significant pain relief, going from 6/10 to 0/10 on the VAS scale. There were no complications. The authors report that their approach may be even less invasive than the mini-open technique, resulting in faster recovery. Further, in cases of foraminal tumors, the MIS approach bypasses the need for facetectomy, decreasing postoperative deformity and eliminating the need for subsequent fusion surgery.[33]

20.9 Complications in Minimally Invasive Surgery

Complications from MIS are similar to those that can be expected from an open procedure and may relate to the approach used. The selected MIS studies yielded an overall complication rate of 22% (▶ Table 20.2). There was one reported intraoperative complication, which was a small dural tear repaired within the same operation. Transient complications included wound infections,[28] urinary tract infection,[19] pulmonary atelectasis,[8] pleural effusion,[8] intercostal neuralgia,[8] and pain flares.[18] One study noted asymptomatic vertebral compression fractures as a long-term complication.[18] Fang et al reported a 28.2% complication rate for mini-open corpectomies compared to the 11.8% rate of the TES group, though this

Table 20.2 Breakdown of complications and overall postoperative outcomes: aggregate data from minimally invasive surgery (MIS) and open tumor resection studies[8,14,15,16,18,19,28,29,30,31,32,33,36,38,39]

Complication rate	MIS (%)	Open (%)
Transient intercostal neuralgia	6	–
Asymptomatic vertical compression fractures	5	–
Pain flare	3	–
Urinary tract infection	2	–
Pulmonary atelectasis	2	–
Pleural effusion	2	22
Wound infection/dehiscence	3	9
Pneumothorax	–	7
Pneumonia	–	5
Unintended durotomy	2	4
Instrumentation complications/subsidence	–	4
30-d mortality	–	3
Pulmonary embolism	–	2
Deep vein thrombosis	–	2
Other[a]	–	7
Weighted local recurrence rate (%)	8	6
Weighted MBL (mL)	682	1,791
Weighted mean operative time (min)	203	331
Weighted mean LOS (d)	3.72	10
Weighted overall complication rate (%)	22	27
Weighted mean rate: neurological improvement (%)	84	55[b]
Weighted mean rate: pain improvement (%)	94.7	97
Weighted mean age (y)	59.9	58

Abbreviations: LOS, length of stay; MBL, mean blood loss.

[a]"Other" complications include (higher-frequency complications listed earlier) neurological worsening, hematoma, cerebrospinal fluid leak, ulcer perforation/gastrointestinal bleed, stroke, colitis, and orthostatic headache.

[b]Neurological improvement was weighted down by Xu et al,[36] in which only discrete changes in ambulation were reported (i.e., whether patient improved from nonambulatory to ambulatory, whereas other studies reported subtler improvements using neurological scoring systems); excluding Xu et al's study, neurological improvement for open surgeries is slightly higher (60%).

difference was not statistically significant ($p = 0.185$).[8] While the available MIS studies generally reported minimal intraoperative or postoperative complications, these statistics should be taken with a caveat, as the overall MIS patient population was very small.

20.10 Conclusion of Minimally Invasive Surgery

MIS for the palliative treatment of metastatic spine disease is an emerging field with the potential to be superior to its open counterpart. In order to overtake traditional approaches, however, MIS must be able to treat symptoms as effectively as open procedures, but with reduced muscular and soft-tissue trauma

and physiological stress on the patient. Further, the normal biomechanics of the spine should be maintained, and the perioperative end points achieved with open techniques should be improved upon. Most importantly, MIS must be safe; there should be fewer complications and a lesser need for subsequent surgeries.[22,23] Finally, from the perspective of both patients and hospitals, MIS should be a financially viable option.

Thus far, the strongest study compares mini-open corpectomy with TES; notably, while postoperative pain and neurological improvement were similar, blood loss and operative time were significantly less in the MIS cohort.[8] Based on these results, MIS appears to be a very promising option, especially for those with a more limited life expectancy. The available level IV studies seem to echo the notion that MIS is a feasible option for pain and neurological improvement. In comparing the available low-class evidence literature (▶ Table 20.2) for MIS and open procedures, respectively, the most notable differences were MBL (682 vs. 1,791 mL) and mean LOS (3.72 vs. 10 days). Additionally, the overall operative time for MIS was approximately 130 minutes shorter than its open counterpart. Interestingly, the rate of neurological improvement was superior (84 vs. 55%). These results, however, are likely statistically underpowered and skewed by the fact that long-term follow-ups are not yet available Regardless of its relative palliative benefits to open surgery, MIS is reported to be a feasible, clinically effective option for many symptomatic metastatic patients who are not eligible to undergo traditional surgery. However, due to the lack of higher level evidence regarding the MIS treatment of epidural spinal cord metastases, only a grade 2B recommendation can be assigned to the conclusion that minimally invasive treatment is superior to open surgery in regard to postoperative pain control and disability, neurologic recovery, and instrumentation failure in patients eligible for both procedures.

Unfortunately, due to the paucity of high-class evidence, the majority of surgeons have not adopted MIS and question its benefit and safety.[22,23] In order to accurately gauge the efficacy of one approach over the other, it is necessary to conduct more comparative cohort studies consisting of a large number of patients. Ideally, these studies should be prospective with long follow-up periods in order to provide stronger evidence.

As the field of spinal metastases continues to advance with regard to knowledge and available technologies, MIS may involve more effective methods of tumor control for durable symptom relief. For example, intraoperative stereotactic radiosurgery maybe me employed to more effectively control local recurrence, as demonstrated in recent studies.[34,35]

20.11 Discussion of Open Surgery

20.11.1 Level I Evidence in Open Surgery

There are no level I studies available.

20.11.2 Level II Evidence in Open Surgery

There are no level II studies available.

20.11.3 Level III Evidence in Open Surgery

One current weakness of certain MIS procedures seems to be the extent of tumoral resection undertaken, especially compared to open approaches.[8] Because the patients selected for MIS have relatively less favorable prognoses, the aggressiveness of the operation must be limited. Additionally, since the goals of the procedure are palliation of pain and neurological symptoms until end of life, the need for gross total resection is less pronounced. However, lesser resection increases the risk of local recurrence and, consequently, reoperation. In comparing postoperative outcomes of MIS to that of open TES, Fang et al noted that the most significant advantage to the open procedure was a smaller probability of local recurrence. Of the 24 mini-open anterior corpectomy and 17 posterior TES patient, 20.8% of the former group had recurrence compared to 0% of the latter group ($p = 0.045$). Further, while all patients experienced VAS improvement, 35% of the TES group became pain free compared to 0% of the MIS group. However, the overall change in VAS scores was not statistically significant between the groups.[8]

20.11.4 Level IV Evidence in Open Surgery

There is an abundance of level IV studies analyzing the results of open surgeries for the metastatic spine disease. However, to improve the strength of the comparison to the MIS studies, we have selected four level IV studies published in or after 2000, constrained to thoracolumbar metastases, and predominantly using a posterior approach (similar to our MIS studies). The fact that the overall mean age for the patients in the MIS and open procedure studies are similar (59.9 vs. 58) further improves the validity of the comparison (▶ Table 20.2). There were no postoperative outcomes that were significantly superior for the open approach. Pain relief was only slightly higher for open procedures (97 vs. 94.7%).

Available level IV evidence suggests that the technical difficulty of certain MIS procedures can make open surgery a more favorable option. Taghva et al describe the challenges associated with MIS circumferential spinal decompression and stabilization. Obtaining an adequate working corridor for vertebrectomy and anterior column reconstruction using minimally invasive retractors is the first obstacle that must be overcome. Additionally, the placement of percutaneous screws through small pedicles in the mid- and upper-thoracic spine can be challenging. Lastly, MIS segmental posterolateral arthrodesis is time-consuming and allows for a more limited fusion surface in comparison to traditional procedures. Nonetheless, the authors concede that technological advances mitigate some of these concerns. For instance, the development of expandable minimally invasive retractors has significantly improved the working corridors. Moreover, the advent of expandable cages has allowed for reconstruction with significantly reduced risk of spinal cord damage.[14]

20.12 Complications in Open Surgery

Based on the selected studies, the overall complication rate for open surgeries was 27%, with the top three complications being pleural effusion (22%), wound infection/dehiscence (9%), and pneumothorax (7%; ▶ Table 20.2). While the overall complication rate was 5% higher than that of MIS, it is difficult to evaluate how significant this difference is since this statistic is largely based on heterogeneous, low-class evidence. There was little overlap in the types of complications between MIS and open surgery, largely due to the difference in approaches taken to resect tumor. Xu et al noted, for example, that pulmonary complications were highest in open surgeries involving a combined anterior–posterior approach.[36]

20.13 Conclusion of Open Surgery

In the absence of substantial high-class evidence supporting MIS[24,37] with regard to clinical efficacy or cost, open surgery remains the predominant method of providing palliation to patients with metastatic spine disease. Traditional methods of tumor resection and stabilization are generally reported to be technically easier because of a larger working space. Furthermore, based on the strongest available level III study comparing TES and MIS,[8] the more aggressive option can allow for better local tumor control, preventing the need for reoperation. Interestingly, there was no significant survival difference between posterior TES and MIS patients. Therefore, the overall benefit of TES is questionable, as the progression of systemic disease yields a similar mortality rate but a higher operative risk. On the other hand, the lack of local recurrence likely results in a better QOL. The authors concede that their study was limited by their small cohort sizes.

Using the Guyatt et al grading scale, a grade 1B may be assigned to the evidence supporting the efficacy of open decompression and fusion in providing stability, pain control, and neurologic improvement in patients with MESCC, when compared with decompression or radiation alone. In contrast, only a grade 2B may be assigned to evidence supporting the efficacy of open decompression and fusion over MIS, as lack of literature and small study populations limit our ability to conclude, with certainty, that an open approach is advantageous.

Unfortunately, the controversy of MIS versus open procedures for metastatic spinal tumors remains unresolved. With technological advances making MIS increasingly viable, now more than ever, higher-class studies need to be conducted to firmly determine what roles traditional and minimally invasive techniques serve in the treatment of metastatic spine disease and whether one modality provides superior clinical outcomes to the other.

20.14 Editors' Commentary

20.14.1 Minimally Invasive Surgery

The last decade has seen a revolution in the role surgery plays in the management of metastatic spine disease. Now that the literature has clearly demonstrated the advantages of circumferential spinal cord decompression with spinal stabilization and adjuvant radiotherapy compared to radiotherapy alone for patients with MESCC, efforts have moved on to making surgical intervention safer with less morbidity for these patients with limited life expectancy. The advent of SBRT has further changed surgical thinking as we have moved away from a "gross total resection" approach to metastatic disease, and instead now employ the principles of "separation surgery" to clear tumor away from the neural elements to allow for adjuvant SBRT. By obviating the need for complete vertebrectomies, the new treatment strategy has resulted in shorter surgical times with less blood loss but at the same time has produced very high rates of local tumor control.

In this same vein, the application of MIS techniques to metastatic spine disease seeks first and foremost to reduce approach-related morbidity. The literature abounds with evidence for the reduction of complication rates when using MIS techniques over open for a host of degenerative and traumatic diseases, and it is only a matter of time and larger study cohorts before the same is shown for the metastatic spine tumor population. Reduced blood loss, operative times, LOS, opioid use, surgical site infections, and wound breakdown (particularly salient in cancer patients) can be expected when using MIS techniques. The authors touch on only a portion of the MIS techniques available for treating metastatic disease and focus primarily on vertebrectomy procedures. Stand-alone percutaneous instrumentation, image-guided navigation, vertebral augmentation, radiofrequency ablation, and laser interstitial thermal therapy are but a few of the other MIS approaches to metastatic spine disease that offer benefits over typical open techniques. But at a fundamental level, the evolution of the MIS version of separation surgery through tubular circumferential decompression with percutaneous instrumentation allows surgeons to accomplish the same surgical goals as open surgery and yet further reduce the surgical morbidity associated with these types of procedures for this challenging patient population.

20.14.2 Open Surgery

Of all potential MIS applications, treatment of metastatic tumors may be the riskiest. In many cases, potential for blood loss is difficult to predict prior to surgery and even tumors typically considered to present with a low risk of high-volume blood loss can surprise surgeons during surgery. Furthermore, reactive changes in surrounding tissue can make defining tissue planes more difficult and impair visualization of anatomic structures used as landmarks. These circumstances conspire together to create a surgical environment that is volatile and where intraoperative complications can quickly mount. In this sense, only the most seasoned MIS surgeons should consider applying these techniques to treat metastatic lesions where multiple level stabilization may be necessary.

There is very little evidence that MIS techniques are superior to open techniques in the management of metastatic spinal disease. Literature support composed primarily of case series is at risk of highlighting "cherry picked" cases of successful MIS interventions. Larger series of the more commonly used open technique presents more accurate descriptions of "average" cases. Additionally, use of MIS surgical techniques that are substantially more expensive in a palliative setting raises questions about resource utilization and cost-effectiveness, particularly given the high cost of health care expenses realized in the last 6 months of life in the United States.

References

[1] Byrne TN. Spinal cord compression from epidural metastases. N Engl J Med. 1992; 327(9):614–619

[2] Findlay GF. Adverse effects of the management of malignant spinal cord compression. J Neurol Neurosurg Psychiatry. 1984; 47(8):761–768

[3] Jemal A, Siegel R, Xu J, Ward E. Cancer statistics, 2010. CA Cancer J Clin. 2010; 60(5):277–300

[4] Gerszten PC, Welch WC. Current surgical management of metastatic spinal disease. Oncology (Williston Park). 2000; 14(7):1013–1024, discussion 1024, 1029–1030

[5] Chaichana KL, Woodworth GF, Sciubba DM, et al. Predictors of ambulatory function after decompressive surgery for metastatic epidural spinal cord compression. Neurosurgery. 2008; 62(3):683–692, discussion 683–692

[6] Chaichana KL, Pendleton C, Sciubba DM, Wolinsky JP, Gokaslan ZL. Outcome following decompressive surgery for different histological types of metastatic tumors causing epidural spinal cord compression. Clinical article. J Neurosurg Spine. 2009; 11(1):56–63

[7] Huang TJ, Hsu RW, Liu HP, et al. Video-assisted thoracoscopic surgery to the upper thoracic spine. Surg Endosc. 1999; 13(2):123–126

[8] Fang T, Dong J, Zhou X, McGuire RA, Jr, Li X. Comparison of mini-open anterior corpectomy and posterior total en bloc spondylectomy for solitary metastases of the thoracolumbar spine. J Neurosurg Spine. 2012; 17(4):271–279

[9] Huang TJ, Hsu RW, Li YY, Cheng CC. Minimal access spinal surgery (MASS) in treating thoracic spine metastasis. Spine. 2006; 31(16):1860–1863

[10] Rose PS, Clarke MJ, Dekutoski MB. Minimally invasive treatment of spinal metastases: techniques. Int J Surg Oncol. 2011; 2011:494381

[11] Kaloostian PE, Yurter A, Zadnik PL, Sciubba DM, Gokaslan ZL. Current paradigms for metastatic spinal disease: an evidence-based review. Ann Surg Oncol. 2014; 21(1):248–262

[12] Sciubba DM, Gokaslan ZL, Suk I, et al. Positive and negative prognostic variables for patients undergoing spine surgery for metastatic breast disease. Eur Spine J. 2007; 16(10):1659–1667

[13] Landreneau FE, Landreneau RJ, Keenan RJ, Ferson PF. Diagnosis and management of spinal metastases from breast cancer. J Neurooncol. 1995; 23 (2):121–134

[14] Taghva A, Li KW, Liu JC, Gokaslan ZL, Hsieh PC. Minimally invasive circumferential spinal decompression and stabilization for symptomatic metastatic spine tumor: technical case report. Neurosurgery. 2010; 66(3):E620–E622

[15] Kimball J, Kusnezov NA, Pezeshkian P, Lu DC. Minimally invasive surgical decompression for lumbar spinal metastases. Surg Neurol Int. 2013; 4:78

[16] Deutsch H, Boco T, Lobel J. Minimally invasive transpedicular vertebrectomy for metastatic disease to the thoracic spine. J Spinal Disord Tech. 2008; 21(2):101–105

[17] Uribe JS, Dakwar E, Le TV, Christian G, Serrano S, Smith WD. Minimally invasive surgery treatment for thoracic spine tumor removal: a mini-open, lateral approach. Spine. 2010; 35(26) Suppl:S347–S354

[18] Massicotte E, Foote M, Reddy R, Sahgal A. Minimal access spine surgery (MASS) for decompression and stabilization performed as an out-patient procedure for metastatic spinal tumours followed by spine stereotactic body radiotherapy (SBRT): first report of technique and preliminary outcomes. Technol Cancer Res Treat. 2012; 11(1):15–25

[19] Zairi F, Arikat A, Allaoui M, Marinho P, Assaker R. Minimally invasive decompression and stabilization for the management of thoracolumbar spine metastasis. J Neurosurg Spine. 2012; 17(1):19–23

[20] Kim YB, Hyun SJ. Clinical applications of the tubular retractor on spinal disorders. J Korean Neurosurg Soc. 2007; 42(4):245–250

[21] Laufer I, Madera M, Bydon A, et al. Minimally invasive surgery in the treatment of thoracolumbar metastatic tumors. ArgoSpine News J. 2011; 23 (4):134–138

[22] Smith ZA, Yang I, Gorgulho A, Raphael D, De Salles AA, Khoo LT. Emerging techniques in the minimally invasive treatment and management of thoracic spine tumors. J Neurooncol. 2012; 107(3):443–455

[23] Smith ZA, Fessler RG. Paradigm changes in spine surgery: evolution of minimally invasive techniques. Nat Rev Neurol. 2012; 8(8):443–450

[24] Allen RT, Garfin SR. The economics of minimally invasive spine surgery: the value perspective. Spine. 2010; 35(26) Suppl:S375–S382

[25] Han PP, Kenny K, Dickman CA. Thoracoscopic approaches to the thoracic spine: experience with 241 surgical procedures. Neurosurgery. 2002; 51(5) Suppl:S88–S95

[26] Witham TF, Khavkin YA, Gallia GL, Wolinsky JP, Gokaslan ZL. Surgery insight: current management of epidural spinal cord compression from metastatic spine disease. Nat Clin Pract Neurol. 2006; 2(2):87–94, quiz 116

[27] Patchell RA, Tibbs PA, Regine WF, et al. Direct decompressive surgical resection in the treatment of spinal cord compression caused by metastatic cancer: a randomised trial. Lancet. 2005; 366(9486):643–648

[28] Chou D, Lu DC. Mini-open transpedicular corpectomies with expandable cage reconstruction. Technical note. J Neurosurg Spine. 2011; 14(1):71–77

[29] Mühlbauer M, Pfisterer W, Eyb R, Knosp E. Minimally invasive retroperitoneal approach for lumbar corpectomy and anterior reconstruction. Technical note. J Neurosurg. 2000; 93(1) Suppl:161–167

[30] Lu DC, Chou D, Mummaneni PV. A comparison of mini-open and open approaches for resection of thoracolumbar intradural spinal tumors. J Neurosurg Spine. 2011; 14(6):758–764

[31] Jandial R, Chen MY. Mini-open transpedicular lumbar vertebrectomy reconstructed with double cages and short segment fixation. Surg Neurol Int. 2012; 3 Suppl 5:S362–S365

[32] Jandial R, Kelly B, Chen MY. Posterior-only approach for lumbar vertebral column resection and expandable cage reconstruction for spinal metastases. J Neurosurg Spine. 2013; 19(1):27–33

[33] Nzokou A, Weil AG, Shedid D. Minimally invasive removal of thoracic and lumbar spinal tumors using a nonexpandable tubular retractor. J Neurosurg Spine. 2013; 19(6):708–715

[34] Gerszten PC, Monaco EA, III. Complete percutaneous treatment of vertebral body tumors causing spinal canal compromise using a transpedicular cavitation, cement augmentation, and radiosurgical technique. Neurosurg Focus. 2009; 27(6):E9

[35] Laufer I, Iorgulescu JB, Chapman T, et al. Local disease control for spinal metastases following "separation surgery" and adjuvant hypofractionated or high-dose single-fraction stereotactic radiosurgery: outcome analysis in 186 patients. J Neurosurg Spine. 2013; 18(3):207–214

[36] Xu R, Garcés-Ambrossi GL, McGirt MJ, et al. Thoracic vertebrectomy and spinal reconstruction via anterior, posterior, or combined approaches: clinical outcomes in 91 consecutive patients with metastatic spinal tumors. J Neurosurg Spine. 2009; 11(3):272–284

[37] Molina CA, Gokaslan ZL, Sciubba DM. A systematic review of the current role of minimally invasive spine surgery in the management of metastatic spine disease. Int J Surg Oncol. 2011; 2011:598148

[38] Bilsky MH, Boland P, Lis E, Raizer JJ, Healey JH. Single-stage posterolateral transpedicle approach for spondylectomy, epidural decompression, and circumferential fusion of spinal metastases. Spine. 2000; 25(17):2240–2249, discussion 250

[39] Wang JC, Boland P, Mitra N, et al. Single-stage posterolateral transpedicular approach for resection of epidural metastatic spine tumors involving the vertebral body with circumferential reconstruction: results in 140 patients. Invited submission from the Joint Section Meeting on Disorders of the Spine and Peripheral Nerves, March 2004. J Neurosurg Spine. 2004; 1(3):287–298

Part IV

Other Issues

IV

21 Radiation Exposure: How Does Radiation Exposure Differ between Open and Minimally Invasive Techniques?

MIS: Jonathan Yun and Alfred T. Ogden
Open: Mark L. Prasarn

21.1 Introduction

Since 1980, there has been a 600% increase in medical radiation exposure to the U.S. population which is mostly attributable to radiological diagnostic studies. As compared to 15% in the 1980s, medical imaging comprises 50% of the per capita radiation dose.[1] It has been shown that patients receive extremely high doses of radiation for diagnostic procedures alone during the average trauma admission, and even more during invasive procedures.[2] These imaging modalities have provided much benefit to the patients, but at the same time have likely resulted in cancer in some.

Routine use of fluoroscopy in musculoskeletal procedures became popular beginning in the early 1980s.[3] Studies have shown that the amount of radiation exposure is 10 to 12 times greater during spine surgery than other fluoroscopically assisted musculoskeletal procedures.[4,5] This higher exposure is related to both the amount of energy required to penetrate the torso, which is thicker than the limbs, and the proximity of the surgeon's hand to both the primary and backscatter sources of radiation during operative imaging.[6,7,8,9]

The amount of radiation necessary to image a patient undergoing spinal surgery adequately is also likely increasing, given this is directly related to the patient's size, in particular their torso mass.[5] This has been shown in numerous studies.[10,11,12] It has been shown that fluoroscopy time and overall procedure time are greater in obese patients.[13]

There is an ever-growing dependence of spine surgeons on intraoperative fluoroscopy as technology and procedures advance. The amount of radiation emitted during fluoroscopy during spine surgery is far from negligible.[6,7,8,14,15,16,17] Quality fluoroscopic images are needed for placing instrumentation during open procedures, but even more importantly during minimally invasive surgery (MIS) that is extremely reliant upon intraoperative imaging. The ability to obtain quality spinal images is of paramount importance to safely, and effectively, perform modern-day spine surgery.

The development of minimally invasive approaches to the spine has afforded several advantages over traditional open techniques. Mechanistically, the benefits are in large part derived from the decrease in soft-tissue injury realized through muscle dilation and the use of tubular retractors as compared to subperiosteal dissection of muscle and traditional retractors.[18] These improvements can be quantified clinically in terms of decreased length of hospital stay, decreased perioperative blood loss and transfusion rate, and decreased use of narcotics for pain control when compared to open approaches.[19,20,21,22,23,24] Minimally invasive spine (MIS) surgeries are also associated with a decreased rate of infection.[25,26]

MIS surgery is not, however, a panacea and its potential downsides must be examined critically. MIS surgery, in general, relies more heavily on image guidance than open spine surgery, and this typically means more use of intraoperative fluoroscopy.

Thus, the benefits of less invasiveness notwithstanding, there is appropriate concern regarding the potential health impact of increased radiation exposure that may come with the utilization of MIS techniques.

Traditionally, image guidance in MIS surgery has been achieved with X-ray fluoroscopy. This is a source of ionizing radiation and carries potential long-term health hazards. Today, the use of intraoperative imaging systems integrated with operative instruments has reduced the amount of fluoroscopy needed for a given case, thereby reducing occupational exposure to X-ray radiation. However, since these systems use X-rays to generate their images, their contribution to the cumulative radiation dose a patient receives during their treatment needs to be considered.

21.2 The Dangers of Radiation Exposure

Ionizing radiation is a potential occupational hazard, but also exists as a part of the environment through natural and man-made sources. Radiation sources include naturally occurring substances such as radon gas and uranium, man-made environmental modifications such as power plants and high-altitude aviation, and occupational/medical exposures such as receiving or working near X-ray producing machines or radioactive substances. Man-made exposures are considered to account for 18% of the average person's radiation exposure, with the remainder attributed to natural sources. Thus, the risk of radiation exposure from medical treatment for most people is not considered to be significant. The same has not been true historically for occupational radiation exposure. Indeed, the relationship of cancer to radiation exposure became apparent, in part, after increased rates of cancer were noted in radiologists and radiology technicians who worked with early and improperly shielded X-ray equipment.[27] In addition to cancer, other health problems have also been linked to radiation exposure, including skin damage[27] and cataract formation.[10,28] Today, occupational exposure to radiation and its associated health problems have been greatly reduced because of improved safety measures; however, concern still exists regarding the degree of risk from exposure to low levels of radiation over long periods of time. Similarly, the effects of radiation exposure from computed tomography (CT) scans are a concern for patients. These risks are difficult to quantify and are not really known. In the absence of such data, limits on radiation exposure are based on models that assume a linear drop-off between radiation exposure and cancer, and use this assumption to calculate risk from known cancer rates after much higher amounts of radiation exposure than one would likely ever encounter working in medicine. These models estimate that a threshold single whole-body dose of 100 mSv or 10 rems over background may be sufficient to produce one additional cancer in 100 adults over their lifetimes. The significance of this number with regard to medicine might be best understood in the context of patient exposures to imaging studies requiring radiation. Patient radiation exposure to a mammogram produces around 0.13 mSv or 0.013 rems of radiation exposure, whereas a whole-body CT scan can result in 12 mSv or 1.2 rems of radiation exposure. Thus, although the radiation effects of a mammogram are likely to be exceedingly low, the radiation effects of multiple whole-body CT scans are potentially significant.[27] According to one estimate, the radiation dose threshold for a measurable, statistically significant increase in solid cancer risk among individuals exposed to radiation from atomic bombs is between 50 and 100 mSv, a number that could be accrued over five whole-body CT scans.

The health effects of daily or weekly exposures to much smaller amounts of radiation are even harder to conceptualize with the data that currently exists. The kind of large, long-term population studies that would be required to answer these questions do not exist. Current Occupational Safety and Health Administration (OSHA) guidelines limit occupational exposure of 1.25 rems per quarter or 3 rems in a year to the "whole body" which includes head and trunk, blood-forming organs, lens of the eye and gonads, 18.75 rems/quarter to the extremities (hands/forearms, feet/ankles), and 7.25 rems/quarter to the skin.[29]

Radiation exposure during spine surgery can be thought of separately as the radiation dose received by the patient and the doses received by the operative team. For the patient, the radiation doses are expected to be higher, but these higher doses are tolerated because, with notable exceptions, the patient is unlikely to have considerable radiation exposure outside of their medical treatment. For the operative team, limiting radiation exposure on a daily basis is very important, and is significantly mitigated by wearing appropriate protective gear and removing or distancing oneself from X-ray sources as much as possible. In spine surgery, radiation is generated from two sources: intraoperative fluoroscopy and intraoperative imaging systems that use X-rays to generate three-dimensional (3D) images for navigation. For the latter, images are stored for intraoperative use, making it possible for the operative team to remove itself to an adjacent room while the scan is being performed. Under these conditions, the exposure to the operative team is negligible.[30] The effective radiation dose to the patient during a lumbosacral scan, according to measurements using a popular system's lowest recommended settings, is between 2.25 and 6.83 mSv depending on the size of the patient. This is between 81 and 85% of the amount of a similar scan performed on a 64-slice CT.[31]

When fluoroscopy is used, radiation exposure to the patient is less than if a 3D imaging system is used, but the exposure to the operative team is much more because it is not possible or practical for the operative team to remove itself from the operating room every time an X-ray is taken.[32] Assuming that proper shielding garments are worn, the two most important variables determining occupational X-ray exposure from a spine surgery are the distance of the exposed body part to the side of the fluoroscope that contains the X-ray source and the time of exposure. The area of greatest exposure is the scatter zone on the side of the patient nearest to the X-ray source. The decrease in radiation exposure as distance from the source is increased is logarithmic. Distancing oneself just 35 cm away from the patient–X-ray interface will reduce the exposure three- to sevenfold depending on the size of the patient.[5] Thus, highest radiation exposure occurs when a given surgical technique requires the surgeon to hold an instrument in the operative field while standing on the side of the X-ray source, particularly if the technique requires multiple X-rays or live fluoroscopy.

21.3 Case Illustration

A 55-year-old woman with a several-year history of progressive back and leg pain presented with an acute foot drop and worsening leg pain despite nonoperative management. Magnetic resonance imaging demonstrated grade 1 spondylolisthesis at L4–L5, associated with disc space collapse, and severe central canal and foraminal stenosis (▶ Fig. 21.1). Surgical intervention was recommended to decompress the neural elements and stabilize the L4–L5 motion segment.

21.4 Surgical Technique in Minimally Invasive Surgery

21.4.1 Localization and Retractor Placement

Following prone positioning on a Jackson operating table, fluoroscopic localization was utilized to demarcate the correct level and to place tandem, paramedian 3-cm incisions,

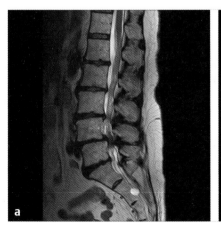
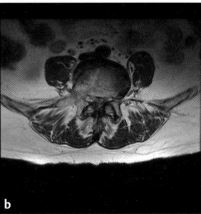

Fig. 21.1 (a) T2-weighted midsagittal image of the lumbar spine demonstrating degenerative spondylolisthesis at L4–L5. **(b)** T2-weighted axial image through the L4–L5 disc space showing severe spinal stenosis in the same patient.

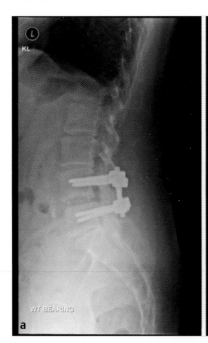 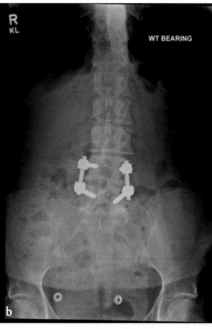

Fig. 21.2 (a) Lateral and (b) anteroposterior radiographs of the lumbar spine showing posterior pedicle screw instrumentation at L4–L5.

approximately 4 cm off midline. The level was localized with X-ray by clamping a Kirschner wire (K wire) to the drape adjacent to the patient's iliac crest, with the surgeon standing behind the X-ray source (surgeon out of field, SOF). After skin incision, the fascia was incised with a monopolar cautery and the facet palpated through the muscle. The K wires were then docked onto the ipsilateral facets and the level confirmed by X-ray (SOF). The turgor of the soft tissue is sufficient to hold the K-wires in place so that the surgeon stepped away during the X-ray. The muscle was dilated and the retractors were inserted, locked into position, and the final retractor position was confirmed by X-ray (SOF).

21.4.2 Decompression and Interbody Fusion

On both sides, soft-tissue dissection was performed to expose the L4 lamina, the L4–5 facet, the L4 pars and transverse process, and the base of the L5 transverse process. A left-sided L4 laminotomy was performed with Kerrison rongeurs. An osteotomy was made in the left L4 pars and the articular process was removed. The osseous component of the stenosis decompression was completed using Kerrison rongeurs on the ipsilateral side. On the contralateral side, a drill was used to remove the base of the L4 spinous process, the ventral L4 lamina, and the medial L4–5 facet. Finally, the ligament was freed from its bony attachments with curettes and removed using pituitaries and Kerrison ronguers. This part of the case required no fluoroscopy.

Next, the transforaminal lumbar interbody fusion (TLIF) was performed. An osteotome was used to remove L5 superior articulating process just superior to the L5 pedicle. The inferior edge of the exiting left L4 root was seen. Superior to the pedicle, the disc space was entered and a total discectomy was performed, and endplates were prepared. The disc space was irrigated. An X-ray was then performed with a rotating shaver in place to assess graft size. Contact with the endplates is enough to hold the shaver in position without needing to be held by the surgeon (SOF). A trial was selected, placed, and evaluated with an X-ray (SOF). The disk space was filled with arthrodesis material and a cage was placed. Several X-rays were used to adjust cage placement (SOF).

21.4.3 Screw Placement and Posterolateral Fusion

We utilized image guidance to place pedicle screws. A reference arc was clamped to the L2 spinous process through a small separate incision, and an O-arm (Medtronic) was performed to generate an intraoperative 3D image with which to navigate pedicle screws. The entire staff vacated the operating room for the 15-second scan. The pedicle screw starting points were clearly seen under direct vision and pedicles were cannulated using a navigated gearshift probe. The cannulations were verified using a ball-tipped probe. K wires were then placed into the cannulations, and cannulated taps were navigated through the pedicle isthmi. A ball-tipped probe again verified cortical integrity. On the right side, a posterolateral fusion was performed by decorticating the L4–5 facet joint and the L4 pars and transverse process. Arthrodesis material was placed. The retractors were collapsed and removed, and the pedicle screws were navigated into place. Rods were passed through the screw extensions and their placement was confirmed with fluoroscopy after provisional tightening of locking screws (SOF). The locking screws were tightened finally. Another 3D spin was performed to confirm construct placement.

Postoperatively, a CT scan was not required because its equivalent had already been performed intraoperatively. The patient will be followed up with plain radiographs (► Fig. 21.2) at 6 weeks, 6 months, 1 year, and 2 years postoperatively. The cumulative fluoroscopy time was 44 seconds and the radiation exposure was 0.29 mSv to the patient. The exposure to the surgeon was not measured, but reasonably expected to be a tiny fraction of this, given the surgeon was at least 3 ft away from the fluoroscope while any X-rays were taken. The two O-arm spins were estimated to produce an exposure of 7 mSv to the patient and negligible exposure to the operative team.

21.5 Surgical Technique in Open Surgery

The patient was taken to the operating room and general endotracheal intubation was performed. The patient was then turned prone using a Jackson table turn with the head placed in a prone view head holder. Pillows were placed under the femurs and tibiae to produce lordosis and prevent decubitus ulcers. The upper extremities were positioned on arm boards that were padded to prevent neuropraxia. Positioning should allow for optimization and ease of intraoperative fluoroscopic imaging to confirm spinal alignment and level and implant position/reduction.

Following a posterior midline exposure over the L4–L5 interspace, using the iliac crests as an external marker, a Kocher clamp was placed on the spinous process of L4. This was confirmed with a single lateral fluoroscopic image. The erector spinous muscles were then subperiosteally elevated to expose the posterior elements of the spine bilaterally out to the transverse processes of L4 and L5. Self-retaining retractors were placed deeply and anatomic landmarks for pedicle screw placement were identified.

Instrument was placed at this point using anatomic technique, although some surgeons prefer to place pedicle screws following decompression and placement of the interbody graft. Using anatomic landmark entry sites, pedicle screws at L4 and L5 were made bilaterally using a high-speed bur and a 5-mm ball tip. Gearshifts were then advanced, cannulating the pedicles and into the vertebral bodies bilaterally to premeasured depths based on preoperative imaging. The holes were probed to ensure there was no breach, and then undertapped. Pedicle screws were placed bilaterally at the level above and below. Adequate and safe positioning was confirmed with a posteroanterior (PA) and lateral image.

At this point, a laminectomy was performed with the removal of the superior and inferior articulating processes of the facet joint unilaterally (in this case, on the patient's right or more affected side clinically). Gentle distraction was performed with a lamina spreader or using the pedicle screws and a distractor. The disc space was exposed, and while protecting the nerve root, an annulotomy was performed. A meticulous discectomy and endplate preparation were carried out, and trial spacers were placed. After determining the appropriate size interbody graft, bone graft material was placed anteriorly into the disc space. An interbody implant was then packed with bone graft and placed. A PA and lateral images were again taken to confirm appropriate position of the interbody spacer.

Following completion of a thorough decompression, appropriate length rods were cut and contoured for lordosis. Gentle compression was performed over the rods and the construct was locked. Final PA and lateral images were obtained with the fluoroscope intraoperatively to document the final position and alignment (▶ Fig. 21.2). During the procedure, a total of four PA

and four lateral images were obtained using an open, anatomic technique.

For this procedure, the following fluoroscopy time and measured doses were observed using a GE OEC 9900 C-arm (General Electric Healthcare, Waukesha, WI):

- PA image: 93 kVP @ 3.1 mA × 0.8 second.
- Lateral image: 97 kVP @ 3.2 mA × 1.0 second.
- Time: 7.2 seconds total.

21.6 Discussion of Minimally Invasive Surgery

Fluoroscopy time and exposure to unshielded areas of the surgeon's body have both been shown to have increased with minimally invasive procedures.[33] However, the clinical significance of these findings is unclear. Furthermore, these results are difficult to extrapolate to all the surgeons, given that there is likely great variability in the amount of fluoroscopy used from practitioner to practitioner.[34]

21.6.1 Level I Evidence in Minimally Invasive Surgery

One meta-analysis and one single-center prospective randomized control trial described increased occupational exposure to ionizing radiation with MIS fusions.[24,35] In the meta-analysis, the authors, Tian et al, examined four level II studies, or level I including the aforementioned RCT (Wang et al) in the context of operative X-ray use. The authors concluded that there was significantly more X-ray time associated with MIS-TLIFs, though the evidence also supported improved short-term patient outcomes. However, the paucity of RCTs in this meta-analysis was a limitation.

21.6.2 Level II Evidence in Minimally Invasive Surgery

Four prospective comparative studies were found in the literature that describe increased radiation exposure with MIS approaches.[21,33,36,37] In one study, whose specific focus was X-ray exposure, Mariscalco et al described an increased radiation exposure to the surgeon performing MIS diskectomies when compared to open surgeries. In their study, surgeons performing MIS diskectomies wore protective gear and used fluoroscopy for retractor placement, while surgeons performing open diskectomies wore no protective gear and stood in the sterile core during localization X-rays. Three radiation detectors were placed outside of any protective gear on the wrist, chest, and collar. The average exposures during an MIS case were 1.72 millirads (mR) to the eye and thyroid, 3.08 mR to the chest, and 0.2 mR to the hand compared to 1.72 mR to the eye and thyroid, 3.08 mR to the chest, and 0.2 mR to the hand during an open discectomy. Despite the fact that X-ray exposure was higher during MIS discectomies, the clinical relevance of this difference was called into question by the authors who estimated that a total of 1,623 MIS surgeries would have to be done in order to reach the yearly total-body exposure limit.[33] A few comparative studies of open and MIS-TLIF report similar clinical and radiologic outcomes but decreased blood loss, earlier rehabilitation, improved pain control, and shorter hospitalization after MIS-TLIF. These studies noted the increased fluoroscopy time required during their MIS procedures.[21,36,37] In these studies, average fluoroscopy times ranged from 17.6 to 39 seconds in the open cohorts versus 49 to 84 seconds in the MIS groups. Another study compared the relative fluoroscopy times of MIS-TLIF if a navigation system was used for screw placement versus fluoroscopy for screw placement. These authors found an average reduction in fluoroscopy time if navigation was used, 57.1 versus 147.2 seconds, although the authors did not elaborate specifically on their technique of fluoroscopy-assisted screw placement.[38]

21.6.3 Level III and Level IV Evidence in Minimally Invasive Surgery

Two retrospective studies described radiation exposure in MIS versus open lumbar fusions, both concluding increased radiation time with MIS approaches.[22,39] The value of other lower level studies involves the specific assessment of radiation exposure during high exposure techniques such as fluoroscopically guided pedicle screw placement. This technique results in higher radiation exposures due to the necessity for multiple X-rays with the practitioner holding the instruments that are being X-rayed. One cadaveric study noted an average of 9.3 seconds of fluoroscopy time per screw placed. Exposures to different parts of the body were as follows: 58.2 mrem/min to hand, reduced to 39.3 mrem/min with leaded gloves, 8.3 mrem/min to unprotected thyroid, 53.3 mrem/min to unprotected waist at the side of the source, 2.2 mrem/min to unprotected waist at the intensifier side, and 0.8 mrem/min to protected waist. Based on these calculations, a one-level lumbar fusion with placement of four percutaneous pedicle screws would result in an exposure of 30 mrem to the hands, 4.7 mrem to the eye lens, and 0.45 mrem to the body. Based on these results, under the assumption that fluoroscopy is used only for pedicle screw placement, 625 surgeries with placement of four percutaneous pedicle screws would have to be performed over a 3-month period to exceed current OSHA limits for hand exposure, 265 of such cases would have to be performed over 3 months to exceed OSHA limits to the lens of the eye, and 2,777 such operations would have to be performed to exceed OSHA limits to the shielded body. If this surgery was performed without body shielding, and the surgeon stayed on the source side of the patient the entire time, 44 operations would have to be performed over the course of 3 months to exceed OSHA guidelines.

21.7 Conclusion of Minimally Invasive Surgery

MIS approaches to the lumbar spine offer short-term advantages to patient recovery and hospitalization, with long-term outcomes that are comparable to traditional open lumbar interbody fusions.[40] The intuition that MIS spine surgery entails increased use of X-rays than open surgeries is supported by the literature. The unanswered question is whether this increase has any occupational or clinical significance whatsoever. There

is a sufficient amount of levels II and III evidence to support a grade 1C recommendation that MIS fusion procedures consistently require greater amounts of fluoroscopy time, and hence expose the surgeon to higher levels of ionizing radiation when compared to open fusion procedures. However, due to the lack of any long-term evidence or observational trials, a grade 2C recommendation may be assigned to the theory that this increased exposure to radiation leads to subsequent increased cancer risk in the surgeon performing minimally invasive procedures or the patient population. Uncertainty regarding the risks of occupational exposure to X-ray radiation during spine surgery stems primarily from an absence of studies that examine the cumulative effects of very low doses of ionizing radiation over long periods of time. Current OSHA guidelines are based on extrapolations from data regarding cancer risk from exposure to atomic bombs. Although radiation exposure is increased for minimally invasive spine procedures, the existing data indicate that OSHA quarterly radiation limits are very unlikely to be exceeded by conscientious and competent spine surgeons for whom minimally invasive procedures comprise the bulk of their surgeries, particularly if these surgeries mostly involve microdiscectomies and short segment lumbar fusions. Safety, however, requires vigilance and compliance. At-risk individuals must comply with their institutions' monitoring practices and endeavor to reduce their exposure when possible. Radiation exposure can be reduced significantly by moving away from the operative field during an X-ray and standing on the side opposite to the X-ray source if a technique requires the surgeon to stay within the operative field during the procedure. Surgeons who use a good deal of intraoperative fluoroscopy should wear leaded eyewear because the lens of the eye is the most vulnerable organ. Image guidance clearly reduces radiation exposure to the surgeon. Although image guidance increases the intraoperative radiation exposure to the patient, it has less of an effect when the overall radiation dose from imaging studies throughout the perioperative period is considered.

21.8 Discussion of Open Surgery

21.8.1 Level I Evidence in Open Surgery

There are no level I studies comparing radiation exposure to the surgeon or patient using MIS versus open surgery.

21.8.2 Level II Evidence in Open Surgery

In a study by Mariscalco et al, patients with isolated lumbar herniated discs were prospectively enrolled following the failure of nonoperative management. A total of five surgeons proficient in both techniques performed the operations, although the type of procedure was at the discretion of the surgeon. Surgeons wore digital dosimeters over their thyroid shields, on their chests, and on their forearms. Surgeons performing the MIS procedures were exposed to 10 to 22 times the ionizing radiation as compared to those using traditional open techniques. It should be noted that the surgeons in the open group who stood in the substerile scrub room were still exposed to radiation (0.2 mrad per case), albeit very small values.[33]

In a prospective study, Wang et al[36] examined the amount of radiation exposure time used to perform MIS versus open TLIF in patients with low-grade degenerative or isthmic spondylolisthesis. The cohort included 85 patients who were treated either by one surgeon with open surgery or another with MIS technique as described in the article. The authors state that the patients were treated "according to random principle" and "one by one." The method of randomization was therefore vague. Patients were followed up to a minimum of 13 months, and the outcomes were assessed with visual analog score (VAS) or Oswestry disability index (ODI) scores. They were able to conclude a lower amount of blood loss with less need for blood transfusion in the MIS group ($p < 0.01$). In addition, patients who underwent MIS surgery had shorter hospital stays ($p < 0.05$). The MIS patients and the operating room staff were exposed to greater amounts of radiation as demonstrated by longer amounts of fluoroscopy time, 84 versus 37 seconds in the open group ($p < 0.05$). Outcomes were similar at latest follow-up between the groups, but there were more intraoperative complications in the MIS group. There was little discussion of the increased fluoroscopy time in the study.[36]

21.8.3 Level III Evidence in Open Surgery

Bronsard et al[39] performed a retrospective study examining radiation exposure during treatment of lumbar fractures without neurological deficits with either an open or MIS technique. Effective radiation dose was threefold higher for the MIS group versus the open group, but was sixfold less than the postoperative CT scan that was performed on all patients. There were no significant differences in length of hospital stay, patient satisfaction, screw malposition, or follow-up kyphosis measurement at an average of 25 months. Postoperative VAS scores were improved in the MIS group.[39]

Ahn et al[41] performed a prospective study to examine the radiation exposure to the surgeon during transforaminal percutaneous endoscopic lumbar discectomy. A total of three surgeons performed 33 disc levels in 30 patients. The procedures were carried out with the surgeons wearing thermoluminescent dosimeters at the level of the neck, chest, arms, and both hands. Dosimeters were placed under the thyroid shield and lead apron at the corresponding level of the externally worn neck and chest badges. The radiation doses per level were as follows: neck, 0.0785 mSv; chest, 0.1718 mSv; right upper arm, 0.0461 mSv; left ring finger, 0.7318 mSv; and right ring finger, 0.6694 mSv. The effective dose to the surgeon was calculated to be 0.0093 mSv per level. The protective effects of lead aprons and thyroid shields were found to be 94.2 and 96.9%, respectively. The authors strongly recommended the use of lead protective equipment in the operating room while using fluoroscopy.

21.8.4 Level IV Evidence in Open Surgery

Mulconrey[42] performed an in vitro investigation on fluoroscopic radiation exposure to personnel involved in spinal surgery. Radiation dosimetry badges were worn on the chests of the operating surgeon and first assistant, and badges were also placed on the cranial and caudal ends of the operating room table. The investigation involved 35 surgeries in total, and included both lumbar and cervical procedures. All procedures were performed in an open fashion. Calculated total fluoroscopic radiation exposure for the surgeon was 1,225 mrem for the surgeon, and 369 mrem for the assistant. Measurements at the cranial and caudal end of the table were less, 92 and 150 mrem, respectively. The total dose to all patients was determined to be 29.2 mrem. The total times for posterior spinal fusion (PSF) with instrumentation averaged 0.89 minutes, while PSF with TLIF averaged 1.9 minutes. To remain below the maximum yearly permissible level of radiation exposure, the total number of minutes per year a surgeon could perform a similar mix of procedures using fluoroscopy would be approximately 453, based on the current study. The author concluded that by using efficient techniques and maintaining surgeon distance from the source in the operating room, open spine surgery can be safely performed below the International Commission on Radiological Protection's (ICRP's) recommended annual limits.[42]

Bindal[43] performed a prospective study on 24 consecutive patients undergoing either one- or two-level MIS-TLIF with pedicle screw instrumentation. The main goal was to report both surgeon and patient radiation exposure during this procedure. There was no open control group. Dosimeters were placed underneath a lead apron at the waist, unshielded at the level of the thyroid and on the operating surgeon's ring finger of the dominant hand. The authors also used an indirect method to calculate patient radiation exposure by "operating the C-arm in manual mode, and setting the system to kVp and mA recorded at the time of the procedure." Mean fluoroscopy time was 1.69 minutes per case (range: 3.73–0.82). Mean exposure per case to the surgeon's hand was 76 mrem, at the waist underneath the apron was 27 mrem, and at the unshielded thyroid level was 32 mrem. The reported average exposure to the skin of the patient using the technique described earlier was 59.5 mGy (range: 8.3–252 mGy) in the PA plane and 78.8 mGy (range: 6.3–269.5 mGy) in the lateral plane. The authors concluded that patient exposures were low, and that surgeons' exposure levels were limited, but could potentially exceed acceptable limits if numerous procedures were performed annually.[43]

Mroz et al[44] examined the amount of radiation exposure to the eyes, hands, and chest under an apron during the placement of percutaneous pedicle screws in a cadaveric study. Percutaneous pedicle screws were placed bilaterally in cadaveric specimens from L2 to S1 while simultaneously using two fluoroscopes to image the anteroposterior and lateral planes. The operating surgeon wore a thermolucent dosimeter on his right hand, and another was placed under the lead apron in the left chest region. Eye exposure doses were calculated by an earlier reported technique reported from a kyphoplasty study using radiation exposure times from the present study.[44] Total fluoroscopic time for the completion of the entire procedure was 4 minutes 56 seconds, or 29 seconds per screw. The dose to the hand was 103 mrem, and that to the chest was not measurable (< 10 mrem). Finally, the indirectly calculated exposure to the eyes was determined to be 2.35 mrem per screw. The main weaknesses of the study include the use of only one cadaver,

Table 21.1 Comparative studies for radiation exposure in MIS versus open spinal surgeries

Author (year)	Level	Study	Type	Patients	Findings
Mroz et al[44] (2011)	III	Cadaveric study	MIS	1	0.29 s per screw flouro time
Rampersaud et al[5] (2000)	III	Cadaveric study	MIS	6	10–12 times greater exposure than other, nonspinal procedures
Bindal et al[43] (2008)	IV	Retrospective	MIS	24	Occupational limit could be surpassed if many cases per year
Wang et al[36] (2011)	II	Prospective, "random"	MIS vs. Open	85	More than twice the fluoro time for MIS-TLIF vs. open
Mariscalco et al[33] (2011)	II	Prospective, controlled	MIS vs. Open	20	10–22 times greater exposure with MIS vs. Open MD
Ahn et al[41] (2013)	III	Prospective cohort	MIS	30	Effective dose to the surgeon 0.0093 mSv per level
Bronsard et al[39] (2013)	III	Retrospective	MIS vs. Open	60	Threefold higher dose for MIS

Abbreviations: MD, microdiscectomy; MIS, minimally invasive surgery; TLIF, transforaminal lumbar interbody fusion.

indirect calculation of exposure to the eyes, and the use of a surgeon proficient in the technique.[43]

Mroz et al[44] also examined the amount of radiation exposure during kyphoplasty in 27 consecutive patients (52 vertebra) using similar techniques. Again, two fluoroscopes were simultaneously employed. Dosimeters were placed in the same positions, but also superficial to the lead apron and at the neck, deep to a thyroid shield. Again, lead protected regions failed to measure any appreciable radiation levels (< 10 mrem), but the hands were exposed to 174.4 mrem/vertebra. Exposure to the eyes was indirectly calculated to be 27.1 mrem/vertebra.[45] In a similar study, Harstall et al examined the radiation exposure during 32 vertebroplasty procedures using two fluoroscopes. Measured with unprotected whole-body dosimeters, the doses to the eyes, hands, and thyroid gland were 2.7, 14.5, and 7.1 mSv, respectively.[15] The risk of a thyroid malignancy over a 20- to 25-year period would be considered high to very high.

Based on the review of the literature presented earlier, the studies evaluated and levels of evidence are summarized in ▶ Table 21.1. There are no level I studies comparing radiation exposure in MIS versus open spinal surgery. There is level II evidence supporting the higher risk of radiation exposure in MIS techniques versus open surgery. This includes the study by Mariscalco et al[33] that showed increased exposure to the surgeon between 10 and 22 times the ionizing radiation during MIS discectomy versus the traditional open approach. In addition, the study by Wang et al[36] demonstrated more than two times the fluoroscopy time during MIS-TLIF as compared to open TLIF. There are numerous other lower quality studies showing similar findings as discussed earlier.

Modern medicine, in particular spinal surgery, is directed toward MIS, or image-guided procedures. The purported advantages of MIS surgery include decreased blood loss, smaller incisions, less soft-tissue damage, less pain, lower infection rates, shorter hospital stays, and faster return to activities. There are few quality studies comparing MIS versus open spine surgeon to validate these potential advantages. The only randomized controlled trial comparing MIS to open surgery was performed by Wang et al. In their study, with 79 patients undergoing either open or MIS single-level TLIF, they were unable to show any benefit with regard to blood loss, creatine phosphokinase levels, hospital stay, or either pain or ODI scores at 2 years. They did demonstrate improved recovery times with MIS surgery,

but at the expense of greater amounts of fluoroscopy to perform the procedure.[37]

From the aforementioned evaluation of the current body of literature, it is clear that MIS surgery involves increased amounts of radiation to the surgeon, the operating room staff, and the patients, with possibly little other benefit than faster rehabilitation. One published study demonstrated that orthopaedic surgeons have an unusually high rate of thyroid malignancy.[4] Another showed a five times higher risk of malignancy in orthopaedic surgeons using fluoroscopy versus other health care professionals.[46] Theocharopoulos et al performed a retrospective analysis of the contribution of various procedures to the effective radiation dose to an orthopaedic surgeon. The lifetime malignancy risk, of course, depends on clinical workload, but the physician who performs 50 hip, spine, and kyphoplasty procedures a year will have an associated risk of development of fatal cancer of 0.75%.[16] Although the risk seems small, it is not insignificant, and we should all be concerned for ourselves, the operating room personnel, and our patients.

21.9 Conclusion of Open Surgery

As previously discussed, only one randomized controlled study has recognized the increased radiation exposure to surgeons performing MIS fusion procedures versus open procedures. Using this study, along with a wealth of level III and level IV studies, a grade 1C recommendation may be assigned to evidence suggesting that surgeons performing MIS fusion procedures are exposed to significantly longer fluoroscopy times and higher ionizing radiation dosages when compared with surgeons performing open fusions. Although historical data have shown that high amounts of occupational radiation exposure may lead to increased risk of several different forms of malignancy, there have been no studies performed concluding that this increased radiation exposure has definitively led to higher malignancy rates in surgeons performing MIS procedures. Therefore, a grade 2C recommendation is assigned to the evidence supporting this increased risk.

Radiation is a known carcinogen that can cause malignancy in patients and operating room personnel. These are stochastic neoplasms that are assumed to be unaffected by dose fractionation. An individual's lifetime risk of developing a malignancy can therefore be significantly reduced by small changes in the amount of cumulative radiation they receive. In other words, small per-case savings in radiation exposure achieved by altering technique or using lower-dose machines can lead to a significant reduction in this risk.[47] One should question the use of MIS surgery, given that it has been shown to result in greater exposures for medical personnel and the patients alike.

21.10 Editors' Commentary

21.10.1 Minimally Invasive Surgery

I will concede that exposure to radiation is greater in MIS than in open surgery. However, the clinical significance of this is unclear. If, as some claim, this is a major health hazard, then why aren't our interventional radiologists all dying of cancer? Same question for the radiology technicians. Is it possible that the risk isn't quite what some are stating? After extensive study of the effects of UNPROTECTED exposure to galactic cosmic radiation and solar particle radiation which our astronauts would be exposed to during a 900-day mission to Mars, NASA concluded that the lifetime risk of death from cancer would only increase 4% in men and 8% in women. Since these are far more powerful sources of radiation than those used in the operating room, combined with the lead and distance safety precautions utilized therein, perhaps a more rational evaluation of the true risk is indicated.

21.10.2 Open Surgery

The development of minimally invasive surgical techniques has been severely limited by reliance on the use of fluoroscopy. Given the general lack of evidence suggesting that minimally invasive techniques are superior to open techniques, it is easy to understand why the majority of spinal surgeons have not adopted MIS because of the associated personal risk. Although some strategies and work processes have been developed to minimize the use of ionizing radiation, a more productive effort for the MIS community would be to focus on developing a paradigm shift that moves away from the routine use of fluoroscopy and toward non–radiation-based techniques. Most open procedures require imaging only for level confirmation and to confirm final position of instrumentation when utilized. Images are most often obtained using conventional radiographs which allow the surgical team to distance themselves from the radiation source. Finally, surgeons utilizing MIS techniques not only expose themselves to ionizing radiation but also the surgical team who has little control over the technique used and may be exposed more frequently given they are subject to surgical procedures on a daily basis when operating with other surgeons who may also use fluoroscopy routinely.

References

[1] Linet MS, Slovis TL, Miller DL, et al. Cancer risks associated with external radiation from diagnostic imaging procedures. CA Cancer J Clin. 2012; 62(2): 75–100

[2] Prasarn ML, Martin E, Schreck M, et al. Analysis of radiation exposure to the orthopaedic trauma patient during their inpatient hospitalisation. Injury. 2012; 43(6):757–761

[3] Giachino AA, Cheng M. Irradiation of the surgeon during pinning of femoral fractures. J Bone Joint Surg Br. 1980; 62-B(2):227–229

[4] Jones DP, Robertson PA, Lunt B, Jackson SA. Radiation exposure during fluoroscopically assisted pedicle screw insertion in the lumbar spine. Spine. 2000; 25(12):1538–1541

[5] Rampersaud YR, Foley KT, Shen AC, Williams S, Solomito M. Radiation exposure to the spine surgeon during fluoroscopically assisted pedicle screw insertion. Spine. 2000; 25(20):2637–2645

[6] Giordano BD, Baumhauer JF, Morgan TL, Rechtine GR. Cervical spine imaging using standard C-arm fluoroscopy: patient and surgeon exposure to ionizing radiation. Spine. 2008; 33(18):1970–1976

[7] Giordano BD, Baumhauer JF, Morgan TL, Rechtine GR, II. Patient and surgeon radiation exposure: comparison of standard and mini-C-arm fluoroscopy. J Bone Joint Surg Am. 2009; 91(2):297–304

[8] Giordano BD, Baumhauer JF, Morgan TL, Rechtine GR, II. Cervical spine imaging using mini–C-arm fluoroscopy: patient and surgeon exposure to direct and scatter radiation. J Spinal Disord Tech. 2009; 22(6):399–403

[9] Giordano BD, Rechtine GR, II, Morgan TL. Minimally invasive surgery and radiation exposure. J Neurosurg Spine. 2009; 11(3):375–376, author reply 376–377

[10] Ding A, Mille MM, Liu T, Caracappa PF, Xu XG. Extension of RPI-adult male and female computational phantoms to obese patients and a Monte Carlo study of the effect on CT imaging dose. Phys Med Biol. 2012; 57(9):2441–2459

[11] Ector J, Dragusin O, Adriaenssens B, et al. Obesity is a major determinant of radiation dose in patients undergoing pulmonary vein isolation for atrial fibrillation. J Am Coll Cardiol. 2007; 50(3):234–242

[12] Hsi RS, Zamora DA, Kanal KM, Harper JD. Severe obesity is associated with 3-fold higher radiation dose rate during ureteroscopy. Urology. 2013; 82(4): 780–785

[13] Smuck M, Zheng P, Chong T, Kao MC, Geisser ME. Duration of fluoroscopic-guided spine interventions and radiation exposure is increased in overweight patients. PM R. 2013; 5(4):291–296, quiz 296

[14] Giordano BD, Grauer JN, Miller CP, Morgan TL, Rechtine GR, II. Radiation exposure issues in orthopaedics. J Bone Joint Surg Am. 2011; 93(12):e69–, 1–10)

[15] Harstall R, Heini PF, Mini RL, Orler R. Radiation exposure to the surgeon during fluoroscopically assisted percutaneous vertebroplasty: a prospective study. Spine. 2005; 30(16):1893–1898

[16] Theocharopoulos N, Perisinakis K, Damilakis J, Papadokostakis G, Hadjipavlou A, Gourtsoyiannis N. Occupational exposure from common fluoroscopic projections used in orthopaedic surgery. J Bone Joint Surg Am. 2003; 85-A (9):1698–1703

[17] Ul Haque M, Shufflebarger HL, O'Brien M, Macagno A. Radiation exposure during pedicle screw placement in adolescent idiopathic scoliosis: is fluoroscopy safe? Spine. 2006; 31(21):2516–2520

[18] Stevens KJ, Spenciner DB, Griffiths KL, et al. Comparison of minimally invasive and conventional open posterolateral lumbar fusion using magnetic resonance imaging and retraction pressure studies. J Spinal Disord Tech. 2006; 19(2):77–86

[19] Isaacs RE, Podichetty VK, Santiago P, et al. Minimally invasive microendoscopy-assisted transforaminal lumbar interbody fusion with instrumentation. J Neurosurg Spine. 2005; 3(2):98–105

[20] Karikari IO, Isaacs RE. Minimally invasive transforaminal lumbar interbody fusion: a review of techniques and outcomes. Spine. 2010; 35(26) Suppl: S294–S301

[21] Lee KH, Yue WM, Yeo W, Soeharno H, Tan SB. Clinical and radiological outcomes of open versus minimally invasive transforaminal lumbar interbody fusion. Eur Spine J. 2012; 21(11):2265–2270

[22] Ntoukas V, Müller A. Minimally invasive approach versus traditional open approach for one level posterior lumbar interbody fusion. Minim Invasive Neurosurg. 2010; 53(1):21–24

[23] Park Y, Ha JW. Comparison of one-level posterior lumbar interbody fusion performed with a minimally invasive approach or a traditional open approach. Spine. 2007; 32(5):537–543

[24] Tian NF, Wu YS, Zhang XL, Xu HZ, Chi YL, Mao FM. Minimally invasive versus open transforaminal lumbar interbody fusion: a meta-analysis based on the current evidence. Eur Spine J. 2013; 22(8):1741–1749

[25] McGirt MJ, Parker SL, Lerner J, Engelhart L, Knight T, Wang MY. Comparative analysis of perioperative surgical site infection after minimally invasive versus open posterior/transforaminal lumbar interbody fusion: analysis of hospital billing and discharge data from 5170 patients. J Neurosurg Spine. 2011; 14(6):771–778

[26] O'Toole JE, Eichholz KM, Fessler RG. Surgical site infection rates after minimally invasive spinal surgery. J Neurosurg Spine. 2009; 11(4):471–476

[27] Committee to Assess Health Risks from Exposure to Low Levels of Ionizing Radiation, National Research Council. Washington, DC: National Academies Press; 2014

[28] Hammer GP, Scheidemann-Wesp U, Samkange-Zeeb F, Wicke H, Neriishi K, Blettner M. Occupational exposure to low doses of ionizing radiation and cataract development: a systematic literature review and perspectives on future studies. Radiat Environ Biophys. 2013; 52(3):303–319

[29] OSHA/Radiation Guidelines. https://http://www.osha.gov/pls/oshaweb/owadisp.show_document?p_table=STANDARDS&p_id=10098. Accessed September 7, 2017

[30] Nottmeier EW, Pirris SM, Edwards S, Kimes S, Bowman C, Nelson KL. Operating room radiation exposure in cone beam computed tomography-based, image-guided spinal surgery: clinical article. J Neurosurg Spine. 2013; 19(2):226–231

[31] O-arm Imaging System Version 3.1 Dosimetry Report. Vol Document Nr Rev2: Medtronic; 2009: B1–150–00155

[32] Tabaraee E, Gibson AG, Karahalios DG, Potts EA, Mobasser JP, Burch S. Intraoperative cone beam-computed tomography with navigation (O-ARM) versus conventional fluoroscopy (C-ARM): a cadaveric study comparing accuracy, efficiency, and safety for spinal instrumentation. Spine. 2013; 38 (22):1953–1958

[33] Mariscalco MW, Yamashita T, Steinmetz MP, Krishnaney AA, Lieberman IH, Mroz TE. Radiation exposure to the surgeon during open lumbar microdiscectomy and minimally invasive microdiscectomy: a prospective, controlled trial. Spine. 2011; 36(3):255–260

[34] Lee KH, Yeo W, Soeharno H, Yue WM. Learning curve of a complex surgical technique: minimally invasive transforaminal lumbar interbody fusion (MIS TLIF). J Spinal Disord Tech. 2014; 27(7):E234–E240

[35] Wang HL, Lü FZ, Jiang JY, Ma X, Xia XL, Wang LX. Minimally invasive lumbar interbody fusion via MAST Quadrant retractor versus open surgery: a prospective randomized clinical trial. Chin Med J (Engl). 2011; 124(23): 3868–3874

[36] Wang J, Zhou Y, Zhang ZF, Li CQ, Zheng WJ, Liu J. Comparison of one-level minimally invasive and open transforaminal lumbar interbody fusion in degenerative and isthmic spondylolisthesis grades 1 and 2. Eur Spine J. 2010; 19(10):1780–1784

[37] Wang J, Zhou Y, Zhang ZF, Li CQ, Zheng WJ, Liu J. Minimally invasive or open transforaminal lumbar interbody fusion as revision surgery for patients previously treated by open discectomy and decompression of the lumbar spine. Eur Spine J. 2011; 20(4):623–628

[38] Kim CW, Lee YP, Taylor W, Oygar A, Kim WK. Use of navigation-assisted fluoroscopy to decrease radiation exposure during minimally invasive spine surgery. Spine J. 2008; 8(4):584–590

[39] Bronsard N, Boli T, Challali M, et al. Comparison between percutaneous and traditional fixation of lumbar spine fracture: intraoperative radiation exposure levels and outcomes. Orthop Traumatol Surg Res. 2013; 99(2):162–168

[40] Kanter AS, Mummaneni PV. Minimally invasive spine surgery. Neurosurg Focus. 2008; 25(2):E1

[41] Ahn Y, Kim CH, Lee JH, Lee SH, Kim JS. Radiation exposure to the surgeon during percutaneous endoscopic lumbar discectomy: a prospective study. Spine. 2013; 38(7):617–625

[42] Mulconrey DS. Fluoroscopic radiation exposure in spinal surgery: in vivo evaluation for operating room personnel. Clin Spine Surg. 2016; 29(7):E331–E335

[43] Bindal RK, Glaze S, Ognoskie M, Tunner V, Malone R, Ghosh S. Surgeon and patient radiation exposure in minimally invasive transforaminal lumbar interbody fusion. J Neurosurg Spine. 2008; 9(6):570–573

[44] Mroz TE, Abdullah KG, Steinmetz MP, Klineberg EO, Lieberman IH. Radiation exposure to the surgeon during percutaneous pedicle screw placement. J Spinal Disord Tech. 2011; 24(4):264–267

[45] Mroz TE, Yamashita T, Davros WJ, Lieberman IH. Radiation exposure to the surgeon and the patient during kyphoplasty. J Spinal Disord Tech. 2008; 21 (2):96–100

[46] Mastrangelo G, Fedeli U, Fadda E, Giovanazzi A, Scoizzato L, Saia B. Increased cancer risk among surgeons in an orthopaedic hospital. Occup Med (Lond). 2005; 55(6):498–500

[47] Prasarn ML, Coyne E, Schreck M, Rodgers JD, Rechtine GR. Comparison of image quality and radiation exposure from C-arm fluoroscopes when used for imaging the spine. Spine. 2013; 38(16):1401–1404

22 Infection Rates: How Do Infection Rates Compare between MIS and Open Spine Techniques?

MIS: Kurt M. Eichholz

Open: Bryce A. Basques, Daniel D. Bohl, Nicholas S. Golinvaux, and Jonathan N. Grauer

22.1 Introduction

The field of minimally invasive spine (MIS) surgery has seen extensive advances over the past 30 years, and MIS procedures have become increasingly common.[1] Following the trends of minimally invasive surgery in other disciplines, MIS aims to provide at least equivalent outcomes while offering benefits, such as decreased soft-tissue disruption, improved cosmesis, reduced blood loss, less postoperative pain, and decreased hospital length of stay following the procedure.[1] The relative rates of complications with open and MIS techniques bear consideration when comparing outcomes with these varying techniques.

Postoperative infection is one complication that is particularly concerning, given that surgical site infection (SSI) of the spine and surrounding structures has significant clinical sequelae. Infection occurs after both open and MIS spine surgery, and there is currently debate over which approach is associated with lower postoperative infection rates.

For the purposes of this chapter, infection was defined according to the Centers for Disease Control and Prevention (CDC)/National Nosocomial Infections Surveillance (NNIS) guidelines.[2] According to these guidelines, an SSI is defined as an infection that involves skin or subcutaneous tissue (superficial), fascia or muscle layers (deep), or any other anatomic components manipulated during surgery (organ space). While SSI definition varies from study to study, each study's findings were correlated with the above-noted definitions in order to most accurately represent SSI occurrences and allow comparison among studies.

Understanding the differences in infection rates between MIS and open spine surgery is important for patients, surgeons, and hospitals, as well as the health system in general. Often, a specific disease state may be the driving factor for determining the best surgical approach. However, there are situations where such decisions are surgeons' or patients' choice. Especially in those situations, the relative risks may sway clinical decisions. With regard to infection, this may be especially true when treating patients at an elevated risk for infection, such as immunocompromised patients. By critically evaluating the quality and results of existing studies, informed discussions of the relative risks of open and MIS techniques can be facilitated.

22.2 Advantages of Minimally Invasive Surgery

There are several factors that may be considered relative risks or benefits of MIS techniques with regard to infection. First, the potential advantages of MIS procedures will be discussed.

The incisions of MIS techniques are smaller than open techniques. Accordingly, there is less exposure of internal structures. In endoscopic and tubular procedures, generally only the area at the base of the tube or trocar is exposed to the outside environment. The larger incisions of open surgeries could expose increased surface area for bacterial colonization.

Muscle ischemia and damage, which can occur during retraction, is believed to be greater during open procedures than MIS procedures.[3] This may lead to compromised tissues at greater risk for infection. Furthermore, there is likely a reduced operative site dead space after the procedure. This may reduce the formation of postoperative seromas or hematomas that could serve as a nidus for an SSI.[4]

Intraoperative blood loss has been consistently reported to be less for MIS versus open transforaminal lumbar interbody fusion (TLIF).[5,6,7,8] As increased intraoperative blood loss has been shown to be a risk factor for postoperative spinal infection,[9] this may be an advantage of MIS techniques with regard to infection.

Hospital length of stay has been repeatedly shown to be less after MIS procedures compared to open surgeries.[5,6,7,8] As increased length of stay has also been considered a risk factor for spinal SSIs due to nosocomial infection, this may be an additional advantage for MIS techniques.

22.3 Advantages of Open Surgery

There are several advantages of open techniques compared to MIS techniques with regard to infection risk. Compared to MIS techniques, most surgeons have more experience with open procedures, which have an easier learning curve.[10] Increased surgeon experience has been shown to lessen risk of complications, including infection.[11]

In addition, perhaps due to better exposure and an easier learning curve, operative time is generally less for open surgery compared to MIS.[5,12] Increased operative time has been shown to be an independent risk factor for postoperative infection after spine surgery.[13]

Open surgery also has the advantage of requiring less operative equipment, which may decrease risk of infection. Studies of operating microscope and C-arm sterility during spine surgery have shown significant bacterial contamination by the end of the surgical case.[14,15,16] Increased exposure to this contaminated equipment, as is necessary with the increased operative time and radiation exposure associated with MIS surgery, has the potential to increase risk of postoperative infection compared to open cases.[5,12,17,18]

22.4 Case Illustration

A 47-year-old man presented with 4 months of pain in the back without radicular pain. He had undergone three prior surgeries—a lumbar microdiscectomy 13 years ago, a lumbar fusion 10 years ago, and then an L4–L5 anterior lumbar interbody fusion (ALIF) with L3–L5 posterior spinal fusion with instrumentation 4 years ago. He was treated conservatively and

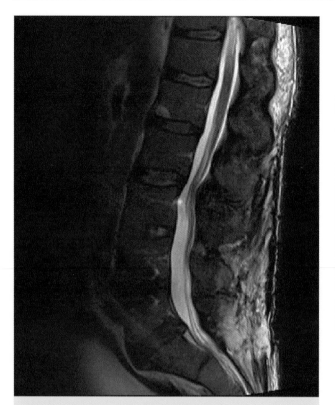

Fig. 22.1 Preoperative T2 sagittal image.

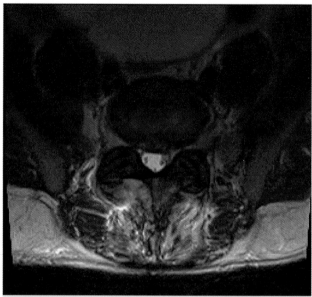

Fig. 22.2 Preoperative T2 axial image.

underwent a series of epidural steroid injections. With this third injection, he had immediate worsening pain that was radiating down the left leg to the lateral aspect of the left foot. He had no right leg radicular pain. On examination, he has weakness in his left hamstrings, anterior tibialis, and extensor hallucis longus at 4/5 with sensory loss in the left S1 distribution. His left Achilles reflex was absent, and his straight leg raise was positive at 30 degrees on the left side. His magnetic resonance imaging (MRI) showed previous instrumentation and interbody graft at L3–L5, and a left paracentral disc herniation causing neural foraminal stenosis at L5–S1 (▶ Fig. 22.1, ▶ Fig. 22.2).

He underwent a minimally invasive left L5–S1 microdiscectomy. The surgery was performed through a muscle-splitting tubular retractor system, using microscopic techniques. The operative time was 43 minutes, and the patient was discharged 3 hours and 50 minutes after surgery. This resulted in immediate improvement in his left leg radicular pain and sensory loss.

The patient presented for his 6-week follow-up visit and continued to have significant improvement in his left leg radicular pain, but had gradual back, buttocks, and upper thigh pain. He was neurologically intact with the exception of mild sensory loss in the left S1 distribution. His incision was well healed with no evidence of infection.

Over the next 2 weeks, the patient had gradually worsening pain that went down to his left leg and to the lateral aspect of his foot, with difficulty walking. He also had some pain in his right leg. On examination, he had full strength in all muscle groups, with increased sensory loss in the left S1 distribution and an absent left ankle jerk. His incision remained clean, dry, and intact.

A postoperative MRI was performed which showed a ring-enhancing epidural mass extending into his hemilaminotomy defect (▶ Fig. 22.3, ▶ Fig. 22.4, ▶ Fig. 22.5, ▶ Fig. 22.6). He was taken to the operating room, and exploration revealed a significant epidural abscess with purulent material in the central canal. This was evacuated and irrigated, and cultures ultimately were negative. A PICC line was placed, and the patient was prescribed intravenous vancomycin for 6 weeks.

Of note, the patient stated that since postoperative day 3, he had spent at least 30 minutes per day soaking in a hot tub, despite postoperative instructions to the contrary.

22.5 Discussion of Minimally Invasive Spine

MIS surgery has several potential advantages compared to open procedures in terms of risk of infection. These potential advantages may be derived from the smaller incisions, decreased tissue ischemia/damage, reduced operative dead space, decreased intraoperative blood loss, and shorter postoperative length of stay of MIS procedures compared to open procedures.[3,4,5,6,7,8] In recent years, there have been a number of studies comparing infection rates between MIS and open spine surgery, with the majority studying fusion cases (▶ Table 22.1). There are also a number of studies examining the complication rates between MIS and open discectomy as well as other types of MIS procedures from which infection data can be extrapolated (▶ Table 22.2, ▶ Table 22.3).

While other studies have reported infection rates in a single cohort of MIS or open surgery patients, it was felt to be most

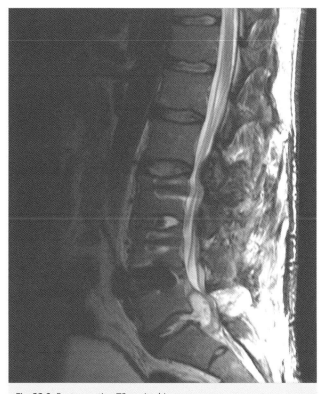

Fig. 22.3 Postoperative T2 sagittal image.

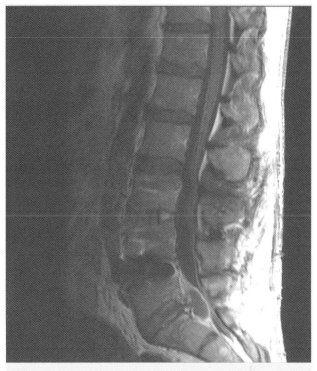

Fig. 22.5 Postoperative T1 with contrast sagittal image.

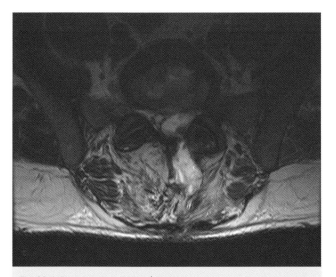

Fig. 22.4 Postoperative T2 axial image.

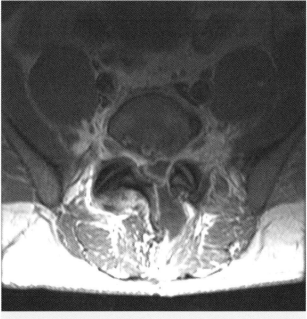

Fig. 22.6 Postoperative T1 with contrast axial image.

Table 22.1 Studies comparing infection rates between MIS and open fusion procedures

Author	Year	Level	Design	Procedure	MIS		Open	
					Number	%	Number	%
Wang et al[27]	2012	II	Pro	MIS-TLIF vs. open in obese patients	2/43	4.7%	3/39	7.7%
Wang et al[28]	2011	II	Pro	MIS-TLIF vs. open as revision surgery after open discectomy and decompression	0/25	0.0%	2/27	7.4%
Shunwu et al[29]	2010	II	Pro	MIS-TLIF vs. open for one-level degenerative disease	3/32	9.4%	2/30	6.7%
Wang et al[18]	2010	II	Pro	MIS-TLIF vs. open for spondylolisthesis	0/42	0.0%	0/43	0.0%
Ghahreman et al[30]	2010	II	Pro	MIS-PLIF vs. open for radicular pain from spondylolisthesis	0/23	0.0%	0/24	0.0%
Peng et al[5]	2009	II	Pro	MIS-TLIF vs. open	2/29	6.9%	1/29	3.4%
Park and Ha[31]	2007	II	Pro	MIS-TLIF vs. open for predominantly axial pain	1/32	3.1%	3/29	10.3%
Seng et al[38]	2013	III	Retro	MIS-TLIF vs. open	1/40	2.5%	1/40	2.5%
Kepler et al[48]	2013	III	Retro	MIS posterior fusion vs. open posterior fusion after open anterior lumbar fusion	3/81	3.7%	1/53	1.2%
Adogwa et al[36]	2011	III	Retro	MIS-TLIF vs. open for spondylolisthesis	0/15	0.0%	0/15	0.0%
McGirt et al[33]	2011	III	Retro	MIS-PLIF/TLIF vs. open	65/1,436	4.5%	138/3,734	3.7%
Lau et al[47]	2011	III	Retro	MIS-TLIF vs. open	1/10	10.0%	0/12	0.0%
Schizas et al[8]	2009	III	Retro	MIS-TLIF vs. open for spondylolisthesis or degenerative disc disease	0/18	0.0%	0/18	0.0%
Dhall et al[6]	2008	III	Retro	Mini-open vs. open TLIF for spondylolisthesis or degenerative disc disease	0/21	0.0%	0/21	0.0%
Bagan et al[49]	2008	III	Retro	MIS-PLIF/TLIF vs. open	1/28	3.6%	0/19	0.0%
Scheufler et al[37]	2007	III	Retro	Percutaneous TLIF vs. mini-open TLIF pseudolithiasis or degenerative disc disease	0/53	0.0%	0/67	0.0%
Villavicencio et al[7]	2006	III	Retro	MIS-TLIF vs. open	2/73	2.7%	0/51	0.0%
Isaacs et al[34]	2005	III	Retro	Microendoscopic TLIF (METLIF) vs. open for spondylolisthesis and/or pure axial pain	0/20	0.0%	1/24	4.2%
Villavicencio et al[35]	2005	III	Retro	MIS-TLIF vs. open for degenerative disc disease	1/43	2.3%	1/31	3.2%
Saraph et al[50]	2004	III	Retro	MIS vs. conventional extraperitoneal ALIF for spondylolisthesis, lumbar instability, or failed back syndrome	1/23	4.3%	0/33	0.0%
Average infection rate for all fusion studies						*2.9%*		*2.5%*

Abbreviations: ALIF, anterior lumbar interbody fusion; MIS, minimally invasive surgery; PLIF, posterior lumbar interbody fusion; Pro, prospective study; TLIF, transforaminal lumbar interbody fusion; Retro, retrospective study.

appropriate to use only those studies that included both cohorts in order to provide accurate comparisons. Most of the following studies looked at complications after various procedures and collected infection data as one of the complication measures. Many of these studies are limited by small patient numbers, making it difficult to accurately compare a rare outcome such as postoperative infection. As such, the quality of studies for each type of procedure varies.

22.5.1 Level I Evidence in Minimally Invasive Surgery

To our knowledge, only two level I studies have been conducted comparing outcomes between MIS and open surgery.[19,20] There have been several other randomized, prospective studies comparing MIS and open spine surgery approaches; however, these other studies did not meet the full criteria for level I evidence, mostly due to inadequate blinding.[21,22,23,24,25,26]

Both level I studies compared MIS and open approaches for discectomy and found no infections in either treatment group (▶ Table 22.2). Arts et al included 325 patients in their study, and Ryang et al included 60 patients in their study.[19,20]

22.5.2 Level II Evidence in Minimally Invasive Surgery

There have been a number of prospective, level II studies comparing MIS and open techniques in recent years. As mentioned earlier, several of these studies were randomized; however, they are considered level II evidence because of methodological limitations.[21,22,23,24,25,26]

We identified seven prospective studies that directly compare MIS and open techniques for fusion (six TLIF and one posterior lumbar interbody fusion [PLIF]), which all show no statistically significant difference in infection rates between MIS and open procedures.[5,18,27,28,29,30,31] Nonetheless, of these

Table 22.2 Studies comparing infection rates between MIS and open discectomy procedures

Author	Year	Level	Design	Procedure	MIS		Open	
					Number	%	Number	%
Arts et al[19]	2009	I	RCT	Tubular vs. conventional microdiscectomy for sciatica	0/166	0.0%	0/159	0.0%
Ryang et al[20]	2008	I	RCT	MIS trocar microdiscectomy vs. open microdiscectomy	0/30	0.0%	0/30	0.0%
Teli et al[21]	2010	II	Pro	Microendoscopic lumbar discectomy vs. microlumbar discectomy vs. open lumbar discectomy	0/70	0.0%	7/144	4.9%
Franke et al[22]	2009	II	Pro	Microscopically assisted percutaneous nucleotomy vs. microsurgical discotomy	0/50	0.0%	0/50	0.0%
Ruetten et al[23]	2008	II	Pro	Full-endoscopic interlaminar and transforaminal lumbar discectomy vs. microsurgical discectomy	0/91	0.0%	1/87	1.1%
Hermantin et al[24]	1999	II	Pro	Arthroscopic lumbar microdiscectomy vs. open lumbar laminotomy and discectomy	0/30	0.0%	0/30	0.0%
Lee et al[39]	2011	III	Retro	MIS vs. open single-level lumbar discectomy	0/64	0.0%	1/45	2.2%
Harrington and French[40]	2008	III	Retro	MIS vs. open lumbar microdiscectomy	0/31	0.0%	0/35	0.0%
Wu et al[41]	2006	III	Retro	Microendoscopic discectomy vs. open lumbar discectomy	9/873	1.0%	5/358	1.4%
Average infection rate for all discectomy studies						*0.1%*		*1.1%*

Abbreviations: MIS, minimally invasive surgery; Pro, prospective study; RCT, randomized controlled trial; Retro, retrospective study.

Table 22.3 Studies comparing infection rates between MIS and open for other/multiple procedures

Author	Year	Level	Design	Procedure	MIS		Open	
					Number	%	Number	%
Ruetten et al[25]	2009	II	Pro	Full-endoscopic transforaminal or interlaminar decompression vs. microsurgical technique for lumbar lateral recess stenosis	0/80	0.0%	2/81	2.5%
Ruetten et al[26]	2008	II	Pro	Full-endoscopic posterior cervical foraminotomy vs. microsurgical technique for lateral cervical disc herniation	0/100	0.0%	0/100	0.0%
Regan et al[32]	1999	II	Pro	Laparoscopic transperitoneal vs. open retroperitoneal approach for lumbar interbody fusion	3/215	1.4%	6/305	2.0%
Ee et al[43]	2013	III	Retro	MIS vs open TLIF, laminectomy, and discectomy	5/83	6.0%	22/106	20.8%
Siddaraju et al[13]	2011	III	Retro	MIS vs. open TLIF, laminectomy, laminotomy, and discectomy	5/791	0.6%	23/1,275	1.8%
Smith et al[44]	2011	III	Retro	MIS vs. open procedures for degenerative disease, spondylolisthesis, fracture, kyphosis, scoliosis, and tumor	78/14,301	0.5%	2,280/94,115	2.4%
Shih et al[12]	2011	III	Retro	Microendoscopic decompression of stenosis vs. open lumbar decompression	0/23	0.0%	1/26	3.8%
Rahman et al[42]	2008	III	Retro	MIS vs. open lumbar laminectomy	1/38	2.6%	2/33	6.1%
Average infection rate for all other/multiple procedure studies						*1.4%*		*4.9%*

Abbreviations: MIS, minimally invasive surgery; Pro, prospective study; TLIF, transforaminal lumbar interbody fusion; Retro, retrospective study.

studies, three show a greater absolute percentage of infections after open surgery,[27,28] two studies show a greater absolute percentage of infections after MIS procedures,[5,29] and two studies show no infections in either group (no difference).[18,30] It is worth noting that the two infections in the MIS group from the Peng et al[5] study were from iliac crest donor sites, not from the primary surgical site. Peng et al found the overall complication rate significantly higher in the open group versus the MIS group.

There have been four prospective studies comparing MIS and open discectomy. Microscopically assisted percutaneous nucleotomy (MAPN) and microsurgical discotomy were compared by Franke et al[22] and video-assisted arthroscopic lumbar microdiscectomy was compared with open laminotomy and discectomy by Hermantin et al.[24] Both Franke et al[22] and Hermantin et al[24] found no infections in both MIS and open cohorts. Ruetten et al[23] compared full-endoscopic interlaminar and transforaminal lumbar discectomy to the conventional microsurgical technique and found zero infections in the MIS cohort and one infection in the microsurgical cohort (1.1%), with the overall complication rate being significantly higher with the microsurgical "open" approach ($p < 0.05$). Teli et al compared outcomes after microendoscopic lumbar discectomy, micro lumbar discectomy, and open lumbar microdiscectomy and found no statistically significant difference in infection rates between groups.[21]

Prospective studies comparing other MIS and open procedures have also found no significant difference in infection rates between the two approaches. Ruetten et al[26] compared full-endoscopic posterior cervical foraminotomy with conventional microsurgical anterior decompression and fusion and found no infections in either cohort. In a different study, Ruetten et al[25] compared full-endoscopic transforaminal or interlaminar decompression to the traditional microsurgical approach and found no infections in the MIS cohort, while there were 2 out of 81 infections in the open cohort (2.5%). This difference, however, was not statistically significant. Regan et al found no significant difference in incidence of infection between a laparoscopic transperitoneal (1.4%) and open retroperitoneal approach (2.0%) for lumbar interbody fusion.[32]

22.5.3 Level III Evidence in Minimally Invasive Surgery

There have been many retrospective studies comparing MIS and open techniques; however, most studies available are limited by a relatively small sample size.

We identified 13 retrospective, level III studies that compared MIS and open techniques for fusion (nine TLIF only, two TLIF plus PLIF, one posterior fusion, and one ALIF) and found no statistically significant difference in infection rates between the two procedures for any study. One study was a database review,[33] while the other 12 studied single-institution patient cohorts. Seven of the 13 studies showed similar or superior infection rates in the MIS cohort versus the open cohort.[6,8,34,35,36,37,38]

Three studies have looked at the difference in infection rates between MIS and open discectomy procedures. Lee et al[39] compared techniques for single-level lumbar discectomy and found no infections in the MIS group and one infection out of 45 patients (2.2%) in the open group, a finding that was not

significant. Harrington and French[40] compared open and MIS lumbar microdiscectomy and found no infections in either group. Wu et al[41] compared microendoscopic discectomy with the open procedure and also found similar infection rates (1.0 and 1.4%, respectively).

MIS and open techniques for decompressive surgery have been compared by two retrospective studies. Shih et al[12] compared microendoscopic decompression of stenosis versus open lumbar decompression and found no infections in the MIS group and one infection out of 26 patients in the open group (3.8%), a difference that was not significant. Rahman et al[42] looked at MIS versus open lumbar laminectomy in 71 patients and found an insignificant difference in infection rates (2.6 and 6.1%, respectively).

There have been several retrospective studies that compared infection rates between MIS and open techniques for multiple procedures simultaneously. Ee et al[43] identified a cohort of TLIF, laminectomy, and discectomy patients with postoperative infections and performed a nested case–control analysis. This study used multivariate analysis to determine that open surgery is associated with a five times greater risk of postoperative infection compared to the MIS approach. Siddaraju et al[13] looked at TLIF, laminectomy, laminotomy, and discectomy procedures and also found the open approach to be significantly associated with increased risk of postoperative SSI. Finally, Smith et al[44] used the Scoliosis Research Society database, which collects morbidity and mortality data from its members, to assess rates of postoperative wound infection after all types of spine surgery (indications include scoliosis, degenerative disease, spondylolisthesis, fracture, kyphosis, and tumor). This study included the most cases out of all studies identified (108,419). They found that a minimally invasive approach was associated with a lower rate of infection for lumbar discectomy (0.4 vs. 1.1%; $p = 0.001$), TLIF (1.3 vs. 2.9%; $p = 0.005$), and all procedures combined (0.5 vs. 2.4%; $p < 0.001$).

22.6 Conclusion of Minimally Invasive Surgery

MIS techniques have been increasingly utilized in spine surgery for several reasons. Across many different spine procedures, MIS surgery has been shown to offer reduced blood loss, decreased postoperative pain, and decreased hospital length of stay when compared to open spine surgery.[3,5,6,7,8,9]

It is important to remember that SSIs are a multifactorial phenomenon, and that an open or minimally invasive approach is only one aspect that may or may not contribute to an SSI in any particular patient. Risk factors for SSIs can be either patient related, surgical, or physiologic. Patient-related risk factors include preexisting infection, low serum albumin concentration, advanced age, history of smoking, diabetes mellitus, vascular disease, and irradiation of the area of surgery. Physiologic factors include trauma, shock, blood transfusion, hypoxia, hyperglycemia, and hypothermia. In addition, surgical risk factors including prolonged length of operating time, inadequate surgical scrub, inadequate skin preparation, and contamination of surgical instruments may increase the risk of SSIs, which are independent of using an open versus minimally invasive approach.[45]

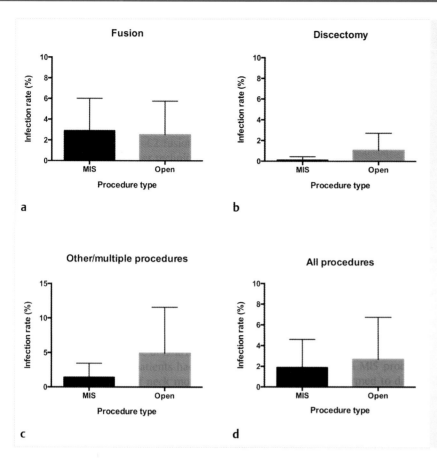

As seen in ▶ Table 22.1, ▶ Table 22.2, ▶ Table 22.3, the majority of the level I, level II, and level III evidences suggest that there is no difference in infection rates between MIS and open approaches for all types of spine surgery. However, there are several level III studies that identify the open technique as a risk factor for developing postoperative infection after spine surgery.[13,43,44] In deciding on the most appropriate surgical approach for an individual patient, the surgeon must take into account his or her training and experience level in using an open or minimally invasive approach for the patient's specific pathology. Considering that operative time and blood loss are independent risk factors for SSI, the potential benefit of using a minimally invasive approach may be negated if the surgeon is less comfortable with that approach for a given pathology.

▶ Fig. 22.7 shows that for discectomy, other/multiple procedures, and all procedures combined, the average infection rate is less for MIS compared to open. Across all studies identified, the infection rate is 1.9% for MIS and 2.5% for open. We used paired-sample t-tests to compare average infection rates between MIS and open procedures grouped by procedure type, and found no significant difference in infection rates for fusion ($p = 0.680$), discectomy ($p = 0.122$), other/multiple procedures ($p = 0.073$), and all procedures combined ($p = 0.228$).

This evidence, combined with the lower morbidity associated with the procedure, makes MIS spine surgery a very attractive approach for patients and surgeons and supports the increasing utilization of MIS over open techniques. However, despite differences in absolute infection rates between all studies, the vast majority of high-quality studies did not find any statistically significant difference in infection rates between MIS and open procedures. Furthermore, when looking at studies in aggregate, no statistically significant difference in infection rates was found between MIS and open procedures. Based on the grading guidelines presented in this book's introduction, the evidence available allows us to give a grade 2A recommendation that MIS techniques are equivalent to open spine surgery with regard to infection risk. This recommendation indicates that there is no clear benefit in terms of infection risk for either the MIS or open approach despite multiple high-quality studies. Further research is unlikely to alter this finding.

22.7 Discussion of Open Surgery

As detailed earlier, there are a number of possible benefits to using open procedures versus MIS procedures in terms of infection risk. Numerous studies have compared complications for each technique, and ▶ Table 22.1, ▶ Table 22.2, ▶ Table 22.3 show the differing infection rates for fusion, discectomy, and other/multiple procedures, respectively. Because there are many different MIS techniques, when looking at each study it is important to note the specific MIS procedure that is being compared to the corresponding open procedure. In addition, it is important to consider the size and quality of the patient sample, the pathology treated, and the study methodology when evaluating results.

22.7.1 Level I Evidence in Open Surgery

As mentioned earlier, to our knowledge there are only two randomized controlled trials available that compare outcomes after MIS and open procedures and meet the criteria for level I evidence. These studies looked at different techniques for microdiscectomy and both studies had no infections in either treatment group. Arts et al compared tubular and conventional microdiscectomy and Ryang et al compared MIS trocar microdiscectomy versus open microdiscectomy.[19,20] Arts et al[19] also found that the MIS approach resulted in less favorable results for leg pain, back pain, and recovery.

22.7.2 Level II Evidence in Open Surgery

There have been several prospective studies evaluating MIS versus open surgery. Despite claims to the contrary,[4,43] of the seven level II studies that compare MIS and open surgery for lumbar fusion, none show a statistically significant difference in infection rates.[5,18,27,28,29,30,31] In fact, a greater number of the available level II studies show an increased risk of infection in MIS compared to open surgery.

The infection risk of MIS and open approaches for discectomy have also been compared by four prospective studies, and none of these level II studies showed a significant difference. As mentioned earlier, both Franke et al[22] and Hermantin et al[24] had no infections in both the MIS and open cohorts, while Ruetten et al[23] and Teli et al found no significant difference in infection rates.[21] Interestingly, Teli et al found that overall complications were higher in the microendoscopic (MIS) group, including dural tears. Dural tear has been previously identified as a risk factor for infection after spine surgery.[46]

For other procedures, the level II evidence also demonstrates no difference in infection risk. Full-endoscopic posterior cervical foraminotomy has similar infection risk as conventional microsurgical anterior decompression and fusion,[26] and full-endoscopic transforaminal or interlaminar decompression compared with the traditional microsurgical approach also yielded no difference in infection risk.[25] The laparoscopic transperitoneal approach and the open retroperitoneal approach for lumbar interbody fusion also had similar infection rates.[32]

22.7.3 Level III Evidence in Open Surgery

There is much level III evidence for similar infection rates between MIS and open surgery; however, most of the evidences come from studies that are significantly limited by sample size or other methodological concerns.

Thirteen retrospective, level III studies compared MIS to open techniques for lumbar fusion and found no statistically significant difference in infection rates between the two procedures for any study. Only two studies found a greater percentage of infections in the open group versus MIS group,[34,35] while six studies showed a greater percentage of infections in the MIS group compared to open (Lau et al[47] also found a significantly greater overall complication rate for MIS).[7,33,47,48,49,50] The remaining five studies had identical infection rates between MIS and open surgery. Four of these studies had zero infections in either group[6,8,36,37] and one study (Seng et al)[38] had the same rate of infections (2.5%) in both groups, due to one iliac crest donor-site infection in each group.

The level III evidence for infection rates after discectomy echoes the same results. Three retrospective studies compared various techniques for discectomy and found no difference in infection rates between MIS and open techniques.[39,40,41] Similar infection rates were also reported for decompressive surgery.[12,42]

The only evidence for increased infection risk is from three level III studies that have compared infection rates for multiple procedures; however, there are problems with each study. Ee et al[43] used multivariate analysis to determine that open surgery is associated with a five times greater risk of postoperative infection compared to the MIS approach. However, this odds ratio was borderline significant (p-value of 0.048), and as the authors admit, even one more infection in either group could resulted in findings that were not statistically significant. Siddaraju et al[13] did not use the MIS approach as a variable in their multivariate analysis (only having tested the association of MIS and infection risk in univariate analysis), leaving its effect on infection risk open to the effects of possible confounding variables. Smith et al[44] used the Scoliosis Research Society database to conclude that infection rates were higher with an open approach; however, this database is not validated and relies on self-reported complication rates submitted by each member surgeon, which increases the chance for selection bias.

22.8 Conclusion of Open Surgery

Open techniques have been the mainstay of spine surgery since they were developed. While MIS procedures have seen increasing use in recent years, it is important to assess the evidence behind using these procedures. Newer techniques do not necessarily mean that they have improved outcomes, especially in the case of postoperative complications such as infection.

In one of the largest randomized controlled trials comparing minimally invasive discectomy with open discectomy, no improvements in outcomes were observed in those treated with minimally invasive techniques as opposed to open techniques, with the clinical results favoring open surgery over the minimally invasive approach.[19]

Looking at every available study (▶ Table 22.1, ▶ Table 22.2, ▶ Table 22.3) comparing the two types of procedures, there is not a clear difference in infection rates after MIS and open spine surgery. While a few flawed level III studies have described decreased infection rates after MIS, the vast majority of level I, II, and III studies have found no difference in infection rates after each type of procedure. It is interesting to note that we did find a higher absolute infection rate for MIS compared to open for fusion procedures (▶ Fig. 22.7a). However, as mentioned in section "Conclusion (Minimally Invasive Spine Surgery)," we found no significant difference in overall infection rates for fusion procedures ($p = 0.680$), discectomy procedures ($p = 0.122$), other/multiple procedures ($p = 0.073$), and all procedures ($p = 0.228$).

These data provide a grade 2A recommendation that MIS and open surgery are equivalent in terms of infection risk. As noted in section "Conclusion (Minimally Invasive Spine Surgery)," this recommendation is based on the findings from multiple high-quality studies, and further research is unlikely to alter this recommendation.

The procedures discussed earlier, including microdiscectomy, lumbar decompression, and even interbody fusion, have been performed with success for decades. Currently, the techniques used to perform these procedures have improved, and the rate of complications has improved. Minimally invasive techniques for lumbar decompression and fusion have evolved only over the past 10 to 15 years, and are a natural progression of reduced intraoperative exposure. As can be seen earlier, minimally invasive techniques have achieved equivalent results to open techniques that have been performed with good results over a much longer period of time. However, the decision of which surgical technique to use must take into account several factors. The surgeon must decide whether open or minimally invasive techniques will allow adequate approach to the compressive pathology, and also decide which technique he or she is most comfortable in using to achieve the surgical goals. This decision is highly surgeon dependent, as no single approach may be appropriate for every type of surgical disease states.

22.9 Editors' Commentary

22.9.1 Minimally Invasive Surgery

Infection as a complication of surgery is one of the most clear-cut demonstrations of the advantage of MIS technique over open surgery. To be blunt, MIS technique has all but eliminated infection as a complication of surgery. This is due to several factors: (1) dilation rather than dissection of soft tissues eliminates the creation of dead space; (2) dilation rather than dissection of soft tissues maintains living, viable soft tissue in the surgical bed; (3) tubular retraction minimizes "air-flow" deep in the wound; (4) once the tubular retractor is placed, no instruments *ever* touch the edges of the wound; and (5) fingers never enter the wound. As a result of these factors, I have not had a deep wound infection using MIS technique in the past 14 years, and I have had only one in the past 20 years. Even superficial infections in compromised patients (e.g., obese, diabetics) are extremely rare. These results alone are so compelling that I believe they argue strongly for the adoption of MIS technique for most spinal surgery.

22.9.2 Open Surgery

Infection is a relatively rare complication of spinal surgery and one that is difficult to study in a manner that can detect differences unless very large groups of patients are studied. The best available evidence suggests that infection rates are not improved by MIS techniques. From previous studies that have identified risk factors associated with infection, there is little to suggest that infection rates will be substantially different in MIS surgery versus open surgery: the length of the skin incision is less important than the protection of the soft-tissue envelope, periodic release of retractors, the use of instrumentation which allows biofilm to form, adherence to proper prophylactic protocols, and patient-related factors. Strategies to prevent infection will be similarly effective in patients undergoing both MIS and open surgery. With the introduction of adjunctive medicinal methods to minimize postsurgical infection such as the addition of vancomycin powder, differences in infection rates between open and MIS procedures will most likely be indistinguishable.

References

[1] Kane J, Kay A, Maltenfort M, et al. Complication rates of minimally invasive spine surgery compared to open surgery: a systematic literature review. Seminars in Spine Surgery. 2013; 25(3):191–199

[2] Mangram AJ, Horan TC, Pearson ML, Silver LC, Jarvis WR, Centers for Disease Control and Prevention (CDC) Hospital Infection Control Practices Advisory Committee. Guideline for prevention of surgical site infection, 1999. Am J Infect Control. 1999; 27(2):97–132, quiz 133–134, discussion 96

[3] Rantanen J, Hurme M, Falck B, et al. The lumbar multifidus muscle five years after surgery for a lumbar intervertebral disc herniation. Spine. 1993; 18(5):568–574

[4] O'Toole JE, Eichholz KM, Fessler RG. Surgical site infection rates after minimally invasive spinal surgery. J Neurosurg Spine. 2009; 11(4):471–476

[5] Peng CW, Yue WM, Poh SY, Yeo W, Tan SB. Clinical and radiological outcomes of minimally invasive versus open transforaminal lumbar interbody fusion. Spine. 2009; 34(13):1385–1389

[6] Dhall SS, Wang MY, Mummaneni PV. Clinical and radiographic comparison of mini-open transforaminal lumbar interbody fusion with open transforaminal lumbar interbody fusion in 42 patients with long-term follow-up. J Neurosurg Spine. 2008; 9(6):560–565

[7] Villavicencio AT, Burneikiene S, Bulsara KR, Thramann JJ. Perioperative complications in transforaminal lumbar interbody fusion versus anterior-posterior reconstruction for lumbar disc degeneration and instability. J Spinal Disord Tech. 2006; 19(2):92–97

[8] Schizas C, Tzinieris N, Tsiridis E, Kosmopoulos V. Minimally invasive versus open transforaminal lumbar interbody fusion: evaluating initial experience. Int Orthop. 2009; 33(6):1683–1688

[9] Pull ter Gunne AF, Cohen DB. Incidence, prevalence, and analysis of risk factors for surgical site infection following adult spinal surgery. Spine. 2009; 34(13):1422–1428

[10] McLoughlin GS, Fourney DR. The learning curve of minimally-invasive lumbar microdiscectomy. Can J Neurol Sci. 2008; 35(1):75–78

[11] Silva PS, Pereira P, Monteiro P, Silva PA, Vaz R. Learning curve and complications of minimally invasive transforaminal lumbar interbody fusion. Neurosurg Focus. 2013; 35(2):E7

[12] Shih P, Wong AP, Smith TR, Lee AI, Fessler RG. Complications of open compared to minimally invasive lumbar spine decompression. J Clin Neurosci. 2011; 18(10):1360–1364

[13] Siddaraju VSM, Yeo W, Yap V, et al. Comparison of surgical site infections and risk factors for minimally invasive versus open spinal surgery. Society for Minimally Invasive Spinal Surgery 2011 Annual Conference. Las Vegas, NV; October 21–23, 2011

[14] Bible JE, O'Neill KR, Crosby CG, Schoenecker JG, McGirt MJ, Devin CJ. Microscope sterility during spine surgery. Spine. 2012; 37(7):623–627

[15] Biswas D, Bible JE, Whang PG, Simpson AK, Grauer JN. Sterility of C-arm fluoroscopy during spinal surgery. Spine. 2008; 33(17):1913–1917

[16] Li CH, Yew AY, Kimball JA, McBride DQ, Wang JC, Lu DC. Comparison of operating field sterility in open versus minimally invasive microdiscectomies of the lumbar spine. Surg Neurol Int. 2013; 4 Suppl 5:S295–S298

[17] Bronsard N, Boli T, Challali M, et al. Comparison between percutaneous and traditional fixation of lumbar spine fracture: intraoperative radiation exposure levels and outcomes. Orthop Traumatol Surg Res. 2013; 99(2):162–168

[18] Wang J, Zhou Y, Zhang ZF, Li CQ, Zheng WJ, Liu J. Comparison of one-level minimally invasive and open transforaminal lumbar interbody fusion in degenerative and isthmic spondylolisthesis grades 1 and 2. Eur Spine J. 2010; 19(10):1780–1784

[19] Arts MP, Brand R, van den Akker ME, Koes BW, Bartels RH, Peul WC, Leiden-The Hague Spine Intervention Prognostic Study Group (SIPS). Tubular diskectomy vs conventional microdiskectomy for sciatica: a randomized controlled trial. JAMA. 2009; 302(2):149–158

[20] Ryang YM, Oertel MF, Mayfrank L, Gilsbach JM, Rohde V. Standard open microdiscectomy versus minimal access trocar microdiscectomy: results of a prospective randomized study. Neurosurgery. 2008; 62(1):174–181, discussion 181–182

[21] Teli M, Lovi A, Brayda-Bruno M, et al. Higher risk of dural tears and recurrent herniation with lumbar micro-endoscopic discectomy. Eur Spine J. 2010; 19(3):443–450

[22] Franke J, Greiner-Perth R, Boehm H, et al. Comparison of a minimally invasive procedure versus standard microscopic discotomy: a prospective randomised controlled clinical trial. Eur Spine J. 2009; 18(7):992–1000

[23] Ruetten S, Komp M, Merk H, Godolias G. Full-endoscopic interlaminar and transforaminal lumbar discectomy versus conventional microsurgical technique: a prospective, randomized, controlled study. Spine. 2008; 33(9): 931–939

[24] Hermantin FU, Peters T, Quartararo L, Kambin P. A prospective, randomized study comparing the results of open discectomy with those of video-assisted arthroscopic microdiscectomy. J Bone Joint Surg Am. 1999; 81(7):958–965

[25] Ruetten S, Komp M, Merk H, Godolias G. Surgical treatment for lumbar lateral recess stenosis with the full-endoscopic interlaminar approach versus conventional microsurgical technique: a prospective, randomized, controlled study. J Neurosurg Spine. 2009; 10(5):476–485

[26] Ruetten S, Komp M, Merk H, Godolias G. Full-endoscopic cervical posterior foraminotomy for the operation of lateral disc herniations using 5.9-mm endoscopes: a prospective, randomized, controlled study. Spine. 2008; 33(9): 940–948

[27] Wang J, Zhou Y, Feng Zhang Z, Qing Li C, Jie Zheng W, Liu J. Comparison of clinical outcome in overweight or obese patients after minimally invasive versus open transforaminal lumbar interbody fusion. J Spinal Disord Tech. 2014; 27(4):202–206

[28] Wang J, Zhou Y, Zhang ZF, Li CQ, Zheng WJ, Liu J. Minimally invasive or open transforaminal lumbar interbody fusion as revision surgery for patients previously treated by open discectomy and decompression of the lumbar spine. Eur Spine J. 2011; 20(4):623–628

[29] Shunwu F, Xing Z, Fengdong Z, Xiangqian F. Minimally invasive transforaminal lumbar interbody fusion for the treatment of degenerative lumbar diseases. Spine. 2010; 35(17):1615–1620

[30] Ghahreman A, Ferch RD, Rao PJ, Bogduk N. Minimal access versus open posterior lumbar interbody fusion in the treatment of spondylolisthesis. Neurosurgery. 2010; 66(2):296–304, discussion 304

[31] Park Y, Ha JW. Comparison of one-level posterior lumbar interbody fusion performed with a minimally invasive approach or a traditional open approach. Spine. 2007; 32(5):537–543

[32] Regan JJ, Yuan H, McAfee PC. Laparoscopic fusion of the lumbar spine: minimally invasive spine surgery. A prospective multicenter study evaluating open and laparoscopic lumbar fusion. Spine. 1999; 24(4):402–411

[33] McGirt MJ, Parker SL, Lerner J, Engelhart L, Knight T, Wang MY. Comparative analysis of perioperative surgical site infection after minimally invasive versus open posterior/transforaminal lumbar interbody fusion: analysis of hospital billing and discharge data from 5170 patients. J Neurosurg Spine. 2011; 14(6):771–778

[34] Isaacs RE, Podichetty VK, Santiago P, et al. Minimally invasive microendoscopy-assisted transforaminal lumbar interbody fusion with instrumentation. J Neurosurg Spine. 2005; 3(2):98–105

[35] Villavicencio AT, Burneikiene S, Nelson EL, Bulsara KR, Favors M, Thramann J. Safety of transforaminal lumbar interbody fusion and intervertebral recombinant human bone morphogenetic protein-2. J Neurosurg Spine. 2005; 3(6):436–443

[36] Adogwa O, Parker SL, Bydon A, Cheng J, McGirt MJ. Comparative effectiveness of minimally invasive versus open transforaminal lumbar interbody fusion: 2-year assessment of narcotic use, return to work, disability, and quality of life. J Spinal Disord Tech. 2011; 24(8):479–484

[37] Scheufler KM, Dohmen H, Vougioukas VI. Percutaneous transforaminal lumbar interbody fusion for the treatment of degenerative lumbar instability. Neurosurgery. 2007; 60(4) Suppl 2:203–212, discussion 212–213

[38] Seng C, Siddiqui MA, Wong KP, et al. Five-year outcomes of minimally invasive versus open transforaminal lumbar interbody fusion: a matched-pair comparison study. Spine. 2013; 38(23):2049–2055

[39] Lee P, Liu JC, Fessler RG. Perioperative results following open and minimally invasive single-level lumbar discectomy. J Clin Neurosci. 2011; 18(12):1667–1670

[40] Harrington JF, French P. Open versus minimally invasive lumbar microdiscectomy: comparison of operative times, length of hospital stay, narcotic use and complications. Minim Invasive Neurosurg. 2008; 51(1):30–35

[41] Wu X, Zhuang S, Mao Z, Chen H. Microendoscopic discectomy for lumbar disc herniation: surgical technique and outcome in 873 consecutive cases. Spine. 2006; 31(23):2689–2694

[42] Rahman M, Summers LE, Richter B, Mimran RI, Jacob RP. Comparison of techniques for decompressive lumbar laminectomy: the minimally invasive versus the "classic" open approach. Minim Invasive Neurosurg. 2008; 51(2): 100–105

[43] Ee WW, Lau WL, Yeo W, Von Bing Y, Yue WM. Does minimally invasive surgery have a lower risk of surgical site infections compared with open spinal surgery? Clin Orthop Relat Res. 2014; 472(6):1718–1724

[44] Smith JS, Shaffrey CI, Sansur CA, et al. Scoliosis Research Society Morbidity and Mortality Committee. Rates of infection after spine surgery based on 108,419 procedures: a report from the Scoliosis Research Society Morbidity and Mortality Committee. Spine. 2011; 36(7):556–563

[45] Cheadle WG. Risk factors for surgical site infection. Surg Infect (Larchmt). 2006; 7 Suppl 1:S7–S11

[46] Koutsoumbelis S, Hughes AP, Girardi FP, et al. Risk factors for postoperative infection following posterior lumbar instrumented arthrodesis. J Bone Joint Surg Am. 2011; 93(17):1627–1633

[47] Lau D, Lee JG, Han SJ, Lu DC, Chou D. Complications and perioperative factors associated with learning the technique of minimally invasive transforaminal lumbar interbody fusion (TLIF). J Clin Neurosci. 2011; 18(5):624–627

[48] Kepler CK, Yu AL, Gruskay JA, et al. Comparison of open and minimally invasive techniques for posterior lumbar instrumentation and fusion after open anterior lumbar interbody fusion. Spine J. 2013; 13(5):489–497

[49] Bagan B, Patel N, Deutsch H, et al. Perioperative complications of minimally invasive surgery (MIS): comparison of MIS and open interbody fusion techniques. Surg Technol Int. 2008; 17:281–286

[50] Saraph V, Lerch C, Walochnik N, Bach CM, Krismer M, Wimmer C. Comparison of conventional versus minimally invasive extraperitoneal approach for anterior lumbar interbody fusion. Eur Spine J. 2004; 13(5):425–431

23 Cost: Which Costs More, Open or Minimally Invasive Surgery?

MIS: Matthew J. McGirt
Open: Scott L. Parker

23.1 Introduction

The current growth in health care cost is unsustainable. Current health care costs are nearly 18% of the U.S. gross domestic product (GDP), with the cost of surgical care alone comprising approximately 7% of GDP.[1] Without reform, health care costs are expected to surpass half of the U.S. GDP within the next few decades. As a result, cost–utility and other forms of value analyses are becoming central aspects of health care reform initiatives. At the heart of this evidence-driven reform process is safety, effectiveness, and cost of care, each of which affects the value of healthcare. To improve the efficiency and reduce the cost of health care delivery, value-based purchasing has emerged as a payment methodology that rewards quality of care. In value-based purchasing, providers are held accountable for both the quality and the cost of the health care services they provide. As we move forward, it will become standard that more costly medical treatments are required to prove their value by demonstrating a health benefit that is greater than its added cost. To achieve a sustainable health care system, reform strategies ranging from bundled payments to accountable care organizations aim to eliminate or minimize the purchasing of low value or cost-ineffective care.

When interpreting cost and value, it is imperative to consider the perspective of the stakeholder or the decision maker. In a complex medical market, the perspective will define the health care consumer and the provider. Cost to a payer may represent profit to a hospital system. Added cost to a hospital may not translate to added cost to the payer or health care system, but merely a decreased profit to the hospital. The preferred perspective for U.S. health care policy remains the societal perspective. From the societal perspective, both direct costs (all health care expenditures) and indirect costs (occupational productivity losses of patient and caregivers) are considered. From the hospital perspective, only the hospital's direct costs are concerned, which represent the expenditures of the hospital to deliver care rather than their billing or payment from the payer.

23.2 Cost-Related Advantages of Minimally Invasive Technique

Minimally invasive approaches for spine surgery have many theoretical cost advantages. The concept that the greatest variability in cost lies within operating room expenses and implant costs is a common misunderstanding. Growing evidence suggests that by far the greatest variability in surgical cost lies within the post–acute care episode, in the immediate days to weeks following hospital discharge after surgery.[2,3,4,5,6,7] It is during this post–acute care episode that the potential value of minimally invasive technologies is greatest. Length of hospital stay, surgical complication, hospital readmission, acute need for reoperation (infection, hematoma, etc.), and need for inpatient rehab or skilled nursing care are significant factors that can greatly reduce cost in the post–acute care episode. Any technology or surgical approach which can reduce the prevalence of any of these events will have a dramatic effect on direct health care cost. Much of these costs are currently the burden of third-party payers; however, with emerging health care payment models, these risks and cost variables are increasingly shifting to the hospital. With more vertical alignment of hospitals and payers in the near future, the theoretical cost benefits of minimally invasive surgery will benefit both stakeholders: hospital and payer. Finally, lost occupational productivity is a significant variable in cost which is largely the burden of health care purchasers, employers, and policymakers. Minimally invasive approaches theoretically allow for a quicker recovery during the post–acute care episode, which may allow for accelerated return to work and reduced indirect costs. The minimally invasive surgery (MIS) value question, which only evidence can answer, is whether the greater upfront operating room costs of MIS are offset by downstream cost reduction benefits. The following section will summarize the evidence to date to help answer this question.

23.3 Cost-Related Advantages of Open Technique

The open techniques for spine surgery are well known to the vast majority of practicing spine surgeons. These techniques have a long track record and provide an effective tool for the treatment of a variety of spinal disorders. An advantage of the open technique is avoidance of the steep learning curve needed to master the MIS approaches, as there is an increased risk for complications during these initial cases. This is important given surgical complications can be a primary driver of increased health care resource utilization in the postoperative period. Finally, due to the lack of anatomic landmarks necessary for placing pedicle screws, the use of MIS technology necessitates a significant amount of radiation exposure via fluoroscopy for both the patient and the surgical team. The use of open surgical techniques and anatomic landmarks for spinal instrumentation has been shown to result in a high success rate of accurately placed pedicle screws.[8]

23.4 Case Illustration

The following case illustration is a representative population-based example of outcomes and associated costs expected

Table 23.1 Case illustration estimates for comparable patients undergoing MIS versus open-TLIF

Variable	MIS-TLIF	Open-TLIF	Statistically significant
Length of hospitalization	3 d	4 d	Yes
In-hospitalization costs	$23,000	$25,000	Yes
• Implants/instruments	$17,000	$15,000	
• Operating room services	$2,000	$3,000	
• Surgical supplies	$1,000	$2,000	
• Room/Board	$1,000	$2,000	
Meds, Labs, PT/OT, Misc	$2,000	$3,000	
Time to narcotic independence	3 wk	7 wk	Yes
Time to return to work	7 wk	11 wk	Yes
CSF leak	7	5	No
Surgical site infections	1	4	Yes
Total direct costs	$30,000	$34,000	No
• In-hospitalization costs	$23,000	$25,000	
• Health care visits	$2,000	$2,500	
• Diagnostic imaging	$1,500	$1,500	
• Medications	$3,500	$5,000	
Total indirect costs	$10,000	$18,000	Yes
Total health care costs	$40,000	$52,000	Yes

Abbreviations: CSF, cerebrospinal fluid; Labs, laboratories; Meds, medications; Misc, miscellaneous; MIS-TLIF, minimally invasive surgery-transforaminal lumbar interbody fusion; PT/OT, physical therapy/occupational therapy.

following MIS versus open transforaminal lumbar interbody fusion (TLIF). The numbers used in this case illustration are based on estimations of the published literature to date.

23.5 Minimally Invasive Surgery

In Practice A, 100 patients undergo MIS-TLIF (▶ Table 23.1). The mean length of postoperative hospital stay was 3 days. The mean total in-hospitalization cost for these patients was $23,000. It is important to note that each 1-day reduction in length of stay results in a direct cost savings of $1,500. The mean length of time to narcotic independence was 3 weeks and the mean time to return to work was 7 weeks (▶ Fig. 23.1). By 3 months postoperatively, cerebrospinal fluid leak occurred in seven patients. One patient experienced a surgical site infection requiring operative intervention and long-term antibiotics. Patient-reported pain, disability, and quality of life significantly improved from baseline status (▶ Fig. 23.2).

Two years postoperatively, significant improvement in patient-reported outcomes was maintained. For this patient population, mean total direct costs were $30,000 (including costs of surgery, hospitalization, health care visits, diagnostic imaging, and medications). Total indirect cost (comprising time of missed work and caregiver hours) was $10,000. Consequently, the total health care cost (direct and indirect) associated with MIS-TLIF at 2 years was $40,000.

23.6 Open Surgery

In Practice B, 100 patients with similar demographic, comorbid, and socioeconomic backgrounds to those in Practice A undergo open-TLIF, ▶ Table 23.1. The mean length of postoperative hospital stay was 4 days. The mean total in-hospitalization cost for these patients was $25,000. The mean length of time to narcotic independence was 9 weeks and the mean time to return to work was 11 weeks (▶ Fig. 23.1). By 3 months postoperatively, cerebrospinal fluid leak occurred in 5 patients. Four patients experienced a surgical site infection requiring operative intervention and long-term antibiotics. Patient-reported pain, disability, and quality of life significantly improved from baseline status (▶ Fig. 23.2).

Two years postoperatively, the significant improvement in patient-reported outcomes was maintained. For this patient population, mean total direct costs were $34,000 (including costs of surgery, hospitalization, health care visits, diagnostic imaging, and medications). Total indirect cost (comprising time of missed work and caregiver hours) was $18,000. Consequently, the total health care cost (direct and indirect) associated with open-TLIF at 2 years was $52,000.

23.7 Discussion of Minimally Invasive Surgery
23.7.1 Level I Evidence in Minimally Invasive Surgery

There are currently no level I studies available that assess cost for MIS versus open spine surgery.

23.7.2 Level II Evidence in Minimally Invasive Surgery

While there have recently been several prospective cohort studies comparing minimally invasive versus open spine surgery reported in the literature, only a few studies evaluate the health care resource utilization and costs associated with these procedures.

The largest cost comparison study to date compared 50 consecutive MIS and 50 consecutive open-TLIF patients at a single institution.[7] The authors reported similar improvement in patient-reported outcome metrics for the two techniques at both short-term (3-month) and long-term (24-month) follow-ups. MIS versus open-TLIF was associated with a 1-day decrease in hospital stay which correlated into a mean hospital cost reduction of $1,758 per case. In this study, measures of surgical quality (morbidity, readmission, and reoperation) and 2-year resource use were similar between the two cohorts, resulting in similar overall direct health care costs for MIS and open-TLIF: $27,621 ± 6,107 versus $28,442 ± 6,005; $p = 0.50$. However, for patients employed preoperatively, the mean time to return to work was accelerated in patients undergoing MIS-TLIF, resulting in a reduction of the indirect cost by almost half for MIS versus open-TLIF: $10,942 ± 9,102 versus $19,416 ± 22,727; $p = 0.06$. This led to significantly reduced total (direct + indirect) cost for MIS versus open-TLIF: $38,563 ± 10,594 versus $47,858 ±

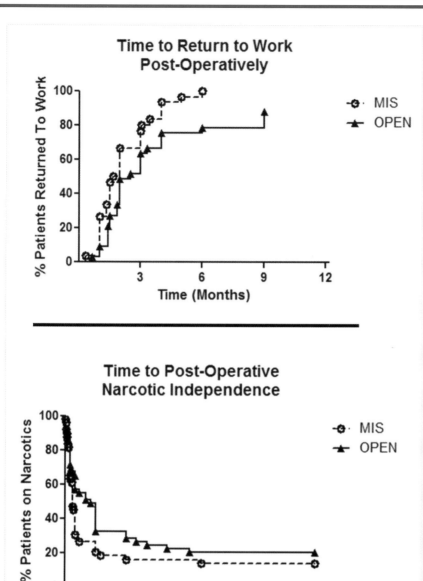

Fig. 23.1 Case illustration example. Kaplan–Meier graph demonstrating reduced time to narcotic independence and return to work for patients undergoing MIS versus open-TLIF.

20,148; $p = 0.03$. It is important to appreciate the various perspectives from which cost saving was demonstrated in this study. Due to the reduction in length of stay, MIS surgery was able to provide cost savings from the hospital perspective. Because surgical quality and resource utilization were similar for each cohort, from the payer perspective (direct cost only), there was no difference in cost for MIS versus open-TLIF. Finally, because of the reduced indirect cost associated with an accelerated return to work after MIS-TLIF, MIS surgery also represented a cost saving technology from the societal perspective (total cost, direct + indirect).

In another prospective comparison study, Pelton et al analyzed perioperative direct hospital costs following MIS versus open-TLIF in both worker's compensation and nonworker's compensation cohorts.[9] The results were similar for both worker's compensation and nonworker's compensation cohorts. MIS-TLIF was associated with reduction in hospital cost of

$5,802 ($p = 0.015$) in the worker's compensation cohort and $3,569 ($p = 0.0001$) in the nonworker's compensation cohort. The authors attribute the reduction in hospital cost associated with the use of MIS technique to lowered resource utilization and improved perioperative outcome measures such as early ambulation and reduced length of stay.

23.7.3 Level III and IV Evidence in Minimally Invasive Surgery

In a retrospective cohort comparison study, Lucio et al examined the differences in perioperative hospital costs associated with MIS and open lumbar fusion procedures.[10] For the purposes of this study, perioperative costs were divided into four categories: (1) index surgical procedure and initial hospital stay; (2) blood transfusions; (3) reoperations; and (4) residual

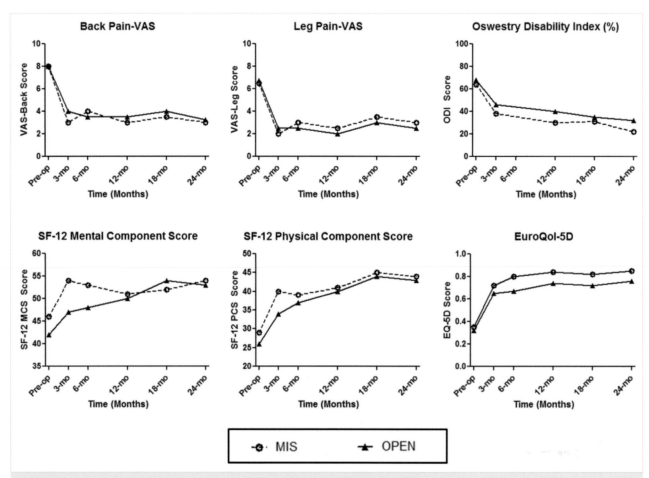

Fig. 23.2 Case illustration example. Patient-reported pain, disability, and quality of life improved similarly for patients undergoing MIS versus open-TLIF.

events (emergency room visits, hospital readmissions [excluding reoperations], postoperative rehabilitation, and additional diagnostics). The authors demonstrated that MIS fusion was associated with a mean total hospital cost savings of $2,825 per patient ($p = 0.03$), which represented a 10.4% reduction in total hospital cost. Further subanalysis revealed that although the MIS implant/instrumentation costs exceeded those of the open cohort by $3,810 (27% increase), this cost was more than offset in the MIS cohort with savings in operating room services ($2,756, 56% decrease), surgical supplies ($955, 45% decrease), and room/board ($788, 52% decrease). Perhaps most importantly, the authors revealed that perioperative residual events represented the most consequential cost category after the original procedure. In this series, there were significantly fewer residual events in the MIS versus open cohort ($p = 0.02$). The total costs for residual events in the MIS and open cohorts were $34,677 and $134,652, respectively, which represented cost savings of $99,974 overall and $2,131 (58.6% decrease) per patient experiencing a residual event for MIS versus open lumbar fusion.

In another retrospective analysis, Cahill et al analyzed hospital charges associated with tubular versus open microdiscectomies in a consecutive series of patients.[11] The authors noted that there was no difference in operative times or postoperative complications between the two groups. However, patients in the tubular cohort had a significantly shorter postoperative length of stay compared to the open cohort: 0.93 versus 1.53 days; $p = 0.01$. With regard to cost, total hospital charges in the tubular group were on average $5,453 less than in the open group ($p = 0.02$). In the open cohort, the mean total charge was $27,811 versus $22,358 for the tubular cohort. Further subanalysis of the data revealed that operating room charges were similar for the two groups, and the cost reduction in the tubular cohort was generated from lower charges for laboratory studies, medications, and therapy. Based on these data, the authors concluded that the hospital cost savings were primarily attributable to the reduced length of stay in the tubular cohort which resulted in less in-patient resource utilization.

In a similar analysis, Wang et al retrospectively reviewed hospital charges for one- and two-level MIS and open posterior lumbar interbody fusions.[12] The authors found that MIS fusion was associated with a hospital cost savings for both one- and two-level fusions. For single-level surgery, MIS fusion was associated with an average hospital charge of $70,159 compared with $78,444 for open fusion ($p = 0.03$). For two-level surgery, the mean charges were $87,454 for MIS fusion versus $108,843 for open fusion ($p = 0.07$). The reduction in hospital charges associated with MIS fusion in this study was secondary to decreases in length of stay, blood transfusions, laboratory tests, postoperative imaging, and physical therapy sessions.

Importantly, the authors noted that this study likely underestimates the cost differences between MIS and open surgery, given that they did not account for the additional cost of discharge to inpatient rehabilitation or skilled nursing facility, which was more common following open fusion.

Rampersaud et al performed a cost–utility analysis comparing minimally invasive fusion with conventional open fusion for lumbar spondylolisthesis.[7] Of note, there were significantly fewer complications in the MIS group (11%) than in the open cohort (29%; $p = 0.02$), and the mean length of stay postoperatively was 2.3 days shorter for the MIS cohort ($p = 0.01$). Both techniques resulted in similar significant improvements in disability and health utility at 1 year postoperatively; however, MIS technique was associated with a 28% reduction in total 1-year direct cost compared to conventional open technique (Can$14,183 vs. 18,633; $p = 0.0009$).

Two studies in the literature have used an administrative database to assess direct hospital costs for MIS versus open lumbar interbody fusion.[13,14] McGirt et al demonstrated that minimally invasive technique was associated with a decreased incidence of perioperative surgical site infection, which resulted in a direct cost savings of $38,400 per 100 procedures when used in two-level fusion.[13] There was no significant difference in the incidence of surgical site infection between the MIS and open cohorts for one-level fusion procedures. Similarly, Wang et al demonstrated that total acute hospitalization costs were similar for one-level MIS and open posterior lumbar interbody fusion. With regard to two-level fusion, minimally invasive technique was associated with an acute hospitalization cost savings of $2,106 per patient ($p = 0.002$). Cost savings were attributable primarily to lower room and board costs, operating room costs, pharmacy use, and laboratory tests in the MIS cohort.

In a retrospective cohort comparison study, Smith et al compared perioperative charges and outcome between open and mini-open (lateral, retroperitoneal, transpsoas) approaches for anterior lumbar discectomy and fusion.[15] The authors found that mean total charges for patients who underwent one-level mini-open procedures were decreased by 9.9% compared to the open cohort ($91,995 vs. $102,146, $p = 0.049$). For patients undergoing two-level procedures, the mini-open approach was associated with a 13.6% decrease in charges ($124,540 vs. $144,183, $p = 0.005$). These cost savings were seen in the setting of similar improvement in functional outcomes in each cohort, leading the authors to conclude that the mini-open approach for anterior lumbar discectomy and fusion provides cost savings with similar long-term outcomes to the traditional open approach.

In a systematic review of the literature to assess the effect of minimally invasive technique on return to work and narcotic use following posterior interbody fusion, Parker et al[6] demonstrated that the literature to date suggests that MIS technique may be associated with an accelerated time to narcotic independence and return to work. For studies assessing U.S. patients, a mean return to work of 8.0 weeks was observed in the MIS cohort versus 17.1 weeks in the open cohorts. Assuming average hourly compensation for U.S. workers, MIS fusion was associated with an indirect cost savings of $10,147 per patient.

In a literature review and cost analysis, Parker et al[16] demonstrated that the published literature suggests that MIS-TLIF is associated with a reduction in postoperative infection compared with open-TLIF. The cumulative published incidence of

surgical site infection was significantly lower for MIS (0.6%) versus open-TLIF (4.0%; $p = 0.0005$). Based on cost estimations from their institution, the authors demonstrated that this 3.4% decrease in surgical site infection would result in a direct cost savings of $98,974 per 100 MIS-TLIF procedures performed.

23.8 Conclusion of Minimally Invasive

While there can be a steep learning curve associated with MIS techniques, these techniques may be associated with reduced surgical costs while maintaining at least equivalent outcomes compared to open surgical techniques for spine surgery. While there is no Level-I evidence to date, a multitude of Level II and Level III studies have demonstrated comparable clinical and radiographic outcomes with reduced length of hospital stay, utilization of perioperative health care resources, time to return to work, and health care costs (both direct and indirect). It is important to note that these cost savings occur only in a setting of high-quality care. If, in an individual surgeon's hands, MIS techniques result in reduced quality of care (increased complications), the cost savings demonstrated in the literature will not be reproducible. In fact, surgical procedures performed with low quality regardless of MIS versus open technique will inevitably result in less patient improvement and greater cost of care.

When interpreting health care costs and the value of care, it is imperative to consider the perspective of the stakeholder or decision maker. The various perspectives include that of the hospital, payer, employer, and society. While the preferred perspective for U.S. health care policy remains the societal perspective, the other perspectives remain important to various other stakeholders in a complex medical market. Based on the literature presented earlier, MIS technique for lumbar spinal fusion may result in cost savings from the hospital perspective (hospital cost), employer perspective (indirect cost), and societal perspective (total cost, direct + indirect). MIS and open technologies appear cost equivalent from the payer perspective (direct cost).

In the literature to date, there is consistent evidence that suggests MIS technique can result in cost savings for lumbar fusion, while the evidence remains inconclusive for lumbar decompression and discectomy procedures. Cost-effectiveness data for minimally invasive approaches to tumor, trauma, and deformity surgeries are lacking.

23.9 Discussion of Open Surgery

23.9.1 Level I Evidence in Open Surgery

There are currently no level I studies available that assess cost for MIS versus open spine surgery.

23.9.2 Level II Evidence in Open Surgery

In a prospective comparison study, Parker et al[17] compared MIS versus open hemilaminectomy for patients with degenerative lumbar spinal stenosis. This analysis revealed that improvement in pain, disability, and quality of life was similar for each surgical technique. Additionally, both direct and indirect costs were similar between the two surgical techniques, leading the authors to conclude that MIS and open hemilaminectomy represent cost-equivalent technology for patients with lumbar stenosis.

23.9.3 Level III and IV Evidence in Open Surgery

There are no Level III or IV studies in the literature that suggest a cost advantage with open surgical technique versus minimally invasive technique when utilized in spine surgery.

23.10 Conclusion of Open Surgery

While a vast majority of studies in the literature to date suggest that the MIS technique is associated with equivalent effectiveness and reduced cost compared to the traditional open technique, it is important to note that there is a significant learning curve associated with mastering minimally invasive spinal surgical skills, especially in the setting of spinal fusion. There may be an inherent bias in the literature with regard to the outcomes of MIS technology, given that published results are often a by-product of experienced surgeons who are extremely proficient with minimally invasive techniques. As such, the clinical outcomes and resultant cost savings reported in the literature may not be reproducible in the hands of surgeons with less experience in minimally invasive techniques.

23.11 Editors' Commentary

23.11.1 Minimally Invasive Surgery

Cost-effectiveness must be viewed on a scale determined by the magnitude of the surgery performed. If one repeatedly analyzes the cost of the smallest operation done either open or MIS, and then generalizes that comparison to all surgeries, the conclusion will be that there is minimal difference in cost between MIS and open technique. After all, most patients with routine discectomy are discharged on the day of surgery whether performed using open or MIS technique. This has been the technique of most publications arguing for cost equivalence between open and MIS surgery. However, most recent data comparing cost of fusions have demonstrated that MIS technique is more cost-effective than open fusion technique. Furthermore, a very recent publication analyzing the cost of adult degenerative deformity correction demonstrated an average savings of $120,000/case when performed using MIS technique compared to open technique. Thus, data are now suggesting that "the bigger the procedure, the greater the cost savings with MIS technique." As our experience in MIS increases, and the complexity of the cases treated using MIS technique grows, it will become increasingly more difficult to argue for either cost-equivalence or cost–benefit of open surgery.

23.11.2 Open Surgery

Cost-effectiveness of a discrete treatment hinges on two factors —sustained differential clinical benefit of an intervention and upfront cost of that intervention. Recent studies have demonstrated small differences in the upfront cost of treatment using MIS because of reduced hospital length of stay for a procedure with otherwise similar direct costs. The shortcoming of promoting MIS surgery as a cost saving strategy comes when considering long-term results. Even surgeons who exclusively utilize MIS surgical techniques do not claim to have superior long-term results. The likely equivalence of results has been borne out recently by studies showing similar outcomes at medium-term follow-up when open and MIS techniques are compared. Additionally, because of the relatively small community of experts who are responsible for the majority of literature describing MIS surgery, the results suggesting equivalence may be more optimistic than can be expected if MIS surgery was to be widely adopted by a larger group of surgeons. Finally, any small cost savings shown in short-term follow-up for procedures expected to have similar long-term outcomes will likely become insignificant with longer follow-up.

References

[1] National Health Expenditure Projections 2011–2021. Centers of Medicare and Medicaid Services, 2009 https://www.cms.gov/Research-Statistics-Data-and-Systems/Statistics-Trends-and-Reports/NationalHealthExpendData/Downloads/Proj2012.pdf. Accessed September 15, 2017

[2] Adogwa O, Parker SL, Bydon A, Cheng J, McGirt MJ. Comparative effectiveness of minimally invasive versus open transforaminal lumbar interbody fusion: 2-year assessment of narcotic use, return to work, disability, and quality of life. J Spinal Disord Tech. 2011; 24(8):479–484

[3] Ntoukas V, Müller A. Minimally invasive approach versus traditional open approach for one level posterior lumbar interbody fusion. Minim Invasive Neurosurg. 2010; 53(1):21–24

[4] Parker SL, Adogwa O, Bydon A, Cheng J, McGirt MJ. Cost-effectiveness of minimally invasive versus open transforaminal lumbar interbody fusion for degenerative spondylolisthesis associated low-back and leg pain over two years. World Neurosurg. 2012; 78(1–2):178–184

[5] Parker SL, Fulchiero EC, Davis BJ, et al. Cost-effectiveness of multilevel hemilaminectomy for lumbar stenosis-associated radiculopathy. Spine J. 2011; 11(8):705–711

[6] Parker SL, Lerner J, McGirt MJ. Effect of minimally invasive technique on return to work and narcotic use following transforaminal lumbar inter-body fusion: a review. Prof Case Manag. 2012; 17(5):229–235

[7] Rampersaud YR, Gray R, Lewis SJ, Massicotte EM, Fehlings MG. Cost-utility analysis of posterior minimally invasive fusion compared with conventional open fusion for lumbar spondylolisthesis. SAS J.. 2011 Jun; 5(2):29–35

[8] Parker SL, McGirt MJ, Farber SH, et al. Accuracy of free-hand pedicle screws in the thoracic and lumbar spine: analysis of 6816 consecutive screws. Neurosurgery. 2011; 68(1):170–178, discussion 178

[9] Pelton MA, Phillips FM, Singh K. A comparison of perioperative costs and outcomes in patients with and without workers' compensation claims treated with minimally invasive or open transforaminal lumbar interbody fusion. Spine. 2012; 37(22):1914–1919

[10] Lucio JC, Vanconia RB, Deluzio KJ, Lehmen JA, Rodgers JA, Rodgers W. Economics of less invasive spinal surgery: an analysis of hospital cost differences between open and minimally invasive instrumented spinal fusion procedures during the perioperative period. Risk Manag Healthc Policy. 2012; 5:65–74

[11] Cahill KS, Levi AD, Cummock MD, Liao W, Wang MY. A comparison of acute hospital charges after tubular versus open microdiskectomy. World Neurosurg. 2013; 80(1–2):208–212

[12] Wang MY, Cummock MD, Yu Y, Trivedi RA. An analysis of the differences in the acute hospitalization charges following minimally invasive versus open posterior lumbar interbody fusion. J Neurosurg Spine. 2010; 12(6):694–699

[13] McGirt MJ, Parker SL, Lerner J, Engelhart L, Knight T, Wang MY. Comparative analysis of perioperative surgical site infection after minimally invasive versus open posterior/transforaminal lumbar interbody fusion: analysis of hospital billing and discharge data from 5170 patients. J Neurosurg Spine. 2011; 14(6):771–778

[14] Wang MY, Lerner J, Lesko J, McGirt MJ. Acute hospital costs after minimally invasive versus open lumbar interbody fusion: data from a US national database with 6106 patients. J Spinal Disord Tech. 2012; 25(6): 324–328

[15] Smith WD, Christian G, Serrano S, Malone KT. A comparison of perioperative charges and outcome between open and mini-open approaches for anterior lumbar discectomy and fusion. J Clin Neurosci. 2012; 19(5):673–680

[16] Parker SL, Adogwa O, Witham TF, Aaronson OS, Cheng J, McGirt MJ. Post-operative infection after minimally invasive versus open transforaminal lumbar interbody fusion (TLIF): literature review and cost analysis. Minim Invasive Neurosurg. 2011; 54(1):33–37

[17] Parker SL, Adogwa O, Davis BJ, et al. Cost-utility analysis of minimally invasive versus open multilevel hemilaminectomy for lumbar stenosis. J Spinal Disord Tech. 2013; 26(1):42–47

24 Success Rates and Time: Can Three-Dimensional Navigational Imaging Improve the Success and Time Required for Minimally Invasive Surgery and Minimize Radiation Exposure to Those in the OR Suite?

Eric W. Nottmeier

24.1 Introduction

Image-guided spinal surgery was introduced in the mid-1990s.[1,2,3,4] Image guidance technology allows the surgeon to navigate the patient's anatomy on preoperative or intraoperative images by tracking surgical instruments in three-dimensional (3D) space using infrared light. Given the reported 14 to 55% misplacement rate for pedicle screws using standard insertion techniques,[5,6,7,8] along with neurologic injury rates that can approach 7%,[9] the desire to develop techniques for more precise spinal instrumentation placement helped advance the evolution of spinal image guidance. Accordingly, over the past two decades this technology has progressed, making it more user-friendly and efficient for the spine surgeon. A significant step forward in this process was the introduction of cone beam computed tomography (CBCT) registration for spinal image guidance. During CBCT acquisition, multiple fluoroscopic images are obtained while the device rotates around the patient. These images are then reconstructed into a 3D data set, basically a CT scan, which can then be navigated after these data are transferred to the image-guided system. Advantages of 3D CBCT image guidance include the ability to register multiple vertebral segments at a time without the need to expose the bony dorsal elements, which has made a presence in minimally invasive spinal surgery procedures. This chapter reviews the spinal image guidance literature. Though the use of image guidance is increasing in spinal surgery, this technology is still not used by a majority of spine surgeons. Subsequently, a large part of the literature concerning spinal image guidance describes its use in open procedures, with a smaller part of the literature reporting on minimally invasive procedures.

24.2 The Accuracy of Spinal Image Guidance

Spinal image guidance has been used as an adjunct for instrumentation placement from the ileum to the occiput.[10,11,12,13,14,15,16,17,18] Kosmopoulos and Schizas[19] reported their meta-analysis of the spinal image guidance literature and found a median accuracy of 90.3% in 12,299 pedicle screws placed in vivo without navigation versus a median accuracy of 95.2% in 3,059 pedicle screws placed in vivo with navigation. Verma et al[20] reported a 93.3% accuracy rate in 3,555 pedicle screws placed using navigation versus an 84.7% accuracy rate in 2,437 pedicle screws placed without navigation in their meta-analysis of the spinal image guidance literature. In another meta-analysis by Tian et al,[21] pedicle screw insertion accuracy between conventional methods of pedicle screw placement and three methods of spinal image guidance (3D point matching image guidance,

2D image guidance, and 3D CBCT image guidance) was compared. They concluded that higher pedicle screw insertion accuracy occurred when image guidance was used and that 3D CBCT image guidance was the most accurate image guidance technique. Shin et al[22] performed a meta-analysis of the literature comparing image-guided pedicle screw insertion to nonnavigated techniques. Twenty studies were included in this meta-analysis which included a total of 8,539 screws (4,814 navigated and 3,725 nonnavigated). A 6% breach rate was noted in the navigated screws as compared to a 15% breach rate in the nonnavigated screws. Additionally, no neurologic complications were found in the navigated group, whereas three neurologic complications were noted in the nonnavigated group.

Four randomized clinical trials comparing image guidance to conventional techniques of pedicle screw placement have reported better screw placement accuracy with image guidance.[23,24,25,26] Rajasekaran et al[23] assessed the accuracy of thoracic pedicle screws placed in spinal deformity cases using either fluoroscopic assistance or 3D CBCT image guidance and reported a 2% breach rate in the 3D CBCT image guidance group versus a 23% breach rate in the fluoroscopic group. In a randomized trial comparing screws placed with the freehand technique to screws placed using 3D point matching image guidance, Laine et al[24] reported a breach rate of 13.4 and 4.6%, respectively. Randomized studies by Wu et al[25] and Yu et al[26] reported significantly higher accuracy in pedicle screws placed using 3D CBCT image guidance as compared to screws placed using fluoroscopic guidance. One randomized study has not demonstrated the advantage of spinal image guidance in which Li et al[27] reported no significant difference in breach rate in pedicle screws placed using the freehand technique versus pedicle screws placed using 3D point matching image guidance.

24.3 Radiation Exposure with Spinal Image Guidance

Fluoroscopy is frequently used to assist in spinal instrumentation placement. The amount of fluoroscopy time required to place a pedicle screw in open procedures ranges in the literature from 3.4 to 66 seconds per screw.[28,29,30,31,32] The use of fluoroscopy requires the surgeon to wear a lead apron and to move around the device during instrumentation placement.[33] Also, a 10- to 12-fold increase in surgeon radiation exposure can occur when fluoroscopy is used for spinal instrumentation cases when compared to nonspinal cases in which fluoroscopy is used.[34] In a prospective study measuring surgeon radiation exposure in 24 patients undergoing one- and two-level minimally invasive transforaminal lumbar interbody fusion (TLIF), Bindal et al[35] reported that the mean fluoroscopy time per case was 1.69 minutes and the mean radiation exposure per case to the surgeon's torso (under a lead apron) was 27 mrem. It was concluded in this study that a surgeon could exceed the recommended maximum annual radiation exposure of 5 rem to the torso if he/she performed more than 194 of these procedures annually.

When comparing image-guided pedicle screw placement to pedicle screw placement using fluoroscopy, several in vitro studies have reported less surgeon radiation exposure with the use of image guidance.[28,31,33,36] In an in vivo study assessing instrumentation placement in cases of less invasive correction for adult degenerative scoliosis, Scheufler et al[37] reported no surgeon radiation exposure using intraoperative CT image guidance. Another in vivo study by Nottmeier et al[38] reported no surgeon radiation exposure in 25 consecutive spinal surgery cases using CBCT image guidance. Izadpanah et al[39] reported significantly lower radiation time and patient radiation exposure in patients undergoing CBCT image-guided kyphoplasty, as compared to patients undergoing fluoroscopically assisted kyphoplasty. Obviously, no surgeon radiation exposure occurs with the use of image guidance as compared to fluoroscopic techniques because active fluoroscopy is not used during instrumentation placement. The patient's spine has to be registered using the CBCT device; however, during acquisition of these images, the surgeon and operating room (OR) staff can stand back from the operative field, which limits or eliminates their radiation exposure. Nottmeier et al[40] measured radiation scatter during intraoperative CBCT registration in 25 spinal surgery cases and determined that radiation exposure to the surgeon and OR staff was minimal if standing at least six feet from the CBCT device. Despite that, it was still emphasized in that study that the surgeon and OR staff should shield themselves during CBCT acquisition or should leave the room. However, radiation exposure to the patient still occurs in 3D CBCT image-guided spinal surgery cases during CBCT registration. Though radiation exposure to the patient must be considered, it should be emphasized that the surgeon and the OR staff will be participating in multiple fusion procedures per year, and the patient will hopefully be undergoing one fusion procedure during that time period. Furthermore, Zhang et al[41] reported that the patient radiation dose delivered by O-ARM (Medtronic) was approximately half of that delivered by a 64-slice CT scanner.

24.4 The Operating Room Time and Learning Curve in Spinal Image Guidance

Though a multitude of authors describe increased accuracy of spinal instrumentation placement with the use of image guidance as compared to standard techniques,[9,23,24,25,26,42,43,44] some authors have reported no benefit when using this technology.[27] Spinal image guidance is an aid to spinal instrumentation placement and not a substitute for knowledge of the spinal anatomy. Additionally, as with all new technologies and methods, a skill set needs to be developed by the surgeon to successfully apply image guidance to spinal surgery procedures. Learning curves are well documented with new technology in other surgical fields, including laparoscopic and robotic surgery.[45,46]

Spinal image guidance technology has been demonstrated to be highly accurate in vitro[47,48]; so, it is the in vivo application by surgeons that determines its success in the clinical setting. Learning curves have been described with the use of spinal image guidance.[49,50,51,52] When assessing the OR time associated with spinal image guidance, both increased OR time[24,27,42,53,54,55] and decreased OR time[23,25,52,56] have been reported. Several steps have to be performed during registration when using 3D CBCT image guidance (reference arc application, draping and undraping the patient, CBCT device positioning, performing the CBCT spin, and data transfer), and the reported time required to accomplish this ranges from 6.5 to 8.5 minutes.[40,57] The relationship between image guidance and OR time is partly dependent on the efficiency of the surgeon and OR staff in accomplishing these steps. Subsequently, studies that report the OR time added or saved in spinal image guidance cases may not be assessing the technology itself, but the OR team's efficiency in applying this technology. As surgeons overcome the learning curve and gain experience with this technology, OR times can decrease. When assessing the use of spinal image guidance versus standard techniques, Sasso and Garrido[52] and Johnson et al[56] found a decrease in OR time with the use of image guidance. Additionally, the authors noted in their studies that OR times decreased as the surgeon became more experienced with image guidance. When compared to traditional techniques, Wu et al[25] and Yu et al[26] reported a significant decrease in screw insertion time with the use of 3D CBCT image guidance.

24.5 Minimally Invasive Applications of Spinal Image Guidance

The placement of percutaneous spinal instrumentation has increased with the increasing popularity of minimally invasive spinal surgery. Advantages of 3D CBCT image guidance in minimally invasive spinal procedures include the ability to place percutaneous instrumentation with no active fluoroscopy.[58,59,60,61,62,63] Additionally, percutaneous placement of pedicle screws without the use of Kirschner's wires has been reported with 3D CBCT image guidance.[64,65] Another advantage of 3D CBCT image guidance is the ability to register the patient in the surgical position prior to exposing the spine and this has aided some surgeons in more focused approaches to spinal lesions. Kim et al[55] described their experience in eight patients who underwent successful 3D CBCT image-guided anterior cervical microforaminotomy. Additionally, Rajasekaran et al[66] have described a minimally invasive approach for removal of osteoid osteomas using 3D CBCT image guidance.

24.6 Case Illustration

A 33-year-old woman presented with a 5-year history of progressive mechanical back pain. After failing extensive conservative therapy, a discogram was accomplished that revealed significant disc derangement with concordant pain at L3–L4 and L4–L5. The patient underwent a two-level extreme lateral interbody fusion (XLIF) at the L3–L4 and L4–L5 levels through a minimally invasive retroperitoneal approach. Posteriorly, 3D CBCT image guidance was used for instrumentation placement. Translaminar facet screws were planned. Preoperative CT revealed thin L4 laminae that would not accommodate translaminar facet screws. The incision for the reference arc was made through the center of her tattoo over the L4–L5 level and the reference arc was attached to the L5 spinous process. The image-guided probe was then used to ascertain the trajectory of the left L3 translaminar facet screw on the skin. Through a stab incision, the image-guided probe was inserted down to the spinolaminar junction and a virtual plan for the translaminar facet screw was set (▶ Fig. 24.1). This area was exposed with a

small tubular retractor and a pilot hole was made at the entry point of the screw as determined by the virtual plan. An image-guided drill guide was then used to drill a hole down the virtual plan (▶ Fig. 24.2). The hole was then probed to confirm that no bony breach existed and the translaminar facet screw was placed. The right translaminar facet screw was placed in the same fashion. An intraoperative CBCT scan confirmed excellent placement of both screws (▶ Fig. 24.3). The reference arc was removed and an interspinous plate was used to fixate the L4–L5 level through the same incision. Postoperative AP and lateral radiographs revealed excellent placement of all instrumentation (▶ Fig. 24.4). At 4-month follow-up, the patient was

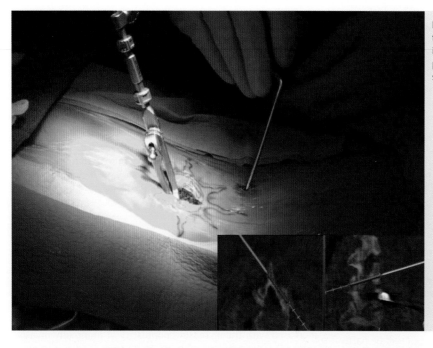

Fig. 24.1 Insertion of the image-guided probe to the spinolaminar junction through a small incision. Inset picture is from the image-guided platform; the probe tip is seen at the spinolaminar junction and a virtual plan is set.

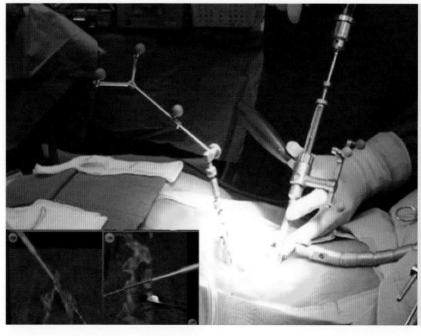

Fig. 24.2 Drilling the hole for the translaminar facet screw using the image-guided drill guide. Inset picture is from the image-guided platform; the drill tip is seen at the spinolaminar junction.

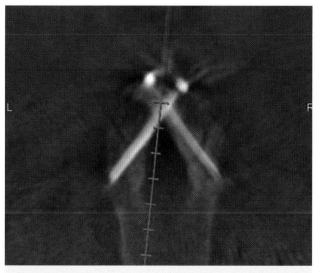

Fig. 24.3 Intraoperative CT confirming excellent placement of the translaminar facet screws.

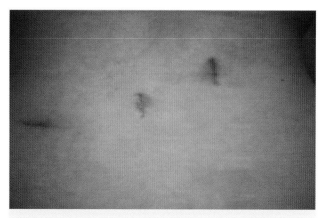

Fig. 24.5 Photograph of patient's incisions at the 4-month postoperative visit.

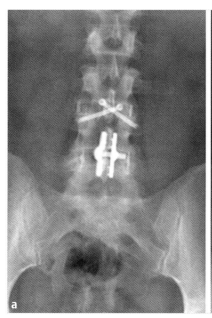
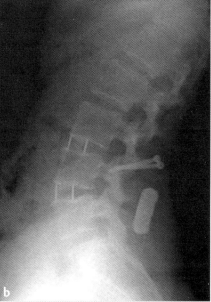

Fig. 24.4 Postoperative **(a)** anteroposterior and **(b)** lateral radiographs show adequate placement of instrumentation.

satisfied with the appearance of her incisions (▶ Fig. 24.5) and she reported near-complete abatement of her preoperative low back pain. In addition, CT scan revealed solid interbody fusion.

24.7 Conclusion

Image guidance has distinct advantages over fluoroscopy when used as an aid to spinal instrumentation placement, including more accurate screw placement and decreased radiation exposure to the surgeon and OR staff. Advances in image-guided technology have expanded its applications to minimally invasive surgery. As the surgeon becomes more experienced with this technology, a decrease in OR time can be realized.

24.8 Editors' Commentary

24.8.1 Minimally Invasive Surgery

Image guidance in many ways is "the promise which has not yet delivered," not unlike the theme of the theatrical play "Waiting for Godot." Its theoretical advantage is clear. If we could acquire accurate images of the 3D anatomy of the spine and then safely guide our instruments and implants through that anatomy using those images alone, our life as surgeons would be easier and the safety of our patients would improve. Unfortunately, despite the many advances in image guidance over the past two decades, we have not yet arrived at that ideal situation. The problem is that the images tell us where the anatomical structures were at the time the images were acquired, not necessarily where they are at the time we perform the surgery. Hence, a false sense of security could lead to disaster. Absolute accuracy, even with image guidance, still requires "real-time" imaging. Furthermore, a second potential pitfall is if the array is inadvertently "bumped." If undetected, all hope of accuracy is lost.

As a case example, in a recent adolescent idiopathic scoliosis correction, image guidance was elected to decrease radiation exposure and to increase accuracy of pedicle screw placement. After acquiring the images, multilevel facetectomies were performed after which posterior instrumentation was placed. Unfortunately, the spine was so mobile following the facet releases that nearly every pedicle screw was misplaced despite the image guidance predicting perfect pedicle screw placement. All pedicle screws were removed and replaced using real-time fluoroscopy.

That being said, there are cases and anatomical locations where image guidance works well. Lumbar spine surgery in adults, especially adults with advanced degenerative changes, and where the array is within three vertebral bodies of the operative site, gives acceptable accuracy for placement of pedicle screws, and does reduce the radiation exposure to the surgeon (although not necessarily the patient). In such cases, image guidance is a reasonable option. However, as the surgical site moves further away from the array, replacement and repeat image acquisition becomes necessary. This may decrease the time and work flow advantages of image guidance, not to mention the increased radiation exposure to the patient.

As a vociferous proponent of advancing surgical technique and technology, I will not say that image guidance will never be a better technique than real-time fluoroscopy. However, it seems evident to me that we are not there yet.

24.8.2 Open Surgery

Moving away from the intraoperative use of ionizing radiation will make minimally invasive surgery (MIS) more attractive to surgeons who consider adopting these techniques. Furthermore, the use of image guidance instead of fluoroscopy addresses the critical issue of unnecessarily exposing operating room staff to radiation, adhering to the principle of "As Low As Reasonably Achievable" (ALARA). MIS has been relatively stagnant from an imaging standpoint for a number of years—a paradigm shift toward nonfluoroscopy systems may be the trigger that MIS needs to achieve more widespread adoption.

References

[1] Nolte LP, Visarius H, Arm E, Langlotz F, Schwarzenbach O, Zamorano L. Computer-aided fixation of spinal implants. J Image Guid Surg. 1995; 1(2): 88–93

[2] Merloz P, Tonetti J, Eid A, et al. Computer assisted spine surgery. Clin Orthop Relat Res. 1997(337):86–96

[3] Lavallée S, Sautot P, Troccaz J, Cinquin P, Merloz P. Computer-assisted spine surgery: a technique for accurate transpedicular screw fixation using CT data and a 3-D optical localizer. J Image Guid Surg. 1995; 1(1):65–73

[4] Kalfas IH, Kormos DW, Murphy MA, et al. Application of frameless stereotaxy to pedicle screw fixation of the spine. J Neurosurg. 1995; 83(4):641–647

[5] Bolger C, Carozzo C, Roger T, et al. A preliminary study of reliability of impedance measurement to detect iatrogenic initial pedicle perforation (in the porcine model). Eur Spine J. 2006; 15(3):316–320

[6] Laine T, Schlenzka D, Mäkitalo K, Tallroth K, Nolte LP, Visarius H. Improved accuracy of pedicle screw insertion with computer-assisted surgery. A prospective clinical trial of 30 patients. Spine. 1997; 22(11):1254–1258

[7] Vaccaro AR, Rizzolo SJ, Balderston RA, et al. Placement of pedicle screws in the thoracic spine. Part II: An anatomical and radiographic assessment. J Bone Joint Surg Am. 1995; 77(8):1200–1206

[8] Xu R, Ebraheim NA, Ou Y, Yeasting RA. Anatomic considerations of pedicle screw placement in the thoracic spine. Roy-Camille technique versus open-lamina technique. Spine. 1998; 23(9):1065–1068

[9] Amiot LP, Lang K, Putzier M, Zippel H, Labelle H. Comparative results between conventional and computer-assisted pedicle screw installation in the thoracic, lumbar, and sacral spine. Spine. 2000; 25(5):606–614

[10] Garrido BJ, Wood KE. Navigated placement of iliac bolts: description of a new technique. Spine J. 2011; 11(4):331–335

[11] Nottmeier EW, Foy AB. Placement of C2 laminar screws using three-dimensional fluoroscopy-based image guidance. Eur Spine J. 2008; 17(4): 610–615

[12] Nottmeier EW, Seemer W, Young PM. Placement of thoracolumbar pedicle screws using three-dimensional image guidance: experience in a large patient cohort. J Neurosurg Spine. 2009; 10(1):33–39

[13] Nottmeier EW, Young PM. Image-guided placement of occipitocervical instrumentation using a reference arc attached to the headholder. Neurosurgery. 2010; 66(3) Suppl Operative:138–142

[14] Bledsoe JM, Fenton D, Fogelson JL, Nottmeier EW. Accuracy of upper thoracic pedicle screw placement using three-dimensional image guidance. Spine J. 2009; 9(10):817–821

[15] Holly LT, Foley KT. Percutaneous placement of posterior cervical screws using three-dimensional fluoroscopy. Spine. 2006; 31(5):536–540, discussion 541

[16] Welch WC, Subach BR, Pollack IF, Jacobs GB. Frameless stereotactic guidance for surgery of the upper cervical spine. Neurosurgery. 1997; 40(5):958–963, discussion 963–964

[17] Nottmeier EW, Pirris SM, Balseiro S, Fenton D. Three-dimensional image-guided placement of S2 alar screws to adjunct or salvage lumbosacral fixation. Spine J. 2010; 10(7):595–601

[18] Lekovic GP, Potts EA, Karahalios DG, Hall G. A comparison of two techniques in image-guided thoracic pedicle screw placement: a retrospective study of 37 patients and 277 pedicle screws. J Neurosurg Spine. 2007; 7(4):393–398

[19] Kosmopoulos V, Schizas C. Pedicle screw placement accuracy: a meta-analysis. Spine. 2007; 32(3):E111–E120

[20] Verma R, Krishan S, Haendlmayer K, Mohsen A. Functional outcome of computer-assisted spinal pedicle screw placement: a systematic review and meta-analysis of 23 studies including 5,992 pedicle screws. Eur Spine J. 2010; 19(3):370–375

[21] Tian NF, Huang QS, Zhou P, et al. Pedicle screw insertion accuracy with different assisted methods: a systematic review and meta-analysis of comparative studies. Eur Spine J. 2011; 20(6):846–859

[22] Shin BJ, James AR, Njoku IU, Härtl R. Pedicle screw navigation: a systematic review and meta-analysis of perforation risk for computer-navigated versus freehand insertion. J Neurosurg Spine. 2012; 17(2):113–122

[23] Rajasekaran S, Vidyadhara S, Ramesh P, Shetty AP. Randomized clinical study to compare the accuracy of navigated and non-navigated thoracic pedicle screws in deformity correction surgeries. Spine. 2007; 32(2):E56–E64

[24] Laine T, Lund T, Ylikoski M, Lohikoski J, Schlenzka D. Accuracy of pedicle screw insertion with and without computer assistance: a randomised controlled clinical study in 100 consecutive patients. Eur Spine J. 2000; 9(3): 235–240

[25] Wu H, Gao ZL, Wang JC, Li YP, Xia P, Jiang R. Pedicle screw placement in the thoracic spine: a randomized comparison study of computer-assisted navigation and conventional techniques. Chin J Traumatol. 2010; 13(4):201–205

[26] Yu X, Xu L, Bi LY. [Spinal navigation with intra-operative 3D-imaging modality in lumbar pedicle screw fixation]. Zhonghua Yi Xue Za Zhi. 2008; 88(27):1905–1908

[27] Li SG, Sheng L, Zhao H, Zhang JG, Zhai JL, Zhu Y. [Clinical applications of computer-assisted navigation technique in spinal pedicle screw internal fixation]. Zhonghua Yi Xue Za Zhi. 2009; 89(11):736–739

[28] Linhardt O, Perlick L, Lüring C, Stern U, Plitz W, Grifka J. Extrakorporale Einzeldosis und Durchleuchtungszeit bei bildwandler-kontrollierter und fluoroskopisch navigierter Implantation von Pedikelschrauben [in English]. Z Orthop Ihre Grenzgeb. 2005; 143(2):175–179

[29] Perisinakis K, Theocharopoulos N, Damilakis J, et al. Estimation of patient dose and associated radiogenic risks from fluoroscopically guided pedicle screw insertion. Spine. 2004; 29(14):1555–1560

[30] Sagi HC, Manos R, Benz R, Ordway NR, Connolly PJ. Electromagnetic field-based image-guided spine surgery part one: results of a cadaveric study evaluating lumbar pedicle screw placement. Spine. 2003; 28(17): 2013–2018

[31] Sagi HC, Manos R, Park SC, Von Jako R, Ordway NR, Connolly PJ. Electromagnetic field-based image-guided spine surgery part two: results of a cadaveric study evaluating thoracic pedicle screw placement. Spine. 2003; 28(17):E351–E354

[32] Slomczykowski M, Roberto M, Schneeberger P, Ozdoba C, Vock P. Radiation dose for pedicle screw insertion. Fluoroscopic method versus computer-assisted surgery. Spine. 1999; 24(10):975–982, discussion 983

[33] Kim CW, Lee YP, Taylor W, Oygar A, Kim WK. Use of navigation-assisted fluoroscopy to decrease radiation exposure during minimally invasive spine surgery. Spine J. 2008; 8(4):584–590

[34] Rampersaud YR, Foley KT, Shen AC, Williams S, Solomito M. Radiation exposure to the spine surgeon during fluoroscopically assisted pedicle screw insertion. Spine. 2000; 25(20):2637–2645

[35] Bindal RK, Glaze S, Ognoskie M, Tunner V, Malone R, Ghosh S. Surgeon and patient radiation exposure in minimally invasive transforaminal lumbar interbody fusion. J Neurosurg Spine. 2008; 9(6):570–573

[36] Smith HE, Welsch MD, Sasso RC, Vaccaro AR. Comparison of radiation exposure in lumbar pedicle screw placement with fluoroscopy vs computer-assisted image guidance with intraoperative three-dimensional imaging. J Spinal Cord Med. 2008; 31(5):532–537

[37] Scheufler KM, Cyron D, Dohmen H, Eckardt A. Less invasive surgical correction of adult degenerative scoliosis, Part I: Technique and radiographic results. Neurosurgery. 2010; 67(3):696–710

[38] Nottmeier EW, Bowman C, Nelson KL. Surgeon radiation exposure in cone beam computed tomography-based, image-guided spinal surgery. Int J Med Robot. 2012; 8(2):196–200

[39] Izadpanah K, Konrad G, Südkamp NP, Oberst M. Computer navigation in balloon kyphoplasty reduces the intraoperative radiation exposure. Spine. 2009; 34(12):1325–1329

[40] Nottmeier EW, Pirris SM, Edwards S, Kimes S, Bowman C, Nelson KL. Operating room radiation exposure in cone beam computed tomography-based, image-guided spinal surgery: clinical article. J Neurosurg Spine. 2013; 19(2):226–231

[41] Zhang J, Weir V, Fajardo L, Lin J, Hsiung H, Ritenour ER. Dosimetric characterization of a cone-beam O-arm imaging system. J Xray Sci Technol. 2009; 17(4):305–317

[42] Silbermann J, Riese F, Allam Y, Reichert T, Koeppert H, Gutberlet M. Computer tomography assessment of pedicle screw placement in lumbar and sacral spine: comparison between free-hand and O-arm based navigation techniques. Eur Spine J. 2011; 20(6):875–881

[43] Kotani Y, Abumi K, Ito M, et al. Accuracy analysis of pedicle screw placement in posterior scoliosis surgery: comparison between conventional fluoroscopic and computer-assisted technique. Spine. 2007; 32(14):1543–1550

[44] Sakai Y, Matsuyama Y, Nakamura H, et al. Segmental pedicle screwing for idiopathic scoliosis using computer-assisted surgery. J Spinal Disord Tech. 2008; 21(3):181–186

[45] Neo EL, Zingg U, Devitt PG, Jamieson GG, Watson DI. Learning curve for laparoscopic repair of very large hiatal hernia. Surg Endosc. 2011; 25(6): 1775–1782

[46] Mayer EK, Winkler MH, Aggarwal R, et al. Robotic prostatectomy: the first UK experience. Int J Med Robot. 2006; 2(4):321–328

[47] Fitzpatrick JM, West JB, Maurer CR, Jr. Predicting error in rigid-body point-based registration. IEEE Trans Med Imaging. 1998; 17(5):694–702

[48] Holly LT, Bloch O, Johnson JP. Evaluation of registration techniques for spinal image guidance. J Neurosurg Spine. 2006; 4(4):323–328

[49] Kim KD, Patrick Johnson J, Bloch BS O, Masciopinto JE. Computer-assisted thoracic pedicle screw placement: an in vitro feasibility study. Spine. 2001; 26(4):360–364

[50] Bai YS, Zhang Y, Chen ZQ, et al. Learning curve of computer-assisted navigation system in spine surgery. Chin Med J (Engl). 2010; 123(21):2989–2994

[51] Nakanishi K, Tanaka M, Misawa H, Sugimoto Y, Takigawa T, Ozaki T. Usefulness of a navigation system in surgery for scoliosis: segmental pedicle screw fixation in the treatment. Arch Orthop Trauma Surg. 2009; 129(9): 1211–1218

[52] Sasso RC, Garrido BJ. Computer-assisted spinal navigation versus serial radiography and operative time for posterior spinal fusion at L5-S1. J Spinal Disord Tech. 2007; 20(2):118–122

[53] Mirza SK, Wiggins GC, Kuntz C, IV, et al. Accuracy of thoracic vertebral body screw placement using standard fluoroscopy, fluoroscopic image guidance, and computed tomographic image guidance: a cadaver study. Spine. 2003; 28 (4):402–413

[54] Lee TC, Yang LC, Liliang PC, Su TM, Rau CS, Chen HJ. Single versus separate registration for computer-assisted lumbar pedicle screw placement. Spine. 2004; 29(14):1585–1589

[55] Kim JS, Eun SS, Prada N, Choi G, Lee SH. Modified transcorporeal anterior cervical microforaminotomy assisted by O-arm-based navigation: a technical case report. Eur Spine J. 2011; 20 Suppl 2:S147–S152

[56] Johnson JP, Stokes JK, Oskouian RJ, Choi WW, King WA. Image-guided thoracoscopic spinal surgery: a merging of 2 technologies. Spine. 2005; 30 (19):E572–E578

[57] Nottmeier EW, Crosby T. Timing of vertebral registration in three-dimensional, fluoroscopy-based, image-guided spinal surgery. J Spinal Disord Tech. 2009; 22(5):358–360

[58] Acosta FL, Jr, Thompson TL, Campbell S, Weinstein PR, Ames CP. Use of intraoperative isocentric C-arm 3D fluoroscopy for sextant percutaneous pedicle screw placement: case report and review of the literature. Spine J. 2005; 5(3):339–343

[59] Villavicencio AT, Burneikiene S, Bulsara KR, Thramann JJ. Utility of computerized isocentric fluoroscopy for minimally invasive spinal surgical techniques. J Spinal Disord Tech. 2005; 18(4):369–375

[60] Scheufler KM, Cyron D, Dohmen H, Eckardt A. Less invasive surgical correction of adult degenerative scoliosis. Part II: Complications and clinical outcome. Neurosurgery. 2010; 67(6):1609–1621, discussion 1621

[61] Sasso RC, Best NM, Potts EA. Percutaneous computer-assisted translaminar facet screw: an initial human cadaveric study. Spine J. 2005; 5(5):515–519

[62] Kakarla UK, Little AS, Chang SW, Sonntag VK, Theodore N. Placement of percutaneous thoracic pedicle screws using neuronavigation. World Neurosurg. 2010; 74(6):606–610

[63] Ravi B, Zahrai A, Rampersaud R. Clinical accuracy of computer-assisted two-dimensional fluoroscopy for the percutaneous placement of lumbosacral pedicle screws. Spine. 2011; 36(1):84–91

[64] Nottmeier EW, Fenton D. Three-dimensional image-guided placement of percutaneous pedicle screws without the use of biplanar fluoroscopy or Kirschner wires: technical note. Int J Med Robot. 2010; 6(4):483–488

[65] Shin BJ, Njoku IU, Tsiouris AJ, Härtl R. Navigated guide tube for the placement of mini-open pedicle screws using stereotactic 3D navigation without the use of K-wires: technical note. J Neurosurg Spine. 2013; 18(2):178–183

[66] Rajasekaran S, Kamath V, Shetty AP. Intraoperative Iso-C three-dimensional navigation in excision of spinal osteoid osteomas. Spine. 2008; 33(1):E25–E29

Index

Note: Page numbers set **bold** or *italic* indicate headings or figures, respectively.